Comprehensive Glossary of Terms Used in Toxicology

Comprehensive Glossary of Terms Used in Toxicology

John Duffus
The Edinburgh Centre for Toxicology, UK
Email: j.h.duffus@btinternet.com

Douglas M. Templeton
University of Toronto, Canada
Email: doug.templeton@utoronto.ca

and

Michael Schwenk
Federal Public Health Department, Germany
Email: mike.schwenk@gmx.net

ROYAL SOCIETY OF CHEMISTRY

IUPAC
INTERNATIONAL UNION OF PURE AND APPLIED CHEMISTRY

THE QUEEN'S AWARDS FOR ENTERPRISE: INTERNATIONAL TRADE 2013

Print ISBN: 978-1-78262-137-9
PDF eISBN: 978-1-78262-372-4
EPUB eISBN: 978-1-78801-199-0

A catalogue record for this book is available from the British Library

The Royal Society of Chemistry is a charity, registered in England and Wales, Number 207890, and a company incorporated in England by Royal Charter (Registered No. RC000524), registered office: Burlington House, Piccadilly, London W1J 0BA, UK, Telephone: +44 (0) 207 4378 6556.

Visit our website at www.rsc.org/books

Printed in the United Kingdom by CPI Group (UK) Ltd, Croydon, CR0 4YY, UK

Preface

This book represents a culmination, or at least a resting point, in the long-term project that has resulted in five glossaries published as IUPAC Recommendations in Pure and Applied Chemistry.[1–5] The project was initiated in 1989 by the IUPAC Commission on Toxicology to provide a glossary of definitions of terms used in toxicology. The impetus was the recognition that toxic substances (indeed all substances) are "chemicals", and that there is a need for chemists to understand the mechanisms of toxicity of the substances with which they deal. Both industrial and academic research chemists are faced with an ever-increasing burden in ensuring a safe environment. Even those who may not be trained as chemists must use chemical and toxicological principles in formulating and enforcing the current legislation introduced to ensure safe handling of substances throughout their life cycle. Thus, there is a need for an unambiguous vocabulary of terms, both for specialist interpretation of the relevant literature and for warning about hazard and risk that must be controlled and eliminated or minimized.

The starting point of the project was a general glossary of terms in toxicology that collected relevant terms from a variety of sources and revised many of them, with contributions from specialists covering the wide range of knowledge required. IUPAC specialists in terminology advised on details of presentation of terms and definitions. The resultant glossary was submitted to Pure and Applied Chemistry for publication following the normal refereeing process for an IUPAC Recommendation.[6] This procedure has been the foundation for future glossary development.

The original glossary was followed by a glossary of terms in toxicokinetics.[7] These two glossaries were later combined and revised,[1] taking into account more recent developments in toxicological science and regulatory activity. Thereafter, it became clear that there were gaps in coverage of terms related to specialized aspects of toxicology that were becoming increasingly important in their own right. These areas of toxicology were covered in new IUPAC glossaries of terms used in ecotoxicology,[2] immunotoxicology,[2] neurotoxicology,[4] and reproductive toxicology and teratology.[5] This book consolidates all these documents, and expands their contents with the addition of terms that have been newly introduced in toxicology or whose absence in the previous publications we felt should be addressed. We have taken the opportunity to harmonize definitions between the various sub-disciplines of toxicology, and to correct a few errors and oversights in our earlier work. Retrospection has also resulted in a uniform syntax and formatting for the construction and presentation of

Comprehensive Glossary of Terms Used in Toxicology
By John Duffus, Douglas M. Templeton and Michael Schwenk

Published by the Royal Society of Chemistry, www.rsc.org

definitions that we believe is an improvement on that used in the earlier glossaries; we hope that the current document will thus contribute to the continuing development of the IUPAC standard for such documents.

In a compilation of terms that intends to be anything short of a complete word list of the language, decisions of inclusion and exclusion must be made. The vocabulary of toxicology necessarily overlaps with those of medicine, physiology, biochemistry and ecology, to name a few, and this takes us on occasion into the more specialized realms of cognate disciplines such as anatomy, histology, immunology, neuroscience, molecular biology, epidemiology and population biology. We have also included a number of terms in regulatory toxicology and jurisdictional matters relating to harmful substances. In each case, where we have drawn the line on inclusion reflects our personal preferences, based on decisions about what we think will be a reasonable collection of terms, hoping both to achieve internal consistency and to meet the needs of most readers who may consult the glossary as they explore the relevant toxicological literature. Our aim has been to provide a one-stop glossary of terms commonly used in toxicology so that chemists reading the toxicological literature will not often need to consult secondary sources in order to understand terms with which they are unfamiliar.

All headwords are listed in the singular, in bold type, with the definition following in plain text. When the plural may be a nonstandard form, it is listed and designated (pl), *e.g.*, "**meninx/meninges** (pl)". When the form of speech may be unclear it is specified as (n), (v) or (adj) after the headword, and when more than one form of speech is indicated, the definition is written so as to apply to the first part of speech listed. When a definition includes a term that is itself another defined term in the glossary, the term is italicized for cross-referencing, but only at first use in the individual entry. However, we realize that complete cross-referencing in this manner is nearly impossible to achieve – nor is it desirable, as italicizing too many general terms in a definition detracts from its readability, and here judgment has been exercised. Italicizing of individual words does not always mean they combine to form a defined term. For instance, under "**optimal stress response**", *somatic growth rate* appears in italics. This grouping does not itself occur as a headword, but rather the three words 'somatic', 'growth', and 'rate' are defined individually, and would be consulted in sequence for a full explanation of the term. Because Latin names of biological species are italicized by convention, they are additionally in bold here to avoid confusion with cross-referencing.

Notes are included for many terms; these are not intended to be encyclopedic, but rather to provide clarification or remove ambiguity when a strict definition may not be entirely clear. Notes are also used to indicate when a term may be in common use but its use is to be discouraged (*e.g.*, "heavy metal"). In general, commonly preferred or American spelling has been adopted for the main entry terms; thus, for example, anesthetic (not anaesthetic), neuron (not neurone), disc (not disk), and tumor (not tumour). Further, somewhat arbitrary decisions have necessarily been made in listing alternative forms of terms as the headword (*e.g.*, vasospasm instead of angiospasm, β-blocker instead of β-antagonist, and intervertebral disc instead of spinal disc). We have generally tried to use the form we consider to be in most common usage, and to cross-reference the less-used term if it seems also to be common; but, if a desired entry is not found under one construction, it may have to be sought under another.

We attempt to give a correct IUPAC name for all chemical structures mentioned, and the manuscript has been passed by the IUPAC Interdivisional Committee on Terminology, Nomenclature and Symbols (ICTNS). This, too, can become a daunting task when particularly lengthy names for complex natural products or pharmaceuticals are involved. And, in some cases different 'correct' IUPAC conventions may lead to alternative names, with the Preferred IUPAC Name (PIN) not always available in the literature. When a drug name is given as the International Nonproprietary Name, it is indicated as such by '(INN)'. Enzyme Commission (EC) numbers are provided for enzymes.

In existing glossaries, dictionaries, or other compilations of words, compound or multi-word terms are often listed consistently under the final word (*e.g.*, "compound term: See term, compound") without regard to what component of the term the user may be most likely to be searching. Here, we do so judiciously. For instance, we suppose it is helpful to list various antibodies (anti-idiotypic, blocking, cross-reacting, enhancing, ...) or mazes (Barnes, Biel water, elevated plus, radial arm, ...) together under "antibody" or "maze", respectively. But we have decided the same is not true of various "models", and "biotic ligand model", "biphasic dose-effect model", "conceptual site model" and "two-compartment model" are alphabetized as written here. In most cases we have included cross-referencing for compound terms to the form associated with the definition. Our decisions are necessarily somewhat arbitrary, and may not suit the needs of all users. We can't give specific guidance in these cases, but suggest that for such multi-word terms, the reader should consider possible variants.

A note on sources: All definitions taken from the earlier sources[1–5] are indicated as [ref. 1], [ref. 2], *etc.* Modifications are designated as "[After ref. X]", and new terms or those substantially modified from our previous glossaries are designated "[*]". Several of the approximately 5,000 definitions are taken from the IUPAC Gold Book[8] on chemical terminology, and are designated as "[ref. 8]". When a definition is cited as being from any of [ref. 1–5], the reader may look to that publication to see whether it originated there, or is attributed to, or modified from, an earlier source. All references (1–8) are currently open access online.

Acknowledgments

A large number of reviewers, some identified and some anonymous, have made invaluable contributions to the development of this work, and many (when known) have been acknowledged in the individual documents.[1–7] Early encouragement was provided by successive Chairs of the IUPAC Commission on Toxicology (COMTOX), Profs. Philippe Grandjean and Rita Cornelis, and their support has continued throughout the years. The meticulous work of Dr. Karl-Heinz Hellwich in reviewing all the nomenclature was invaluable. We would particularly like to single out our coauthors on the foundation publications, Profs. Monica Nordberg,[1,2] Ole Andersen[2] and Reinhild Klein.[3]

References

1. J. H. Duffus, M. Nordberg and D. M. Templeton, Glossary of terms used in toxicology, 2nd edition, *Pure Appl. Chem.*, 2007, **79**, 1153–1344.
2. M. Nordberg, D. M. Templeton, O. Andersen and J. H. Duffus, Glossary of terms used in ecotoxicology, *Pure Appl. Chem.*, 2009, **81**, 829–97.
3. D. M. Templeton, M. Schwenk, R. Klein and J. H. Duffus, Glossary of terms used in immunotoxicology, *Pure Appl. Chem.*, 2012, **84**, 1113–1295.
4. D. M. Templeton, M. Schwenk and J. H. Duffus, IUPAC Glossary of terms used in neurotoxicology, *Pure Appl. Chem.*, 2015, **87**, 841–927.
5. J. H. Duffus, M. Schwenk and D. M. Templeton, IUPAC Glossary of terms used in developmental and reproductive toxicology, *Pure Appl. Chem.*, 2016, **88**, 713–830.
6. J. H. Duffus, Glossary for chemists of terms used in toxicology, *Pure Appl. Chem.*, 1993, **65**, 2003–2122.
7. M. Nordberg, J. H. Duffus and D. M. Templeton, Glossary of terms used in toxicokinetics, *Pure Appl. Chem.*, 2004, **76**, 1033–1082.
8. IUPAC Compendium of Chemical Terminology – the Gold Book, Version 2.3.3, 2005-2014, http://goldbook.iupac.org/pdf/goldbook.pdf.

Contents

Alphabetical List of Terms

Comprehensive Glossary of Terms Used in Toxicology
By John Duffus, Douglas M. Templeton and Michael Schwenk

Published by the Royal Society of Chemistry, www.rsc.org

Alphabetical List of Terms

ABC transporter

See *transporter, ABC.*

ABL oncogene

See *oncogene, ABL.*

ABO blood group system

See *blood group system, ABO.*

Ad4BP

See *adrenal 4 binding protein.*

A/D ratio

Ratio of the *adult toxic dose* to the developmentally toxic dose.
[ref. 5]

AMPA receptor

See *receptor, 2-amino-3-(3-hydroxy-5-methyl-1,2-oxazol-4-yl)propanoic acid (AMPA).*

ANCA-associated vasculitis

See *vasculitis, antineutrophil cytoplasmic autoantibody-associated vasculitis.*

APECED syndrome

See *polyendocrinopathy, autoimmune.*

ATP

See *adenosine triphosphate.*

abdomen (n)/abdominal (adj)

1. Part of the body between the *thorax* and the pelvis in *vertebrates.*
2. Most posterior segment of the insect body.

[*]

abdominal cavity

See *cavity, abdominal.*

abiological

See *abiotic.*

abiotic

abiological
Opposite term: *biotic.*

Not associated with living organisms.
[ref. 1]

Comprehensive Glossary of Terms Used in Toxicology
By John Duffus, Douglas M. Templeton and Michael Schwenk

Published by the Royal Society of Chemistry, www.rsc.org

abiotic degradation

See *degradation, abiotic.*

abiotic transformation

See *transformation, abiotic.*

ablepharia (n)/ablepharous (adj)

Congenital absence of the eyelids.
[ref. 5]

abortifacient

Substance that causes *pregnancy* to end prematurely and causes an *abortion.*
[ref. 1]

abortion, induced

Intentional termination of a *pregnancy* with death of the *embryo* or *fetus.*
[ref. 5]

abortion, spontaneous
miscarriage

Unintentional termination of *pregnancy* before the *embryo* or *fetus* has developed to the stage of independent *viability*, or in humans before the 20th week of *gestation.*
[ref. 5]

absolute bioavailability

See *bioavailability, absolute.*

absolute fitness

See *fitness.*

absolute lethal concentration (LC_{100})

See *lethal concentration, absolute*

absolute lethal dose (LD_{100})

See *lethal dose, absolute.*

absolute risk

See *risk, absolute.*

absorbance (A)

Logarithm of the ratio of incident to transmitted *radiant power* through a sample (excluding the effects of sample cell walls).
Note 1: Depending on the base of the logarithm, decadic and Napierian absorbances are used. Symbols: A, A_{10}, A_e.
Note 2: Absorbance is sometimes called extinction, although the term "extinction", better called *attenuance*, is reserved for the quantity that takes into account the effects of luminescence and scattering as well.
Note 3: When natural logarithms are used, the Napierian absorbance is the logarithm to the base e of the incident *spectral radiant power*, essentially monochromatic, divided by the transmitted spectral radiant power, P_λ.
[ref. 1]

absorbate

Substance that enters and is retained inside a solid or semisolid *matrix* (*absorbent*).
[ref. 2]

absorbed dose (of a substance)

See *dose, absorbed*.

absorbed dose (of ionizing radiation)

Energy imparted by *ionizing radiation* to a specified volume of matter divided by the mass of that volume.
[ref. 1]

absorbent

Solid or semisolid *matrix* that is able to accommodate and retain an *absorbate*.
[ref. 2]
See also *sorbate; sorbent*.

absorptance (in chemistry), α

Absorbed radiant power divided by the incident radiant power. Also called *absorption factor*. When $\alpha \leq 1$, $\alpha \approx A_e$, where A_e is the Napierian absorbance.
[ref. 1]
See also *absorbance*.

absorption (general)

1. Process of one material (*absorbate*) being retained by another (*absorbent*). Note: Absorption may be the physical solution of a gas, liquid, or solid in a liquid, attachment of molecules of a gas, vapor, liquid, or dissolved substance to a solid surface by physical forces, *etc.*
2. Transfer of some or all of the energy of radiation to matter that it traverses. Note: Absorption of light at bands of characteristic wavelengths is used as an analytical method in spectrophotometry to identify the chemical nature of molecules, atoms, or ions and to measure the concentrations of these *chemical species*.

[ref. 2]
See also *adsorption; sorption*.

absorption (in biology)

uptake

Penetration of a substance into an organism and its cells by various processes, some specialized, some involving expenditure of energy (*active transport*), some involving a *carrier* system, and others involving passive movement down an electrochemical gradient (*passive transport*).
Note: In mammals, absorption is usually through the respiratory tract, *gastrointestinal tract*, or skin into the circulatory system and from the circulation into *organs, tissues,* and *cells.*
[ref. 2]

absorption (of radiation)

Phenomenon in which radiation transfers some or all of its energy to matter that it traverses.
[ref. 1]

absorption, systemic

Uptake to the blood and transport via the blood of a substance to one or more organs or *compartments* in the body distant from the site of *absorption*.
[ref. 2]

absorption coefficient (in biology)

absorption factor

Absorbed quantity (*uptake*) of a substance divided by the administered quantity (intake).
Note: For *exposure* by way of the respiratory tract, the absorption coefficient is the ratio of the absorbed amount to the amount of the substance (usually particles) deposited (adsorbed) in the lungs.
[ref. 1]

absorption factor

See *absorptance* (in chemistry); *absorption coefficient* (in biology).

abundance

1. Total number of individual organisms in a *population*, seen over a defined period of time in a certain place.
   Note: For abundance of fish, an estimate of total weight may replace number.
2. Total number of organisms per unit of *habitat* space seen over a defined period.
3. Amount of an element that exists in nature, usually expressed in relative terms as a percentage of the total amount of all elements in a given medium (*e.g.*, the Earth's crust).
4. Amount of an isotope of an element that exists in nature, usually expressed in relative terms as a percentage of the total amount of all isotopes of the element.

[ref. 2]

abundant element

See *element, abundant*.

abundant metal

See *element, abundant*.

abuse (of substances)

Improper use of *drugs*, solvents or other substances.
[ref. 1]

abzyme

Antibody or antibody construct with catalytic activity.
[ref. 3]

acaricide

Substance intended to kill mites, ticks, or other ***Acaridae***.
[ref. 1]

acceptable daily intake

See *daily intake, acceptable*.

acceptable daily intake (ADI) not allocated

See *no-acceptable-daily-intake-allocated.*

acceptable daily intake, temporary

Value for the *acceptable daily intake* (ADI) proposed for guidance when data are sufficient to conclude that use of the substance is safe over the relatively short period of time required to generate and evaluate further safety data, but are insufficient to conclude that use of the substance is safe over a lifetime.
Note: A higher-than-normal *safety* factor (see *uncertainty factor*) is used when establishing a temporary ADI, and an expiration date is established by which time appropriate data to resolve the safety issue should be available.
[ref. 1]

acceptable residue level of an antibiotic

See *residue level of an antibiotic, acceptable.*

acceptable risk

See *risk, acceptable.*

accepted risk

See *risk, accepted.*

accessible

Capable of being entered or reached; easy of access; such as one can go to, come into the presence of, reach, or lay hold of.
[ref. 2]

accessibility

See *bioaccessibility.*

accessory cell

Cell that assists in the *adaptive immune response* but does not directly mediate specific *antigen* recognition.
Note 1: Accessory cells include *phagocytes, mast cells, dendritic cells*, and *natural killer cells.*
Note 2: The term accessory cell is often used to describe *antigen-presenting cells.*
[ref. 3]

accessory molecule

Molecule other than *immunoglobulin, T-cell receptor*, or *major histocompatibility complex molecule* that participates in *T-lymphocyte* recognition and response to *antigen.*
[ref. 3]

accessory rib

Rib arising from a cervical *vertebra* (*cervical rib*), or *supernumerary* rib arising from a *thoracic* or lumbar vertebra.
[ref. 5]

accessory sex gland

Any gland, other than a *gonad*, associated with the genital tract, such as the *bulbourethral* gland and *prostate*.
[ref. 5]

accessory sex organ
secondary sex organ

Organ or structure other than the *gonads* that matures at *puberty* and assists indirectly in *sexual reproduction* by nurturing and transporting *gametes*.
Note 1: In the human female the accessory sex organs include the *Fallopian tubes, uterus, vagina*, and the external genitalia.
Note 2: In the human male, the accessory sex organs include the *epididymis, vas deferens*, ejaculatory *duct, urethra, seminal vesicles, bulbourethral glands, prostate*, and penis.
[ref. 5]

accidental cell death

Death of a cell by a catastrophic process such as acute physical, mechanical, chemical or osmotic injury, in contrast to *programmed cell death*.
[*]

accidental exposure

See *exposure, accidental.*

acclimation (n)/acclimate (v)
acclimatization (n)/acclimatize (v)
biological acclimatization

1. Modification or adjustment of a biological process or structure that helps to maintain *homeostasis* in response to a change in environment.
   Note: The modification occurring in acclimation may be physiological, in response to changes in the physical environment (*e.g.*, thermoregulation), including changes in the concentration of a *toxicant*. It may also refer to behavioral changes reflecting psychological adjustment.
2. Processes, including selection and *adaptation*, by which a *population* of microorganisms develops a *tolerance* to a substance that may follow acquisition of the ability to degrade the substance.
3. Experimental manoeuvre of allowing an organism to adjust to its environment prior to undertaking a *study*.

[*]

acclimatization, biological

See *acclimation.*

accumulation (in biology)

See *bioaccumulation*.

accumulation factor (AF)

See *biota-sediment accumulation factor*.
See also *bioaccumulation factor*.

accuracy

Quantity referring to the differences between the mean of a set of results or an individual result and the value that is accepted as the true or correct value for the quantity measured.
[ref. 1]

acetylcholine (ACh)

2-acetoxy-*N,N,N*-trimethylethanaminium
2-(acetyloxy)-*N,N,N*-trimethylethan-1-aminium (PIN)

Substance that functions as a *neurotransmitter* between *nerve cells* and between nerves and muscles.
[ref. 4]

acetylcholine receptor

See *receptor, acetylcholine.*

acetylcholinesterase (AChE)

acetylcholine hydrolase

Enzyme (EC 3.1.1.7) that hydrolyzes *acetylcholine.*
[ref. 4]

acetylcholinesterase inhibitor

Substance that inhibits the action of acetylcholinesterase (EC 3.1.1.7) and related enzymes that catalyze the hydrolysis of choline esters, causing hyperactivity in *parasympathetic* nerves.
Note: Examples include *organophosphate* and carbamate *pesticides.*
[*]

β-*N*-acetylhexosaminidase

Hydrolytic enzyme (EC 3.2.1.52) that acts on *ganglioside* G_{M2}, producing *N*-acetyl-D-galactosamine and ganglioside G_{M3}.
Note: Deficiency of β-*N*-acetylhexosaminidase is associated with *Tay-Sachs disease.*
[ref. 5]

acetyltransferase

acyltransferase

Any of a group of enzymes (EC 2.3.x.y) that transfers an acyl group from a donor (*e.g.*, acetyl-coenzyme A) usually to a hydroxyl or amino (aminoacyltransferase) group of a substrate.
Note: Acetylation of xenobiotics is classified as a *phase II biotransformation* reaction.
[*]

achondroplasia (n)/achondroplastic (adj)

Inherited *disorder* where *ossification* of cartilage is retarded, especially affecting growth of long bones, resulting in very short limbs and a comparatively large head. Type of dwarfism.
Note: Achondroplasia results from a *mutation* in the *fibroblast* growth factor *receptor* FGFR3 gene, increasing its activity in suppressing *endochondral ossification.*
[ref. 5]

acid dissociation constant, *K*a

Equilibrium constant for the following reaction of an acid, HB:

$$HB(aq) \rightleftharpoons H^+(aq) + B^-(aq)$$

$$K_a = [H^+][B^-] / [HB]c^o$$

where $c^o = 1$ mol dm^{-3} is the standard amount concentration and activity coefficients have been neglected.
Note 1: The acid dissociation constant, because activity coefficients are neglected, is valid at a specified ionic strength. The thermodynamic dissociation constant is found by suitable extrapolation of the conditional constant to zero ionic strength. Note that it is defined as a dimensionless quantity, but sometimes it is given dimensions by omitting the standard amount concentration.
Note 2: Because the acid dissociation constant differs for each acid, and varies over many degrees of magnitude, the acidity constant is often represented by the additive inverse of its common logarithm, represented by the symbol pK_a (using the same mathematical relationship as $[H^+]$ is to pH), viz.:

$$pK_a = -\log_{10} K_a$$

Note 3: In general, a larger value of K_a (or a smaller value of pK_a) indicates a stronger acid, since the extent of dissociation is larger at the same concentration.
[ref. 8]

acid precipitation

Rain, fog, snow, sleet, or other particulate matter from the atmosphere with a pH below 5.6 deposited from the air.
Note 1: Rain under clean air conditions has a pH slightly under 6, caused by dissolved carbon dioxide dissociating to form carbonate and hydrogencarbonate ions. "*Acid rain*" has a pH of about pH 4.2 to 4.4.
Note 2: Acid precipitation is partly due to volcanic emissions, but, more importantly, results from human activities, such as incineration of sulfur-containing fossils (emission of SO_2) and emission of nitrogen-oxides (NO_x) that are formed in combustion engines.
Note 3: Acid precipitations may fall at a distance remote from emission sources owing to atmospheric transport.
Note 4: Acid precipitation causes acidification of soils and surface waters, with adverse effects on ecosystems.
[After ref. 2]

acid rain

Subtype of *acid precipitation*.
[ref. 2]

acid-volatile sulfide (AVS)

Soil- and *sediment*-associated solid-phase sulfide extractable with cold hydrochloric acid.
Note: AVS may be chemically *available* by acid extraction without being *bioavailable*. Thus, AVS can decrease metal *toxicity* by binding metals in anoxic soils or sediments, thereby rendering them unavailable to most living organisms.
[ref. 2]

acidosis
Opposite term: *alkalosis*

Abnormal increase in hydronium ion activity (decrease in pH below the reference interval measured in the arterial blood) usually caused either by an accumulation of carbon dioxide or acidic metabolites, or by a depletion of alkaline reserve (*i.e.*, bicarbonate).
Note 1: In humans, the blood pH is tightly regulated within a range of 7.35 to 7.45.
Note 2: Acidosis may occur as a result of accumulation of ketones in uncontrolled *diabetes mellitus* (diabetic acidosis) or after calory deprivation (starvation acidosis), or with accumulation of keto-acids at the expense of bicarbonate (*metabolic* acidosis). Suppression of respiration can produce a respiratory acidosis.
Note 3: Some intoxications can produce metabolic and (or) respiratory acidosis.
[ref. 5]

acinus

1. Small sac-like *cavity* in a *gland*, surrounded by secretory cells.
2. Terminal region of the airways of the lung where gas exchange occurs.

[ref. 5]

acoustic meatus

Either of two passages in the ear, one leading to the *tympanic* membrane (external acoustic meatus), and one for passage of nerves and blood vessels (internal acoustic meatus).
[ref. 5]

acoustic neuroma
acoustic neurinoma
vestibular Schwannoma

Noncancerous intra*cranial tumor* of the eighth *cranial nerve.*
Note 1: An acoustic neuroma arises from the *Schwann cells.*
Note 2: The eighth cranial (vestibulocochlear) nerve is involved in both hearing and balance.
[ref. 4]

acquired immunity

See *immunity, acquired.*

acquired immunodeficiency syndrome (AIDS)

Disease caused by infection with the *human immunodeficiency virus*, assuming clinical relevance when an infected patient has lost most of his/her *CD4+ T-cells*, so that infections with *opportunistic pathogens* occur.
[ref. 3]

acrania

Rare *congenital disorder* that occurs in the human *fetus* in which the flat bones in the *cranium* are either completely or partially absent.
[ref. 5]

acrocephaly
acrocephalia
oxycephaly

Type of *cephalic disorder* where the top of the skull is pointed or conical due to premature closure of the *coronal suture* plus any other suture.
Note: Acrocephaly should be differentiated from *Crouzon syndrome*, which involves the *maxilla* and *mandible*.
[ref. 5]

acromegaly

acromegalia

Abnormal enlargement of the hands, feet, and face in adults, caused by overproduction of *growth hormone* by the *pituitary* gland.
Note: Overproduction of growth hormone by the pituitary gland in children causes *gigantism*.
[ref. 5]

acroparesthesia

Abnormal feeling of numbness, tingling, or burning of the skin, typically in the extremities.
[ref. 4]

acrosome

Organelle that develops over the anterior half of the head in the *spermatozoon*.
Note: The acrosome is a cap-like structure derived from the *Golgi apparatus*.
[ref. 5]

acrosome reaction

Process that occurs in the *acrosome* of the *sperm* as it contacts the *egg*, leading to structural changes that facilitate fusion.
[ref. 5]

action level

1. *Concentration* of a substance in air, soil, water, or other defined medium at which specified emergency counter-measures, such as the seizure and destruction of contaminated materials, evacuation of the local population or closing down the sources of pollution, are to be taken.
2. Concentration of a *pollutant* in air, soil, water, or other defined medium at which some kind of preventive action (not necessarily of an emergency nature) is to be taken.

[ref. 1]

action potential

Brief, spike-like *depolarization* associated with the passage of an impulse without decrement along the membrane of a muscle cell or *nerve cell*.
Note 1: An action potential is used for rapid signaling over a distance.
Note 2: Action potentials also occur in many endocrine cells.
[ref. 4]

activated sludge

Product of treatment of industrial *sludge* with microorganisms and aeration, facilitating its *biodegradation*.
[*]

activation (abiotic)

Conversion of a substance to a more biologically active derivative by modification not involving biological catalysis.
Note: Examples of *abiotic* activation could include activation of a *xenobiotic* to a more *toxic* form, activation of a *prodrug* to an active *drug*, and generation of *photochemical smog* from air *pollutants*.
[*]

activation (biotic)

See *bioactivation.*
See also *activation, complement; activation, lymphocyte; activation, neutrophil.*

activation, complement

Cascade of protein cleavages, releasing *cytokines* that start a further amplifying cascade of cleavages. The result is *complement* activation that, in turn, activates *phagocytes* to degrade foreign and damaged cells or substances, and starts *inflammatory* processes that attract more phagocytes and further activate the cell-killing membrane-destroying complex.
[*]

activation, lymphocyte

Sum of the biochemical processes necessary to stimulate a resting *lymphocyte* to become an immune effector cell, requiring *antigen* and co-stimulatory molecules.
[ref. 3]
See also *costimulation; activation, neutrophil.*

activation, metabolic

Formation of one or more chemically *reactive intermediate*(s) as a result of modification of a molecule by the *xenobiotic*-metabolizing enzymes of liver and other organs.
Note 1: Metabolic activation may lead to acute cell damage and recognition of the damaged cell by the *immune system* as *self.*
Note 2: The reactive intermediate in metabolic activation can also act as a *hapten.*
[ref. 3]

activation, neutrophil

Change in morphology and behavior of a *neutrophil* resulting from exposure to a *cytokine, chemokine*, cellular *ligand*, or soluble factor.
[ref. 3]
See also *activation, lymphocyte.*

activation-induced cell death

Process by which *immune responses* end in the death of most of the responding *lymphocytes*, leaving only a small number of resting *memory cells.*
[ref. 3]
See also *apoptosis.*

active avoidance test

See *avoidance test, active.*

active immunization

See *immunization, active.*

active ingredient

Component of a *mixture* responsible for the biological effects of the mixture.
[ref. 1]
Compare *inert ingredient.*

active metabolite

See *metabolite, active.*

active systemic anaphylaxis (ASA) test

Test for determining whether a *drug* can cause *anaphylactic reactions* in an animal following *immunization* with the drug.
[ref. 3]

active transport

See *transport, active.*

activin

Growth factor of the transforming growth factor β superfamily, originally identified as a gonadal factor that stimulated secretion of *follicle stimulating hormone*, also involved in many aspects of development including *mesodermal* induction (see *mesenchyme*), *hematopoiesis*, and *neuronal* differentiation.
[ref. 5]

acute

Opposite term: *chronic.*

1. Of short duration, in relation to *exposure* or effect; the effect usually shows a rapid onset.
   Note 1: In regulatory *toxicology*, "acute" refers to studies where dosing is either single or limited to one day although the total study duration may extend to two weeks to permit appearance of *toxicity* in susceptible organ systems.
   Note 2: In aquatic *ecotoxicology*, acute exposure of the test organisms is typically continuous and of four days or less.
2. In clinical medicine, sudden and severe, having a rapid onset.

[ref. 2]

acute effect

See *effect, acute.*

acute exposure

See *exposure, acute.*

acute lymphoblastic (lymphocytic) leukemia (ALL)

See *leukemia, acute lymphoblastic.*

acute myelogenous leukemia (AML)

See *leukemia, acute myelogenous.*

acute-phase protein

One of a group of serum proteins, mostly produced in the liver, which rapidly changes in concentration (some acute-phase proteins increase, some decrease) during the initiation of an *inflammatory response.*
[ref. 3]

acute-phase response (APR)

Physiological response stimulated by *cytokines* including *interleukin*-1, interleukin-6, *interferons*, and *tumor necrosis factor*, characterized by increased vascular permeability, fever, and increased levels of proteins (thus called *acute-phase proteins*) such as *C-reactive protein*, occurring within a few hours of initiation.
Note: Infection, *inflammation*, tissue injury, and occasionally *neoplasms* may trigger the APR.
[ref. 3]

acute rejection

See *rejection, acute.*

acute respiratory distress syndrome (ARDS)

Acute lung failure characterized by *alveolar* and interstitial *edema*, perivascular *pulmonary* edema, and *hyalin membrane* formation, resulting from a variety of underlying causes, including inhalational *toxicities*, that result in increased pulmonary vascular *permeability.*
[ref. 3]

acute-to-chronic toxicity ratio (ACR)

Numerical dimensionless quantity by dividing an *acute toxicity* test result (*e.g.*, LC_{50}) by a *chronic toxicity* test result (*e.g., maximum acceptable toxicant concentration*) where both are expressed in the same units (*e.g.*, substance concentration). Ideally, the data are for the same *chemical species.*
Note 1: The ACR is in principle the inverse of an *application factor* and is used in a similar manner, commonly for estimating chronic toxicity of a substance on the basis of its acute toxicity.
Note 2: The ACR should be greater than one because the ratio compares an acute to a chronic value.
[ref. 2]

acute toxicity

See *toxicity, acute.*

acute toxicity test

See *toxicity test, acute.*

acyclicity

Irregular or absent *estrous cycles.*
[ref. 5]
Compare *anestrus.*

adactyly
adactylia
adactylism

Congenital absence of fingers or toes.
[ref. 5]

adaptation
physiological adaptation

Process by which an organism stabilizes its physiological condition after an environmental change.
Note: If adaptation exceeds the *homeostatic* range, it becomes pathological and results in symptoms of *disease* (*adverse effects*).
[After ref. 1]

adaptation, genetic

Result of random genetic variation due to *mutation* and (or) to changes in *allele* frequencies, causing variation in the survival and reproductive success of individuals and hence of groups of organisms, with the consequence that those best adjusted to their *environment* flourish.
Note: Genetic *adaptation* underlies the concept of *natural selection* leading to Darwinian *evolution*.
[ref. 2]

adaptive immune response

See *immune response, adaptive*.

adaptive immune system

That part of the *immune* system responsible for the *adaptive immune response*.
[ref. 3]

adaptive response

See *response, adaptive*.

added risk

See *risk, added*.

addiction

Compulsive, uncontrolled reward-seeking behavior, especially referring to substance *abuse*.
Note: An addiction may be psychological, referring to a craving or felt need for a behavior that produces a desired mental state without a known physiological basis, or it may be a physical (physiological) dependence in which discontinued use of a substance leads to symptoms of *withdrawal*.
[ref. 4]
See also *habituation*.

Addison disease (autoimmune)

Adrenocortical hypofunction characterized by *hypotension*, weight loss, *anorexia*, and weakness.

Note 1: The most common form is *idiopathic* Addison *disease*, mediated by *autoimmune* mechanisms. *Autoantibodies* specific to the adrenal cortex are specific diagnostic markers of this form.
Note 2: *Steroid 21-monooxygenase* (EC 1.14.14.16; 21-hydroxylase), a cytochrome P450 steroidogenic enzyme, is one of the major targets of adrenal autoantibodies in idiopathic Addison disease as well as in Addison disease in the context of autoimmune polyglandular *syndromes* (*polyendocrinopathies, autoimmune*).
Note 3: Hypofunction or failure of the adrenal gland may also be a manifestation of *antiphospholipid syndrome* due to *thrombosis* of the blood vessels of the adrenal glands.
[ref. 3]

additive effect

See *effect, additive.*

additive index

Quantification of the joint action of *toxicants* in a *mixture* by adding measures of their *toxicity* calculated in relation to the toxicity of a reference toxicant.
[ref. 2]

additivity (in toxicology)

Property of the toxicities of substances whereby the *toxicity* of a *mixture* of the substances reflects the simple sum of the individual *toxicant* effects.
[ref. 2]
See also *effect, additive.*

addressin

Extracellular protein of the venular *endothelium* serving as a *ligand* to a *homing receptor* for *lymphocytes.*
Note: Addressins are *glycoproteins* recognized by *L-selectin.*
[ref. 3]

addressin, vascular

Cell *adhesion molecule* present on the luminal surface of blood and *lymph* vessel endothelium, recognized by *homing* molecules that direct *leukocytes* to tissues with the appropriate "address".
[ref. 3]

adduct

New *chemical species* AB, each molecular entity of which is formed by direct combination of two separate molecular entities A and B in such a way that there is change in connectivity, but no loss, of atoms within the moieties A and B.
Note 1: Adduct stoichiometries other than 1:1 are also possible, for example, a bis-adduct (2:1). An "intramolecular adduct" can be formed when A and B are groups contained within the same molecular entity.
Note 2: Adduct is a general term that, whenever appropriate, should be used in preference to the less explicit term "complex". It is also used specifically for products of an addition reaction.
[ref. 8]
Note 3: In toxicology, adducts of *reactive intermediates* or bioactivated substances to DNA and proteins often cause cell damage.
[*]

adenocarcinoma

Malignant tumor formed from *glandular epithelial* tissue or formed in a glandular pattern.
[ref. 5]

adenoma

Benign *tumor* arising from *epithelial* cells in glandular tissue.
[ref. 4]

adenosine deaminase (ADA) deficiency

Lack of the enzyme adenosine deaminase (EC 3.5.4.4), which catalyzes the deamination of adenosine and deoxyadenosine to produce inosine and deoxyinosine, respectively. Affected individuals have a form of *severe combined immunodeficiency*.
[ref. 3]

adenosine receptor

Any of four types of purinergic *receptors* that respond to the nucleoside adenosine, two of which are involved in release of the *neurotransmitters, dopamine* and *glutamate*.
Note: The stimulatory effects of caffeine are thought to be due to caffeine's blockade of adenosine receptors.
[ref. 4]

adenosine triphosphate (ATP)

Major molecular component in the energy currency of the *cell*.
Note 1: In *eukaryotes*, ATP is produced mainly in the *mitochondria* through *oxidative phosphorylation* under *aerobic* conditions. *Toxic substances* that interfere with delivery of dioxygen to the cell, *poison* the *electron transport chain, uncouple* oxidative phosphorylation from ATP synthesis, or interfere with mitochondrial structure or function, compromise the cell's energy utilization.
Note 2: Under conditions of decreased dioxygen, *glycolysis* can become a secondary, though less efficient, source of ATP.
[*]

adenylate energy charge (AEC)

Index reflecting the balance of energy transfer between catabolic and anabolic processes, calculated from the equation

$$\mathrm{AEC} = ([\mathrm{ATP}] + 1/2[\mathrm{ADP}])/([\mathrm{ATP}] + [\mathrm{ADP}] + [\mathrm{AMP}])$$

where ATP, ADP, and AMP are the substance concentrations of adenosine tri-, di-, and monophosphate, respectively.
[ref. 2]

adermia

Congenital absence of skin.
[ref. 5]

adhesion factor

Substance contributing to selective cell-cell and cell-matrix binding.
[ref. 5]
See also *extracellular matrix*.

adhesion molecule

Molecule belonging mainly to the *immunoglobulins, integrin superfamily* (*e.g.*, LFA-1, ICAM-1) or *selectins*, expressed on the cell membrane of various cells including those of the *immune system.*
Note: Interaction of adhesion molecules with each other as *receptor* and corresponding *ligand* facilitates cooperation (cross-talk) of cells, *signal transduction*, and information transfer between cells.
[ref. 3]

aditus

Entrance or opening to some interior space or *cavity*.
[ref. 5]

adjuvant

1. In *pharmacology*, a substance added to a *drug* to speed or increase the action of the main component.
2. In *immunology*, a substance (such as aluminum hydroxide) or a suspension in oil of a dead organism (such as fragments of killed ***Mycobacterium***) that increases the response to an *antigen.*

[ref. 3]
See also *Freund's adjuvant.*

adjuvant arthritis

See *arthritis, adjuvant.*

administration (of a substance)

Application of a known amount of a substance to an organism in a reproducible manner and by a defined route.
[ref. 1]

adolescence (n)/**adolescent** (adj)

Stage of human development beginning with *puberty* and ending with *adulthood.*
[ref. 5]

adoptive transfer

Transfer, by *transplantation* of *immunocompetent* cells, of the capacity to mount an *immune response.*
[ref. 3]

adrenal 4 binding protein (Ad4BP)

Transcription factor that regulates the *expression* of the enzymes of *steroid* synthesis and is expressed primarily in steroidogenic cells.
[ref. 5]

adrenal gland

paranephric gland
suprarenal gland

Either of two small *endocrine glands*, one located above each kidney, consisting of a cortex, which secretes several *steroid hormones*, and a *medulla,* which secretes *adrenaline* and *noradrenaline*.
[ref. 5]

adrenaline

adrenalin
epinephrine (INN)
4-[(1*R*)-1-hydroxy-2-(methylamino)ethyl]benzene-1,2-diol

Catecholamine hormone secreted by the *adrenal glands* that increases heart rate, breathing rate, blood pressure, and carbohydrate metabolism.
[ref. 5]
See also *noradrenaline.*

adrenergic

1. Relating to or denoting secretion of and (or) response to *adrenaline, noradrenaline* or related substances; in particular referring to *sympathetic* nerve fibers.
2. Relating to or denoting an agent that mimics the activity of *adrenaline, noradrenaline* or related substances.

[ref. 4]
Compare *cholinergic.*
See also *sympathomimetic.*

α-adrenergic receptor

See *receptor, α-adrenergic.*

β-adrenergic antagonist

See *β-blocker.*

β-adrenergic blocking agent

See *β-blocker.*

β-adrenergic receptor

See *receptor, β-adrenergic.*

adrenoceptor

See *receptor, β-adrenergic.*

adrenocortocotropic hormone (ACTH)

Hormone secreted by the *pituitary gland* and stimulating the adrenal cortex (see *adrenal gland*).
[ref. 5]

adrenogenital syndrome

See *congenital adrenal hyperplasia.*

adsorbate

Molecular species of gas, dissolved substance, or liquid that adheres to or is adsorbed in an extremely thin surface layer of a solid substance.
[ref. 2]

adsorbent

Condensed phase at the surface of which *adsorption* may occur.
[ref. 2]

adsorption

Increase in the *concentration* of a substance at the interface of a condensed and a liquid or a gaseous layer owing to the operation of surface forces.
[ref. 1]
See also *absorption; interfacial layer; sorption.*

adsorption factor

Amount of substance adsorbed at the interface of a condensed and a liquid or gaseous phase divided by the total amount of the substance available for *adsorption*.
[ref. 1]

adstringent

See *astringent*.

adult

Person or animal that is fully grown, developed, and sexually mature.
[ref. 5]

adulthood

State of being *adult*.
[ref. 5]

adult respiratory distress syndrome (ARDS)

See *acute respiratory distress syndrome.*

adult stem cell

See *stem cell.*

advanced glycation endproduct (AGE)

Protein or lipid that becomes non-enzymatically and stably *glycosylated*.
Note 1: Circulating protein AGEs bind to cell-surface receptors for AGE (RAGE) present on *endothelial cells, macrophages*, and renal mesangial cells, resulting in increased vascular permeability and *cytokine* production.
Note 2: Important sources of AGEs include reaction with methyl glyoxal (produced nonenzymatically from triose phosphate intermediates of *glycolysis*, glyceraldehyde 3-phosphate and dihydroxyacetone phosphate, especially under hyperglycemic conditions) and glyoxal (produced by *lipid peroxidation*). Both are more potent than glucose in the formation of AGE.
Note 3: Production of AGE and occupancy of RAGE have been strongly implicated in the microvascular *pathology* occurring from hyperglycemia due to *diabetes mellitus*.
[*]
See also *glycosylation; nonenzymatic glycosylation.*

advection (in ecotology)

Process of transport of a substance and its properties (*e.g.*, heat) in air or water solely by bulk motion (in water or air currents).
Note: In open-ocean marine systems, advective transport of chemicals into the water column from *sediments* is small compared with that by *diffusion*. In *estuarine* systems, freshwater rivers, and lakes, advective processes can contribute substantially to system transport.
[After ref. 2]

adverse drug reaction

Harmful or unpleasant reaction following administration of a pharmaceutical product.
[*]

adverse effect

adverse outcome

Change in biochemistry, physiology, growth, development morphology, or behavior of an organism, including the effects of aging, that results in impairment of functional capacity or impairment of capacity to compensate for additional stress or increase in susceptibility to other environmental influences.
[After ref. 1]
See also *adverse event*.

adverse event

Occurrence that causes an *adverse effect*.
Note: An adverse event in clinical studies is any untoward reaction in a human subject participating in a research project; such an adverse event, which may be a psychological reaction, must be reported to an institutional review board.
[ref. 1]

adverse immunostimulation

Antigen-nonspecific, inappropriate, or unintended activation of a component of the *immune system*.
Note: The distinction from *pseudoallergy* is subtle.
[ref. 3]

adverse outcome

See *adverse effect*.

adverse outcome pathway (AOP)

Ordered sequence of *key events* linking an initiating molecular event to an *adverse effect* in an individual organism, population of organisms or an ecosystem, relevant to a specific *risk assessment*.
Note: The causal links between key events in the AOP are referred to as "key event (KE) relationships".
[*]
Compare *toxicity pathway*.

aeroallergen

Any airborne particle, such as a pollen grain or spore, that triggers an *allergic* reaction in sensitive individuals.
[ref. 3]

aerobe

Organism that requires dioxygen for respiration and hence for life and growth.
[ref. 1]

aerobic

Opposite term: anaerobic.

Requiring dioxygen.
[ref. 1]

aerodynamic diameter (of a particle)

Diameter of a spherical particle with relative density equal to unity that has the same settling velocity in air as the particle in question.
[ref. 1]

aerosol

Mixture of small particles (solid, liquid, or a mixed variety) and a *carrier* gas (usually air).
Note 1: Owing to their size, aerosol particles (usually less than 100 μm and greater than 0.01 μm in diameter) have a comparatively small sedimentation velocity and hence exhibit some degree of stability in the earth's gravitational field.
Note 2: An aerosol may be characterized by its chemical composition, its radioactivity, the particle size distribution, the electrical charge, and the optical properties.
[ref. 1]

aetiology

See *etiology*.

afferent

Opposite term: *efferent*.

Inflowing. Of nerves, those that conduct impulses toward the *central nervous system*.
[ref. 4]

affinity

intrinsic affinity

Strength of binding (affinity constant) between a *receptor* (*e.g.*, one *antigen*-binding site on an *antibody*) and a *ligand* (*e.g., epitope* on an antigen).
[ref. 3]
See also *avidity*.

affinity chromatography

Chromatography in which immobilized *antibody* (or *antigen*) is used to select specific antigen (or antibody) from a mixture. The purified *ligand* is then released by disrupting the antibody–antigen interaction, *e.g.*, by changing the pH.
[ref. 3]

affinity maturation

Increase in *antibody affinity* for an *antigen* observed as the *humoral immune response* progresses.
[ref. 3]

agammaglobulinemia

See *agammaglobulinemia, X-linked*.

agammaglobulinemia, X-linked

Bruton syndrome

X-linked impairment of the ability to produce *mature B-cells*, thus characterized by recurrent infections.
[ref. 3]

aganglionic megacolon, congenital

See *Hirschsprung disease.*

age class

Group of organisms of the same age within a *population.*
[ref. 2]

age composition

Distribution of organisms among the various age classes present in the *population.*
Note: The sum of the number of individuals in all *age classes* equals the population size.
[ref. 2]

age distribution

Composition of a *population* in terms of how its *abundance* is distributed across *age classes.*
[ref. 2]

age sensitivity

Quantitative and qualitative age dependence of susceptibility to an *adverse effect.*
[ref. 1]

age-specific birth rate

age-specific fecundity
age-specific fertility rate

Mean number of offspring born to a female in a specific *age class* in a given year, expressed per 1000 females in that age class.
[ref. 2]

age-specific death rate

age-specific mortality
age-specific number of individuals dying

Mean number of deaths as tabulated for a life table interval or for a specific *age class* in a given year, expressed per 1000 in that interval or age class.
[ref. 2]

age-specific fecundity

See *age-specific birth rate.*

age-specific fertility rate

See *age-specific birth rate.*

age-specific mortality

See *age-specific death rate.*

age-specific number of individuals dying

See *age-specific death rate.*

agenesis

Absence or partial development of an organ or body part observed at *birth.*
[ref. 5]

agglutination (n)/**agglutinate** (v)

Clumping of particles, such as *erythrocytes* or bacteria, caused by bivalent binding of *antibodies* to *antigens* on the surfaces of adjacent particles.
Note: When the particles that agglutinate are erythrocytes, the phenomenon is called hemagglutination.
[ref. 3]
See also *hemagglutinin; prozone effect.*

aggregation chimera

Organism made by combining cells from two *embryos* of different *genotypes*.
[ref. 5]

aggregation error

Error in *Bayesian probability* analysis of model systems resulting from the use of a single set of parameters to represent a collection of distinct entities, such as individuals, in a *population*.
[ref. 2]

aging (of a contaminant)

Decrease in *bioavailability* of a *contaminant* with time.
Note: Generally aging of a contaminant is due to increased *absorption* by solid particles.
[ref. 2]

aging (of acetylcholinesterase)

Property of the complex formed by reaction of *organophosphate* (OP) pesticide with *acetylcholinesterase* whereby the reversible enzyme-OP complex dealkylates to form an irreversibly inhibited *enzyme*.
[ref. 2]

aging, rate-of-living theory of

Idea that the total *metabolic* expenditure of a *genotype* is generally fixed, and longevity depends upon the rate of energy expenditure.
[ref. 2]

agnathia

Congenital absence or partial absence of the lower jaw.
[ref. 5]
See also *macrognathia; otocephaly; synotia.*

agnosia

Impaired ability to recognize or comprehend the meaning of various sensations, not attributable to faulty sensory input or general intellect.
Note: Generally agnosia involves several sensory forms, such as *auditory (acoustic),* gustatory, *olfactory,* tactile, and visual agnosias.
[ref. 4]

agonist

Opposite term: *antagonist.*

Substance, naturally occurring or otherwise, that binds to cell *receptors* that normally respond to a naturally occurring substance, and produces an effect similar to the natural substance.

Note 1: A partial agonist activates a receptor but does not cause as much of a physiological change as does a full agonist.
Note 2: A co-agonist works together with other co-agonists to produce an altered effect.
[ref. 5]

agonist, inverse

Ligand that binds to a *receptor*, thereby inhibiting receptor reactivity to an *agonist* without having itself a negative effect on the receptor response.
[*]

agranulocytosis

Failure of the *bone marrow* to make sufficient *granulocytes*, especially *neutrophils*.
Note: Agranulocytosis is normally identified by a *neutrophil* count less than 0.5×10^9 L^{-1} of blood.
[ref. 3]

air pollution

Presence of substances in the atmosphere resulting either from human activity or natural processes, in sufficient concentration, for a sufficient time and under circumstances such as to interfere with comfort, *health*, or welfare of persons, or to harm the environment.
[ref. 1]

air pollution control system

1. Network of organizations carrying out the various aspects of *monitoring*, regulating and reducing air pollution.
2. Group of measures or processes used to minimize or prevent air pollution.

[After ref. 1]

air pollution tolerance index (APTI)

See *tolerance index, air pollution*.

alar plate

Part of the *dorsal* side of *neural tube* in the *embryo*, involved in general *somatic* and *visceral* sensory communication.
[ref. 5]

albedo (in astronomy)

Amount of light reflected by the surface of a body (typically a planet or moon) divided by the amount of incident light, usually expressed as a percentage but sometimes on a scale from zero to 1.
Note: Albedo depends on the wavelength of light, but usually refers to an average across the spectrum of visible light.
[*]

albinism

achromasia
achromatosis
hypomelanism
hypomelanosis

Congenital disorder characterized by a lack of melanin pigment in the eyes, skin, and hair.
Note 1: Albinism is known to affect mammals, fish, birds, reptiles, and amphibians.
Note 2: The lack of melanin in albinism is typically due to an absence of or defect in the copper-containing enzyme, tyrosinase (EC 1.14.18.1).
[ref. 2,5]
See also *leucism*.

albuminuria

Presence of albumin, derived from *plasma*, in the urine.
[ref. 1]

alcohol dehydrogenase

One of a group of *enzymes* (EC 1.1.1.1) that uses NAD to convert an alcohol to the respective aldehyde or ketone, with production of NADH.
Note 1: Alcohol dehydrogenase in the liver and *gastrointestinal tract* is important in human ethanol *metabolism*, producing acetaldehyde.
Note 2: Alcohol dehydrogenase oxidizes methanol to the *toxic substance*, formaldehyde.
Note 3: Acetaldehyde dehydrogenase (EC 1.2.1.10) potentially oxidizes the resultant acetaldehyde further, producing acetic acid, which is available for energy metabolism; additional aldehyde dehydrogenases can convert formaldehyde into formic acid that can produce an *acidosis*.
Note 4: *Allelic* variations in aldehyde dehydrogenases, and possibly alcohol dehydrogenase, give rise to variable ethanol *tolerance* in human *populations*.
[*]

alcohol-related neurodevelopmental disabilities (ARND)

Spectrum of functional neurologic (behavioral) defects resulting from exposure *in utero* to alcohol.
[ref. 5]
See also *fetal alcohol syndrome*.

alga (n)/algae (pl)/algal (adj)

Any of various chiefly aquatic, eukaryotic, photosynthetic organisms, ranging in size from single-celled forms to the giant kelp.
Note 1: Algae of various species, often unicells, are used for *toxicity* testing in *ecotoxicology*.
Note 2: Algae are important components of aquatic *food webs*.
[ref. 2]

algal bloom

Rapid increase in the abundance of *phytoplankton* or *benthic algae* in a given area, often as a result of increased availability of nutrients or light, or increased temperature (*e.g.*, the spring bloom).
[ref. 2]

algicide
algaecide

Substance intended to kill *algae*.
[ref. 1]

algistatic

Inhibiting algal *population* growth.
[ref. 2]
See also *algicide*.

alimentary canal

See *gastrointestinal tract*.

aliquot (in analytical chemistry)

Known amount of a homogeneous material, assumed to be taken with negligible *sampling error*.
Note 1: The term "aliquot" is usually applied to fluids.
Note 2: The term "aliquot" is usually used when the fractional part is an exact divisor of the whole; the term "aliquant" has been used when the fractional part is not an exact divisor of the whole (*e.g.*, a 15-mL portion is an aliquant of 100 mL).
Note 3: When an aliquot is taken of a laboratory sample or test sample or the sample is otherwise subdivided, the samples have been called split samples.
[ref. 1]

alkalinity

Opposite term: acidity.

Capacity of natural water to neutralize acid (proton-accepting capacity) as measured by titration of a water sample with a dilute acid to a specific pH endpoint.
Note: Most often, alkalinity is a function of carbonate (CO_3^{2-}), hydrogencarbonate (HCO_3^-), and hydroxide (OH^-) concentrations, *i.e.*, the carbonate-hydrogencarbonate buffering of the water. However, dissolved organic compounds, borates, phosphates, and silicates can also contribute to alkalinity.
[ref. 2]

alkalosis

Opposite term: *acidosis*.

Abnormal decrease in hydronium ion activity (increase in pH above the reference interval of 7.35 to 7.45 in humans) measured in the arterial blood.
Note: Common causes of alkalosis include a decrease in CO_2, deficiency of chloride, and decreased bicarbonate.
[ref. 5]

alkylating agent

Substance that introduces an alkyl substituent into a compound.
[ref. 1]

all-or-none effect

See *quantal effect*.

allantois (n)/allantoic (adj)

Extra-*embryonic membrane* formed early in development as an outpouching of the *yolk sac* into the area of the future *umbilical cord*.
Note: Blood vessels of the allantois become the *umbilical artery* and *umbilical veins*.
[ref. 5]

allele (n)/**allelic** (adj)

One of several alternate forms of a *gene* that occur at the same relative position (*locus*) on *homologous chromosomes*.
Note: Paired alleles become separated during *meiosis* and can be recombined following fusion of *gametes*.
[ref. 5]

allelic exclusion

Phenomenon whereby, following successful rearrangement of one *allele* of an *antigen receptor* gene, rearrangement of the other parental allele is suppressed, thereby ensuring each *lymphocyte* expresses only a single specificity of antigen receptor.
Note: Allelic exclusion does not occur for α chains in *T-lymphocytes*.
[ref. 3]

allergen (n)/**allergenic** (adj)

Immunostimulant (see *immunostimulation*) *antigenic* substance that may or may not cause a clinically significant effect but is capable of producing an immune reaction, often *immediate-type hypersensitivity*.
[ref. 3]
See also *allergen, contact; allergen, latex.*

allergen, contact

Substance that causes a skin *hypersensitivity* reaction by direct contact.
[ref. 3]

allergen, latex

Allergen found in natural rubber latex (NRL).
Note: Major latex (NRL-specific) allergens are Hev b 1, Hev b 3, Hev b 5, and Hev b 6.02. These four major allergens account for the allergenic potential of NRL products such as gloves, condoms, teats, and balloons.
[ref. 3]

allergic

Immunologically hypersensitive.
[ref. 3]
See also *hypersensitivity*.

allergy

Symptoms or signs occurring in sensitized individuals (see *sensitization*) following exposure to a previously encountered substance (*allergen*) that would otherwise not cause such symptoms or signs in nonsensitized individuals. The most common forms of allergy are *rhinitis, urticaria, asthma*, and *contact dermatitis*.
Note: Except in the case of exposure to *contact allergens*, allergy is often an *immunoglobulin E-mediated hypersensitivity, e.g.*, asthma, *eczema, hay fever*, or food allergy.
[ref. 3]
See also *pseudoallergy*.

alloantibody

Antibody produced against an *antigen* from another member of the same species.
[ref. 3]
See also *alloantigen*.

alloantigen

Antigen, present in some but not all individuals of a particular species, that arises from polymorphisms at the *major histocompatibility complex* loci and stimulates intense reactions to *allograft* tissues from other individuals of the same species that do not produce it.
Note: The human *ABO blood group* system antigens and *Rhesus (Rh) factor* are important examples of alloantigens.
[ref. 3]

allogeneic
allogenic

Genetically different, referring to individuals of the same species.
Note: In *immunotoxicology* allogeneic generally refers to the use of genetically dissimilar cells to elicit a *cell-mediated immune response* in *in vitro* assays.
[ref. 3]
Compare *xenogeneic.*

allogenic succession

See *succession, allogenic.*

allograft

Tissue or organ *graft* between *allogeneic* individuals.
[ref. 3]

allometric

1. Pertaining to a systematic relationship between growth rates of different parts of an organism and its overall growth rate.
2. Pertaining to a systematic relationship between size, shape, and metabolism in different species.

[ref. 1]

allometric growth

Regular and systematic pattern of growth such that the mass or size of any *organ* or part of a body can be expressed in relation to the total mass or size of the entire organism according to the *allometric* equation:

$$Y = bx^{\alpha}$$

where Y = mass of the organ, x = mass of the organism, α = growth coefficient of the organ, and b is a constant.
[ref. 1]

allometric scaling

See *scaling, allometric.*

allometry (in biology)

Measurement of the rate of growth of a part or parts of an organism relative to the growth of the whole organism.
[ref. 1]

allomone

Semiochemical that is produced by an organism inducing a response in an organism of another species that is favorable to the emitter.
[ref. 1]
See also *kairomone; synomone.*

alloreactivity

Reactivity of an *antibody* with an *alloantigen.*
[ref. 3]

allotype

Allelic variant of an *antibody* that, because it is not present in all individuals, may be *immunogenic* in members of the same species that have a different version of the *allele.*
[ref. 3]

alopecia

Loss of hair; absence or thinning of hair from areas of skin where it is usually present.
Note: Alopecia is often associated with *autoimmune disease, e.g.*, autoimmune thyroid diseases, *pernicious anemia, Addison disease, diabetes mellitus type 1*, or *systemic lupus erythematosus.*
[1,3]

alopecia, neonatal

See *neonatal occipital alopecia.*

alternative pathway (of complement activation)

Activation pathway involving *complement* components C3, Factor B, Factor D, and *properdin* that, in the presence of a stabilizing activator surface such as microbial polysaccharide, generates the alternative pathway C3 convertase (EC 3.4.21.43) C3bBb.
[ref. 3]
See also *classical pathway (of complement activation).*

alternative test (in toxicology)

Any toxicological test that is suitable to reduce or replace animal studies, often using microorganisms (*e.g., Ames Test*), lower organisms, or cell lines.
Note: Alternative tests are often simple to perform and standardize. They may provide valuable information about mechanisms, but may differ significantly from the situation in the living higher organism.
[*]

alveolar period

alveolar phase

Phase in lung development beginning *in utero* (about 32 to 36 weeks in the human *fetus*) and lasting until about 8 years of age.
Note: In the alveolar period, the terminal alveolar saccules subdivide several more times, giving rise to the mature *alveoli.*
[ref. 5]

alveolus (n)/**alveoli** (n, pl)/**alveolar** (adj) (*pulmonary*)

Any of the many terminal air sacs of the airways in the lungs necessary for rapid gaseous exchange with the blood.
[ref. 5]

alveolar macrophage

Macrophage found in the lung *alveoli*; it may remove and sometimes retain inhaled particulate matter.
[ref. 3]

alveolitis

1. Inflammation of *alveoli*.
2. Inflammation of a tooth socket.

[ref. 3]

alveolitis, exogen allergic

See *atypical interstitial pneumonia.*

Alzheimer disease

Common and progressive *neurodegenerative disease* leading to loss of memory, orientation, and judgment (*dementia*).
[ref. 4]
See also *b-amyloid; amyloid plaque; neurofibrillary tangle; tau protein.*

amastia

Congenital absence of one or more *mammary glands.*
[ref. 5]

ambient

Surrounding (applied to environmental media such as air, water, sediment, or soil).
[ref. 1]

ambient monitoring

Continuous or repeated measurement of agents in the environment to evaluate ambient *exposure* and *health risk* by comparison with appropriate reference values based on knowledge of the probable relationship between exposure and resultant *adverse* health *effects.*
[ref. 1]

ambient standard

See *environmental quality standard.*

ambisexual

bisexual

1. Pertaining to or characterized by *hermaphroditism.*
2. Denoting sexual characteristics common to both sexes, *e.g., pubic* hair.

[ref. 5]

amelia

Lacking one or more limbs or having a shrunken or deformed limb as a *birth defect.*
[ref. 5]
See also *phocomelia.*

ameloblast

Epithelial cell that deposits enamel during tooth development.
[ref. 5]

amelogenesis imperfecta

hereditary yellow, brown or grey tooth enamel
Developmental *disorder* of the teeth in which they are covered with thin, abnormal enamel resulting from defective structure or processing of enamel proteins.
[ref. 5]

amenorrhea

menostasis

Absence or abnormal stoppage of *menstruation.*
[ref. 5]

Ames test

Method for assessing *mutagenicity* in vitro using mutant (see *mutation*) strains of the bacterium ***Salmonella typhimurium*** that cannot grow in a given histidine-deficient medium
Note 1: Mutagens cause reverse mutations that enable the bacterium to grow on the histidine-deficient medium used in the Ames test.
Note 2: The Ames test can be carried out in the presence of differentially centrifuged liver homogenates, providing enzymes that catalyze the *metabolic transformation* of mutagen precursors to active derivatives.
[ref. 5]

γ-aminobutyric acid (GABA)

4-aminobutanoic acid

Major *neurotransmitter* at inhibitory *synapses* in the *central nervous system* of mammals.
Note: GABA is often referred to as an "inhibitory neurotransmitter".
[ref. 4]

γ-aminobutyric acid (GABA) receptor

See *receptor, γ-aminobutyric acid.*

2-amino-3-(3-hydroxy-5-methyl-1,2-oxazol-4-yl)propanoic acid (AMPA) receptor

See *receptor, 2-amino-3-(3-hydroxy-5-methyl-1,2-oxazol-4-yl)propanoic acid.*

δ-aminolevulinic acid dehydrase (ALAD)

5-aminolevulinate dehydrase
porphobilinogen synthase

Enzyme (EC 4.2.1.24) that catalyzes the condensation of two molecules of 5-aminolevulinic acid (IUPAC name: 4-oxopentanoic acid) to porphobilinogen, a precursor of porphyrin, and hence of heme, cytochromes, and hemoproteins.

Note: ALAD is inhibited by lead at low blood concentrations (less than 100 μg L^{-1}), leading to anemia, excess production of erythropoietin, and an increased number of immature erythrocytes.
[*]

amnesia

Partial or total, transient or permanent loss of memory.
[ref. 4]

amnesic shellfish poisoning (ASP)

Human illness caused by consumption of the marine *toxin domoic acid* that may lead to dizziness, confusion, motor weakness and seizures, with permanent cognitive impairment and short term memory loss.
Note 1: Domoic acid is produced by marine diatoms belonging to the genus ***Pseudo-nitzschia*** and the species ***Nitzschia navis-varingica.*** It is passed on to humans by consumption of bivalve shellfish (mollusks) such as mussels, oysters, and clams that have accumulated it during filter feeding.
Note 2: ASP is often characterized by *excitotoxicity* and loss of *hippocampal neurons.*
[ref. 4]

amniocentesis

Transabdominal procedure in which *amniotic fluid* is sampled by means of a needle inserted into the *amniotic sac.*
Note: Amniocentesis is used to screen for infections and abnormalities in the developing *fetus.*
[ref. 5]

amniochorionic membrane

Composite *membrane*, formed by fusion of the *amnion* interiorly and the outer *chorion*, that surrounds the developing *fetus.*
[ref. 5]

amnion (n)/amniotic (adj)

Membrane that lines the *amniotic cavity* (*amniotic sac*) and encloses the *embryo* of a mammal, bird, or reptile.
[ref. 5]

amniote

Any *vertebrate* animal, such as a reptile, bird, or mammal, that possesses an *amnion, chorion*, and *allantois* during *embryonic* development.
[ref. 5]
Compare *anamniote.*

amniotic cavity

Fluid-filled space that surrounds the developing *embryo* of a mammal, bird, or reptile, bounded by the *amniotic sac.*
[ref. 5]

amniotic fluid

Fluid surrounding an *embryo* or *fetus* in the *amniotic cavity.*
[ref. 5]

amniotic sac

Membranous structure in *amniotes*, within which the *embryo* and *fetus* develop.
Note: The amniotic sac consists of a thin but tough, transparent pair of membranes, the *amnion* and *chorion*, that hold the developing *embryo* (and later *fetus*) until shortly before *birth*.
[ref. 5]

amphibian metamorphosis assay

Procedure in which a frog (often ***Xenopus laevis***) is exposed to a substance starting at the tadpole stage, and the growth and development of the animals is studied.
[ref. 5]
See also *FETAX*.

amplification (of genes)

See *gene amplification*.

ampulla

Flask-like dilatation of a *canal* or *duct*.
[ref. 5]

amygdala

Brain nucleus located in the median *temporal lobe* that is part of the *limbic system* and plays an important role in emotional responses.
[ref. 4]

amyloid

Fibrous protein secreted into the extracellular space where it forms amorphous deposits in multiple organs in some pathological states.
[ref. 3]
See also *β-amyloid*.

β-amyloid

Extracellular aggregate of *misfolded* fibrous proteins, typically with cross-linked β-sheet structure.
Note: β-Amyloid occurs naturally with aging, but it is found in increased amounts in a number of tissue pathologies including *Alzheimer disease*.
[ref. 4]
See also *amyloid plaque*.

amyloid plaque
neuritic plaque
senile plaque

Structure representing extracellular deposition of *β-amyloid* protein in the *grey matter* of the *brain* that occurs with aging and in increased amount in *Alzheimer disease*.
[ref. 4]

amyotrophic lateral sclerosis (ALS)
Lou Gehrig's disease
motor neuron disease

Debilitating degenerative *disease* of the *motor neurons* characterized by progressive muscle weakness, muscle *atrophy* and *fasciculations*, muscle *spasticity*, difficulty

speaking (*dysarthria*), difficulty swallowing (*dysphagia*), and difficulty breathing (*dyspnea*).
[ref. 4]

anabolism

Opposite term: *catabolism.*

Complete set of biochemical processes that use energy to build complex molecules from simpler precursors.
[*]

anadromous

Showing *anadromy.*
[ref. 2]

anadromy

Life-history pattern that is characterized by egg incubation and early juvenile development in freshwater, migration to seawater for adult development, and a return to freshwater for spawning.
Note: Obligatory anadromy is the term applied where migration to seawater is required for survival.
[ref. 2]
See also *catadromy.*

anaemia

See *anemia.*

anaerobe (n)/anaerobic (adj)

Opposite term: *aerobe/aerobic.*

Organism that does not require dioxygen for life.
Note: Obligate (strict) anaerobes grow only in the absence of dioxygen. Facultative anaerobes can grow either in the presence or in the absence of dioxygen.
[ref. 1]

anaesthetic

See *anesthetic.*

anal canal

Terminal part of the large intestine between the rectum and anus.
Note: The anal canal arises as the *dorsal cavity* of the *cloaca* after division of the cloaca by the urorectal septum, the *ventral* cavity becoming the *urogenital sinus.*
[ref. 5]
See also *anal membrane.*

anal membrane

In the *embryo, dorsal* part of the *cloacal membrane* after its division of the urorectal septum.
[ref. 5]

anal pit

See *proctodeum.*

analgesic
anodyne
painkiller

Substance that relieves *pain* without causing loss of *consciousness*.
[ref. 4]

analogue metabolism

Process by which a normally nonbiodegradable compound is biodegraded in the presence of a structurally similar compound that can induce the necessary enzymes.
[ref. 1]

analytic study

See *study, analytic*.

anamnestic (in immunology)

Describing *immunological memory* that gives rise to a rapid increase in *immunological response* after reexposure to *antigen*.
Note: Literal meaning, "does not forget".
[ref. 3]

anamniote

Any *vertebrate* animal, such as a fish or amphibian, that lacks an *amnion, chorion*, and *allantois* during *embryonic* development.
[ref. 5]
Compare *amniote*.

anaphase

Stage of *mitosis* and *meiosis* in which the *chromosomes* move from the equatorial plate toward opposite ends of the *nuclear spindle*.
[ref. 5]

anaphase lag

Slowing or stopping of normal migration of *chromosomes* during *anaphase*, resulting in chromosomes being excluded from one of the daughter cells causing *aneuploidy*.
[ref. 5]

anaphrodisiac

Anything tending to reduce *libido*.
[ref. 4]

anaphylactic shock

Immediate overreaction of the *immune system* to a *drug* or other agent in an individual who has previously encountered the agent and has produced *antibodies* to that agent.
Note: The major manifestation of anaphylactic shock is *angioedema*, leading to hypovolemia, obstruction of the airway, and bronchospasm; these in turn may lead to coma or death.
[ref. 3]
See also *anaphylaxis*.

anaphylactoid

Of or resembling *anaphylaxis*.
[ref. 1]

anaphylatoxin

Complement-derived protein fragment (*e.g.*, C3a, C4a, or C5a) capable of directly triggering *mast cell degranulation, chemotaxis*, smooth muscle contraction, and *inflammation*.
[ref. 3]

anaphylaxis

Life-threatening *type I hypersensitivity allergic reaction* (see *allergy*) occurring in a person or animal exposed to an *antigen* or *hapten* to which they have previously been sensitized.
Note: Consequences of the reaction may include *angioedema*, vascular collapse, shock (see *anaphylactic shock*), and respiratory distress.
[ref. 3]

anaplasia (n)/anaplastic (adj)

Loss of normal cell differentiation, a characteristic feature of most *malignancies*.
[ref. 1]

anasarca
hydrosarca
dropsy

Generalized *edema* in the subcutaneous *connective tissue*.
Note: Anasarca may be *congenital* (whole body edema) caused by liver failure, renal failure, right-sided heart failure, or severe malnutrition with resultant protein deficiency.
[ref. 5]

anastomosis

Connection creating continuity between two tubular body structures, *e.g.* blood vessels or loops of bowel.
Note: An anastomosis may be a surgical construction (as when the two cut ends are joined following resection of a loop of bowel), may result from trauma, or may occur as a natural anatomic feature, typically involving blood vessels (as in an arteriovenous anastomosis bypassing a capillary bed; see *arteriovenous shunt*).
[ref. 5]

anatomic position, fetal

Usual positioning of the developing *fetus* with the back curved forward, head bent forward, and limbs drawn in towards the body.
Note: This anatomic position arises from the natural positioning of the *embryo* as the *germ layers* develop.
[ref. 5]

anchoring villus

Chorionic villus that is attached to the region of the *endometrium* (see also *decidua*) that interacts with the *trophoblast* during development of the *placenta*.
[ref. 5]

androblastoma
arrhenoblastoma
Sertoli cell tumor

Rare benign *tumor* of the *testis* histologically resembling the *fetal* testis: the *epithelium* contains *Sertoli cells* that may produce *estrogen* and cause feminization.
[ref. 5]

androgen (n)/androgenic (adj)

Substance, such as a naturally occurring *steroid hormone*, that binds to *androgen receptors* to activate the male *accessory sex organs* and induce male *secondary sexual characteristics*.
[ref. 5]
See also *androgenic*.

androgen receptor (AR)

Nuclear receptor that is activated by binding of *testosterone* or dihydrotestosterone.
[ref. 5]
See also *androgen*.

androstenedione

Steroid hormone produced in the *adrenal glands* and *gonads* as a common precursor of male (*testosterone*) and female (*estrogen*) sex hormones.
[ref. 5]

anemia

Decrease in the number of *erythrocytes* or total *hemoglobin* in the blood that results in a decrease in the oxygen-carrying capacity of the blood, sometimes pallor and fatigue.
[ref. 5]

anemia, aplastic

Greatly decreased formation of *erythrocytes* and *hemoglobin*, usually associated with pronounced *granulocytopenia* and *thrombocytopenia*, as a result of hypoplastic or aplastic *bone marrow*.
Note: The diagnosis of aplastic anemia requires *bone marrow* biopsy to demonstrate replacement of blood cell precursors with fat cells and rule out other causes of *pancytopenia* such as neoplastic infiltration.
[ref. 3]

anencephalus

1. *Fetus* lacking all or most of the neural tissues of brain.
2. *Anencephaly*.

[ref. 5]

anencephaly (n)/anencephalic (adj)
anencephalia

Congenital absence of a major portion of the brain and its *meninges*, skull, and scalp that results from abnormal *embryonic* development.
[ref. 5]

anergy

Lack of an *immune response*, usually taken as lack of response to common *recall antigens*.
Note: The failure of *B*- or *T-cells* to proliferate in response to defined *autoantigens* (*clonal anergy*) is a primary mechanism of *self-tolerance*.
[ref. 3]

anesthetic
anaesthetic

Substance that reduces the experience of *pain* systemically (general anesthetic) or locally, with or without loss of *consciousness*.
[ref. 1,4]

anestrus

Interval of sexual inactivity between two periods of *estrus*.
[ref. 5]

aneugen (n)/**aneugenic** (adj)

Agent inducing *aneuploidy*.
[ref. 5]

aneuploid

Referring to a cell or organism with missing or extra *chromosomes* or parts of chromosomes, and thus an abnormal number of chromosomes that is not an exact multiple of the *haploid* number.
[ref. 5]
See also *euploid; ploidy*.

aneuploidy

State of being *aneuploid*.
[ref. 5]

aneurysm

Abnormal bulging of the wall of an artery or a chamber of the heart.
Note: An aneurysm may present a risk of *hemorrhage* if it ruptures.
[ref. 5]

angioblast
vasoformative cell

1. Cell taking part in blood vessel formation.
2. Primordial *mesenchymal* tissue from which *embryonic* blood cells and vascular *endothelium* are differentiated.

[ref. 5]

angioedema
angioneurotic edema

Swelling that occurs in the tissue just below the surface of the skin, most often around the lips and eyes, the mucous membranes and occasionally the viscera.

Note 1: Angioedema may be genetic, when it is referred to as hereditary angioedema (HAE), but is more usually caused by an *allergic* reaction to either food or medication, and is then called acquired angioedema (AAE).
Note 2: Angioedema may take from minutes to hours to develop. Severe angioedema can compromise the airway, and can be life-threatening.
Note 3: Angioedema is often associated with *dermatographism, urticaria, erythema,* and *purpura.* It may sometimes be a sign of a condition such as *leukemia* or *Hodgkin disease.*
Note 4: Angioedema is similar to *hives*, but hives involve itchy red welts on the surface of the skin, whereas angioedema is a deeper swelling under the skin.
[ref. 3]

angiogenesis (n)/**angiogenic** (adj)

Development of new blood vessels in the *embryo* or from pre-existing vessels; formation of capillary networks.
[ref. 5]
Compare *arteriogenesis; vasculogenesis.*

angiography

Radiography of blood or *lymph* vessels, following the introduction of a radio-opaque substance.
[ref. 4]

angiospasm

See *vasospasm.*

angiotensin

Peptide *hormone*, produced as a prohormone in liver, that circulates in the *blood*, increases aldosterone secretion, and raises blood pressure by *vasoconstriction.*
[*]
See also *angiotensin converting enzyme.*

angiotensin converting enzyme (ACE)

Enzyme (EC 3.4.15.1) that converts *angiotensin* I to angiotensin II, causing blood vessels to constrict thus increasing blood pressure.
Note: ACE inhibitors are used clinically to lower blood pressure.
[ref. 5]

ankyloglossia

Congenital oral anomaly, in which the lingual frenulum (the membrane connecting the underside of the tongue to the floor of the mouth) is unusually short and thick.
Note: As a result of ankyloglossia, mobility of the tongue tip is decreased.
[ref. 5]

ankylosing spondylitis

Chronic inflammatory *disease* affecting the spine, sacroiliac joints, and large peripheral joints, having a major genetic predisposition.
[ref. 3]

annulus (of intervertebral disc)

Tough outer ring of an *intervertebral disc.*
[ref. 4]

anodontia

Congenital absence of all primary or permanent teeth.
[ref. 5]

anodyne

See *analgesic.*

anogenital distance (AGD)

Distance along the *perineum* between the *anus* and the base of the *vagina* or penis, or in the *fetus* between the anus and the base of the *genital tubercle.*
Note 1: The anogenital distance is relatively longer in males than females. This in part relates to dihydro*testosterone* levels, and abnormal distances may indicate birth defects, *feminization* in males, *etc.*
Note 2: In some species where gender is not obvious at birth, anogenital distance can be used for a tentative determination of the sex of the *neonate.*
[ref. 5]

anoikis

Mechanism of *programmed cell death*, resembling *apoptosis*, initiated in anchorage-dependent cells when they lose contact with *extracellular matrix.*
Note: As a consequence of anoikis, cells that become anchorage-independent following *malignant transformation* should die before they successfully *metastasize.*
[*]

anomaly, developmental

congenital anomaly

Deviation in structure or function arising in the *embryo* or *fetus*, due to genetic or other causes.
[ref. 5]
See also *congenital malformation; variation.*

anonychia

Absence of nails.
Note: The rare *disorder* of anonychia may be the result of a *congenital* defect of *ectoderm, ichthyosis*, severe infection, severe allergic contact dermatitis, self-inflicted trauma, Raynaud phenomenon, *lichen planus*, epidermolysis bullosa, or severe *exfoliative diseases.*
[ref. 5]

anophthalmia

Congenital absence of one or both eyeballs.
[ref. 5]

anorchism

Congenital absence of one or both testes.
[ref. 5]

anorectal

Relating to the *anus* and rectum.
[ref. 5]

anorexia

Eating *disorder* characterized by self-imposed food restriction.
[ref. 4]
Compare *anorexia nervosa.*

anorexia nervosa

Eating *disorder* characterized by obsessive desire to lose weight by reducing food intake or by repeated vomiting.
[ref. 4]
Compare *anorexia.*

anosmia (n)/anosmic (adj)

Loss of the sense of smell, either total or selective.
[ref. 4]

anotia

Congenital absence of the (outer ear) *pinna*, often with narrowing or absence of the ear canal.
[ref. 5]

anovulation

Failure of the *ovaries* to produce, to facilitate maturation of, or to release *ova.*
[ref. 5]

anoxia

Total absence of dioxygen.
Note: Sometimes anoxia is incorrectly used instead of *hypoxia* to mean a decreased dioxygen supply to the tissues.
[ref. 5]

antagonism (in toxicology)

Combined effect of two or more agents that is smaller than the solitary effect of any one of those agents.
Note: In *bioassays*, the term "antagonism" may be used when a specified effect is produced by *exposure* to either of two factors but not by exposure to both together.
[After ref. 1]

antagonist (in toxicology)

1. Any substance that competes for effect with, or blocks the biological action of, another.
2. At a cell *receptor*, substance that binds to the receptor without activating it, and prevents a response to the natural ligand (the *agonist*).

[ref. 5]
See also *inhibitor.*

antemortem

Opposite term: *postmortem.*

Before death.
[ref. 5]

antepartum
Opposite term: *postpartum*.

Before *birth*.
[ref. 5]

anthelmint(h)ic
antihelminth
helminthagogue
helminthic
vermifuge

1. (n) Substance that kills or causes the expulsion of parasitic intestinal worms, such as helminths.
2. (adj) Acting to expel or kill parasitic intestinal worms.

[ref. 1]

anthracosis
coal miners' pneumoconiosis
Form of *pneumoconiosis* caused by accumulation of anthracite carbon deposits in the lungs due to *inhalation* of smoke or coal *dust*.
[ref. 1]

anthropogenic
1. Caused by or influenced by human activities.
2. Describing a conversion factor used to calculate a *dose* or *concentration* affecting a human that has been derived from data obtained with another species (*e.g.*, the rat).

[ref. 1]

anthropogenic enrichment factor
See *enrichment factor*.

anti-adrenergic
See *sympatholytic*.

anti-DNA antibody
See *antibody, anti-DNA*.

antibiotic
Substance produced by, and obtained from, certain living cells (especially bacteria, yeasts, and molds), or an equivalent synthetic substance, which is *biostatic* or *biocidal* to bacteria.
[*]

antibody
Protein (*immunoglobulin*) produced by the *immune system* in response to exposure to an *antigenic* molecule and characterized by its specific binding to a site on that molecule (*antigenic determinant* or *epitope*).
[ref. 3]

antibody, anti-DNA

Antibody directed against single-stranded or double-stranded *DNA.*
[ref. 3]
See also *antinuclear antibody; systemic lupus erythematosus.*

antibody, anti-erythrocyte

Antibody against molecules of the red blood cell, usually against membrane proteins, causing lysis of the red blood cells.
Note: Maternal *IgG* antibodies specific for the *Rhesus (Rh) factor blood group antigen* expressed against the *erythrocytes* of the fetus may lead to hemolytic *disease* of the newborn.
[ref. 3]
See also *hemolytic anemia.*

antibody, anti-idiotypic

Antibody raised against *antigenic determinants* unique to the *variable region* of a single antibody.
[ref. 3]
See also *idiotope; idiotype; idiotypic network.*

antibody, antinuclear (ANA)

antinuclear factor (ANF)
Antibody, detectable in the blood, that has the capability of binding to a substance, *e.g.*, DNA, within the nucleus of the cells.
Note: ANAs are found in patients whose *immune system* may be predisposed to cause *inflammation* against their own body tissues. ANAs indicate the possible presence of *autoimmunity* and are an indication of *autoimmune disease*, such as *rheumatoid arthritis, scleroderma, Sjögren syndrome, systemic lupus erythematosus*, and *mixed connective tissue disease.*
[ref. 3]

antibody, autologous

Antibody derived from a specific individual, acting within that individual.
[ref. 3]
See also *heterologous antibody.*

antibody, bispecific

Artificially produced hybrid *antibody* in which each of the two *antigen*-binding arms is specific for a different antigenic *epitope*.
Note: Bispecific antibodies, which can be produced either by chemical cross-linkage or by recombinant DNA techniques, can be used to link together two different antigens or cells, *e.g.*, a *cytotoxic T-lymphocyte* and a tumor cell.
[ref. 3]

antibody, blocking

Antibody that prevents other antibodies from combining with a specific *antigen* but does not itself produce an *immunological response* when combined with that antigen.
[ref. 3]

antibody, cross-reacting

Antibody that is able to react with an *antigen* that did not specifically stimulate its production.

Note: Cross-reacting antibody reactions are usually weaker than the reaction of the antibody with the antigen that caused its production.
[ref. 3]

antibody, enhancing

Antibody that binds to an antibody-*antigen* complex or idiotypic-*anti-idiotypic antibody* complex and strengthens the interaction.
[ref. 3]

antibody, fluorescent

Antibody conjugated to a fluorescent dye such as *fluorescein isothiocyanate*.
[ref. 3]

antibody, heterologous

Antibody derived from another individual of the same species or another species.
[ref. 3]
See also *antibody, autologous*.

antibody, heterophile
heterophilic antibody

Antibody raised against an *antigen* from one species, which also reacts against antigens from other species.
Note 1: Heterophile antibodies are usually of low affinity and are a common cause of problems with *immunoassays*.
Note 2: The existence of heterophile antibodies explains observations of the presence of antibody against antigens from a variety of species without *immunization*.
Note 3: Heterophile antibodies commonly arise from viral infection.
[ref. 3]
See also *Forssman antigen*.

antibody, homocytotropic

Antibody that binds preferentially to cells from the same species rather than to cells from other species.
[ref. 3]
See also *autologous antibody; heterologous antibody; heterophile antibody*.

antibody, humanized

Genetically engineered *monoclonal antibody* of nonhuman origin in which all but the *antigen*-binding *complementarity-determining region* sequences have been replaced with sequences derived from human antibodies.
Note: Antibodies are humanized with the aim of minimizing the *immunogenicity* of *therapeutic, monoclonal antibodies*.
[ref. 3]

antibody, islet cell (ICA)

Any *autoantibody* reacting with endocrine (pancreatic islet) cells and detectable by *indirect immunofluorescence* on pancreatic cryostat sections.
Note: Islet cell antibodies are diagnostic markers of *diabetes mellitus type 1*.
[ref. 3]

antibody, liver-kidney microsomal (LKM)

Any *autoantibody* directed against cytochrome P450 and uridine diphosphate (UDP)-*glucuronosyltransferase* (EC 2.4.1.17) (UGT) *antigens* typically found in patients with immune-mediated hepatitis.
Note: LKM antibodies include LKM-1 antibodies (against cytochrome P4502D6) in patients with *autoimmune* hepatitis type 2 (AIH-2) and *autoimmunity* associated with hepatitis C; LKM-2 (against cytochrome P4502C9) in patients with *drug*-induced hepatitis caused by tienilic acid; and LKM-3 (UGT-1) in patients with chronic hepatitis D and AIH-2.
[ref. 3]

antibody, monoclonal

Antibody derived from a single *B-cell clone* and therefore bearing identical *antigen*-binding sites and *isotype* to other members of the clone.
[ref. 3]

antibody, nondepleting

Cell surface *antibody* that does not provoke attack by *killer cells* and thus does not provoke depletion of a group of cells in the body, usually referring to *B-cells.*
[ref. 3]

antibody, polyclonal

Mixture of antibody molecules, produced by a number of different B-cell lineages (*clones*), that are all directed against the same antigen, but may have different antigen-binding sites.
[*]

antibody, precipitating

Antibody that is capable of reacting with a soluble *antigen* with the formation of an insoluble antigen-antibody complex.
[ref. 3]
See also *precipitin.*

antibody, recombinant

Antibody fragment manufactured by use of genetically modified microorganisms (see *genetically modified organism*).
[ref. 3]

antibody, single-chain (SCA)

Small *antibody* construct in which the variable fragment (*Fv*) [see *variable (V) region*] of a *heavy chain* is linked via a synthetic peptide to the variable fragment of a *light chain.*
[ref. 3]

antibody, therapeutic

Antibody administered with the aim of treating a *disease.*
[ref. 3]

antibody-dependent cellular cytotoxicity (ADCC)

antibody-dependent cell-mediated cytotoxicity
Cytotoxic reaction in which an *antibody*-coated *target cell* is directly killed by an *Fc receptor*-bearing *leukocyte, e.g., natural killer cell, macrophage, neutrophil*, or *eosinophil.*
[ref. 3]

antibody-forming cell (AFC) assay

hemolytic plaque assay
Jerne plaque assay
plaque-forming cell (PFC) assay

Assay that measures the humoral immune response mediated by the concerted actions of *antigen-presenting cells, T-lymphocytes*, and *B-lymphocytes*, generally by determination of murine primary *IgM* or *IgG* antibodies directed against the T-cell-dependent sheep red blood cell (SRBC) surface antigens after in vivo sensitization.
Note: Due to involvement of multiple cell populations in mounting an antibody response, the AFC assay actually evaluates several immune parameters simultaneously. It is considered to be one of the most sensitive indicator systems for *immunotoxicology* studies.
[ref. 3]

antibody therapy

Use of an *antibody* to target specific cells (often tumor cells) or *signal transduction* pathways (often via *chemokines/cytokines*) in the treatment of *disease*.
Note: The main objectives of antibody therapy are stimulation of the patient's *immune system* to attack malignant tumor cells and the prevention of tumor growth by blockage of specific cell *receptors*.
[ref. 3]

anticholinergic

1. (n) Substance that prevents transmission of parasympathetic nerve impulses.
2. (adj) Preventing transmission of *parasympathetic* (acetylcholine releasing) nerve impulses.

[ref. 1]

anticholinesterase

See *cholinesterase inhibitor.*

anticoagulant

Substance that prevents blood *clotting* (*e.g.*, warfarin, heparin), usually intended for *therapeutic* purposes but also posing an increased risk of *hemmorhage*.
[*]

anticoagulant, lupus

antibody, lupus

Autoantibody that binds to phospholipids and/or proteins of the cell membrane in *systemic lupus erythematosus*, and can interfere with blood *clotting* and tests of clotting function.
[ref. 3]

anticonvulsant

Substance used to prevent or reduce the severity of *convulsions*.
[ref. 4]

antidepressant

Substance used to alleviate *depression*.
[ref. 4]

antidiuretic hormone

See *vasopressin.*

antidote

Substance capable of specifically counteracting or reducing the effect of a potentially *toxic* substance in an organism by a relatively specific chemical or pharmacological action.
[ref. 1]

antiemetic

Substance used to prevent nausea and vomiting (*emesis*).
[ref. 4]

anti-erythrocyte antibody

See *antibody, anti-erythrocyte.*

antigen (n)/antigenic (adj)

Substance or a structural part (*epitope*) of a substance that is recognized by an *antibody*.
Note: An antigen often causes the *immune system* to produce a specific *antibody* or specific cells and combines with a specific binding site (*paratope*) on the antibody or cells.
[ref. 3]

antigen, blood group

Surface *antigen* on *erythrocytes*, detectable with a specific *antibody* from other individuals.
Note: The major blood group antigens ABO and Rh (Rhesus) are used in routine blood banking to type blood, but there are many other blood group antigens that can also be detected in *cross-matching.*
[ref. 3]
See also *blood group; blood group system, ABO; Rhesus factor.*

antigen, carcinoembryonic (CEA)

Membrane *glycoprotein epitope* normally present in the *fetal gastrointestinal tract* and elevated in many patients with various *carcinomas*.
[ref. 3]

antigen, cross-reacting

1. *Antigen* that is able to react with an *antibody* induced by a different antigen.
   Note: The two cross-reacting antigens may share the same *antigenic determinants* or carry determinants that are sufficiently alike stereochemically to enable the *antibody* to react with both.
2. Antigen that has an identical structure in two strains of microorganism, so that antibody raised against one strain will react with the other strain.

[ref. 3]

antigen, differentiation

Cell surface molecule expressed at a particular stage of development or on cells of a given lineage.
[ref. 3]

antigen, fetal

Human *cancer* cell *antigen* that *cross-reacts* serologically (see *serology*) with antigens normally expressed by *embryonic* tissue.
Examples: Carcinoembryonic antigen, α-fetoprotein.
[ref. 3]

antigen, Forssman

Glycolipid *heterophile antigen* (globopentosylceramide) expressed on cell surfaces during *embryonic* and adult life.
Note 1: The Forsmann antigen is found in dogs, horses, sheep, cats, turtles, eggs of some fish, in certain bacteria (some strains of enteric organisms and pneumococci), and varieties of maize; with the exception of guinea pigs and hamsters, Forssman antigen is not found in rodents, nor in frogs, hogs, and most primates.
Note 2: The antibody that develops in infectious mononucleosis of humans reacts specifically with the Forssman antigen.
Note 3: Anti-Forssman *antibodies* directed against the terminal sugar moiety of the Forssman antigen are commonly found in plasma and may be involved in *Guillain–Barré syndrome.*
Note 4: Antibodies against the Forssman antigen reportedly disrupt tight junction formation, apical-basal *polarization*, and cell adhesion.
Modified from [ref. 3]

antigen, heterologous

Antigen that reacts with an *antibody* other than the one whose formation it induced.
[ref. 3]
See also *antibody, autologous.*

antigen, heterophile
heterophilic antigen

Antigen that stimulates production in a *vertebrate* of *antibodies* capable of reacting with tissue components having related antigens in a wide range of other species.
[ref. 3]
See also *Forssman antigen.*

antigen, human leukocyte

See *human leukocyte antigen.*

antigen, Ia
I region-associated antigen
immune response-associated antigen

Isooantigen encoded by the Ia region of the mouse *major histocompatibility complex (H-2 complex).*
Note 1: Ia *antigens* are defined by serological methods (see *serology*) and are found predominantly on *B-lymphocytes* and *macrophages.*
Note 2: Ia antigen is also used as a generic term for any *major histocompatibility complex class II* antigen.
[ref. 3]
See also *immune response-associated protein.*

antigen, minor histocompatibility

Non *major histocompatibility complex* (MHC)-encoded cell surface processed peptide that, in association with MHC-encoded molecules, contributes to *graft rejection*, albeit not usually as severe as that due to MHC mismatch.
[ref. 3]

antigen, oncofetal

Antigen whose expression is normally restricted to the fetus but that may be expressed during malignancy in adults.
[ref. 3]

antigen, Qa

"Nonclassical" *major histocompatibility complex class I molecule* in mice.
[ref. 3]

antigen, recall

Substance recognized by *memory cells* that stimulates rapid *(secondary) immune responses*, often associated with *hypersensitivity*.
[ref. 3]

antigen, sheep red blood cell (SRBC)

T-cell-dependent target *antigen* often used in hemolytic plaque assays of *immune responsiveness*.
[ref. 3]

antigen, thymus(T)-dependent (TD)

Antigen that requires the participation of *helper T-lymphocytes* to elicit an *immune response* in *B-lymphocytes*.
[ref. 3]

antigen, thymus(T)-independent (TI)

Antigen that does not require the participation of *helper T-lymphocytes* to elicit an *immune response* in *B-lymphocytes*.
[ref. 3]

antigen, tumor

Antigen whose expression is associated with *tumor* cells.
[ref. 3]

antigen, tumor rejection (TRA)

Antigen present specifically on a tumor cell that may target it for destruction by the *immune system* or for *antibody therapy*.
[ref. 3]

antigen, tumor-specific transplantation (TSTA)

Antigen, present only on a tumor cell, and targetable by the immune system or by antibody therapy in order to destroy the tumor.
[ref. 3]

antigen-binding groove

See *antigen-presenting groove.*

antigen presentation

Display of *antigen* as peptide fragments bound to *major histocompatibility complex molecules* on the surface of a cell.
Note: *T-cells* recognize antigen only when it is presented in this way.
[ref. 3]

antigen-presenting cell (APC)

Cell, such as a *dendritic cell* or *macrophage*, that is responsible for making *antigens* accessible to *lymphocytes* and other immune effector and regulatory cells, making possible specific recognition by *receptors* on the cell surface.
Note: In a more restricted way, used to describe *major histocompatibility complex class II*-positive cells (*accessory cells*) that internalize and degrade an antigen (generally by *phagocytosis*), before a fragment of the antigen molecule is presented on the APC cell surface in association with an MHC molecule. This complex is recognized by either *B-cells* via surface-bound *immunoglobulin* molecules, or by *T-cells* via the *T-cell receptor* for the antigen. Induction of a specific *immune response* then proceeds.
[ref. 3]

antigen-presenting groove

1. Pocket in a *major histocompatibility complex molecule* that binds *antigen* for *antigen presentation.*
2. Hydrophobic binding region in the CD1 protein that anchors lipid-containing antigens causing exposure of the peptide or carbohydrate moiety in a position enabling *T-cell receptor* contact.

[ref. 3]

antigen processing

Cleavage of protein *antigens* in *antigen-presenting cells (APCs).*
Note: In antigen processing, the *immunogenic* peptides interact with the binding sites of *major histocompatibility complex (MHC) class II* products (exogenous antigens) or with those in *MHC class I* products (endogenous antigens, including viruses). The processed antigen-MHC complex is recognized by the *antigen receptor* complex of *T-lymphocytes.*
[ref. 4]
See also *antigen presentation.*

antigen receptor

See *receptor, antigen.*

antigen recognition

Ability of highly specialized proteins of the *immune system* to recognize *antigens* and specifically bind to them.
Note: Types of antigen recognition include that by *antibodies, T-cell receptors (TCRs)*, and *toll-like receptors (TLRs).*
[ref. 3]

antigenic

Capable of stimulating *lymphocytes* to produce *antibodies*.
[ref. 3]

antigenic determinant

See *determinant, antigenic*.

antigenicity

Ability of an *antigen* to bind to a specific *antibody* or *T-cell receptor*; often a measure of its ability to produce *immunity*.
[ref. 3]

antihistamine

Substance that blocks or counteracts the action of *histamine*.
[ref. 1]

antihelminth

See *anthelmint(h)ic*.

anti-idiotypic antibody

See *antibody, anti-idiotypic*.

anti-isotypic antibody

Antibody against universal features of a given *constant (C) region isotype* (such as γ or μ) of one species that is made by immunizing a member of another species with that isotype.
Note: Anti-isotypic antibodies will bind any antibody of that isotype, and are thus useful for detecting bound antibody molecules in *immunoassays* and other applications.
[ref. 3]

antimetabolite

Substance that competes with a structurally similar *metabolite*, or replaces it, and so prevents or reduces its normal utilization.
[ref. 1]

antimitochondrial antibody (AMA)

Autoantibody producing a *mitochondrial* staining pattern on sections of various tissues and on tumor cell monolayers.
Note 1: According to the fluorescence pattern, different subtypes of AMA can be differentiated. Antimitochondrial antibodies of the subtype 2 are directed against *antigens* of three related 2-oxo acid dehydrogenase complexes (*e.g.*, the E2 subunit of the pyruvate dehydrogenase complex, EC 1.2.4.1) localized to the inner mitochondrial membrane.
Note 2: AMA-M2 is a specific marker of *primary biliary cirrhosis*.
[ref. 3]

antimitotic (n, adj)

(Substance) inhibiting *mitotic* cell division.
[After ref. 5]

anti-Müllerian hormone (AMH)

Müllerian inhibiting factor (MIF)
Müllerian-inhibiting hormone (MIH)
Müllerian-inhibiting substance (MIS)

Protein that inhibits the development of the *Müllerian ducts* (paramesonephric ducts) in the male *embryo*.
Note: Without AMH, the Müllerian ducts would otherwise differentiate into the *uterus* and *Fallopian tubes*.
[ref. 5]

antimuscarinic (n, adj)

(Substance) inhibiting or preventing the actions of muscarine and muscarine-like agents (*e.g.*, atropine) on the *muscarinic receptors* for *acetylcholine*.
[After ref. 1]

antimycotic (n, adj)

fungicide

(Substance) intended to kill a fungus or to inhibit its growth.
[After ref. 1]

antineuralgic (n, adj)

(Substance) used to alleviate the *pain* of *neuralgia*.
[ref. 4]

antineutrophil cytoplasmic autoantibody (ANCA)

Antibody against *antigens* in the cytoplasm of *neutrophils*.
[ref. 3]
See also *antineutrophil cytoplasmic autoantibody-associated vasculitis*.

antineutrophil cytoplasmic autoantibody (ANCA)-associated vasculitis

See *vasculitis, antineutrophil cytoplasmic autoantibody-associated vasculitis*.

antinicotinic (n, adj)

(Substance) inhibiting or preventing the actions of nicotine and nicotine-like agents (*e.g.*, suxamethonium chloride) on *nicotinic receptors* for *acetylcholine*.
[After ref. 1]

antinociception

Blockage of the perception of *pain*.
[ref. 4]
See also *nociception*.

antinuclear antibody (ANA)

See *antibody, antinuclear*.

antioxidant (biological)

Agent that prevents or reverses oxidation reactions, notably by counteracting the effects of *reactive oxygen species*.

Note: Antioxidants include endogenous thiols such as *glutathione* and lipoic acid; dietary components such as vitamins A, C and E; food additives such as butylated hydroxy toluene [2,6-bis(1,1-dimethylethyl)-4-methylphenol]; natural products such as resveratrol [3,5,4′-trihydroxy-*trans*-stilbene], quercetin [2-(3,4-dihydroxyphenyl)-3,5,7-trihydroxy-4*H*-chromen-4-one], and other phenolics and flavonoids; and enzymes such as *catalase, superoxide dismutase*, and *glutathione peroxidase*.
[*]

antiphospholipid syndrome (APS)

One of the most common *autoimmune diseases*, characterized by *thrombosis*, recurrent spontaneous abortions, and the presence of antiphospholipid *antibodies*.
Note: APS may occur as an isolated *disease* (primary APS) or in combination with another autoimmune disease, especially *systemic lupus erythematosus* (secondary APS).
[ref. 3]

antipsychotic (n, adj)

(*Psychoactive* substance) relieving or reducing *psychotic* behavior or psychotic ideation.
[After ref. 4]

antipyretic (n, adj)

(Substance) relieving or reducing fever.
[ref. 1]

antiresistant

Substance used as an additive to a *pesticide* formulation in order to reduce the resistance of insects to the pesticide (*e.g.*, an antimetabolite that inhibits *metabolic* inactivation of the pesticide).
[ref. 1]

antispasmodic (n, adj)

(Substance) preventing muscle *spasms*.
[ref. 1]

antiserum

Blood serum from an immunized animal that contains *polyclonal antibodies* against the agent used for *immunization*.
[ref. 3]

anti-sheep red blood cell IgM response (SRBC) **assay**

Test to determine *T-cell*-dependent *antibody* response, usually by *enzyme-linked immunosorbent assay*. Sheep red blood cells are used as an *antigen*. Often referred to as the *plaque assay*.
Note: A test similar to the SRBC assay is often performed with the *tetanus toxoid* as the antigen.
[ref. 3]

antisymmetry (in population biology)

Quality of a *population* of bilaterally symmetrical individuals in which the difference in measurement of a trait made from the right and left sides of individuals from that population produces a bimodal distribution.
[ref. 2]
See also *fluctuating asymmetry*.

antitoxin

Antibody specific for *exotoxins* produced by certain microorganisms such as the causative agents of diphtheria and tetanus.
[ref. 3]

antiviral

Substance used to control viruses.
[ref. 1]

antrum

Cavity or chamber, often in bone, with specific meanings in some hollow organs.
Examples: The nasal antrum, the pyloric (gastric) antrum of the stomach.
[4,5]

anus (n)/**anal** (adj)

External opening of the rectum to the body surface, controlled by the anal *sphincter*.
[ref. 5]
See also *imperforate anus*.

anxiolytic (n, adj)

(Agent) reducing anxiety without causing excessive sedation (see *sedative*).
Note: Most, if not all, anxiolytics show at least some degree of sedation.
[ref. 4]
Compare *sedative*.

aorta (n)/**aortic** (adj)

Great artery arising from the left *ventricle*, being the main trunk from which the systemic arterial system proceeds
[ref. 5]

aorta-gonad-mesonephros (AGM) **region**

Region of the *vertebrate embryonic mesoderm* that gives rise to the *genitourinary* tract and its blood supply.
Note: The AGM region is the first embryonic site for autonomous *hematopoiesis* and production of hematopoietic stem cells.
[ref. 5]

aortic arch

Curved portion of the *aorta* between its ascending portion exiting the heart and its descending portion that proceeds to the arteries of the *thoracic* and *abdominal cavities* and the lower body.
[ref. 5]

aortopulmonary septum

aorticopulmonary septum
Spiral *septum* that, during development, separates the *truncus arteriosus* into a *ventral pulmonary* trunk and the ascending *aorta dorsally*.
[ref. 5]

aphakia

Absence of the lens of the eye, occurring as a *congenital* defect or as a result of trauma or surgery.
Note: Aphakia causes a loss of visual accommodation, far sightedness (hyperopia), and a deep anterior chamber of the eye.
[ref. 5]

aphasia

Difficulty with, or loss of the use of language in reading, writing or speaking owing to specific lesions in the *brain*.
[ref. 4]
Compare *aphonia*.
See also *dysphasia*.

aphicide

Substance intended to kill *aphids*.
[ref. 1]

aphid

Common name for a harmful plant parasite in the family ***Aphididae***, some species of which are *vectors* of plant virus *diseases*.
[ref. 1]

aphonia

Loss of the voice.
[ref. 4]

aphrodisiac

Anything that stimulates *libido*.
[ref. 4]

apical endpoint

Observable final adverse outcome in an intact organism following exposure to a potentially toxic substance.
Note: The apical endpoint is often death, reproductive failure, or a failure of normal development.
[*]

apical surface (of a cell)

See *cell polarity*.

aplasia

Lack of development of an organ or tissue, or of the cellular products from an organ or tissue.
[ref. 1]

aplastic anemia

See *anemia, aplastic*.

apneusis
apneustic respiration

Abnormal breathing pattern consisting of a pause at full inspiration.
Note*:* Apneusis characterized by a prolonged inspiratory *cramp* is caused by a lesion in the *brainstem.*
[ref. 4]

apneustic breathing

See *apneusis.*

aponecrosis

See *necrapoptosis.*

apoptosis (n)/**apoptotic** (adj)

Active process of programmed cell death, characterized by cell shrinkage, nuclear condensation, and fragmentation and loss of individual cells; usually involving activation of *caspase* enzymes and requiring energy provided by hydrolysis of ATP.
Note 1: Other factors trigger cell death with characteristics of apoptosis but independent of caspase activation, an example being release of apoptosis-inducing factor (AIF) from the *mitochondrion.* Here the term caspase-independent apoptosis is used.
Note 2: While ATP is generally necessary to sustain the apoptotic program, depletion of ATP during the course of apoptosis may cause cells to default to death by *necrosis* (see *necrapoptosis, aponecrosis*), or proceed to apoptotic death with features common to necrosis, sometimes called "late apoptosis". Alternatively, in some circumstances apoptosis may proceed without ATP ("ATP-independent apoptosis").
[ref. 5]
See also *anoikis; autophagy; extrinsic pathway; intrinsic pathway; parthanatos.*

appendix (in anatomy)

1. Tube-shaped sac of lymphoid tissue ("vermiform appendix") attached to and opening into the upper end of the large intestine (*cecum*) in humans and some other mammals.
2. Appendage, blind sac, or diverticulum.

[ref. 3,5]
See also *epididymal appendix; gut-associated lymphoid tissue.*

application factor (AF)

See *uncertainty factor.*

apraxia

Neurological condition characterized by loss of the ability to perform skilled or purposeful movement that a person is nevertheless physically able and willing to do.
[ref. 4]

arachnodactyly

Extreme length and slenderness of the fingers or toes.
[ref. 5]

arachnoiditis

Inflammation of the *arachnoid membrane*, often characterized by perception of burning pain in the legs.
[ref. 4]

arachnoid mater

See *arachnoid membrane.*

arachnoid membrane

arachnoid mater

Weblike *membrane* that lies between the outer (and much thicker) *dura mater* and the deeper *pia mater,* together forming the meninges (see *meninx*) and covering the *brain.*
Note: The arachnoid membrane is separated from the pia mater by the subarachnoid space, in which the *cerebrospinal fluid* flows and is absorbed by the arachnoid villi.
[ref. 5]

arachnoid villus

arachnoid granulation

Small projection of the *arachnoid membrane* into some of the venous sinuses of the *dura mater.*
[ref. 5]

arboricide

Substance intended to kill trees and shrubs.
[ref. 1]

arborization

Terminal treelike branching of an anatomical structure, *e.g.*, of a neuron into *dendrites* or the airways into their terminal branches.
[*]

arcsine square root transformation

Arcsin $\sqrt{P}$, where P is the value of a measured effect, *e.g.*, the proportion of *exposed* organisms in a *population.*
Note: The arcsin $\sqrt{P}$ *transformation* of effects data often results in the data conforming to an assumption of homogeneous variances in the proportions of exposed individuals responding to a stimulus.
[ref. 2]

area source

Widespread origin of *emissions.*
[ref. 1]

area under the concentration–time curve

See *area under the curve.*

area under the curve (AUC)

Area between a curve and the abscissa (horizontal axis) in a plot of *concentration* vs. time.
[*]

area under the moment curve (AUMC)

Area between a curve and the abscissa (horizontal axis) in a plot of (*concentration* × time) vs. time.
[ref. 1]

areola (n)/areolar (adj)/areolate (adj)

1. Circular area of different color surrounding a central point, such as that surrounding the nipple of the breast, the part of the iris surrounding the pupil of the eye, or an area surrounding a *vesicle*.
2. Any minute space or interstice in a tissue.

[ref. 5]

argyria

argyrosis

Pathological condition characterized by gray-bluish or black pigmentation of tissues (such as skin, retina, mucous membranes, internal organs) caused by the accumulation of metallic silver, due to reduction of a silver compound that has entered the organism during (prolonged) administration or *exposure*.
[ref. 1]

arhinencephaly

See *holoprosencephaly*.

arm bud

See *limb bud*.

Arnold-Chiari malformation

Chiari malformation

Congenital herniation of the brainstem and lower cerebellum through the *foramen magnum* into the cervical *vertebral canal*.
Note: The Arnold-Chiari malformation is often associated with *meningocele* and *spina bifida*.
[ref. 5]
See also *neural tube defect*.

aromatase

estrogen synthetase

Enzyme (EC 1.14.14.1) of the *cytochrome P450* superfamily that converts *testosterone* to 17β-estradiol and androstenedione to estrone.
Note: Inhibiting the action of aromatase is one approach to the management of breast *cancer*.
[ref. 5]

arrhenoblastoma

See *Sertoli-Leydig cell tumor*.

arrhythmia

Condition in which there is an irregular or abnormal heart beat.
[ref. 4]

arseniasis
arsenism

Chronic arsenical poisoning.
[ref. 1]

arteriogenesis
Increase in the diameter of arterial vessels that leads to the formation of large conductance arteries from pre-existing arterioles.
[ref. 5]

arteriography
See *angiography*.

arteriolovenular anastomosis
Communication in which blood is shunted from arterioles to venules without passing through capillaries.
[ref. 4]
See also *arteriovenous anastomosis*.

arteriosclerosis
Hardening, thickening and diminished elasticity of the walls of the arteries.
[After ref. 1]
See also *atherosclerosis.*

arteriovenous (AV)
Relating to both arteries and veins.
Note: Arteriovenous also refers to relations between arteries and veins, *e.g., arteriovenous malformation, arteriovenous fistula.*
[ref. 4]

arteriovenous (AV) anastomosis
Communication (*anastomosis*) between an artery and a vein by collateral channels.
Note: AV anastamosis is generally between arterioles and venules, in which case the term *arteriolovenular anastomosis* is preferred.
[ref. 4]

arteriovenous malformation (AVM)
Web of blood vessels with one or more abnormal communications between arteries and veins that bypass the capillary system.
Note: AVM may cause *hemorrhage*, seizures, *headache*s, *paralysis* or loss of speech, memory or vision.
[ref. 4]

arteriovenous (AV) fistula
Abnormal channel connecting an artery and a vein.
[After ref. 4]

arteriovenous (AV) shunt
See *shunt, arteriovenous.*

arthralgia

Pain in a joint.
[ref. 1]

arthritis

Inflammation of a joint or joints.
[ref. 3]

arthritis, adjuvant

Experimental model of *immunopathology* with features of *rheumatoid arthritis (RA)*, induced in rats by injection with bacterial products, which may be used to study anti-*inflammatory* therapies.
[ref. 3]

arthritis, rheumatoid (RA)

Episodic *inflammatory systemic disease* with *autoimmune pathogenic* mechanisms.
Note 1: RA primarily affects the joints, causing symmetrical lesions and severe damage to the affected joints.
Note 2: RA is the most common form of inflammatory joint disease (prevalence about 0.5 to 1 %).
[ref. 3]

arthropathy

Disease of a joint.
[ref. 1]
See also *arthrosis*.

arthrosis

1. Degeneration of a joint or articular surface, usually caused by chronic wear of the cartilage.
   Synonym: osteoarthritis.
2. Joint or articulation.

[*]

Arthus reaction

Gell and Coombs Type III reaction
Local *antibody*-mediated *hypersensitivity* reaction in which *antigen-antibody* complexes that fix *complement* are deposited in the walls of small vessels, often in the skin, causing acute *inflammation* with an infiltration of *neutrophils*.
[ref. 3]
See also *Gell and Coombs classification*.

artifact, scientific

Effect, result or phenomenon that is not naturally present, arising as a result of the investigational procedures or from experimental error.
[*]

artificial insemination

Introduction of *semen* into the *cervix, uterus* or *Fallopian tubes* by means other than the natural one.
[ref. 5]
See also *insemination*.

artificial soil test

Test with earthworms in which the *toxicity* of a substance by skin and gut uptake is determined by adding the earthworms to an artificial *soil* made of sand, clay mineral, and peat, containing the substance of concern.
[ref. 2]

artisol test

Test with earthworms in which the *toxicity* of a substance by skin and gut uptake is determined by placing the worms in an artificial substrate consisting of silica, water, and glass balls, containing the substance of concern.
Note: In the artisol test, the earthworms ingest the silica paste as they do *soil*.
[ref. 2]

aryl hydrocarbon hydroxylase (AHH)

cytochrome P450 1A1

Enzyme (EC 1.14.14.1) whose activity is often measured in units of benzo[α]pyrene hydroxylation.
[After ref. 2]

aryl hydrocarbon receptor (AHR)

See *receptor, aryl hydrocarbon*.

aryl hydrocarbon receptor nucleotide translocator protein (ARNT)

Protein coded for by a gene on *chromosome* 1q21 that forms a complex with ligand-bound *aryl hydrocarbon receptor*, resulting in translocation of the ligand-binding subunit to the nucleus.
Note: A t(1;12)(q21;p13) *chromosomal translocation*, which results in a translocated ETS leukemia (TEL)-ARNT fusion protein, is associated with acute myeloblastic leukemia.
[ref. 5]

as low as reasonably achievable (ALARA)

Describing the situation in which everything practicable is done to reduce *risks* to a minimum with the approval of the regulatory authorities.
[ref. 2]
See also *precautionary principle*.

asbestosis

Form of *pneumoconiosis* caused by *inhalation* of asbestos fibers.
[ref. 1]

ascaricide

Substance intended to kill roundworms (***Ascaridae***).
[ref. 1]

asepsis (n)/aseptic (adj)

Opposite of *sepsis/septic*.
[*]

asphyxia

Condition resulting from insufficient intake of dioxygen.
Note: Symptoms of asphyxia include difficulty breathing, impairment of senses, and, in extreme cases, convulsions, unconsciousness and death.
[ref. 1]

asphyxiant

Substance that blocks the transport or use of dioxygen by living organisms.
Note: Examples of asphyxiants include both physical (nitrogen gas) and chemical (carbon monoxide) asphyxiants.
[ref. 1]

assay

1. (n) Process of quantitative or qualitative analysis of a component of a *sample*.
2. (n) Results of a quantitative or qualitative analysis of a component of a sample.
3. (v) Carry out quantitative or qualitative analysis of a component of a sample.

[ref. 1]

assessment endpoint (in ecological risk assessment)

Ecological property that is to be protected and the precise parameter to be measured for this property.
[ref. 2]
See also *measurement endpoint.*

assessment factor

See *uncertainty factor*.

assimilation

Uptake and incorporation of substances by a living organism.
[ref. 1]

association study

See *study, association.*

associative avoidance test

See *avoidance test, associative*.

associative learning

Process in which a new behavior arises as a consequence of association with a particular stimulus, sometimes restricted to learning through *classical conditioning*.
[ref. 4]

assymmetry, directional

Deviation within a *population,* from a mean of zero, for the difference between a trait measured from the right and left sides of bilaterally symmetrical individuals from that population.
Example: Measurement of the difference in muscle mass of left and right arms of humans would display directional asymmetry because most humans are right-handed and have larger right arms.
[ref. 2]
See also *antisymmetry; asymmetry, fluctuating.*

asymmetry, fluctuating

Deviation from perfect bilateral symmetry for a *population* of a bilaterally symmetrical *species* that is thought to reflect developmental instability.
Note: A trait is measured from the right and left sides of each individual, and the variance in the difference (right–left) for the population is a measure of fluctuating asymmetry.
[ref. 2]
See also *antisymmetry; asymmetry, directional.*

asymptomatic

Showing no *symptoms*.
Note: An asymptomatic individual is not necessarily free of *disease*.
[*]

asthenia

Weakness; lack or loss of strength.
[ref. 1]

asthma (n)/asthmatic (adj)

Chronic inflammatory *disease* of the airways characterized by bronchoconstriction and excessive mucus secretion, resulting in wheezing and difficulty in breathing out.
[*]

astringent

1. (adj) Causing contraction, usually locally after topical application.
2. (n) Substance causing tissues to contract, decreasing the blood supply at the small vessels, or stopping secretions and discharges.

Note: Astringent substances may be applied to skin or mucus membranes to dry or harden them.
[*]

astrocyte

Glial cell of ectodermal origin in the *central nervous system*, characterized by *filamentous* protoplasmic extensions.
[ref. 4]

astrocyte, reactive

Astrocyte that, after injury or excessive neural activity, undergoes morphological (including extension of pseudopodia) and biochemical (notably increased synthesis of *glial fibrillary acidic protein*) changes and participates in *astrocytic scar* formation.
[ref. 4]

astrocytic scar

glial scar

Clustering of *reactive astrocytes* separating a localized *brain* injury from surrounding uninjured tissue.
[ref. 4]

astrocytoma

Tumor within the substance of the *brain* or *spinal cord* made up of *astrocytes*.
Note 1: Astrocytomas are classified from Grade I (least aggressive) to Grade IV (most aggressive).

Note 2: Astrocytomas do not usually spread outside the brain and spinal cord and do not usually affect other organs.
[ref. 4]

astrogliosis

Localized site of *reactive astrocytes*, distinct from an *astrocytic scar*.
[ref. 4]
See *astrocyte, reactive*.

asymptomatic

Showing no *symptoms*.
Note: An asymptomatic individual is not necessarily free of *disease*.
[*]

asymptotic threshold concentration (ATCN)

Concentration of a chemical at which some percentage of a *population* of test organisms is in a state of approximate *homeostasis* for a prolonged period of time (48 h or more).
Note: Occurrence of an ATCN can be demonstrated as the concentration at which the *toxicity* curve is approximately asymptotic (parallel) to the time axis.
[ref. 2]

ataxia

Loss of muscular coordination (see *motor coordination*) resulting in abnormal clumsiness.
[ref. 4]

ataxia telangiectasia (AT)

Disease characterized by staggering gait, multiple disorganized blood vessels, and an *immunodeficiency*, associated with a protein called ataxia telangiectasia-mutated (ATM), a *protein kinase* thought to be important in detection of double-stranded DNA breaks.
[ref. 3]

atelectasis

1. Total or partial collapse of the lung.
2. *Congenital* condition characterized by the incomplete expansion of the lungs at *birth*.

[ref. 5]

athelia

Congenital absence of one or both nipples.
[ref. 5]

atherosclerosis

Pathological condition characterized by *arteriosclerosis*, and representing a major risk for heart attack and stroke.
Note: Biochemical features of atherosclerosis include a variable combination of changes of the innermost layer of the vessel (tunica intima) consisting of local accumulation of lipids, complex carbohydrates, *macrophages*, fibrous tissue, and calcium deposits, constituting an atheroma. In addition, the outer layer (tunica

externa) becomes thickened and there is fatty degeneration of the middle layer (tunica media).
[*]
See also *arteriosclerosis*.

athetosis

Condition in which inappropriate muscle contraction causes involuntary writhing movements.
[ref. 4]

athymia

1. *Congenital* absence of functioning thymus tissue.
2. Absence of affect; suppressed emotion.

[ref. 5]

atmospheric deposition

See *deposition, atmospheric*

atony (n)/atonic (adj)

(State of) lacking muscular tone.
[ref. 4]

atopic allergy

Immunoglobulin E-mediated hypersensitivity, including *asthma, eczema, hay fever*, and food allergy.
[ref. 3]
See also *atopy*.

atopic dermatitis

Inflammation of the skin in *atopic* individuals.
Note: The term "atopic dermatitis" is broader than *atopic eczema*.
[ref. 3]

atopic eczema

Chronic skin *disease*, often localized on flexural surfaces, in individuals with propensity to develop *immunoglobulin E*-mediated *allergy*.
Note: Atopic eczema describes *eczema* occurring in *atopic* individuals and does not imply mechanisms.
[ref. 3]

atopy (n)/atopic (adj)

Of, relating to, or caused by a hereditary predisposition toward developing certain *hypersensitivity* reactions, such as *hay fever, asthma*, or chronic *urticaria*, upon exposure to specific *antigens*.
[ref. 3]

atresia
clausura

Congenital absence or abnormal narrowing of a normal opening or normally patent *lumen*.
[ref. 5]

atresia, follicular

Degeneration of those *ovarian follicles* that do not *ovulate* during the *menstrual cycle*.
[ref. 5]

atrial-septal defect (ASD)

Defect in the septum between the atria of the heart, due to failure of normal closure of the *foramen ovale* in the *perinatal* period.
[ref. 5]

atrichia congenita

Congenital baldness caused by an abnormality of the hairless *gene*.
Note: Atrichia congenita may include loss of hair in early childhood that never regrows.
[ref. 5]

atrioventricular

Relating to the atrial and ventricular chambers of the heart.
[ref. 5]

atrioventricular bundle

See *bundle of His*

atrium (n) /atria (n, pl)/ atrial (adj)

Each of the two upper chambers of the heart from which blood is passed to the *ventricles*.
Note: The right atrium receives deoxygenated blood from the veins of the body, the left atrium oxygenated blood from the *pulmonary* vein.
[ref. 5]

atrophy

Pathological decrease in tissue, organ or body mass.
Note: Atrophy may be a consequence of decreased cell volume, cell number, or both.
[ref. 4]

attention deficit hyperactivity disorder (ADHD)

hyperkinetic disorder

Neuropsychiatric *disorder* of childhood characterized by decreased attention span, impulsiveness and hyperactivity.
Note: Both genetic and environmental factors (such as lead exposure) are implicated in increased risk of occurrence of ADHD.
[ref. 4]

attenuated vaccine

See *vaccine, attenuated.*

attenuation

Reduction in amount, *e.g.*, attenuation of light is a decrease in energy per area due to *absorption* or scattering.
Note: In reference to *pollution*, attenuation is mostly applied to reduction in amount of organic *contamination* following microbial *mineralization*.
[ref. 2]
See also *attenuation (in genetics)*.

attenuation (in genetics)

Regulation of *gene* expression in bacteria by premature termination of *transcription* of a biosynthetic *operon*.
[ref. 1]

attractant

Substance that attracts animals. Some attractants support natural biological functions such as mating or predation; others may be used to attract animals for monitoring or for control.
[ref. 1]
See also *pheromone*.

attributable risk

Part of a *risk* that is identified as due to *exposure* to a defined substance.
[ref. 1]

atypical interstitial pneumonia

Acute or chronic respiratory distress in cattle, in the absence of toxemia or other *systemic* signs that are characteristic of other pneumonias.
Examples: Bovine *pulmonary* emphysema, enzootic bovine adenomatosis, pulmonary adenomatosis, mold *hypersensitivity*, fog fever, panters.
Note: The causes of atypical interstitial pneumonia are often unclear, but may include *allergic* reactions or toxicity due to conversion of *tryptophan* to toxic 3-methylindole by gut flora.
[After ref. 3]

auditory tube
Eustachian tube

Narrow channel connecting the middle ear and the naso*pharynx*.
[ref. 5]

aufwuchs

Floral and (or) or faunal *community* attached to submerged surfaces in aquatic *ecosystems*.
[ref. 2]
See also *periphyton*.

aura

Constellation of symptoms experienced before a *migraine headache* or *seizure*.
Note: An aura may consist of flickering light, blurred vision, an odor, numbness, weakness, difficulty in speaking, or the feeling of a wind blowing.
[ref. 4]

auricle

1. See *pinna* of the ear.
2. An appendage to the *atrium* of the heart.

[ref. 5]

auscultation

Process of listening for sounds within the body by ear, unassisted or using a stethoscope.
[*]

autism

Neurodevelopmental *disorder*, present from early childhood, characterized by great difficulty in communicating and forming relationships with other people and in using abstract concepts.
Note: Autism is now considered part of a range of conditions (autism spectrum disorders) that includes Asperger *syndrome*, Rett syndrome, and childhood disintegrative disorder.
[ref. 4]

autoantibody

Immunoglobulin antibody that is directed against the organism's own *antigen(s).*
[ref. 3]

autoantibody, natural (NAA)

Part of the naturally occurring repertoire of polyreactive *antibodies* that bind to *autoantigens* with low *affinity*. They are mainly of *immunoglobulin M isotype* and produced by *CD5+ B-lymphocytes.*
Note 1: Natural autoantibodies and the cells that produce them may have a physiological role in the following processes: (i) first line of protection against external invaders, (ii) elimination of degraded autoantigens and senescent cells, and (iii) tolerization (see *tolerance*) of *T-cells* by presenting autoantigens, and thereby in protecting human beings from development of pathological *autoimmunity.*
Note 2: In contrast to their physiological function, natural autoantibodies may become *pathogenic* in clonal B-cell *disorders, e.g., monoclonal* anti-I *antibodies* in cold agglutinin *disease* cause *autoimmune hemolytic anemia.*
[ref. 3]

autoantibody, warm type

Autoantibody that reacts optimally at higher temperatures (37 °C) with surface *antigens* of *erythrocytes* and mediate *autoimmune hemolytic anemia.*
[ref. 3]

autoantigen

Antigenic component of an individual's tissues that may be a target of *autoimmune* responses by autoreactive *B-cells* (*autoantibodies*) or *T-cells*, including proteins (*e.g.*, enzymes, structural proteins), *glycoproteins* (*e.g.*, 2-glycoprotein I), nucleic acids, (*e.g.*, double-stranded *DNA*), phospholipids (*e.g., cardiolipin*), and glycosphingolipids (*e.g.*, gangliosides).
[ref. 3]
See also *self-tolerance.*

autochthonous

Indigenous inhabitant of a place; not an immigrant or colonist.
[*]

autocrine

Type of signaling in which a cell secretes a chemical messenger that binds to *receptors* on the same cell, leading to changes in the cell.
[ref. 3]
See also *paracrine.*

autogenic succession

See *succession, autogenic.*

autograft

Tissue transplant (see *transplantation*) from one site to another in an individual.
[ref. 3]

autoimmune

Of or relating to an *immune response* by the body against one of its own cells or tissues.
[ref. 3]

autoimmune disease

Pathological condition resulting when an organism produces *antibodies* or specific cells that bind to constituents of its own tissues (*autoantigens*) and cause tissue injury.
Examples: Rheumatoid arthritis, myasthenia gravis, systemic lupus erythematosus, scleroderma.
[ref. 3]

autoimmune disease, systemic

Autoimmune disease affecting a number of organs or tissues, or the whole body.
[ref. 3]

autoimmune hemolytic anemia

Autoimmune disease in which *antibodies* initiate *complement* lysis of *erythrocytes.*
Note: Autoimmune hemolytic anemia may be *idiopathic*, secondary to lymphoproliferative, autoimmune (*e.g., systemic lupus erythematosus*), or chronic inflammatory *disorders*, either postinfectious or *drug*-induced.
[ref. 3]

autoimmune hepatitis (AIH)

Chronic *autoimmune*-mediated hepatic *inflammation* usually characterized by *antinuclear (ANA)*, smooth muscle (SMA)/anti-F-actin, *liver-kidney microsomal (LKM)*, and/or soluble liver antigen (SLA) *antibodies.*
[ref. 3]

autoimmune lymphoproliferative syndrome (ALPS)

Canale–Smith syndrome

Disease characterized by *lymphadenopathy, hepatosplenomegaly, autoimmune cytopenias*, and *hypergammaglobulinemia.*
[ref. 3]

autoimmune nephritis

See *nephritis, autoimmune.*

autoimmune polyendocrine syndrome (APS), type 1 or type 2

Heterogeneous group of rare *diseases* characterized by *autoimmune* activity against more than one endocrine organ, although nonendocrine organs can also be affected.

Note 1: APS type 1 is known as the *candidiasis*-hypoparathyroidism-*Addison disease syndrome* after its main features:

(a) A mild immune deficiency, leading to persistent *mucosal* and cutaneous infections with ***Candida*** yeasts. There is also decreased function of the *spleen* (asplenism).
(b) Autoimmune dysfunction of the parathyroid gland (leading to hypocalcemia) and the adrenal gland (Addison disease).

Note 2: APS type 2 (also known as Schmidt syndrome) is more heterogeneous, occurs more often and has not been linked to one gene. Features of this syndrome are Addison disease, hypothyroidism (*Hashimoto thyroiditis*), and *diabetes mellitus type 1*. Patients are at a higher risk when they carry a particular *human leukocyte antigen* genotype (*e.g.*, DQ2, DQ8, and DRB1*0404).
[ref. 3]

autoimmune regulator (AIRE)

DNA-binding protein involved in immunoregulation (probably in the establishment and maintenance of *tolerance*).
[ref. 3]

autoimmune syndrome, paraneoplastic

Any of several *autoimmune diseases* (*e.g., cancer*-associated retinopathy, paraneoplastic neurological *syndromes*, paraneoplastic cutaneous syndromes) that are caused by tumor-induced perturbations of the *immune system* with damaging effects on various organ systems.
Note: In most cases, *autoantibodies* generated by antitumor *immunity* are responsible for the tissue injury in paraneoplastic autoimmune syndrome.
[ref. 3]
See also *Lambert–Eaton myasthenic syndrome*.

autoimmune thyroiditis

See *thyroiditis, autoimmune*.

autoimmunity

Immune response to "self" tissues or components.
Note: Autoimmunity may have pathological consequences leading to *autoimmune diseases*.
[ref. 3]
See also *autoantigen; self-antigen*.

autoimmunity, drug-induced

Immune-mediated *idiosyncratic drug reaction* against *self-antigens*.
[ref. 3]

autoinflammatory disease

Unregulated *inflammation* without significant levels of *autoantibodies* or auto-activated *T-cells*, or evidence of infection, but rather caused by genetic disturbance of the mechanisms that initiate and control inflammation.
[ref. 3]

autologous
autogenous

From the same individual.
[ref. 3]

autologous antibody
See *antibody, autologous.*

autonomic nervous system (ANS)
Part of the *peripheral nervous system* controlling the bodily functions that are not consciously directed, *e.g.*, breathing, heart rate, and digestive processes.
[ref. 4]

autooxidation
See *autoxidation.*

autophagosome
Membrane-bound body (secondary *lysosome*) in which parts of the cell are digested in the process of *autophagy.*
[ref. 1]

autophagy (n)/autophagic (adj)
Digestion and breakdown in *lysosomes* of a cell's own proteins and/or organelles.
Note: Autophagy may be one route by which proteins can be processed for *antigen presentation.*
[ref. 3]
See also *heterophagy; macroautophagy; microautophagy; mitophagy; pexophagy.*

autophagy, chaperone-mediated (CMA)
Type of *autophagy* targeting only those proteins that are recognized by the binding of a heat shock cognate 70 (hsc70) protein-containing chaperone/co-chaperone complex.
[ref. 3]

autopsy
Postmortem examination of the human organs and body tissue to determine cause of death or pathological condition.
[ref. 5]

autoreactivity
Immune response directed at *self-antigens.*
[ref. 3]

autosite
Independent twin of a pair of *conjoined twins*; the other twin is a *parasitic twin.*
[ref. 5]

autosomal dominant mutation

Change in an *autosomal gene* capable of *expression* when carried by only one of a pair of *homologous chromosomes*.
[ref. 5]

autosomal recessive mutation

Change in an *autosomal gene* that produces an effect in the organism only when it is *homozygous*.
[ref. 5]

autosome (n)/**autosomal** (adj)

Any *chromosome* that is not a *sex chromosome*.
[ref. 5]

autotroph

Organism that is independent of outside sources for organic food materials and manufactures its own organic material from inorganic sources.
[ref. 2]
See also *auxotroph*.

autotrophic succession

See *succession, autotrophic*.

autotrophy (n)/**autotrophic** (adj)

Ability of an organism to manufacture its own organic material from inorganic sources, thus surviving independent of outside sources of organic food.
[*]
See also *autotroph*.

autoxidation

Reaction with dioxygen at moderate temperatures.
[ref. 1]

auxotroph

Organism unable to synthesize an organic molecule that is required for its growth; when the compound is given to the organism with the other nutrients it requires, growth of the organism may occur.
[ref. 1]
See also *autotroph*.

auxotrophy (n)/**auxotrophic** (adj)

Inability of an organism to synthesize a particular organic compound required for its growth.
[ref. 1]
See also *auxotroph*.

availability

See *bioavailability*.

availability, environmental

Portion of the total amount of a substance present in the environment that is subject to environmental, physicochemical, and biological modifying influences.
[After ref. 2]
See also *bioavailability, environmental.*

available

See *bioavailable.*

avascularity (n)/avascular (adj)

Absence of a blood supply.
[ref. 5]

avicide

Substance intended to kill birds.
[ref. 1]

avidity

functional affinity

Binding strength between two molecules (*e.g., antibody* and *antigen*) taking into account the valency of the interaction. Thus the avidity will always be equal to or greater than the *affinity*.
[ref. 3]

avoidance test

Associative learning that is paired with an adverse event with a nonspecific stimulus so that the animal learns to respond in a manner to avoid the adverse event.
[ref. 4]

avoidance test, active

Fear-motivated associative *avoidance test* based on presentation of an adverse stimulus (*e.g.*, an electric current) as a source of discomfort, to create an environment from which the animal or subject would prefer to escape.
Note: In an active avoidance test, a mouse or rat learns to associate the occurrence of an aversive event with the presentation of a specific stimulus, and to avoid the event by actively moving to a different location. The number of avoidances (moving to the other location during the stimulus signal), number of nonresponses or errors (failing to move to the other location during the trial), and response latency (time between signal onset and response), are used as an *index* of learning.
[ref. 4]

avoidance test, associative

Avoidance test in which the test animal has learned to develop an association between the stimulus and the delivery of an aversive event.
[ref. 4]

axenic animal

See *germ-free animal.*

axenic culture

Growth of organisms of a single *species* in the absence of cells or living organisms of any other species.
[ref. 2]

axial skeleton

Bones of the body axis, including the skull, *spinal column*, ribs and sternum.
[ref. 5]
See also *appendicular skeleton*.

axon (n)/axonal (adj)

Long thread-like process of a *neuron* along which impulses are conducted from the cell body to the nerve ending.
[ref. 4]
Compare *dendrite*.

axonal degeneration

Progressive loss of structure and function of an *axon*, typically in a peripheral-to-central direction.
[ref. 4]

axonal transport

axoplasmic transport

Movement of organelles and biomolecules to (retrograde) and from (anterograde) a *neuron*'s cell body, within the cytoplasm of its *axon* (the axoplasm).
[ref. 4]

axonal transport, retrograde

Transport of material from the *nerve* ending back to the cell body.
[ref. 4]
See also *axonal transport*.

axonopathy

Disorder of *axons* causing weakness, numbness, and *paresthesia*, particularly involving the *peripheral nerves*.
Note: Axonopathy often starts distally as a symmetrical polyneuropathy involving nerves in roughly the same areas on both sides of the body.
[After ref. 4]
See also *polyneuropathy*.

azoospermia

Absence of viable *spermatozoa* in the *semen*.
[ref. 5]

B1/B2 cells

B1/B2 lymphocytes

Two major subpopulations of *B-lymphocytes*.
Note 1: The majority of *B-cells* are B2 cells that express low levels of surface IgM, higher levels of surface IgD, do not express CD5, and are CD43−, *CD23+*; they are directly generated from precursors in the *bone marrow*, and secrete highly specific antibody.
Note 2: B1 cells bear high levels of surface *immunoglobulin M*, show lower levels of surface *immunoglobulin D*, are CD43+/*CD23−*, and most express the cell surface *antigen* CD5. They are self-renewing, and frequently secrete high levels of *antibody* that binds to a range of antigens ("polyspecificity") with a relatively low *affinity*.
[ref. 3]

B7 molecule

Co-stimulatory molecule (see *co-stimulation*) on the surface of *T-cell*-activating *antigen-presenting cells*, allowing full *activation* of T-cells that are bound to *major histocompatibility complex* (*MHC*)-peptide complexes.
Note: Whereas binding of B7 molecules to CD28 is stimulatory, binding to *cytotoxic T-lymphocyte antigen-4* decreases T-cell activity and contributes to *tolerance*.
[ref. 3]

B-cell

See *B-lymphocyte*.

B-cell linker protein (BLNK)

Adaptor protein operating in *B-cells* that, upon phosphorylation, recruits signaling molecules to *membrane lipid rafts*.
[ref. 3]

B-cell receptor (BCR)

See *receptor, B-cell*.

B-cell stimulatory factor (BSF)

Generic name given to *B-cell*-specific *growth factors* and differentiation factors involved in the *T-cell*-dependent *activation* of B-cells.
Note: Many BSFs are now identified as specific *interleukins*.
[ref. 3]

B-lymphocyte

B-cell

Bone marrow-derived *lymphocyte*, expressing an *antigen-receptor* complex composed of membrane bound *immunoglobulin* and associated molecular chains.
Note 1: B-lymphocyte *receptors* interact with *epitopes* directly (no *major histocompatibility complex* restriction).

Comprehensive Glossary of Terms Used in Toxicology
By John Duffus, Douglas M. Templeton and Michael Schwenk

Published by the Royal Society of Chemistry, www.rsc.org

Note 2: Mature activated B-lymphocytes (*plasma cells*) produce *antibody* and are efficient *antigen-presenting cells.*
[ref. 3]
See also *B1/B2 cells.*

B-lymphocyte chemokine (CXCL13)

Chemokine that attracts *B-cells* and activated *T-cells* into the follicles of peripheral *lymphoid tissues.*
[ref. 3]

B-lymphocyte-induced maturation protein 1 (BLIMP-1)

Transcriptional repressor in *B-cells* that switches off genes required for B-cell proliferation in the *germinal center*, and for *class switching* and *affinity maturation.*
Note: B-lymphocytes in which BLIMP-1 is induced become *plasma cells.*
[ref. 3]

BALB/c mouse

Inbred albino mouse strain, substrains of which produce *plasmacytomas* on injection with mineral oil, useful for the production of *monoclonal antibodies.*
[ref. 3]

Bcl-2

Member of the Bcl protein family that protects cells from *apoptosis* by binding to the *mitochondrial membrane.*
Note: Bcl-2 protein is encoded by the bcl-2 *gene*, which was discovered at the breakpoint of an oncogenic chromosomal translocation in *B-cell leukemia.*
[ref. 3]

BCR-ABL

See *oncogene, ABL.*

bacille Calmette–Guérin (BCG)

Attenuated ***Mycobacterium tuberculosis*** used both as a specific *vaccine* for tuberculosis and as an *adjuvant.*
Note: BCG is also used as an *immunostimulant* in cancer therapy (*e.g.*, in bladder cancer).
[ref. 1]

back mutation

See *mutation, back.*

background concentration

See *concentration, background.*

bacterial artificial chromosome (BAC)

DNA vector based on a functional fertility *plasmid* into which large DNA fragments can be inserted and cloned into a bacterial host.
[*]

bactericide

Substance intended to kill bacteria.
[ref. 1]

bagassosis

Interstitial lung *disease* (*hypersensitivity pneumonitis*) caused by the *inhalation* of *dust* from sugar-cane residues.
[ref. 1]

bar test

Test for *catalepsy* in which a mouse is placed on a bar oriented parallel to and approximately 2.5 cm off the ground. Typically, if the mouse remains immobile on the bar for more than 20 seconds, it is considered to be cataleptic.
Note: The test can also be used for evaluating motor coordination.
[ref. 4]
See also *tetrad test.*

bare lymphocyte syndrome (BLS)

Rare, *recessive* genetic condition in which the products of one or more *genes* required to switch on *major histocompatibility complex* (*MHC*) *class I* or *MHC class II* genes are defective or absent.
Note: As a consequence of the gene defect, MHC class I (BLS1) or MHC class II (BLS2) genes are not expressed, leading to severe *immunodeficiency.*
[ref. 3]

Barnes maze

See *maze, Barnes.*

Barr body

See *sex chromatin.*

barrier

Obstruction to the exchange of materials between body compartments.
[*]
See also *barrier, blood-air; barrier, blood-aqueous; barrier, blood-brain; barrier, blood-testis; barrier, placental; barrier methods.*

barrier, alveolar-capillary

barrier, alveolocapillary
membrane, alveolocapillary
membrane respiratory

Structures through which gases diffuse from air to blood or blood to air.
Note: The relevant structures include *alveolar* fluid and surfactant, alveolar wall tissue, interstitial tissue fluid, and capillary wall tissue.
[*]

barrier, blood-aqueous

Physiological mechanism preventing free exchange of substances between the chambers of the eye and the blood.
[*]

barrier, blood-brain (BBB)

Selectively permeable structure that restricts the exit of blood cells and many substances from the *brain* capillaries into the extracellular space of the brain.

Note 1: The BBB consists of a layer of tightly packed cells (chiefly endothelial cells and *astrocytes*) and basement membrane, continuous along the brain capillaries.
Note 2: The BBB normally keeps cells of the systemic *immune system* outside the brain.
[ref. 3,4]

barrier, blood-cerebrospinal fluid

Functional restriction by cells of the *choroid plexus* of transit of substances from the *cerebrospinal fluid* into the extracellular space of the brain.
[ref. 4]

barrier, blood–placenta

Physiological interface between maternal and fetal blood circulations that filters out some substances that could harm the fetus while favoring the passage of others such as nutrients.
Note 1: Many fat-soluble substances, *e.g.*, alcohols, are not filtered out by the blood-placenta barrier, and several types of virus can also cross this barrier.
Note 2: The effectiveness of the blood-placenta interface as a barrier varies with species and different forms of *placentation*.
Note 3: *Immunoglobulin G antibodies* are specifically transported across the blood-placenta barrier and reach the same levels in the newborn, as in the mother.
[ref. 3]
See also *barrier, placental*.

barrier, blood-retinal

Functional restriction of transit of substances from the blood to the retina by non-fenestrated endothelial cells with tight junctions.
[ref. 4]

barrier, blood-testis

blood-seminiferous tubule barrier
Sertoli cell barrier (SCB)

Occluding barrier, formed by the *Sertoli cells* of the *seminiferous tubules*, that separates the more mature cells of *spermatogenesis* from blood-borne products.
Note: The name "blood-testis barrier" is misleading in that it is not a blood-organ barrier in a strict sense, but is formed between Sertoli cells of the seminiferous tubule and, as such, isolates the further developed stages of *germ cells* from the blood. A more correct term is the "Sertoli cell barrier".
[ref. 5]

barrier, placental

placental membrane

Multilayered *membrane* of *fetal* tissue within the *placenta* that separates the maternal blood from the fetal blood and allows selective passage of substances between the two.
Note: The placental barrier blocks only a few *xenobiotics*.
[ref. 5]
See also *barrier, blood–placenta*.

barrier, skin

Restriction on the uptake of substances through the skin to the blood, probably partly due to the keratinized surface *epithelial* cells and partly due to surface lipids.
[*]

basal ganglia
basal nuclei

Complex structure at the base of the brain consisting of several groups of *neurons*, the *caudate nucleus*, the *putamen*, the *globus pallidus*, and the *substantia nigra*.
Note: The basal ganglia are involved in various functions including voluntary motor movements and involuntary movements such as *tremors*, *bruxism*, *athetosis*, and *chorea*.
[ref. 4]

basal lamina

See *basement membrane*.

base-pairing

Linking of the complementary pair of polynucleotide chains of nucleic acids (*DNA*, *RNA*) by means of hydrogen bonds between complementary purine and pyrimidine bases - adenine with thymine or uracil, cytosine with guanine.
[ref. 1]

baseline

Describing a measurement, calculation, condition or location observed before an intervention and used as a basis for comparison after the intervention.
[*]

baseline toxicity

General, nonspecific, level of toxicity occurring in living organisms resulting from background environmental exposure.
[*]

basement membrane
basal lamina

Thin layer of *connective tissue* underlying an attached *epithelial* cell layer.
Note 1: The basement membrane separates the epithelium from the deeper interstitial *matrix*.
Note 2: The basement membrane is a triple-layered structure consisting of an electron-dense layer (the lamina densa) composed of type IV collagen, sandwiched between two electron-transparent layers (the laminae lucida), rich in the *glycoprotein* laminin.
Note 3: Cancer cells break through the basement membrane in order to migrate to other parts of the body and form metastases.
[ref. 1,5]

basolateral surface (of a cell)

See *cell polarity*.

basophil

Type of *granulocyte* found in the blood and resembling the tissue *mast cell*.
[ref. 3]

basophilic degranulation

Loss of granules in basophilic cells (see *basophil*), associated with the release of active substances from the cells, characteristic of *type I immediate hypersensitivity*.
[ref. 3]

batch-replacement test

See *static-renewal test.*

Bateman function

Equation expressing the build up and decay in *concentration* of a substance (usually in *plasma*) based on first-order *uptake* and *elimination* in a *one-compartment model*, having the form

$$C = [fDk_a/V(k_a - k_e)][\exp(-k_e t) - \exp(-k_a t)]$$

where C is the concentration and D the *dose* of the substance, f the fraction absorbed, and V the *volume of distribution.* k_a and k_e are the first-order *rate constants* of uptake and elimination, respectively, and t is time.
[ref. 1]

Bayesian

Term used to designate concepts relating to *Bayesian probability*, especially involving Bayes' theorem.
Note: Bayes' theorem expresses the probability of one of a number of mutually exclusive events, H_i, given some other event, E, in terms of the probabilities of all the H_i independently of E and the probabilities of E given each H_i.
[After ref. 2]

Bayesian probability

Subjective or objective concept of probability as a "measure of the state of knowledge".
Note 1: Assessment of probability in *Bayesian* theory can be approached as, *e.g.*, odds for one or the other result of a stochastic outcome.
Note 2: Modern machine learning methods are frequently based on Bayesian theory.
[ref. 2]

Bayley scale

Bayley scales of infant development (BSID)

Range of scores on play tasks performed by infants age 0-3 years, intended to assess development of motor, cognitive, and language skills against norms for age-matched normal child development.
[ref. 4]

beading (in *neurites*)

neuritic beading

Focal bead-like swellings in *dendrites* and *axons*.
Note: Beading can be an early neuropathological sign in *neuronal* injury, *e.g.*, in *epilepsy*, trauma, *ischemia*, aging, and *neurodegenerative diseases*.
[ref. 4]

beam walking test

Assessment of the ability of an animal to remain upright and to walk on an elevated and relatively narrow beam.
Note: Unilateral *brain* injury tends to induce a hemi*paresis*-like effect that can cause the animal to slip to one side during the beam waking test, usually to that which is contralateral to the injury site.
[ref. 4]

behavior scenario

See *scenario*.

behavioral teratology

Study of behavioral abnormalities in otherwise apparently developmentally normal individuals after *exposure in utero* to a substance or physical agent.
[After ref. 2]

behavioral toxicology

Study of behavioral abnormalities produced by *exposure* to a substance or physical agent.
[ref. 2]

Behcet disease

Chronic *vasculitis* of unknown origin, characterized by ulcerations and skin rash and treated by *immunosuppression*.
[ref. 3]

bell stage

Period in which the developing tooth takes on a bell shape in cross section, immediately preceding the "advanced bell stage", in which the hard tissues (dentin and enamel) form the crown of the tooth.
[ref. 5]

Bence–Jones protein

Excess circulating *kappa (κ)-light chain* found in the urine of patients with *multiple myeloma*.
[ref. 3]

benchmark concentration (BMC)

See *concentration, benchmark*

benchmark dose (BMD)

See *dose, benchmark*.

benchmark guidance value

Biological monitoring guidance value set at the 90th percentile of available *biological monitoring* results collected from a representative *sample* of workplaces with good occupational hygiene practices.
[ref. 1]

benchmark response (BMR)

See *response, benchmark*.

benefit

Opposite term: *detriment*.

Advantage to, or improvement in *condition* of, an individual, a *population*, a *species*, an *assemblage*, a *community*, or an *ecosystem*.
Note: For *risk*/benefit comparisons, the probability of benefit is the appropriate comparator.
[ref. 2]

benign

Opposite term: *malignant.*

1. Of a *disease*, producing no persisting harmful effects.
2. Of a *tumor* that does not invade other tissues (see *metastasis*), having lost growth control but not positional control, and still may cause mechanical damage to adjacent tissues.

[ref. 1]

benign monoclonal gammopathy

Nonmalignant overproduction of γ-*globulin* by a single *clone* of lymphocytes.
[ref. 3]

benthic

Living on the bottom or in the *sediment* of an aquatic system.
[ref. 2]
See also *epibenthic; nektonic.*

Benton test

Benton visual memory test

Procedure in which patterns on cards are memorized by a test subject who then attempts to recognize them on other cards presented subsequently.
Note 1: The Benton test measures short-term visual memory.
Note 2: Benton test conditions have repeatedly been modified, and variations such as asking the subject to redraw the pattern are in use.
[ref. 4]
See also *neurobehavior core test battery.*

berylliosis

See *beryllium disease.*

beryllium disease

berylliosis

Serious and usually permanent lung damage resulting from chronic *inhalation* of beryllium.
[ref. 1]

bias

Any trend in the collection, analysis, interpretation, publication, or review of data that can lead to results and conclusions that are systematically different from the true situation.
[ref. 1]

biased sample

Opposite term: *random sample*
Any *sample* that is not a *random sample.*
[ref. 1]

bicornate uterus

See *uterus, bicornate.*

Biel water maze

See *maze, Biel water.*

bilaminar embryo

See *embryo, bilaminar.*

bile

Fluid rich in bile acids, phospholipids and cholesterol that is secreted through the *canalicular membrane* of *hepatocytes* into the biliary tract.
Note 1: Bile flows via the gall bladder into the upper small intestine, where it activates enzymes of triglyceride digestion (lipases).
Note 2: *ABC-transporters* in the canalicular membrane of the *hepatocyte* are involved in *elimination* into the bile of a wide range of organic molecules, including *bilirubin*, many *xenobiotics* and their *metabolites,* and copper.
Note 3: Reduced bile flow (*cholestasis*) causes a reflux of biliary substances into the blood, visible as *jaundice* and associated with decreased intestinal fat digestion.
[*]

bilirubin

Breakdown product of heme-containing proteins (*hemoglobin, myoglobin, cytochromes*) to a yellowish pigment that circulates in the blood *plasma* bound to albumin, or as water-soluble glucuronide *conjugates*, and is excreted in the bile by the liver.
[ref. 1]

bioaccessibility

environmental availability

Potential for a substance to come in contact with a living organism and interact with it, with the possibility of *absorption* into the organism.
Note 1: A substance trapped inside an insoluble particle is not *bioaccessible*, although substances on the surface of the same particle are bioaccessible and may also be *bioavailable*. Bioaccessibility, like bioavailability, is a function of both *chemical speciation* and biological properties. Even substances bound to the surface of particles may not be accessible to organisms that require the substances to be in solution. Bioaccessibility is a necessary precursor of *bioavailability* but not, on its own, sufficient for bioavailability to occur.
Note 2: In *ecotoxicology*, bioaccessibility is often measured by assessment of the fraction of a substance (see *fractionation*) released from a *matrix* (usually *soil* or *sediment*) into an aqueous medium under defined laboratory conditions. Such measurements must be interpreted with care as laboratory conditions rarely equate to those in nature.
Note 3: In human toxicology, bioaccessibility may be measured as the amount of a specific compound released from a matrix when exposed *in vitro* to conditions mimicking those in the human gut and small intestine. This gives no measure of bioaccessibility on the skin, in the lung, or in the eye.
[ref. 2]
See also *bioavailability*.

bioaccessible

Able to come in contact with a living organism and perhaps interact with it with the possibility of *absorption* into the organism.

Note: Contact of a bioaccessible substance with a living organism may not result in any interaction of the substance with, or absorption by, the organism.
[ref. 2]
See also *bioaccessibility, bioavailable.*

bioaccumulation

Progressive increase in the amount of a substance in an organism or part of an organism that occurs because the rate of intake from all contributing sources and by all possible routes exceeds the organism's ability to eliminate the substance from its body.
Note: Bioaccumulation of organic molecules usually correlates with lipophilicity. Bioaccumulation of metal ions tends to correlate with strong binding to biomolecules or incorporation into bone and teeth.
[ref. 2]
See also *bioaccessibility; bioavailability; bioconcentration; biomagnification.*

bioaccumulation factor (BAF, BF)

accumulation factor

Ratio of tissue substance residue to substance concentration in an external environmental phase (*e.g.*, *sediment*, water, *soil*, air, or food), measured at a steady state.
Note 1: The concentration of lipophilic substances in the organism is typically expressed per unit mass of body fat (BAF, lipid-based).
Note 2: The concentration in *sediment* may be expressed per dry mass of sediment or per mass of organic carbon and may be referred to as the *biota-sediment accumulation factor* (BSAF).
Note 3: The substance for which a BAF is calculated may have entered the organism by any source of exposure.
[After ref. 2]

bioaccumulation potential

Ability of living organisms to concentrate a substance to which it is *exposed.*
[*]

bioaccumulative chemicals of concern (BCC)

See *persistent organic pollutants.*

bioactivation

Metabolic conversion of an exogenous substance to a more biologically active form.
Examples: Conversion of a *xenobiotic* to a more *toxic* derivative, conversion of a *prodrug* to its *therapeutic* form.
[*]
See also *bioinactivation.*

bioamplification

See *biomagnification.*

bioassay

Procedure for estimating the *concentration* or biological activity of a substance or physical agent by measuring its effect on a living system compared to a standard system.
[ref. 2]

bioavailable

Able to be *absorbed* by living organisms.
[ref. 1]
See also *bioaccessible; bioavailability*.

bioavailability (general)

biological availability
physiological availability

Potential for uptake of a substance by a living organism.
Note 1: Bioavailability may be expressed as a fraction of the total amount of the substance available in the *matrix* of *exposure*, and measured as the extent of *absorption* of the substance by a living organism.
Note 2: Bioavailability, like *bioaccessibility*, is a function of both *chemical speciation* and biological properties. Even surface-bound substances may not be bioaccessible to, and thus not bioavailable to, organisms that require substances to be in solution before they can interact with them.
[After ref. 1,2]
Note 3: Knowledge of bioavailability and the factors affecting it is an essential part of *risk assessment*.

bioavailability, absolute

Systemic exposure from extravascular (ev) exposure divided by that following intravenous (iv) exposure as described by the equation:

$$F = A_{\mathrm{ev}}\, D_{\mathrm{iv}}/B_{\mathrm{iv}}\, D_{\mathrm{ev}}$$

where F (fraction of *dose* absorbed) is a measure of the bioavailability, A and B are the *areas under the* (plasma) *concentration–time curve* following extravascular and intravenous administration, respectively, and Dev and Div are the administered extravascular and intravenous *doses*.
[After ref. 1]

bioavailability, environmental

Clearance rate of an environmental contaminant taken up by an organism divided by the rate at which the organism encounters the contaminant in an environmental medium (*e.g., soil, sediment*, water, food) being processed by the organism.
Note: Environmental bioavailability is a measure of an organism's extraction efficiency, via respiratory, dietary, and surface absorption processes, from the environmentally available (*bioaccessible*, but not necessarily *bioavailable*) portion of a material.
[ref. 2]
See also *availability, environmental*.

bioavailability, relative

Bioavailability estimated for a *dose* administered by any route or formulation, relative to a dose administered in a reference (or alternate) route or formulation.
[ref. 2]
Compare *relative systemic availability*.

biocenosis

biocoenosis
biotic *community*

biological community
ecological community

All the interacting organisms living together in a specified *habitat*.
Note: The area occupied by a biocenosis is defined by a characteristic *assembly* of *species*.
[ref. 2]

biochemical mechanism

Reaction or series of reactions in a living organism, usually enzyme-catalyzed, associated with a specific process, such as a *metabolic*, physiological, pharmacological or toxicological pathway.
[*]

biochemical (biological) oxygen demand (BOD)

Amount *concentration* of dioxygen taken up through the respiratory activity of microorganisms growing on organic compounds when incubated at a specified temperature (usually 20 °C) for a fixed period (usually 5 days).
Note 1: BOD is regarded as a measure of the fraction of organic *pollutants* in water that can be degraded biologically.
Note 2: The empirical test used in the laboratory to determine BOD also measures the oxidation of inorganic material such as sulfide and iron(II). Reduced forms of nitrogen may interfere unless their oxidation is prevented by an inhibitor such as allyl thiourea.
Note 3: Because the test method involves variables limiting reproducibility, BOD measurements may vary plus or minus ten to twenty percent around the mean.
[After ref. 1]

biocide (n)/biocidal (adj)

Substance intended to kill living organisms.
[ref. 1]
Note: More specifically, a biocide is a member of a diverse group of toxic substances including preservatives, *insecticides*, disinfectants, repellants, and *pesticides* used to control organisms that are harmful to human or animal health, feedstocks, or manufactured products.
[*]

biocoenosis

See *biocenosis.*

biocommunity

See *community.*

bioconcentration

Process leading to a higher *concentration* of a substance in an organism than in environmental media to which it is *exposed.*
Note: Bioconcentration is often used as a term for *uptake* by aquatic organisms directly from water.
[ref. 2]
See also *bioaccumulation.*

bioconcentration factor (BCF)

Measure of the tendency for a substance in water to accumulate in aquatic organisms defined as the ratio at equilibrium of the *concentration* of the substance of concern in the organism to its concentration in water.
Note 1: The equilibrium concentration of a substance in an aquatic organism can be estimated by multiplying its concentration in the surrounding water by its BCF in that organism.
Note 2: The BCF is an important determinant of human intake of *contaminants* from water by ingestion of aquatic food.
[ref. 2]

bioconcentration factor, lipid-based

Concentration of a substance of concern in the lipid fraction of the test organism divided by its concentration in the *ambient* water.
[ref. 2]

bioconjugate

See *conjugate.*

bioconversion

See *biotransformation.*

biodegradation

Breakdown of a substance catalyzed by enzymes *in vitro* or *in vivo.*
Note 1: Biodegradation may be characterized for purposes of *hazard assessment* as a) primary (alteration of the chemical structure of a substance resulting in loss of a specific property), b) partial (biodegradation to an extent that removes properties that may be considered environmentally unacceptable), and c) ultimate (complete breakdown of the substance).
Note 2: In *ecotoxicology*, biodegradation is almost entirely due to microbial or fungal activity.
[After ref. 2]
See also *activated sludge; degradation; inherently biodegradable.*

biodiversity

Occurrence of a number of *species* within a given *ecosystem* or *biome*, or the presence of a number of *community* types in a given area.
Note 1: In special cases, biodiversity may include a degree of genetic variation within a single species.
Note 2: Biodiversity is often a measure of the health of biological systems.
Note 3: Biodiversity often refers to the number of different species in a defined area (*species richness*) and is quantified by calculating a *diversity index* that takes into account the relative *abundance* of individuals of each species.
[ref. 2]

biodiversity action plan (BAP)

Internationally recognized program designed to protect and restore biological systems containing threatened *species* and *habitats*.
Note 1: The original impetus for BAPs derives from the 1992 Convention on Biological *Diversity* (CBD).
Note 2: The principal elements of a BAP typically include: (a) preparing inventories of biological information for selected species or habitats; (b) assessing the conservation

status of *species* within specified ecosystems; (c) creation of targets for conservation and restoration; and (d) establishing budgets, timelines, and institutional partnerships for implementing the BAP.
[ref. 2]

bioelimination

Total removal, usually from the aqueous phase, of a test substance by biological processes supplemented by physicochemical reactions.
[After ref. 1]

bioequivalence (n)/bioequivalent (adj)

Property of there being similar efficacy between two preparations of the same *drug* at the same dose.
[*]

biogeochemical cycle

Movement of elements or molecules among organisms and nonliving compartments of the atmosphere, lithosphere, and hydrosphere.
Note 1: Examples of biogeochemical *cycles* are the carbon, nitrogen, phosphorus, and sulfur cycles. These are defined as the global flow of C, N, P, and S atoms, respectively, from plants through animals to the atmosphere, *soil*, water, and back to plants.
Note 2: The water cycle refers to the global flow of water from surface and ground water sources to soil, plants, animals, and the atmosphere, and back to soil and surface water.
[ref. 2]

bioinactivation

Metabolic conversion of a *xenobiotic* to a less *toxic* derivative.
[ref. 1]
See also *bioactivation.*

bioinformatics

Discipline encompassing the development and utilization of computational facilities to store, analyze, and interpret biological data.
[ref. 1]

biokinetics (chemical)

Study of the rates of movement involved in the *distribution* of substances in living organisms and the *biosphere.*
[*]
See also *pharmacokinetics; toxicokinetics.*

biolistics

Use of small particles, *e.g.*, colloidal gold, as a vehicle for carrying agents (*drugs*, nucleic acid, *etc.*) into a cell.
Note: Following coating of particles with the desired agent(s), biolistic refers to their being propelled into the dermis of a recipient.
[ref. 3]

biological absorption

See *absorption, biological.*

biological accessibility

See *bioaccessibility.*

biological acclimatization

See *acclimation*.

biological assessment of exposure

See *monitoring, biological*.

biological availability

See *bioavailability*.

biological determinant

See *determinant, biological*.

biological effect monitoring (BEM)

Continuous or repeated measurement of early biological effects of exposure of an organism to a substance to evaluate ambient *exposure* and *health risk* by comparison with appropriate reference values based on knowledge of the probable relationship between ambient exposure and biological effects.
[ref. 1]

biological exposure indices (BEI)

Guidance values recommended by ACGIH for assessing *biological monitoring* results.
[ref. 1]

biological half-life ($t_{1/2}$)

See *half-life, biological*.

biological half-time

See *half-life, biological*.

biological indicator
bioindicator
indicator species

Any biological *species* or group of species whose performance, *abundance*, or *population* status is used to determine the health of an environment or *ecosystem* by systematic monitoring of biochemical, physiological, or behavioral changes, or of accumulation of a substance by the species.
Note 1: A bioindicator is chosen because an alteration in its performance, abundance, or population status indicates an adverse effect. In a wider sense, the number and abundance of different indicator species (*biodiversity, species richness*) are used to calculate *biotic indices*.
Note 2: Bioindicator is commonly misused as a synonym for the term *biomarker*. Such use is to be deprecated.
[ref. 2]

biological marker

See *biomarker*.

biological monitoring

See *monitoring, biological*.

biological oxygen demand

See *biochemical oxygen demand.*

biological preparation

biological (n)
biopreparation

Substance derived from living organisms and their products, *e.g.*, for use in *medicine* or as a *pesticide*.
[ref. 1]

biological specimen

1. Organ, tissue (including blood), secretion, or excretion product taken from an organism as a *sample* reflecting the state of the whole organism.
2. Organism taken as a sample reflecting the state of a population or their environment.

[ref. 1]

biological warfare

Military operations using any organism (bacterium, virus, or other *disease*-causing organism) or *toxin*, to kill, injure, or incapacitate human beings, animals, or plants.
[ref. 1]

biomagnification

bioamplification
ecological magnification
trophic enrichment

1. Sequence of processes by which higher *concentrations* of a substance are attained in organisms at higher *trophic levels*.
2. Result of these processes of *bioconcentration* and *bioaccumulation* by which tissue concentrations of bioaccumulated chemicals increase as the chemical passes up through two or more trophic levels.

Note: Biomagnification occurs in a food chain as a consequence of efficient transfer of a substance from food to consumer accompanied by the lack of, or very slow, excretion or *degradation* of the substance.
[ref. 2]

biomagnification factor, *B*

Ratio of *concentrations* of a compound at two consecutive trophic levels at steady state.
Note: Biomagnification can also be expressed in terms of a rate constant-based bioaccumulation model

$$B = C_n / C_{n-1} = \alpha f / k_e$$

where α is assimilation efficiency, f is feeding rate, and k_e is the first-order elimination constant. B can be calculated from field data on assumed trophic relations or from laboratory feeding experiments.
[ref. 2]
See also *trophic enrichment factor.*

biomarker (general)

Indicator signaling an event or condition in a biological system or *sample* and giving a measure of *exposure*, effect, or *susceptibility*.
Note: A biomarker may be a measurable substance; a biochemical, physiological, or behavioral change; or any other alteration within an organism.
[ref. 1]

biomarker (in ecotoxicology)

Quantifiable behavioral, physiological, histological, biochemical, or genetic property that is used to measure response to an environmental change.
Note 1: A biomarker may be an analytical measurement of a *pollutant* or group of pollutants, or metabolite(s) at the organismal or suborganismal level in individual members of a *species* that is regarded as a suitable *bioindicator* or *sentinel* species. Ideally, biomarker results should have the possibility of extrapolation to indicate potential *risk* to *populations, communities*, or *ecosystems*.
Note 2: Biomarkers may be used for early warning purposes to indicate either *exposure* before serious irreversible damage occurs or increased *susceptibility* of subpopulations.
Note 3: Biomarkers are used for *biomonitoring* potential effects of environmental factors, either in a time frame or by comparing biomarker intensity between putatively affected and nonaffected areas.
[ref. 2]

biomarker, prognostic

Biomarker used to predict the occurrence, recurrence, or progression of *disease*.
[*]

biomarker of effect

effect biomarker
response biomarker

Biomarker that, depending upon the magnitude, can be recognized as associated with an established or possible *health* impairment or *disease*.
[ref. 1]
Note: Biomarkers used to assess the response to a pharmacological intervention or toxic exposure may be referred to as *pharmacodynamic* or *toxicodynamic* biomarkers, respectively.
[*]

biomarker of exposure

exposure biomarker

Biomarker that relates *exposure* to a *xenobiotic* or other substance of concern, to the levels of the substance or its *metabolite*, or of the product of an interaction between the substance and some *target* molecule or cell that can be measured in a *compartment* within an organism.
[ref. 1]

biomarker of susceptibility

susceptibility biomarker

Biomarker of an inherent or acquired *sensitivity* of an organism to *exposure* to a specific substance.
[After ref. 1]

biomass

1. Total amount of *biotic* material, usually expressed per unit surface area or volume, in a medium such as water.
2. Material produced by the growth of microorganisms, plants, or animals.

[ref. 1]

biome

Set of plants and animals that occupy a certain geographic area.
Note: The term is usually applied to large areas occupied by *climax communities* arising as a result of interactions between *biotic* and *abiotic* factors.
[ref. 2]

biomineralization

1. Formation of mineralized tissue (*e.g.*, bone, teeth or shell) by a living organism. [*]
2. Deposition of minerals in the environment mediated by living organisms.
   Examples: Silicates in algae, carbonates in diatoms and invertebrates, calcium phosphates (*e.g.*, hydroxyapatite in bone), carbonates in vertebrates.
3. Complete conversion of organic substances to inorganic derivatives by living organisms, especially microorganisms.

[ref. 2]
See also *mineralization.*

biominification

bioreduction
See *trophic dilution.*

biomodification

Alteration of the chemical or physical properties of a substance by the action of living organisms.
[ref. 2]

biomolecule

Substance that is synthesized by, and occurs naturally in, living organisms.
[ref. 1]

biomonitor

1. (n) Organism that provides quantitative information on the quality of the environment around it.
   Note: The ideal substance biomonitor would indicate the presence of a specific *pollutant* and provide additional information about the amount present.
2. (v) To use organisms to monitor pollutants and to deduce possible effects on biota or routes of *toxicant exposure* to humans.

[ref. 2]
See also *biological monitoring.*

biomonitoring

See *monitoring, biological.*

biopanning

Technique for selection of peptides with high *affinity* binding to a chosen target.
[ref. 3]

biopesticide

Biological agent with *pesticidal* activity, *e.g.*, the bacterium ***Bacillus thuringiensis*** when used to kill insects.
[ref. 1]

biopharmaceutical

1. *Pharmaceutical* obtained from, or related to, biological sources, *e.g.*, blood-derived products or *vaccines*.
2. Synthetic pharmaceuticals incorporating targeting *biomolecules* such as *antibodies*.

[*]

biopsy

1. (v) Excision of a small piece of tissue for microscopic or biochemical examination; usually performed to establish a diagnosis.
2. (n) Small piece of tissue for microscopic or biochemical examination; usually obtained in order to establish a diagnosis.

[After ref. 1]

bioremediation

Use of biological organisms such as microbes or plants to aid in removing hazardous substances from an area.
[ref. 2]

biosensor

Device that uses specific biochemical reactions mediated by isolated enzymes, immunosystems, tissues, organelles, or whole cells to detect substances usually by electrical, thermal, or optical signals.
[ref. 2]

biosimilar (n)

follow-on biologic

Biological pharmaceutical agent made deliberately to have *therapeutic* properties similar to one that has already been clinically tested and licensed.
Note: Because of their similarity to licensed biologicals, in the USA there is an abbreviated licensing approval process for biosimilars.
[*]

biosphere

ecosphere

Zone of air, land, and water, at the surface of the Earth, that is occupied by biological organisms.
[ref. 2]

biostatic

Adjective applied to a substance that arrests the growth or multiplication of living organisms.
[ref. 1]

biota

All biological organisms as a totality.
[ref. 1]

biota-sediment accumulation factor (BSAF)
accumulation factor (AF)
biota-sediment factor (BSF)

See *bioaccumulation factor* (Note 2).

biotic
Opposite term: *abiotic.*

Associated with biological organisms.
[*]

biotic index

See *index, biotic*.

biotic ligand

Component of a biological organism to which an ion or other substance in aqueous solution can bind, usually with subsequent beneficial or harmful effect on the physiology of the organism.
[ref. 2]

biotic ligand model (BLM)

Model that integrates the interactions of metals with *ligands* in water to calculate the *chemical speciation* (based on hardness, salinity, and presence of other metals) and the *concentration* of ionic species producing *toxicity*.
Note 1: The BLM chemically and mathematically models the organism's target site as ligand(s) competing with nonbiotic ligands, based on the concept that toxicity occurs when a metal-(biotic ligand) complex reaches a critical concentration.
Note 2: The BLM is a development of the *free ion activity model* (FIAM) for calculating free metal ions in relation to water-borne ligands, and the Windermere humic aqueous model (WHAM) for calculating metal speciation in relation to organic species in water.
Note 3: The BLM is a generalization of the FIAM. The difference between the BLM and the FIAM is that the BLM considers competitive binding at the biotic ligand, thus modeling the protective effects of other metal cations, and the direct influence of pH.
Note 4: For fish, the biotic ligand for metal ions is either known or suspected to be the *ion channel* proteins in the gill surface that regulate the ionic composition of the blood. For other organisms, it is hypothesized that a biotic ligand exists and that mortality can be modeled in a similar way.
[After ref. 2]

biotic score

Weighted measurement of biological organisms present—the weighted part is determined by each group's *pollution* tolerance or intolerance.
Note: As pollution increases in a stream, the biotic score value tends to change.
[ref. 2]

biotope

Habitat shared by many *species*, most often an area that is uniform in environmental conditions and in its distribution of animal and plant life.
[ref. 2]

biotransformation

bioconversion

Chemical conversion of a substance that is mediated by biological organisms or *enzyme* preparations derived from them.
[ref. 1]
See also *phase I reaction of biotransformation; phase II reaction of biotransformation; phase III reaction of biotransformation.*

bioturbation

Group of processes whereby biological organisms affect the structure of *sediment*.
Note: Bioturbation consists of two processes, particle mixing and *irrigation*, mainly carried out by *infaunal* organisms, but also by *epifaunal* organisms and bottom-feeding fish.
[ref. 2]

biphasic dose–effect model

1. Model of *adverse effect* vs. *dose* relationship that, owing to *hormesis*, drops below the control level before increasing with the dose; individuals *exposed* to low, but nontoxic concentrations are healthier than individuals not exposed to the chemical.
   Note: Biphasic *dose–effect curves* occur for any nutrient. Hormesis is a phenomenon associated with compounds that have no nutrient properties.
2. Model of adverse effect vs. dose relationship that changes slope owing to a change in the mechanism of toxic action.
   Note: The biphasic dose-effect may, *e.g.*, be due to saturation of a transport or *metabolic* system.

[ref. 2]

bipolar disorder

manic-depressive disorder

Psychiatric illness characterized by mood shifts with periods of severe depressive illness and one or more episodes of exaggerated activity levels (manic behavior).
[ref. 4]

birth

Start of life as a physically separate being, *e.g.*, the emergence of a baby from the body of its mother, or the hatching of an egg.
[ref. 5]

birth defect

congenital defect

Physical or biochemical abnormality that is present at *birth*, and that may either be inherited or be the result of environmental influence.
[ref. 5]
Compare *congenital malformation.*

birth rate

1. (in demography) Number of live births in a defined administrative jurisdiction in a calendar year divided by a midyear *population* of the jurisdiction, with the customary multiplier of 1 000 to produce a whole number rather than a decimal or a fraction.
   Note: An alternative statistic to birth rate is total fertility rate, the average number of children born to each woman over the course of her life. In general, the total fertility rate is a better indicator of fertility rates because, unlike the crude birth rate, it is not affected by the age distribution of the population.
2. (in ecology) Number of births, B, in a population of a defined size, N, during a specified time interval Δt. The rate is calculated from the formula

$$B = \Delta N / \Delta t$$

   where ΔN is the change in the number of births in a limited time period Δt.

[ref. 2]
See also *birth rate, per capita.*

birth rate, per capita

Average number of offspring per *population* member per time unit, calculated from birth rate, B, and population size, N, as $b = B/N$.
[ref. 2]
See also *population growth* rate; *per capita rate of increase.*

bisexual

See *ambisexual.*

bispecific antibody

See *antibody, bispecific.*

blast

Immature stage in cell development, before the appearance of the definitive characteristics of the cell; used also as a word termination, as in erythroblast or *normoblast.*
[ref. 3]
See also *erythroblastosis.*

blastema

Mass of cells from which an organ or a body part develops, either in normal development or in the regeneration of a lost body part.
[ref. 5]

blastocoel
cleavage cavity
segmentation cavity

Fluid-filled *cavity* in the *blastula* of a developing *embryo.*
[ref. 5]

blastocyst

Modified *blastula* that is characteristic of *placental* mammals.

Note: The blastocyst has an outer cell layer, known as the *trophoblast*, which participates in the development of the placenta, and an inner mass of cells in the *blastocoel*, which develops into the *embryo*.
[ref. 5]

blastogenesis assay

See *lymphocyte transformation test.*

blastomere

Any of the cells formed by *cleavage* of a *fertilized egg.*
[ref. 5]

blastula

blastocyst
blastodermic vesicle

Hollow mass of cells formed after a *zygote* has undergone approximately six cell divisions.
[ref. 5]
See also *blastocoel; blastocyst.*

blastulation

Process by which the early *embryo* transforms from the *morula* into the *blastula.*
[ref. 5]
See also *blastocyst.*

Blau syndrome

Rare familial inflammatory *disease* characterized by *arthritis, dermatitis*, and uveitis.
[ref. 3]

β-blocker

β-adrenergic antagonist
β-adrenergic blocking agent
β-adrenergic receptor antagonist
β-adrenoreceptor antagonist
β-antagonist

Any of a class of *drugs* that targets the *β-adrenergic receptor*, interferes with binding of *adrenaline* and other related substances to the receptor, and weakens their effects.
[ref. 4]

blocking antibody

See *antibody, blocking.*

blood

Body fluid consisting of *erythrocytes, leukocytes, platelets*, and *blood plasma* with its *clotting* factors, normally circulating in the *cardiovascular* system.
[*]

blood-brain barrier (BBB)

See *barrier, blood-brain.*

blood-cerebrospinal fluid barrier

See *barrier, blood-cerebrospinal fluid.*

blood dyscrasia

Presence of abnormal material in the blood, usually applied to *diseases* affecting blood cells or *platelets.*
[ref. 3]

blood group

blood type

Any of the various types of blood whose characteristic *erythrocyte* surface *antigens* determine compatibility in *transfusion.*
[ref. 3]
See also *blood group system, ABO.*

blood group antigen

See *antigen, blood group.*

blood group system, ABO

System of *antigens* expressed on *erythrocytes* and used for typing human blood for *transfusion.*
Note: Individuals who do not express A or B antigens on their erythrocytes naturally form *antibodies* against them.
[ref. 3]
See also *blood group.*

blood–placenta barrier

See *barrier, blood–placenta.*

blood plasma

See *plasma (in biology).*

blood-retinal barrier

See *barrier, blood-retinal.*

blood serum

See *serum.*

blood substitution

See *exchange transfusion.*

blood-testis barrier

See *barrier, blood-testis.*

Bloom syndrome

Disease caused by mutations in a DNA helicase and characterized by low *T-cell* numbers, reduced *antibody* levels, and an increased susceptibility to respiratory infections, cancer, and radiation damage.
[ref. 3]

body burden

Total amount of a substance present in the body at a given time.
[ref. 1]

body cavity

See *coelom.*

body-on-a-chip

In vitro diagnostic system with modular, microchip-based technology, connected by microfluidic channels to cultured organ-specific cells, allowing simultaneous study of (often *toxic*) effects on a range of such cells.
Note: The method is in its infancy. The final aim is to develop a system that reflects events in the whole organism.
[*]
See also *organ-on-a-chip; lab-on-a-chip.*

bolus

1. Single *dose* of a substance, originally a large pill.
2. Dose of a substance administered by a single rapid intravenous injection.
3. Concentrated mass of food ready to be swallowed.

[ref. 1]

bone age

Average age at which children reach a given stage of bone maturation, denoting the stage of skeletal development of an individual *fetus* or child.
Note: A child's current height and bone age can be used to predict *adult* height.
[ref. 5]

bone marrow

Soft, fatty, vascularized substance in the *cavity* of bone where blood cells are formed.
[ref. 3]

bone marrow transplantation

Transfer of *bone marrow* from a donor to a recipient whose bone marrow has been ablated.
Note 1: Bone marrow transplantation is used to treat both nonneoplastic and neoplastic conditions not amenable to other forms of therapy.
Note 2: Bone marrow transplantation has been used especially in cases of *aplastic anemia, acute lymphoblastic (lymphocytic) leukemia*, and *acute myelogenous leukemia.*
[ref. 3]

bone morphogenetic protein (BMP)

bone morphogenic protein

Any of a family of *growth factor*s involved in bone and *cartilage* formation and, more generally, in orchestrating tissue architecture through *morphogenetic* signals.
Note: BMPs are considered to be *metabologens*.
[ref. 5]

bone morphogenetic protein-4 (BMP4)

bone morphogenic protein-4 (BMP4)

Bone morphogenetic protein member of the transforming growth factor β (TGF-β) superfamily.
Note: Amongst the multiple functions of BMP4 is a role in early *embryonic* differentiation, where it is secreted from the *notochord* and acts with *sonic hedgehog* protein to establish a *dorsal-ventral* axis.
[ref. 5]
See also *Spemann organizer*.

boomerang effect

Delayed damage from earlier *environmental contamination*.
Note: The boomerang effect is sometimes stated as "what you throw away can come back to hurt you".
[ref. 2]

booster

Portion of an immunizing agent (see *immunization*) given at a later time to stimulate the *effects* of a previous *dose* of the same agent.
[ref. 3]

borderline metal ion

Metal ion intermediate in properties between *class (a)* and *class (b) metal ions*.
[ref. 2]

Boston naming test (BNT)

Neuropsychological test used to study brain function and learning disabilities in children.
Note: The BNT is a procedure in which 60 pictures are shown to a subject who has to name them quickly.
[ref. 4]

botanical

Product that contains plant materials, algae, macroscopic fungi, or combinations of these where ingredients are not (highly) purified; it may be a food, *drug*, nutraceutical or cosmetic.
[*]

botanical pesticide

See *pesticide, botanical*.

bottom-up ecotoxicological study

Approach to investigating ecotoxicological effects that starts with a determination of the presence and nature of any adverse effects via responses at the suborganismal (cellular and biochemical) levels of organization rather than via the *community* and (or) *ecosystem* levels of organization.
[ref. 2]
See also *top-down ecotoxicological study*.

botulism

Acute food poisoning caused by botulinum toxin produced in food by the bacterium, ***Clostridium botulinum***, under anaerobic conditions.

Note: Botulism is characterized by muscle weakness and paralysis, disturbances of vision, swallowing, and speech, and a high mortality rate.
[ref. 1]

brachial plexus

Bundle of *nerve fibers* that begins in the *spine* at the base of the neck, travels through the axilla (armpit region), and into the arm.
Note: Damage to the motor and sensory nerves of the brachial plexus affects muscle function and sensation in the arm and chest.
[ref. 4]

brachydactyly
brachydactylia

Congenital abnormal shortness of fingers and toes.
[ref. 5]

brady-
Opposite term: *tachy-*

Prefix meaning slow as in *bradycardia* or *bradypnoea*.
[ref. 1]

bradycardia

Opposite term: *tachycardia*.
Abnormally slow heart rate.
[ref. 4]

bradykinesia
hypokinesia

Abnormally slow body movement.
[ref. 4]

bradykinin

Vasoactive peptide and inflammatory mediator (see *inflammation*) produced at sites of tissue damage.
[ref. 3]

bradypnoea
Opposite term: *tachypnoea*.

Abnormally slow breathing.
[ref. 1]

brain

That part of the *central nervous system* contained within the *cranium*.
[ref. 4]

brain-derived neurotrophic factor (BDNF)

Protein secreted by the *brain* that acts on *neurons* in the *central* and *peripheral nervous systems*; a member of the *neurotrophin* family of growth factors, related to the *nerve growth factor (NGF)*.
Note: BDNF is also secreted by contracting skeletal muscle and can be classified as a myokine.
[ref. 4]

brain herniation

Movement of part of the *brain* across structures within the skull, *e.g.*, a shift across structures such as the *falx cerebri*, the *tentorium cerebelli*, and even sometimes through the *foramen magnum* in the base of the skull (through which the *spinal cord* connects with the brain).
Note: Brain herniation is caused by high *intracranial pressure* and may have fatal results.
[ref. 4]

brain slice

Slice of *brain* tissue immersed in artificial *cerebrospinal fluid*, used in electrophysiology experiments to allow study of a *synapse* or *neural* circuit in isolation from the rest of the *brain*, and in *metabolic* studies, under controlled physiological conditions.
[ref. 4]

brainstem

Unpaired subdivision of the *brain*, continuous with the *spinal cord*, that includes the *thalamus, hypothalamus,* pons, *medulla oblongata*, and the *mesencephalon.*
[ref. 4]

branchial

Of, relating to, or resembling the gills of a fish, or the *homologous embryonic* structures and their derivatives in higher animals.
[ref. 5]

branchial arch

gill arch

1. (in *embryology*) One of several arches, resembling the gill arches of a fish, found in the *embryo* of a higher *vertebrate*; these arches develop into structures of the ear and neck.
2. (in biology) One of several bony or *cartilaginous* arches located on either side of the *pharynx* and supporting the gills in fish and amphibians.

[ref. 5]

branchial cyst, congenital

branchiogenic cyst

Congenital cyst arising in the lateral aspect of the neck, from *epithelial* remnants of a *pharyngeal groove.*
[ref. 5]

breathing zone

Space around a worker's nose and mouth, from which air is drawn into the lungs.
[*]

brevicollis

Shortness of the neck.
[ref. 5]

Brillouin index, H_B

See *index, Brillouin.*

British anti-Lewisite (BAL)

2,3-bis(sulfanyl)propan-1-ol
dimercaprol (INN)
2,3-dimercapto-1-propanol

Metal chelator that has been used in the treatment of metal or semi-metal poisoning, *e.g.*, with arsenic, antimony, gold, mercury, or lead.
[ref. 1]

Broca area

Broca speech area

Region in the *frontal lobe* of one of the *hemispheres* (the speech-dominant *hemisphere,* usually the left) of the hominid *brain* that is involved in motor functions of speech production.
Note: Destruction of the Broca area results in a characteristic type of *aphasia.*
[ref. 4]

bronchial provocation test

Test of altered lung function induced by *inhalation* of an *allergen* or airway-constricting agent, providing information on bronchial responsiveness.
[ref. 3]

bronchoconstriction

Opposite term: *bronchodilation.*

Narrowing of the air passages the bronchi of the lungs.
[ref. 1]

bronchodilation

Opposite term: *bronchoconstriction.*

Expansion of the air passages (the bronchi) of the lungs.
[ref. 1]

bronchopulmonary segment

Largest subdivision of a lobe of the lung with its air supply from a major branch of the bronchus and having its own arterial blood supply.
[ref. 5]

bronchospasm

Intermittent violent contraction of the air passages of the lungs.
[ref. 1]

bronchus-associated lymphoid tissue (BALT)

See *mucosa-associated lymphoid tissue.*

broodstock

Adult fish producing either *eggs* or *sperm.*
[ref. 2]

brownfield
brownfield land

Former industrial area that has been abandoned and often has a contaminated environment.
[*]

Bruton agammaglobulinemia

See *X-linked agammaglobulinemia*.

bruxism

Involuntary habitual grinding of the teeth, frequently during sleep.
[ref. 4]

buccopharyngeal membrane
oropharyngeal membrane

Membrane present in *fetal* life that separates the *nasal* cavities from the *pharynx*.
[ref. 5]

bud

Small protuberance, resembling the bud of a plant and having the potential for growth and differentiation.
[ref. 5]

Buehler assay (BA)
Buehler test

Skin sensitization test for *contact allergic dermatitis* in which a test substance is applied to the shaved flank of a guinea pig in an occlusive patch for 6 h at 0, 1, and 2 weeks, followed by *challenge* of the untreated flank at 4 weeks.
[ref. 3]

builder (in chemistry)

Material that enhances or maintains the cleaning efficiency of a surfactant in a detergent, principally by counteracting water hardness.
Note: Complex phosphates (especially sodium tripolyphosphate, *i.e.*, pentasodium triphosphate), sodium carbonate, and sodium silicate are the builders most commonly used.
[ref. 1]

bulb, olfactory

Region of the frontal lobe of the brain, receiving input from *neurons* of the *nasal mucosa* and involved in the sense of smell.
[ref. 5]

bulbourethral gland
Cowper's gland

One of two small *glands,* draining to the *urethra,* located on each side of, and inferior to, the *prostate* gland.
Note: Bulbourethral glands secrete a fluid component of the *seminal fluid*.
[ref. 5]

bulbus cordis

Outflow tract of the *embryonic* heart between the primitive *ventricle* and the *aorta*.
[ref. 5]

bullous skin disease, autoimmune

Any of several *autoimmune diseases* characterized by intraepidermal or subepidermal blisters (*e.g., pemphigus vulgaris*, bullous pemphigoid) and highly specific *autoantibodies* against components of the desmosome or hemidesmosome (*e.g.*, desmoglein 3, BP180).
[ref. 3]

bundle of His

atrioventricular bundle

Band of specialized cardiac muscle fibers connecting the *atria* with the *ventricles* of the heart.
Note: The bundle of His conducts the electrical impulse that regulates the heartbeat from the right atrium to the ventricles.
[ref. 5]

Burkitt lymphoma

Lymphoma caused by *Epstein–Barr virus (EBV)*, occurring mainly in sub-Saharan Africa.
[ref. 3]

burr hole surgery

trepanning
trephination
trephining

Medical intervention in which a hole is drilled or scraped into the human skull, exposing the *dura mater*, to gain access during surgery, to relieve *intracranial pressure, e.g.*, to evacuate a subdural hematoma.
[ref. 4]

bursa

Padlike fluid-filled sac or sac-like *cavity*, especially one reducing friction at a joint.
[ref. 5]

bursa of Fabricius

Primary *lymphoid* organ in avian species, located at the cloacal-hind gut junction; it is the site of *B-cell maturation*.
[ref. 3]

butyrylcholinesterase

plasma cholinesterase
pseudocholinesterase

Enzyme (EC 3.1.1.8), found mainly in the liver, that hydrolyzes choline esters; it is nonspecific and distinct from *acetylcholinesterase* (EC 3.1.1.7).
Note: Measurement of plasma cholinesterase activity mainly reflects butyrylcholinesterase activity, although the inhibitory action of many neurotoxic substances on the two enzymes acetyl- and butyrylcholinesterase, is correlated.
[ref. 4]

byssinosis

Pneumoconiosis caused by *inhalation* of *dust* and associated microbial contaminants, observed in cotton, flax, and hemp workers.
[ref. 1]

bystander effect (in immunology)

See *effect, bystander*.

bystander exposure

See *exposure, bystander*.

bystander suppression

See *suppression, bystander*.

C1 esterase inhibitor

See *C1 inhibitor*.

C1 inhibitor

C1 esterase inhibitor

Plasma glycoprotein secreted primarily by the liver and acting as a serine proteinase inhibitor (serpin), inhibiting C1 components of the *complement system*.
Note 1: C1 inhibitor also inhibits coagulation factors XI and XII and *kallikrein*.
Note 2: Patients with C1 inhibitor deficiency may manifest *systemic lupus erythematosus*, *glomerulonephritis*, or pyogenic infections.
[ref. 3]
See also *edema, hereditary angioneurotic*.

CA1-pyramidal cell

Pyramidal neuron located in the *cornu ammonis* area 1, in the *hippocampus*.
Note 1: CA1-pyramidal cells provide an output pathway from the hippocampus involved in long-term learning and memory.
Note 2: CA1-pyramidal cells are more susceptible to ischemia and hypoxia than the neighbouring *CA3-pyramidal cells*.
[ref. 4]

CA3-pyramidal cell

Pyramidal neuron located in the *cornu ammonis* area 3, in the *hippocampus*.
Note: CA3-pyramidal cells receive information from neurons of the *dentate gyrus* and sends information to the *CA1-pyramidal cells*.
[ref. 4]

CC chemokine

See *chemokine*.

CD1

Cell surface protein of *antigen-presenting cells* involved in presentation of lipopeptide or glycolipid *antigens*.
[ref. 3]
See also *antigen-presenting groove*.

CD3

Molecule composed of five polypeptide chains associated with the heterodimer *T-cell receptor*, forming the T-cell receptor complex (TCR/CD3).
Note: CD3 transduces the activating signals when *antigen* binds to the TCR.
[ref. 3]

CD4

Cell surface *antigen* belonging to the *immunoglobulin superfamily* of molecules and a marker of *helper T-cells*.

Comprehensive Glossary of Terms Used in Toxicology
By John Duffus, Douglas M. Templeton and Michael Schwenk

Published by the Royal Society of Chemistry, www.rsc.org

Note: As an adhesion molecule, CD4 interacts with the nonpolymorphic part of *major histocompatibility complex class II gene product.*
[ref. 3]

CD4+/CD25+ T-cell

Subtype of *CD4+ regulatory T-cell* with potential role in the regulation of *immune homeostasis.*
Note 1: CD4+/CD25+ T-cells seem to be important in preventing the development of *autoimmune diseases* (depletion leads to the spontaneous development of various autoimmune diseases in genetically susceptible animals; transfer prevents the development of organ-specific *autoimmunity*).
Note 2: Activated (see *activation*) *T-cells* may also have the CD4+/CD25+ phenotype. Regulatory T-cells may be further distinguished by positivity for a protein marker *Foxp3.*
[ref. 3]

CD5+ B-lymphocyte

Lymphocyte of type B1a, which is predominant in fetal *lymphoid* organs and in *neonatal* cord blood.
Note 1: In adults, CD5+ B-lymphocytes range from 2 to 6 % of total mononuclear cells in peripheral blood. They utilize an *immunoglobulin variable (V) gene* repertoire different from that of CD5– *B-cells* and they produce *natural autoantibodies.*
Note 2: The expansion of autoreactive B1-a cells has been reported in peripheral blood of patients with autoimmune *diseases* (*e.g., rheumatoid arthritis, Sjögren syndrome, antiphospholipid syndrome*). In rheumatoid arthritis, CD5+ B-lymphocytes can account for up to 60 % of circulating B-cells and may produce *rheumatoid factor.*
[ref. 3]

CD8

Cell surface molecule belonging to the *immunoglobulin superfamily* of molecules found, among others, on *cytotoxic T-cells*, which binds to *major histocompatibility complex class I molecules.*
[ref. 3]

CD8+ T suppressor cell

Outdated term for CD8+ *cytotoxic T-lymphocyte* (CTL, Tc). The term "*suppressor T-cell*" is nowadays reserved for *regulatory T-cell.*
[ref. 3]

CD16

Low-*affinity Fc-γ receptor* (Fc-γ-RIII) expressed mainly on natural *killer cells, granulocytes*, and *macrophages*, mediating *antibody-dependent cellular cytotoxicity.*
[ref. 3]

CD23

Low-*affinity Fc-ε receptor* induced by *interleukin*-4 and expressed on activated *B-cells* (see *activation, lymphocyte*) and *macrophages.*
[ref. 3]

CD25

α-Chain of the *interleukin*-2 *receptor.*
[ref. 3]

CD40 ligand (CD40L)

Essential molecule for normal signaling of *class switching* through binding to CD40 on *B-cells*.
Note: The interaction of CD40L and CD40 is also critical for optimal *T-cell* function.
[ref. 3]
See also *hyperimmunoglobulin M syndrome*.

CD45

See *leukocyte common antigen*.

C domain

See *constant (C) region*.

C gene

See *constant (C) gene*.

C-reactive protein (CRP)

Serum protein produced by liver cells as part of the *acute-phase response*, which acts as a stimulus of the *classical pathway of complement activation*.
Note: CRP binds to the phosphorylcholine component of the C-polysaccharide, a component of the surface of many bacteria and fungi, resulting in *opsonization* for enhanced *phagocytosis*.
[ref. 3]

C region

See *constant (C) region*.

C-type lectin

Any of a large family of Ca^{2+}-dependent *lectins*; members of this family share primary structural homology in their carbohydrate-recognition domains and include many endocytic *receptors*, many proteoglycans, and all known *collectins* and *selectins*.
Note: The C-type lectins are involved in many *immune system* functions, such as *inflammation* and *immunity* to tumor and virally infected cells, whereas the *collectins* are involved in *innate immunity*.
[ref. 3]

CXC chemokine

See *chemokine*.

CX3C chemokine

See *chemokine*.

cacosmia

Related terms: parosmia, troposmia
Opposite term: euosmia.

Imagined perception of vile odors, including coprosmia (smelling feces) and necrosmia (the smell of death).
[ref. 1]

cadherin

Calcium-dependent, transmembrane *glycoprotein* occurring in cell-cell contacts (desmosomes) and functioning as an *adhesion molecule*.
Note: Cadherins may mediate *lymphocyte homing* and are also important elements in cellular *signal transduction*.
[ref. 3]

Caenorhabditis elegans

Nematode with a well-defined number of cells, and a small *neural network* with homologues of human *neurotransmitters*, used as a model organism for studying normal and abnormal development, as well as *neurotoxic*ity.
Note: Neurotoxic *endpoints* studied in ***C. elegans*** include locomotion, reaction to touch and temperature-*sensitivity*.
[After ref. 4]

Caesarian section

Caesarian delivery
C-section

Surgical operation for delivering a child by opening the mother's abdominal wall and *uterus*.
[ref. 5]

calcification

Form of *mineralization* in which organic tissue becomes hardened by deposition of calcium salts within its substance.
[ref. 1]

calcineurin inhibitor

Any member of a group of immunomodulating (see *immunomodulation*) *drugs* that bind to the cytosolic protein cyclophilin of *T-lymphocytes*, thus inhibiting the phosphatase calcineurin, an inducer of *interleukin*-2 formation.
Note: Calcineurin inhibitors include potent *immunomodulating* drugs, such as cyclosporin, tacrolimus, pimecrolimus, and voclosporin.
[ref. 3]

calcinosis

Any *pathological* condition characterized by the deposition of calcium salts in tissues.
[ref. 2]

calcium sink

Tissue such as arthropod cuticle, molluscan shell, or vertebrate bone that renders calcium or elements with similar biological behavior (such as lead or cadmium) less *bioavailable* during trophic interactions, thus providing a mechanism for *trophic dilution*.
[ref. 2]

calibration

Operation that, under specified conditions, in a first step establishes a relation between the quantity values with measurement *uncertainties* provided by measurement *standards* and corresponding *indications* with associated measurement uncertainties

and, in a second step, uses this information to establish a relation for obtaining a measurement result from an indication.
[ref. 1]

calibration material

See *reference material.*

California verbal learning test

Procedure in which some common words are read aloud and the test subject is asked to recall as many of these as possible.
Note: The California verbal learning test is a neuropsychological test is used to assess the verbal memory.
[ref. 4]

canal

In biology and medicine, a relatively narrow tubular passage or channel.
[ref. 5]

Canale–Smith syndrome

See *autoimmune lymphoproliferative syndrome.*

canalicular membrane

Part of the *hepatocyte membrane* that faces the *lumen* of the biliary tract (canaliculus) and produces *bile* by transporting its constituents into the lumen.
[*]

cancer

Disease resulting from the development of a *malignant tumor*, characterized by uncontrolled growth, invasiveness of surrounding tissues, and the potential for *metastasis.*
[ref. 1]

candidiasis
candidosis
moniliasis

Infection with a fungus of the genus ***Candida***, especially ***C. albicans***, that usually occurs in the skin and mucous membranes of the mouth, respiratory tract, or vagina but may invade the bloodstream, especially in *immunocompromised* individuals.
[ref. 3]
See also *thrush.*

capacitation (of sperm)

Sum of biochemical changes undergone by mammalian *spermatozoa* in the female *genital tract* that enables them to penetrate and *fertilize* an *egg.*
[ref. 5]

capping (in cell biology)

Active process whereby cross-linking of cell surface molecules (*e.g.*, by *antibody*) leads to aggregation and subsequent migration of the molecules to one pole of the cell.
[ref. 3]

caput epididymis
globus major
head of epididymis

Upper and larger extremity of the *epididymis*.
[ref. 5]

carbohydrate kinase

Kinase enzyme that phosphorylates carbohydrates, often facilitating important *metabolic* pathways.
Example: Hexokinase (EC 2.7.1.1), which converts D-glucose to glucose-6-phosphate, preventing the glucose moiety from leaving the *cell*, and facilitating *glycolysis*.
[*]

carbonmonoxyhemoglobin

See *carbonylhemoglobin*.

carbonylhemoglobin
carbonmonoxyhemoglobin
carboxyhemoglobin

Compound that is formed when *hemoglobin* binds carbon monoxide instead of dioxygen in the blood, and becomes incapable of transporting dioxygen.
[After ref. 1]

carboxyhemoglobin

See *carbonylhemoglobin.*

carcinoembryonic antigen (CEA)

See *antigen, carcinoembryonic*.

carcinogen (n)/carcinogenic (adj)

Agent (chemical, physical, or biological) that is capable of increasing the *incidence* of *malignant neoplasms*, thus causing *cancer*.
[ref. 1]

carcinogen, transplacental

Substance that crosses the *placenta* and subsequently causes *cancer* in the child or young *adult*.
[ref. 5]

carcinogenesis (n)/carcinogen(et)ic (adj)

Induction, by chemical, physical, or biological agents, of *malignant neoplasms* and thus of *cancer*.
[ref. 1]

carcinogenic mutagenic reprotoxic (CMR) substance

Substance that produces long lasting *toxic* effects on the *genome*, leading to, *mutagenesis,* cancer, and (or) effects on reproductive health.
Note: When identified in industrial use or manufactured products, a CMR substance is a priority candidate for replacement by a less toxic compound.
[*]

carcinogenicity

Ability of chemical, physical, or biological agents, to induce or promote *malignant neoplasms*, and thus *cancer*.
[*]

carcinogenicity test

Test carried out over a sufficient time to detect any possible carcinogenic effect of a test substance.
[After ref. 1]

carcinoma
epithelioma

Malignant tumor of an *epithelial* cell.
[ref. 1]

cardiac

Pertaining to the heart.
[ref. 5]

cardiac jelly

Gelatinous substance, present between the *endothelium* and *myocardium* of the heart in early *embryos*, that develops into the *connective tissue* of the *endocardium*.
[ref. 5]

cardiogenesis

Development of the heart in the *embryo*.
[ref. 5]

cardiogenic

1. Originating in the heart; describing anything caused by normal or abnormal function of the heart.
2. Pertaining to *cardiogenesis*.

[ref. 5]

cardiolipin
1,3-bis(3-*sn*-phosphatidyl)-*sn*-glycerol

Main target of antiphospholipid *antibodies*.
[ref. 3]
See also *antiphospholipid syndrome*.

cardiotoxic

Harmful to the cells of the heart.
[ref. 1]

cardiovascular

Pertaining to the heart and blood vessels.
[ref. 5]

carotid artery

One of two paired large arteries on either side of the neck that supplies most of the *cerebral hemisphere*.
[ref. 4]

carpel tunnel syndrome (CTS)

Median *nerve* entrapment *neuropathy* that causes *paresthesia, pain*, and *numbness* due to compression of the nerve at the wrist in the carpal tunnel.
[ref. 4]

carrier

1. Substance in appreciable amount that, when associated with a trace of a specified substance, will carry the trace with it through a chemical or physical process.
2. Gas, liquid, or solid substance (often in particulate form) used to absorb, adsorb, dilute, or suspend a substance to facilitate its transfer from one medium to another.

[ref. 1]

carrier (in genetics)

Person who is heterozygous (*e.g.*, carries only one *allele*) for a recessive genetic character leading to *disease*, and hence does not, under most circumstances, display the disease *phenotype* but can pass it on to the next generation.
[ref. 1]

carrier (in immunology)

Molecule that, when *conjugated* to a non*immunogenic* molecule (*e.g.*, a *hapten*), makes the latter immunogenic by providing *epitopes* for *helper T-lymphocytes* that the hapten lacks.
[ref. 3]

carrier-linked prodrug
carrier prodrug

Compound that contains a temporary linkage between a given active substance and a transient *carrier* group, the latter producing improved physicochemical or *pharmacokinetic* properties and easily removable *in vivo*.
[ref. 1]

carrier protein

1. Protein to which a specific *ligand* or *hapten* is *conjugated.*
2. Unlabeled protein introduced into an assay at relatively high *concentrations* that distributes in a *fractionation* process in the same manner as labeled protein analyte, present in very low concentrations.
3. Protein added to prevent nonspecific interaction of reagents with surfaces, *sample* components, and each other.
4. Protein found in cell membranes that facilitates transport of a *ligand* across the membrane.

[ref. 1]
See also *transport, facilitated*.

carrier substance

Substance that binds to another substance and transfers it from one site to another.
[ref. 1]
See also *carrier.*

carrying capacity, *K*

Maximum *population* size expressed as total number of individuals, biomass, or *population density* that a given unit of *habitat* is capable of sustaining.
[ref. 2]

carry-over

1. Transfer in farming and agricultural processing of a component from one system such as soil or feed to another system such as a plant, animal, or human being.
   Note: Carry-over is expressed as the *concentration* of the component in the second system divided by its concentration in the first.
2. Process in analytical studies by which materials are carried into a reaction *mixture* in which they do not belong.
3. Persistence of a substance in soil (*e.g.*, a *pesticide*), such that a subsequent crop may be harmed.
4. Persistence of a test substance in participants undergoing a cross-over clinical trial, in which each participant randomly receives the *placebo* and test substance with an intervening washout period.

[ref. 1]

cartilage (n)/cartilaginous (adj)

Specialized, fibrous *connective tissue*, forming the temporary skeleton in the *embryo*, providing a template in which the bones develop, persistent mainly in the joints throughout life, and constituting a part of the organism's growth mechanism.
[ref. 5]

case-base study

See *study, case-base.*

case-case study

See study, *case-case.*

case-cohort study

See *study, case cohort.*

case comparison study

See *study, case-control.*

case-compeer study

See *study, case-control.*

case-control study

See *study, case-control.*

case-crossover study

See *study, case-crossover.*

case-referent study

See *study, case-control.*

caspase

Any member of a family of intracellular cysteine proteinases that cleave proteins at specific aspartic acid residues, initiating or executing *apoptosis*, or activating pro-inflammatory cytokines.
Note 1: The name caspase derives from **c**ysteine-dependent **asp**artate prote**ase**.
Note 2: In humans, initiator caspases include caspase 8 (EC 4.4.22.61) and caspase 9 (EC 3.4.22,62); executor caspases include caspase 3 (EC 3.4.22.56) and caspase 6 (EC 3.4.22.59); and pro-inflammatory caspases include caspase 1 (EC 3.4.22.36), caspase 4 (EC 3.4.22.57), and caspase 5 (EC 3.4.22.58).
[*]

cassava toxin

See *cassavism.*

cassavism

konzo
mantakassa

Epidemic paralytic *disease*, mainly affecting women and children, occurring in remote rural areas of African and Latin American countries, where cassava root is an important food.
Note: Cassavism is associated with many weeks of consumption of "bitter" (high cyanide) cassava that has not been adequately treated to remove the cyanide.
[ref. 4]

castration

Removal of the *testes* or *ovaries.*
[ref. 5]
See also *sterilization.*

catabolism

Opposite term: *anabolism.*

1. Reactions involving the oxidative *degradation* of organic substrates to provide energy (mostly in the form of ATP) and to generate *metabolic* intermediates.
2. Generally, process of breakdown of complex molecules into simpler ones, often providing biologically useful energy.

[ref. 1]

catadromous

Describing a species exhibiting *catadromy.*
[ref. 2]

catadromy

Life-history pattern that is characterized by egg incubation and early juvenile development in seawater, migration to freshwater for adult development, and return to seawater for spawning.

Note: Obligatory catadromy is the term applied where migration to freshwater is required for survival.
[ref. 2]
See also *anadromy.*

catagenesis

Long-term geochemical alteration to organic matter, involving high temperatures and pressures deep below the surface of the Earth.
[ref. 2]

catalase

Peroxysomal enzyme (EC 1.11.1.6), found in most cells, that catalyzes the efficient decomposition of peroxide to water and dioxygen, thus protecting the cell against *reactive oxygen species.*
[*]

cataract

Partial or complete opacity (clouding) of the lens of the eye.
[ref. 5]

catatonia

Behavior marked by excessive and sometimes violent motor activity and excitement, or by generalized inhibition or stupor, that may occur in schizophrenia, mood *disorders*, or organic brain *syndromes.*
[ref. 1]

catchment area

See *drainage basin.*

catecholamine

Any one of a group of bioactive molecules that contains a catechol (benzene-1,2-diol) moiety and usually affects the *sympathetic* nervous system.
Note: The common catecholamines include the *neurotransmitters* dopamine, *adrenaline*, and *noradrenaline.*
[ref. 5]

cathartic

See *laxative.*

cauda epididymis

globus minor

Tail of the *epididymis* that opens into the ductus deferens; part of the reservoir of *spermatozoa.*
[ref. 5]

cauda equina

Bundle of long spinal *nerve roots* arising from the end of the *spinal cord* and filling the lower part of the spinal canal (from approximately the thoraco-lumbar junction downwards).

Note 1: The cauda equina contributes to the innervation of the pelvic organs and lower limbs to include motor innervation of the hips, knees, ankles, feet, and internal and external anal sphincter.
Note 2: The cauda equina also extends to sensory innervation of the perineum and, partially, *parasympathetic* innervation of the bladder.
[ref. 4]

caudal

Situated more toward the cauda, or tail, than some specified reference point; toward the inferior (in humans) or posterior (in animals) end of the body.
[ref. 5]

caudate nucleus
caudatum

Crescent-shaped mass of *grey matter* forming part of the *corpus striatum* and part of the *basal ganglia*.
[ref. 4]

caveola/caveolae (pl)

Invagination on the cell surface (*plasma membrane*), enriched in caveolin proteins, cholesterol, and glycosphingolipids, important in various processes including *pinocytosis* and *signal transduction*.
Note: Caveolae are a type of *lipid raft*.
[ref. 3]

cavitation (in biology)

Formation of a *cavity*, as in formation of the *amnion* in mammalian development.
[ref. 5]

cavity

1. Empty space within an object.
2. Decayed space in a tooth.

[*]

cavity, abdominal

Body *cavity* between the *diaphragm* and pelvis that contains the abdominal organs.
[ref. 5]

cecum

Pouch connected to the junction of the small and large intestines.
[ref. 1]
See also *appendix, vermiform*.

ceiling value (CV)

Airborne *concentration* of a potentially *toxic substance* that should never be exceeded in a worker's breathing zone.
[ref. 1]

celiac disease
gluten enteropathy
nontropical sprue

Autoimmune disorder occuring in genetically predisposed individuals, characterized by *immune intolerance* to the α-gliadin component of gluten, a protein found in wheat, barley, and rye.
Note: If gluten intake continues in an individual with celiac *disease*, resultant *inflammation* of the *mucosa* of the upper small intestine produces malabsorption of nutrients and a wasting illness.
[ref. 3]

cell (in biology)

Smallest structural and functional unit of living organisms; it contains an inner *cytoplasmic* compartment, it is surrounded by a delimiting semi-permeable lipid membrane that controls exchange of substances with the surrounding environment, it is capable of *metabolic* activity, and it often contains its own genetic material.
Note 1: While the ability to reproduce itself through division is an important property distinguishing most cells, it is not universal. Examples of nondividing cells include the mature *erythrocyte* that lacks a *nucleus*, and cells that have undergone terminal differentiation, such as *neurons*.
Note 2: Some organisms (*e.g.*, bacteria, yeast) consist of single cells, whereas in higher organisms cells are involved in a hierarchical organization that progresses from the cell to *tissue, organ*, and whole organism.
Note 3: Cells of higher organisms contain organelles (*e.g. mitochondria, ribosomes*, *endoplasmic reticulum*, and at least one *nucleus* (some cells, *e.g., osteoclasts* and skeletal muscle cells are multinucleate) and make structural and chemical (*e.g., paracrine*) contacts with other cells and extracellular structures.
Note 4: Higher animals possess more than 100 different cell types, each characterized by unique structural and functional properties, and a given toxic substance may show cell-type specificity in its toxicity.
[*]

cell, effector

effector lymphocyte

Cell that carries out an immune function, *e.g., cytokine* release, *cytotoxicity*.
[ref. 3]

cell cycle

Regulated series of biochemical and physiological steps including *DNA* replication, chromosome separation, and cell division, usually depicted as a sequential cyclical series of events.
[ref. 1]

cell line

Defined unique population of cells obtained by culture from a primary source through numerous generations.
[ref. 1]
See also *transformed cell line.*

cell-mediated cytotoxicity

Lysis of a *target cell,* initiated by a *T-lymphocyte* binding to surface *antibodies* or *antigen*-bound *major histocompatibility complex molecules.*
[ref. 3]

cell-mediated hypersensitivity

See *hypersensitivity, type IV.*

cell-mediated immune response

See *immune response, cell-mediated.*

cell-mediated immunity (CMI)

Immune response mediated by *antigen*-specific *T-lymphocytes*, either through the release of *cytokines* or through *cytotoxicity*, in contrast with *humoral immunity*, which is *antibody*-mediated.
Note: Cell-mediated immunity may be expressed as immune regulatory activity (primarily mediated by *CD4+ helper T-lymphocytes*, possibly important in preventing *autoimmune diseases*) or immune effector activity (mediated largely by *CD8+ cytotoxic T-cells*).
[ref. 3]
See also *immune regulation.*

cell-mediated response

See *cell-mediated immune response.*

cell membrane

See *plasma membrane.*

cell polarity

Asymmetry in shape or in distribution of molecular components of a *cell* that contributes to its function.
Note 1: Cell polarity is typical of *epithelial* cell layers, with the cells having an *apical surface* or pole facing the *lumen* of a tubule or *cavity*, and a *basolateral surface* directed away from the lumen. This facilitates directional (*e.g.*, apical-to-basolateral) *transcellular transport.*
Note 2: Describing a cell as polarized, referring to cell polarity, is not to be confused with *membrane polarization.*
[*]

cell proliferation

Increase in cell number.
[ref. 1]

cell strain

Cells having specific properties or markers derived from a primary culture or *cell line.*
[ref. 1]

cellular immunity

See *cell-mediated immunity.*

censored data

Sample observations for which the complete distribution is not known: for example, a *cohort study* in which some persons cannot be followed to the predetermined end of the study ("right-censored data") or environmental assay data in which some results are less than the sample detection limit ("left-censored data").
[ref. 1]

central nervous system (CNS)

Part of an animal's *nervous system* that exerts control over the rest of the nervous system; in vertebrates, the *brain* and *spinal cord* protected within the dorsal *cavity* (cranial and spinal cavities).
[ref. 4]

central tolerance

See *tolerance, central.*

centromere

Constricted region of a *chromosome* that joins the two *chromatids* to each other and attaches to spindle fibers in *mitosis* and *meiosis.*
[ref. 5]

centromere, acrocentric

Having the *centromere* very close to one end.
[ref. 5]

cephalic

In or relating to the head.
[ref. 4]

ceramide

Family of lipid molecules, each one composed of *sphingosine* and a fatty acid.
Note: Ceramides are lipids making up *sphingomyelin*, one of the major components of the lipid bilayer.
[ref. 4]

cerebellar tonsillar herniation

Abnormal protrusion of a portion of the *cerebellum* through the *foramen magnum* of the skull.
[ref. 4]

cerebellum

Lower part of the *brain* that is beneath the posterior portion of the *cerebrum*, regulating the *unconscious* coordination of movement.
[ref. 4]
See also *inferior cerebellar peduncle.*

cerebral cortex

See *cortex, cerebral.*

cerebral hemisphere

Right or left half of the brain in *sagittal* section.
[ref. 5]

cerebral herniation

See *brain herniation.*

cerebral palsy
spastic paralysis

Condition marked by lack of muscle control, resulting from brain damage before, at, or shortly after *birth.*
[ref. 5]

cerebroside

Member of a group of *glycosphingolipids* called *monoglycosylceramides* that are important components in animal *nerve* and muscle cell membranes and the *myelin sheath.*
[ref. 4]

cerebrospinal fluid (CSF)

Clear colorless extracellular fluid found in the *brain* and spinal cord, filling the *ventricles* and *subarachnoid* spaces.
Note 1: CSF is produced in the *choroid plexus* of the brain from arterial blood by a combined process of diffusion, pinocytosis and active transfer.
Note 2: CSF acts as a cushion or buffer for the *cortex*, providing mechanical and immunological protection to the brain, is involved in autoregulation of blood flow in the *cerebrum,* and plays an important role in the *homeostasis* and metabolism of the *central nervous system.*
[ref. 4]

cerebrum (n)/cerebral (adj)

Principal part of the *brain* in vertebrates, located frontwards in the skull, consisting of the two *hemispheres* of the *cerebral cortex* separated by a fissure, and certain subcortical structures such as the *hippocampus, basal ganglia*, and the *olfactory bulb.*
[ref. 4]

certified reference material (CRM)

Reference material, accompanied by documentation issued by an authoritative body and referring to valid procedures used to obtain a specified property value with *uncertainty* and *traceability.*
[ref. 1]

cervical rib
costa cervicalis

Supernumerary rib arising from a cervical *vertebra.*
[ref. 5]

cervical spine (in vertebrates)

Part of the spine, made up of seven *vertebrae*, immediately inferior to the skull and connecting to the *thoracic spine.*
[ref. 4]

cervical vertebra

Any of seven *vertebrae* that provide strength and structure to the *cervical spine* and support the head, allowing for its rotation and flexion.
[ref. 4]

cervix

cervix uteri
uterine cervix

Narrow lower end of the *uterus* that opens into the *vagina*.
[ref. 5]

cetacean

Animal in the order ***Cetacea***; this order includes whales, dolphins, and porpoises.
[ref. 2]

chain of custody

Sequence of responsibility for a substance from the manufacturer to the distributor, to the user, or to the person(s) ultimately responsible for *waste* disposal; also used in controlled transmission of *samples* from collection to analysis, especially of samples of materials used for medico-legal or forensic purposes.
[ref. 1]

challenge (in immunology)

Induction and evaluation of an *immune response* in an organism by administration of a specific *antigen* to which it has been sensitized.
[ref. 3]

chaperone-mediated autophagy (CMA)

See *autophagy, chaperone-mediated.*

Chapman mechanism

Series of reactions by which ozone is formed in the stratosphere.
[ref. 2]
See *ozone hole; ozone layer.*

checkpoint pathway

Type of pathway used in intracellular signaling, activated in response to a *cell's* own internal imbalance or to errors in its synthetic activities.
Note: Activation of checkpoint pathways leads to a delay in certain synthetic processes until other processes are complete, thereby averting damage.
[ref. 5]

cheiloschisis

See *cleft lip.*

chelation therapy

Treatment with a chelating agent to enhance the *elimination* or reduce the *toxicity* of a metal ion.
[ref. 1]

chemesthesis

Sensations that arise when chemical compounds activate *receptor* mechanisms for other effectors, such as light, pain, pressure, and heat, in the eye, skin, nose, mouth, and throat.

Examples: The burning feeling from chili pepper, the cooling from the menthol in mouthwash, and the stinging feeling of carbonated drinks.
[ref. 1]

chemical etiologic agent

See *toxic substance.*

chemical conversion

Change from one *chemical species* to another.
[ref. 1]

chemical oxygen demand (COD)

Measure of the amount of dioxygen, divided by the volume of the system, giving the concentration of dioxygen required to oxidize the organic (and inorganic) matter in wastewater using an oxidizing agent.
[ref. 1]

chemical safety

Practical certainty that there will be no *exposure* of organisms to toxic amounts of any substance or group of substances, implying attainment of an acceptably low *risk* of exposure to potentially toxic substances.
[ref. 1]

chemical species (of an element)

Specific form of an element defined as to isotopic composition, electronic or oxidation state, and (or) complex or molecular structure.
[ref. 1]

chemical time bomb

Substance or substances in a component of the environment that are not currently *bioavailable* but that may become so in the future, with harmful consequences.
[ref. 2]

chemical warfare

Military operations using the *toxic* properties of chemical agents to kill, injure, or incapacitate human beings, animals, or plants.
[ref. 1]

chemisorption

Sorption that results from chemical bond formation (strong interaction) between the *sorbent* and the *sorbate* in a monolayer on a surface or internal to an absorbent.
[ref. 2]
See also *sorption.*

chemoattractant

Opposite term: chemorepellent.

Substance that induces movement of a motile cell or organism in the direction of higher concentration.
[*]
See also *chemotactic factor.*

chemokine

Any of a large family of small proteins, produced by many types of cells, that attract and guide *lymphocytes* to sites of infection and *inflammation* or to other sites, such as those associated with lymphocyte development and with migration into *lymph nodes.*
Note 1: Chemokines fall into two main categories: CC chemokines (β-chemokines) have two cysteine (C) residues near the amino terminus of the protein, whereas in CXC chemokines (α-chemokines) the two cysteines are separated by a single variable amino acid (X). There are two other groups of chemokines: C chemokines (γ-chemokines) that have two cysteines, one N-terminal cysteine and one cysteine downstream; and CX3C chemokines (or δ-chemokines) that have three amino acids between the two cysteines.
Note 2: Chemokines act in conjunction with other factors, such as *tumor necrosis factor*, to induce the *adhesion* factors that attach lymphocytes to the blood vessel wall before they move through it into the tissues.
[ref. 3]

chemophobia

Irrational fear of chemicals.
[ref. 1]

chemosis

Chemically induced swelling around the eye caused by *edema* of the conjunctiva.
[ref. 1]

chemosterilizer

Substance used to render sterilie mites, insects, rodents, or other animals.
[ref. 1]

chemotactic factor

Biologically active substance, *e.g.*, a *chemokine* or *anaphylatoxin*, that induces a concentration gradient-dependent movement of cells.
[ref. 3]
See also *chemoatttractant; chemotaxis.*

chemotaxis

1. (general) Movement of an organism or cell along a concentration gradient of a chemical.
2. (in immunology) Movement of cells up a concentration gradient of a chemical attractant (*chemotactic factor*), such as a *chemokine* or other *cytokine.*

[ref. 3]

chemotype

chemovar

Character of a plant or microorganism based on a metabolite distinct from that found in other members of the same species.
[ref. 3]

Chernoff-Kavlock assay

Group of testing methods for assessing *parturition, postnatal* growth, and *viability* of *prenatally exposed litters* of test animals.
[ref. 5]

Chiari malformation

See *Arnold-Chiari malformation.*

chimera (n)/chimeric (adj)

1. Animal consisting of genetically different cells derived from two (or more) different *zygotes*, or composed of genetically distinct individuals, *e.g.*, following an *allogeneic bone marrow graft.*
2. Substance, such as an *antibody*, created from the proteins or *genes* of two different *species.*

[ref. 3, 5]

chloracne

Acne-like eruption caused by exposure to certain chlorinated organic substances such as polychlorinated biphenyls, 2,3,7,8-tetrachlorodibenzo[*b,e*][1,4]dioxin, and other polychlorinated dibenzodioxins and dibenzofurans.
Note: The lesions are most frequently found on the cheeks, behind the ears, in the armpits and in the groin region.
[ref. 3]

chloride cell

Specialized cell with a role in ion regulation, characterized by large numbers of mitochondria, an extensive intracellular tubular network and a high concentration of Na^+/K^+ ATPase (EC 3.6.3.9).
Note: The chloride cell is found in salt-secreting glands like the rectal gland of elasmobranchs, the nasal gland of seabirds, and the gills of both seawater and freshwater fish, mainly on the primary lamellae but also on the secondary lamellae.
[ref. 2]

chlorinity

Mass concentration of dissolved chloride ions in water.
[ref. 2]

chlorofluorocarbon (CFC)

Carbon-based chemical containing chlorine and fluorine.
Note: Formerly CFCs were commonly used as aerosol propellants and refrigeration coolants, but now are prohibited in many countries, as they are responsible for ozone depletion in the stratosphere.
[ref. 2]
See also *Montreal Protocol.*

chlorosis

Loss of green color in plants owing to the lack of production or the destruction of chlorophyll.
[ref. 2]

cholestasis

Reduced bile flow.
Note 1: Extrahepatic cholestasis is caused by mechanical obstruction of the biliary tract. Intrahepatic cholestasis is often a consequence of reduced bile formation by *hepatocytes*, sometimes as a side-effect of *drugs.*

Note 2: The reduced bile-flow of cholestasis may increase the half-life of drugs and other xenobiotics.
[*]

cholinergic

1. Relating to or denoting a *nerve* that liberates *acetylcholine* at a *synapse* upon receiving an appropriate nerve impulse; in particular referring to *parasympathetic* nerve fibers.
2. Relating to or denoting an agent that mimics or enhances the activity of acetylcholine.

[ref. 4]
Compare *adrenergic*.

cholinesterase

See *acetylcholinesterase, butyrylcholinesterase*.

cholinesterase inhibitor

Substance that inhibits the action of *acetylcholinesterase* (EC 3.1.1.7) and related enzymes that catalyze the hydrolysis of choline esters: Such a substance causes hyperactivity in *parasympathetic* nerves.
Examples: Organophosphate *pesticides*, carbamates.
[ref. 1]

cholinomimetic

Having an action similar to acetylcholine.
[ref. 4]
See also *parasympathomimetic*.

chondrification

Formation of, or *transformation* into, *cartilage*.
[ref. 5]

chondroblast

Cartilage-producing *mesenchymal* progenitor cell, capable of proliferating and maturing into a *chondrocyte* or *osteoblast*.
[ref. 5]

chondrocyte (n)/chondrocytic (adj)

Any one of the cells embedded in the lacunae of the *cartilage matrix*.
[ref. 5]

chordin

Secreted protein that *dorsal*izes early *vertebrate embryonic* tissues by binding to *ventral*izing *transforming growth factor β*-like *bone morphogenetic proteins*, sequestering them in latent form in the resultant complexes.
[ref. 5]

chorea
choreia

Neurological *disorder* characterized by rapid, jerky involuntary movements affecting especially the limbs or facial muscles.
[ref. 4]

choreoathetosis

Occurrence of involuntary movements in a combination of *chorea* and *athetosis*.
[ref. 4]

chorioallantoic placenta

Placenta developed from the *allantois* and *chorion*, establishing a nutritive and excretory connection between the blood of the *fetus* and that of the mother.
[ref. 5]

chorion

1. (in human *embryology*) Cellular, outermost extra-*embryonic membrane*, composed of *trophoblast* lined with *mesoderm*.
   Note: The chorion develops *villi*, becomes vascularized by *allantoic* vessels, and forms the *fetal* part of the *placenta*.
2. (in mammalian embryology) Cellular, outer extra embryonic membrane, not necessarily developing villi.
3. (in biology, general) Noncellular membrane covering *eggs* of various animals, *e.g.*, fish and insects.

[ref. 5]

chorionic gonadotropin

Hormone secreted by the *chorionic villi* of the *placenta* in mammals, especially *human chorionic gonadotropin*.
Note 1: Chorionic gonadotropin promotes the secretion of *progesterone* by the *corpus luteum*.
Note 2: Human chorionic gonadotropin is the hormone that is detected by *pregnancy* tests.
[ref. 5]

chorionic sac

Outermost *membranous* sac that encloses the *embryo* in higher *vertebrates* (reptiles, birds and mammals), lined by *chorion*.
[ref. 5]

chorionic villus

Any of the tiny extensions from the *chorion* that contain *fetal* blood vessels and combine with the *uterine* tissue to form the *placenta*.
[ref. 5]

chorioretinitis

Inflammation of the choroid layer behind the *retina* of the eye.
[ref. 5]

choroid plexus

Infoldings of blood vessels of the *pia mater*, projecting into the cerebral *ventricles*, covered with ependymal cells, and regulating *intraventricular pressure* by secretion and absorption of *cerebrospinal fluid*.
[ref. 4,5]

chromaffin cell

Cell of the *adrenal* medulla that secretes *epinephrine* and *norepinephrine*, and contains granules that are readily stained with chromate salts.
[ref. 5]

chromate uptake assay

Method used in *immunotoxicology* to quantify the toxic effect of a substance on *leukocytes* by measuring uptake of ^{51}Cr-labeled chromate.
[ref. 3]
See also *chromium release assay*.

chromatid

One of a pair of *chromosomes* arising by duplication during *mitosis* or by pairing during *meiosis*, and joined together at the *centromere*.
Note: Sister chromatid refers to either one of the joined pair arising from the same chromosome by duplication, and nonsister chromatid refers to either of the joined homologous chromosomes of maternal or paternal origin arising during meiosis.
[ref. 5]
See also *sister chromatid exchange*.

chromatin

Stainable complex of *DNA* and proteins present in the nucleus of a *eukaryotic* cell.
[ref. 1]
See also *sex chromatin*.

chromatolysis

1. Disintegration of nuclear *chromatin*.
2. Disintegration of *Nissl bodies* following *neuronal* injury.

[ref. 4]
See also *karyolysis; karyorrhexis*.

chromium release assay
^{51}Cr release assay

Immunotoxicity assay that can be used to assess either *natural killer cell* or *cytotoxic T-cell* activity or *macrophage* activity.
Note 1: When incubated with ^{51}Cr-labeled chicken red blood cells (cRBCs), NK and cytotoxic T-cells lyse the cRBC and thus induce the release of ^{51}Cr into the medium. In contrast, macrophages phagocytose cRBC, and are then lysed to assess the amount of ^{51}Cr they have taken up.
Note 2: The chromium release assay is usually applied to measure parameters of *innate immunity*.
[ref. 3]
See also *chromate uptake assay*.

chromosomal abnormality
chromosomal aberration

Incorrect number or deviant structure of *chromosomes*.
[ref. 5]

chromosomal translocation

See *translocation, chromosomal.*

chromosome (n)/chromosomal (adj)

1. Self-replicating structure consisting of DNA complexed with various proteins and involved in the storage and transmission of genetic information.
2. Physical structure that contains the *genes*.

[ref. 5]

chromosome, acrocentric

See *centromere, acrocentric.*

chromosome deletion

Loss of a *chromosome* or part of a chromosome.
[ref. 5]

chromosome ring

Abnormal *chromosome* in which both ends have been lost and the two broken ends have reunited to form a ring-shaped structure.
[ref. 5]
See also *chromosome deletion.*

chronic

long-term
Opposite term: *acute.*

Occurring over an extended period of time in reference to *exposure* or effect.
Note 1: In experimental toxicology, chronic refers to mammalian studies lasting considerably more than 90 days or to studies occupying a large part of the lifetime of an organism.
Note 2: In clinical medicine, chronic implies long-established or long-lasting.
[ref. 1]

chronic allergic inflammation

Disease of airways, skin, eyes and other organs, resulting from repeated or continuous exposure to an *allergen* and involving *immunoglobulin E* formation, IgE-induced *histamine*-release from *mast cells*, liberation of mediators such as *cytokines* and *prostaglandins*, and local *inflammation* characterized by infiltrating *leucocytes.*
Note: Chronic allergic inflammation results in augmented susceptibility to the allergen.
[ref. 3]

chronic effect

long-term effect
Opposite term: *acute effect.*

Consequence that develops slowly and (or) has a long-lasting course; may be applied to an effect that develops rapidly and is long lasting.
[ref. 1]

chronic exposure

long-term exposure
Opposite term: *acute exposure.*

Continued or repeated exposure(s) occurring over an extended period of time, or over a significant fraction of the life time of the test species, of the group of individuals, or of the population.
[ref. 1]

chronic fatigue syndrome

See *fatigue*.

chronic graft rejection

See *rejection, chronic; rejection, graft*.

chronic granulomatous disease (CGD)

Immunodeficiency disease in which multiple *granulomas* form as a result of defective elimination of bacteria by *phagocytes*.
Note: CGD is caused by deficiency of the *NADPH oxidase* system of enzymes that generates superoxide involved in bacterial killing.
[ref. 3]

chronic lymphocytic leukemia (CLL)

See *leukemia, chronic lymphocytic*.

chronic lymphocytic thyroiditis

See *Hashimoto thyroiditis*.

chronic myelogenous leukemia (CML)

See *leukemia, chronic myelogenous*.

chronic rejection

See *rejection, chronic*.

chronic solvent-induced encephalopathy (CSE)

organic solvent syndrome
toxic solvent syndrome

Constellation of neurological symptoms that may include poly*neuropathies*, *encephalopathy*, memory loss, attention deficit and *dementia* following long-term exposure, often occupational, to organic solvents found in paints, glues, and other industrial products.
[ref. 4]

chronic toxicity

long-term toxicity
Opposite term: *acute toxicity*.

1. *Adverse effects* following *chronic exposure*.
2. Effects that persist over a long period of time, whether or not they occur immediately upon *exposure* or are delayed.

[ref. 1]

chronic toxicity test

long-term toxicity test
Opposite term: *acute toxicity test*.

Study in which organisms are observed during the greater part of their life span, and in which *exposure* to the test agent takes place over the whole observation time or a substantial part thereof.
[ref. 1]

chronotoxicology

Study of the influence of biological rhythms on the *toxicity* of substances, or of a toxicant on biological rhythms.
[ref. 1]

chronotropic

Able to alter the rate of a rhythmic physiological process such as the heartbeat.
[*]
See also *chronotoxicology*.

ciguatera toxin poisoning

Food-borne illness caused by ingesting fish containing ciguatera *toxins*.
Note 1: Gastrointestinal symptoms of ciguatera toxin poisoning may accompany a wide variety of neurological symptoms, including *ataxia, vertigo*, flaccid paralysis, respiratory arrest, and reversed perception of hot and cold; the neurological symptoms may persist for many years.
Note 2: Ciguatera toxins tend to accumulate in *predator* fish, such as the barracuda and other carnivorous reef fish, after eating other fish that consume toxin-producing algae (dinoflagellates, *e.g.*, ***Gambierdiscus toxicus***) living in coral reef waters. The toxins are harmless to fish but poisonous to humans.
Note 3: The ciguatera toxins are heat-resistant, and cooking does not destroy them.
[ref. 1,4]

ciliary muscle

Intrinsic smooth muscle of the eye that contracts to cause the lens to thicken, allowing accommodation to near vision.
[ref. 4]

ciliary neurotrophic factor

Polypeptide hormone and *nerve growth factor* that promotes *neurotransmitter* synthesis and *neurite* outgrowth in certain *neural* populations including *astrocytes*.
[ref. 4]

cilium (n)/cilia (n, pl)/ciliated (adj)

Hair-like *organelles* that project from the surface of most mammalian *cells*.
Note 1: Cilia occur in two types.

- Primary cilia are short, non-motile structures that function in *signal transduction* and in sensing the cell's environment.
- Motile cilia have a *microtubule*-based motor that causes them to beat in waves, assisting in, *e.g.*, movement of the *ovum* along the *Fallopian tube* and clearance of dirt and *mucus* along the *trachea* from the lung.

Note 2: Ciliated epithelium refers to columnar *epithelial cells* that have motile cilia on their *apical* surface.
[*]
See also *mucociliary escalator*.

circadian
nychthemeral

Relating to or exhibiting an approximately 24-h periodicity.
[ref. 1]

cirrhosis (n)/cirrhotic (adj)

1. Liver *disease* defined by histological examination and characterized by increased fibrous tissue in the liver, abnormal morphological and physiological changes such as loss of functional liver cells, and increased resistance to blood flow through the liver (portal *hypertension*).
   Note: Common causes of liver cirrhosis are ethanol and - where still in use - carbon tetrachloride.
2. Chronic interstitial *inflammation* and *fibrosis* of an organ.

[ref. 1]

cis-acting element

Regulatory *DNA* sequence in the vicinity of a coding region (of a *gene*) that is necessary for, or regulates expression of, that gene.
[*]
Compare *trans-acting factor*.

clade (n)/cladistic (adj)

Group of organisms that consists of all the descendents of a common ancestor starting from one point in a *cladogram*.
[*]
See also *cladistics, cladogram*.

cladistics

1. Systematic classification of groups of organisms on the basis of shared characteristics thought to derive from a common ancestor.
2. Study of the branching of evolutionary lines of descent and the relationship between branches.

[ref. 2]
See also *clade*.

cladogram
evolutionary tree
phylogenetic tree

Dendrogram illustrating the supposed evolutionary relationships between *clades*; a diagram showing *cladistic* relationships.
Note: Cladograms are often based on such information as the number of differences in amino acids or nucleic acid bases in common proteins or genes, respectively. From estimated *mutation* rates, the evolutionary time can be estimated. Accordingly, cladograms have two components, branching order (showing group relationships) and branch length (showing extent of evolution).
[ref. 2]

class 'a' metal ion

Metal ion that combines preferentially with *ligands* containing ligating atoms that are the lightest (smallest atomic number) of their periodic group.
[ref. 2]
See also *borderline metal ion; class 'b' metal ion; hard acid; soft acid.*

class 'b' metal ion

Metal ion that combines preferentially with *ligands* containing ligating atoms other than the lightest (smallest atomic number) of their periodic group.
[ref. 2]
See also *borderline metal ion; class 'a' metal ion; hard acid; soft acid.*

class I MHC gene product

See *major histocompatibility complex class I molecule.*

class II MHC gene product

See *major histocompatibility complex class II molecule.*

class switching

Process by which a *B-cell* changes the class but not specificity of a given *antibody* it produces, *e.g.*, switching from an *immunoglobulin M* to an *immunoglobulin G* antibody.
[ref. 3]

classical pathway (of complement activation)

Activation pathway involving *complement* components C1, C2, and C4 that, following fixation of C1q, *e.g.*, by *antigen-antibody* complexes, produces the *classical pathway* C3 convertase C4b2a.
[ref. 3]
See also *alternative pathway (of complement activation).*

clastogen (n)/clastogenic (adj)

Agent causing *chromosome* breakage and (or) consequent gain, loss, or rearrangement of pieces of chromosomes.
[ref. 1]

clastogenesis

Formation (or generation) of chromosomal breaks and (or) consequent gain, loss, or rearrangement of pieces of *chromosomes*.
[ref. 1]

clearance

1. (in physiology and *toxicology*) Volume of blood or *plasma* or mass of an organ effectively cleared of a substance by *elimination* (*metabolism* and *excretion*) divided by time of elimination.
   Note: Total clearance is the sum of the clearances of each eliminating organ or tissue for that component.
2. (in *pulmonary* toxicology) Volume or mass of lung cleared divided by time of elimination; used qualitatively to describe removal of any inhaled substance that deposits on the lining surface of the lung.
3. (in *renal* toxicology) Quantification of the removal of a substance by the kidneys by the processes of filtration and secretion; clearance is calculated by relating the rate of renal excretion to the *plasma concentration*.

Note: In general, clearance, $(c_o/c_i)(\Delta V/\Delta t)$, is the product of the *concentration* c_o of a component in an output system and the volume flow rate of the output fluid, divided by the concentration c_i of this component in the input fluid.
[ref. 1]

cleavage (of a molecule)

Splitting of a molecule into smaller molecular entities.
[ref. 1]

cleavage (in embryology)

First few divisions of a *fertilized egg*.
Note: There is little or no growth during cleavage; the cytoplasm is cleaved into smaller and smaller units with individual biochemistry that contributes to subsequent cell differentiation.
[ref. 5]
See also *blastocyst; blastomere; blastula; gastrulation; holoblastic; inner cell mass; meroblastic; trophoblast; zygote.*

cleavage, meroblastic

Partial *cleavage* of the *egg*, occurring in some animals such as reptiles and birds whose eggs have a large amount of yolk, resulting in unequal *blastomeres* and only part of the egg progressing to further cell division; the yolk mass remains and nourishes the cell mass.
[ref. 5]

cleavage, holoblastic

Total cleavage of the *egg* producing separate, equal *blastomeres.*
[ref. 5]

cleft (n)
fissure

Gap in soft tissue, bone, or both.
[ref. 5]
See also *cleft (adj).*

cleft (adj)

Split, divided, or partly divided into two.
[ref. 5]
See also *cleft lip; cleft palate; cleft sternum.*

cleft lip
cheiloschisis
hare lip

Congenital malformation consisting of one or more *clefts* in the upper lip, the result of failed closure in the *embryo* of the *maxillary* and median *nasal* processes.
[ref. 5]
See also *cleft palate.*

cleft palate

Congenital fissure along the midline of the hard *palate*, sometimes extending into the *soft palate.*
[ref. 5]

cleft sternum

Rare *congenital malformation* resulting from defective fusion in the *embryo* of paired *mesodermal* bands in the *ventral* midline.
[ref. 5]

climax community

Community of plants and animals in a steady state due to ecological *succession* resulting in a composition of the community best adapted to average conditions in the area.
Note: The term "climax community" is sometimes applied to *soil* development.
[ref. 2]

clinical toxicology

Scientific study involving research, analysis, education, prevention, diagnosis, and treatment of *diseases* caused by substances such as *drugs* and *toxicants*.
Note: Clinical toxicology often refers specifically to the application of toxicological principles to the treatment of human *poisoning*.
[ref. 1]

clinical trial

Study in humans to gain information regarding diagnostic or *therapeutic* value, notably in the context of *drug* development or the introduction of other therapeutic procedures.
Note 1: Clinical trials require approval by an ethics committee and informed consent of the participant.
Note 2: Clinical trials are usually preceded by preclinical investigations in nonhuman models or human cell lines.
Note 3: In the development of new therapeutics, clinical trials typically have five phases:

- Phase 0: Single subtherapeutic dose in few volunteers to study pharmacokinetics and other parameters.
- Phase I: Repeated dosing in a small group of healthy volunteers (*e.g.*, 15-30) to get information about a safe and tolerable dose.
- Phase II: Testing of the efficacy of the drug in a larger group of patients (*e.g.*, 100-300)
- Phase III: Confirmation of efficacy and safety in a larger group of patients (*e.g.*, 1000-3000).
- Phase IV: Ongoing post-marketing observation to get information about rare unwanted side effects, possible interactions and other parameters of possible concern.

[*]

clitoral hood

See *prepuce*.

clitoris

Erectile body in the female genitalia, homologous with the penis in the male.
[ref. 5]

cloaca (in zoology)

Common *cavity* at the end of the digestive tract in *vertebrates* (apart from most mammals) into which are released both excretory and *genital* products.
[ref. 5]

cloacal membrane

Membrane that covers the *embryonic cloaca* during the development of urinary and reproductive organs in those *vertebrates* where the cloaca occurs.
[ref. 5]

clonal

See *clone*.

clonal anergy

Form of *self-tolerance* developing as a consequence of negative selection during *thymic* selection processes. *Clones* of *thymocytes* whose antigen receptors (*T-cell receptors*) bind with high *affinity* to *self-antigens* in association with *major histocompatibility complex molecules* are inactivated.
[ref. 3]

clonal deletion

Process by which contact with *antigen* (*e.g.*, self-antigen) at an early stage of *lymphocyte* differentiation leads to cell death by *apoptosis*.
[ref. 3]

clonal expansion

Proliferation of *B-lymphocytes* and *T-lymphocytes* activated by *clonal selection* in order to produce a *clone* of identical cells.
Note: Clonal expansion enables the body to have sufficient numbers of *antigen*-specific *lymphocytes* to mount an effective *immune response*.
[ref. 3]

clonal indifference

clonal ignorance

Failure of *B*- or *T-cells* expressing anti-self-*receptors* to interact with *antigen e.g.*, by low valency, low concentration, or sequestration of antigens; low receptor *avidity*; or lack of co-stimulatory molecules.
Note: Clonal indifference is the primary mechanism involved in the induction and maintenance of *self-tolerance*.
[ref. 3]

clonal selection

Selection and *activation* by *antigen* of a *lymphocyte*, bearing a complementary *receptor*, which then proliferates to form an expanded *clone*.
[ref. 3]

clone (n,v)/clonal (adj)

1. Population of genetically identical cells or organisms having a common ancestor.
2. To produce such a population.
3. *Recombinant DNA* molecules, all carrying the same inserted sequence.

[ref. 1]
See also *cloning, therapeutic*.

clonic

See clonus.

cloning, therapeutic

1. Transfer of the nucleus extracted from a somatic cell into an egg that has had its own nucleus previously extracted.
   Note: *Therapeutic* cloning is also known as somatic cell nuclear transfer (SCNT).
   [*]
2. Generation and manipulation of stem cells with the objective of deriving cells of a particular organ or tissue to treat a *disease*.
   [ref. 1]

See also *clone* (v).

cloning vector

Small circle of *DNA* (*e.g.*, a *plasmid*) or modified bacteriophage that can carry a segment of foreign DNA into an appropriate host organism (*e.g.*, a bacterium, a yeast, or a mammalian cell).
[ref. 1]

clonus (n)/clonic (adj)

1. Alternate involuntary muscular contraction and relaxation in rapid succession.
2. Continuous rhythmic *reflex* tremor initiated by the *spinal cord* below an area of spinal cord injury, set in motion by reflex testing.

[ref. 4]

clot (n,v) (blood)

Coagulated mass of *blood cells* and *plasma* formed upon *activation* of *platelets* and the *coagulation system*.
Note 1: Clotting serves to staunch blood flow from disrupted blood vessels, but may also result in occlusive *thromboemboli*.
Note 2: *Drugs* intended to prevent clot formation are referred to as *anticoagulants*.
[*]

clover disease

estrogenism

Condition caused by the continued ingestion of low but toxic levels of *estrogens*.
Note 1: The most important occurrence of estrogenism is in farm animals pastured on plants containing *phytoestrogens*. The signs are those related to *endometrial* hyperplasia and *vaginal* tumefaction (swelling and puffiness), including long-term *infertility* and *rectal prolapse*, especially in pigs; *uterine* prolapse, especially in ewes; and *feminization* of males that have undergone *castration*.
Note 2: Dogs are particularly susceptible to the *myelotoxic* effects of estrogens and high dose or prolonged administration causes severe bone marrow depression with *thrombocytopenia*, followed by *leukopenia* and *anemia*.
[ref. 5]

clubfoot

talipes

Deformed foot that is twisted out of shape or position, usually *congenital* (congenital talipes equinovarus).
[ref. 5]

cluster determinant (CD)

Cluster of *antigens* representating a cell surface marker with which *antibodies* react.
Note: The term "cluster determinant" is not to be confused with *cluster of differentiation antigen*, although both take the abbreviation "CD".
[ref. 3]

cluster of differentiation (CD) antigen

Any of a family of molecular markers on cell surfaces that may be used operationally to define phenotype, origin, and *activation* state of the cell.
Note 1: The CD antigens expressed by a *T-cell* vary with its stage of development and thus with its role in the *immune response*.
Note 2: The term "cluster of differentiation antigen" is not to be confused with *cluster determinant*, although both take the abbreviation "CD".
[ref. 3]

cluster sampling

1. Method of sampling in which the population is divided into aggregates (or clusters) of items bound together in a certain manner; a *sample* of these clusters is taken at random, and all the items that constitute them are included in the sample.
2. Method of sampling in which each unit selected is a group of persons (*e.g.*, all persons in a city block or a family) rather than an individual.

[ref. 1]

coagonist

See *agonist*.

coagulation system

Proteolytic cascade of *plasma* enzymes that triggers blood clotting when blood vessels are damaged.
[ref. 3]

coarctation

Narrowing or constriction of a short section of a blood vessel, commonly of the *aorta*.
[ref. 5]

cobaltism, arthroplastic

Systemic disease caused by cobalt ions released from cobalt-containing alloys used in metal-on-metal total hip replacement.
[*]

cocarcinogen

Chemical, physical, or biological factor that intensifies the effect of a *carcinogen*.
[ref. 1]

cochlea

Spiral *cavity* of the inner ear containing the *organ of Corti* that transduces sound into nerve impulses.
[ref. 5]

Codex Alimentarius

Collection of internationally adopted food standards drawn up by the Codex Alimentarius Commission, the principal body implementing the joint FAO/WHO Food Standards Program.
[ref. 1]

coelom

Body *cavity*, found in many animals, lined with *mesodermal epithelium* and containing the digestive tract and other *visceral* organs
Note: The principal cavities of the trunk arise from the intra*embryonic* coelom.
[ref. 5]

coexposure

Simultaneous exposure to two or more potentially harmful agents. Interactions may result in *potentiation, additivity, synergism* or other types of interactive effects.
Note: The risks of coexposure to ingredients of chemical *mixtures* are evaluated on a case-by-case basis.
[*]

cognate T-cell

Helper T-lymphocyte primed by the same *antigen* as the *B-cell* that it helps.
[ref. 3]

cognition (n)/**cognitive** (adj)

Sum of the mental processes by which sensory input is stored, recovered, and used by the *conscious brain*, including attention, memory, language usage, learning, reasoning, problem solving, and decision making.
Note: Cognition usually refers to human information processing, but is sometimes used to describe learning and memory in rodents.
[ref. 4]

cognitive function

See *cognition*.

cohort (in epidemiology)

Component of the population born during a particular period and identified by period of birth so that its characteristics (such as causes of death and numbers still living) can be ascertained as it enters successive time and age periods.
Note: Use of the term "cohort" has broadened to describe any designated group of persons followed or traced over a period of time, as in the term *cohort study* (*prospective study*).
[ref. 1]

cohort analysis (in epidemiology)

Tabulation and analysis of *morbidity* or *mortality* rates in relationship to the ages of a specific group of people (*cohort*), identified by their birth period, and followed as they pass through different ages during part or all of their life span.
Note: In certain circumstances such as studies of migrant populations, cohort analysis may be performed according to duration of residence in a country rather than year of birth, in order to relate *health* or mortality to duration of *exposure*.
[ref. 1]
See also *study, cohort*.

cohort study

See *study, cohort.*

cold autoantibody type

Autoantibody that reacts optimally at low temperatures (0-5 °C) with surface *antigens* of *erythrocytes*.
Note: The cold autoantibody mediates *autoimmune hemolytic anemia* by either *cold agglutinins* (cold *hemagglutinin disease*) or cold hemolysins (paroxysmal cold hemoglobinuria).
[ref. 3]

cold condensation theory

Theory that *pollutants* with high vapor pressure, *e.g.*, mercury or *persistent organic pollutants* (POPs), in the air will condense onto *soil*, water, and biota at cool temperatures; consequently, the ratios for POP concentrations in the air and on condensed phases decrease as one moves from warmer to cooler climates.
[ref. 2]

collagen arthritis

Autoimmune model of *rheumatoid arthritis*, arising from combined *cellular immunity* and *humoral immunity* against collagen type II, and characterized by rapid and severe erosions of cartilage and bone.
[ref. 3]

collagenous

Rich in the fibrous *connective tissue* protein, collagen.
[ref. 5]

collectin

Any member of a structurally related family of calcium-dependent carbohydrate-binding proteins, or *lectins,* containing collagen-like sequences, *e.g., mannose-binding lectin.*
[ref. 3]
See also *C-type lectin.*

collembolan reproduction test

Procedure in which collembolans (small soil-inhabiting insects) are *exposed* to soil that has been treated with a test substance, and *adult* mortality and reproductive output are studied.
[ref. 5]

colligative property

Chemical behavior depending only on the number of molecules or ions in solution and not on their identity.
Note: Colligative properties include depression of freezing point, elevation of boiling point, lowering of vapor pressure, and osmotic pressure.
[*]

coloboma

Any defect resulting from incomplete closure of the *retinal* fissure.
Note: Coloboma may be *congenital*, pathological, or artificial.
[ref. 5]

colony-stimulating factor (CSF)

Factor that permits the proliferation and differentiation of *hematopoietic* cells.
[ref. 3]

coma

State of profound *unconscious*ness lasting more than several hours in which one cannot respond to stimuli and from which one cannot be roused.
[ref. 4]

combinatorial diversity

Component of *antibody* and *T-cell receptor (TCR)* diversity that is generated by the recombination of *variable (V), diversity* (*D*, for *immunoglobulin heavy chains*, and for TCR β and δ chains), and *joining (J) gene* segments.
[ref. 3]
See also *V(D)J recombination.*

combinatorial joining

Merging of *DNA* segments generating new genetic information.
[ref. 3]

combined effect (in toxicology)

combination effect

Toxic effect on an organism of simultaneous or successive *exposures* to two or more substances.
[After ref. 1]
See also *additivity; antagonism; coexposure; potentiation; synergism.*

combined immunodeficiency

See *X-linked severe combined immune deficiency.*

combined repeated dose toxicity study

Procedure to evaluate both general *systemic* toxicity, with an emphasis on neurological endpoints, and notably reproductive effects and developmental progression in rodents. Groups of males and females are administered a test substance in graded doses prior to mating, during the mating period, and subsequently (up to two weeks post-mating in males and four days post-delivery in females).
[ref. 5]

comet assay

Method in which a cell is embedded in agar, *exposed* to a *DNA*-damaging agent, then permeabilized with a detergent, and subjected to an electric field. Small genomic DNA fragments will move out of the cell upon electrophoresis and form a streak or "tail" looking like a comet leading away from the cell.
Note: The comet assay is a means of measuring DNA damage, particularly DNA strand breaks.
[After ref. 1]

cometabolism

Microbial *transformation* or *degradation* of a compound that occurs only in the presence of a transformable cosubstrate.

Note: Cometabolism may involve *enzymatic* change of the substrate to a product or products that are not transformed further (*dead-end metabolites*).
[*]
See also *cooxidation; metabolism; secondary substrate metabolism.*

common variable immunodeficiency

Relatively common deficiency in *antibody* production, of unknown *pathogenesis* but strongly associated with genes mapping within the *major histocompatibility complex.*
Note 1: Common variable immunodeficiency is characterized by decreased *γ globulin* levels, generally affecting all the *antibody* classes, but sometimes only *immunoglobulin G.*
Note 2: Most patients with common variable immunodeficiency have normal or near-normal numbers of *B-cells* do not differentiate into *plasma cells.*
[ref. 3]

community (in ecotoxicology)

Assembly of *populations* of usually interdependent *species* of living organisms, interacting with each other within a specified location in space and time.
[ref. 2]
See also *ecosystem.*

community conditioning hypothesis

Hypothesis that ecological communities retain information about events in their history and will not return to their original state after perturbation.
Note: The *community* conditioning hypothesis was derived from the concept of nonequilibrium *community ecology* and was developed as a framework for understanding the persistence of *dose*-related responses in multispecies *toxicity* tests.
[ref. 2]

community resilience
ecological resilience

Ability of a *community* to return to its former state after perturbation.
Note: A community with high resilience will return to its original state faster than one with low resilience.
[ref. 2]
See also *community resistance; community stability.*

community resistance

Ability of a *community* to avoid displacement from its present state by a disturbance.
[ref. 2]

community stability

Tendency of a *community* to return to its original state after a disturbance, *e.g.*, a new competition or a temporary change in environment.
[ref. 2]
See also *community resilience; community resistance.*

community structure

Species present in a *community* and their relative *abundances.*
[ref. 2]

compaction

1. (in reproductive physiology) Complication of *labor* in *twin births* in which there is attempted simultaneous expulsion of both twins, so that the lower part of the mother's pelvis is filled and further descent through the birth canal is prevented.
2. (in *embryology*) Process during which *blastomeres* change their shape and align themselves tightly against each other to form the compact *morula*.

[ref. 5]

comparative genomics

Study of the relationship of *genome* structure and function across different biological *species*.
[ref. 1]

comparative risk

See *relative excess risk*.

comparison group

See *control group*.

compartment

1. Conceptualized part of the body (organs, tissues, cells, or fluids) considered as an independent system for purposes of modeling and assessment of *distribution* and clearance of a substance.
2. Part of an *ecosystem* considered as an independent system for purposes of assessment of uptake, distribution, and dissipation of a substance.

[ref. 2]

compartmental analysis

Mathematical process leading to a model of transport of a substance in terms of *compartments* and rate constants, usually taking the form $C = Ae^{-\alpha t} + Be^{-\beta t} + \ldots$ where each exponential term represents one compartment. C is the substance *concentration;* A, B, ... are proportionality constants; α, β, ... are rate constants; and t is time.
[ref. 1]

compartmentalize

Separate into *compartments*.
[ref. 1]

compensation

pseudo-adaptation

Adaptation of an organism to changing environmental conditions, accompanied by the emergence of stresses in biochemical systems that exceed the limits of normal (*homeostatic*) mechanisms.
Note: Compensation is a temporary concealed *pathology* that later on can result in explicit pathological changes (decompensation).
[ref. 1]

competent bacterium

Bacterium growing in culture, treated in such a way that its ability to take up *DNA* molecules has been enhanced.
[After ref. 1]

competition (in ecology)

General struggle for existence in which living organisms in a *niche* compete for the same limited resources.
[ref. 2]
See also *intraspecific competition; interspecific competition.*

competitive exclusion

Exclusion from a *niche* of one *species* by another that uses the available resources of the niche more efficiently, eventually resulting in the disappearance of the outcompeted species.
[ref. 2]

competitive inhibition assay (in immunology)

Method of measuring an *antigen* in a sample using a labeled species of the antigen as a competitive inhibitor of its binding in a specific *antigen–antibody reaction.*
[ref. 3]

complement

Group of approximately 20 *serum* proteinase precursors, some of which act in an *enzymatic* cascade, producing effector molecules involved in *inflammation* (proteins C3a, C5a), *phagocytosis* (*opsonization*) (C3b), and cell lysis (C5b, C6–C9).
[ref. 3]
See also *complement system.*

complement activation

See *activation, complement.*

complement deficiency

Inherited deficiency in any of the various components of the *complement system.*
Note 1: Rheumatic *disorders* (mainly *systemic lupus erythematosus*) are associated with deficiencies of the early complement system components of the *classical pathway.*
Note 2: More than 30 % of individuals with C2 deficiency and nearly 80 % with either C3 or C4 deficiency have an *autoimmune* manifestation.
[ref. 3]

complement reaction

Physiological response to the presence of a foreign body in which a cascade of *enzymatic* reactions results in lysis or *phagocytosis* of the foreign material.
[After ref. 3]

complement receptor (CR)

See *receptor, complement.*

complement system

Group of *serum* proteins having the capacity to interact with each other when activated in a chain reaction, resulting in formation of a lytic complex and release of several biologically active peptides of low relative molecular mass (*anaphylatoxins*).
Note 1: The complement system can be activated by *antigen-antibody* complexes (*classical pathway*) and by other components, *e.g.*, bacteria (*alternative pathway*).
Note 2: As an effector mechanism of the *humoral immune response*, the activated complement system facilitates *opsonization, phagocytosis*, and lysis of cellular *antigens*.
[ref. 3]

complementarity-determining region (CDR)

Hypervariable amino acid sequence within *antibody* and *T-cell receptor variable (V) regions*, which interacts with complementary residues on the antigen or *major histocompatibility complex*–peptide complex.
[ref. 3]

complementary DNA (cDNA)

DNA generated from an expressed m*RNA* through a process known as reverse transcription.
[ref. 1]

complementary niches

See *niche, complementary*.

comprehensive effect of poisons

Simultaneous or successive effect made on an organism by *poisons* entering from different media, air, water, or food or through the skin.
[ref. 1]
See also *combined effect*.

computational toxicology

Application of mathematical and computer models to predict *adverse effects* and better to understand the mechanism(s) through which a given chemical causes harm.
[ref. 1]

computed tomography (CT)
X-ray computed tomography (X-ray CT)
computerized axial tomography (CAT)

Tomographic technique that images the body in cross-sections, or slices: thereafter, a computer algorithm reconstructs a map from the slices to create a three-dimensional image of soft tissue or bone.
[ref. 4]

conal growth hypothesis

Hypothesis that explains *transposition of the great arteries* of the heart by failure of the *aortopulmonary septum* to follow a spiral course during partitioning of the *bulbus cordis* and *truncus arteriosus* in the process of forming the *aorta* and pulmonary *trunk*.
[ref. 5]

concanavalin A (conA)

Hemagglutinin, isolated from jack bean (***Canavalia ensiformis***) meal, which reacts with polyglucosans in the blood of mammals, causing *agglutination*.
Note: Concanavalin A has been used to activate *T-cells in vitro*.
[ref. 3]

concentration

1. Any one of a group of four quantities characterizing the composition of a mixture and defined as one of mass, amount of substance (chemical amount), or number divided by volume, giving, respectively, mass, amount (of substance), volume, or number concentration.
2. Short form for amount (of substance) concentration (substance concentration in clinical chemistry).

[ref. 1]

concentration, background

Concentration of a substance in a medium prior to a particular action (usually increasing the concentration), or the concentration that would have occurred in the absence of the action.
[ref. 3]

concentration, benchmark

benchmark concentration (BMC)

Statistically calculated lower 95 % confidence limit on the *concentration* that produces a defined *response* (called the *benchmark response* or BMR, usually 5 % or 10 %) for an *adverse effect* compared to background, often defined as 0 % or 5 % (respectively).
[ref. 1]

concentration, effective

Concentration of a substance that causes a defined magnitude of *response* in a given system after a specified *exposure* time, *e.g.*, concentration that affects *x* % of a test *population* after a given time (EC_x).
[ref. 2]
See also *median effective concentration*.

concentration–effect curve

exposure–effect curve

Graph of the relation between *exposure concentration* and the magnitude of the resultant biological change.
[ref. 1]

concentration–effect relationship

exposure–effect relationship

Association between *exposure concentration* and the resultant magnitude of the continuously graded change produced, either in an individual or in a population.
[ref. 1]

concentration factor (CF), C_f

Quantitative expression of the *concentration* of substance n (Cn) at different trophic levels divided by the concentration in the ultimate or lowest defined source, *e.g.*, relative to the concentration in water (C_{water}):

$$C_f = C_n / C_{water}$$

[ref. 2]

concentration–response curve

exposure–response curve

Graph of the relation between *exposure concentration* and the proportion of individuals in a *population* responding with a defined effect.
[ref. 1]

concentration–response relationship

exposure–response relationship

Association between *exposure concentration* and the *incidence* of a defined effect in an *exposed population.*
[ref. 1]

conception

Formation of a viable *zygote* by the union of a *spermatozoon* and an *ovum.*
[ref. 5]
See also *fertilization.*

concept of strategy

See *principle of allocation.*

conceptual model (in ecotoxicology)

Linkage and interrelationship of assessment endpoint(s) and stressors.
Note 1: Establishing a conceptual model includes evaluation of potential *exposure* pathways, effects, and ecological *receptors.*
Note 2: Conceptual models include hypotheses of risk and a diagram of the conceptual model.
[ref. 2]

conceptual model diagram (in ecotoxicology)

Figure showing pathways of *exposure* of organisms and illustrating areas of uncertainty or concern.
[ref. 2]

conceptual site model (CSM)

Integration of information on contaminants of potential concern (COPCs), ecological resources, evaluated *exposure* routes, fate and transport mechanisms, evaluated COPC *toxicity*, identified assessment endpoints, and risk questions and hypotheses, into a description of all that is known and (or) expected about a contaminated site.
[ref. 2]

conceptus

Products of *conception* during intrauterine development from implantation to birth, *i.e.*, the *embryo, fetus*, and associated membranes.
[*]

concordance (n)/**concordant** (adj)

Occurrence of pairs or groups of individuals of identical *phenotype*.
Note: In *twin* studies, concordance is a condition in which both twins exhibit or fail to exhibit a trait under investigation.
[ref. 1]

concurrent study

See *study, concurrent cohort.*

concurrent validity

Situation in which a measurement and its criterion refer to the same point in time.
Note: An example of concurrent validity would be a visual inspection of a wound for evidence of infection validated against bacteriological examination of a specimen taken at the same time.
[ref. 1]

condition (in ecotoxicology)

State of health effecting the potential for reproduction and growth.
Note: Condition in this sense is mainly used in fish, mussel, and oyster *ecology*.
[ref. 2]

condition factor, *K*

Parameter used to describe growth in fish, calculated from the equation

$$K = m\ l^{-3}$$

with mass *m*, and length *l*, of the fish, the usual units being $g\,cm^{-3}$.
Note: *K* reflects real growth and nutritional status better than simple measurement of body mass.
[ref. 2]

condition index

Any quantitative measure of the *condition* in relation to a defined baseline.
Example: In mussels, various shell indexes (volume/length, mass/length), glycogen concentration (w/bw), or relative organ mass are used.
[ref. 2]

conditioned avoidance response (CAR) **test**

Experimental procedure in which an adverse effect (*e.g.*, foot shock, *drug withdrawal*) is delivered to rats or mice after presentation of a *cue* (*e.g.*, light or sound); the rodents are trained to avoid rather than escape the shock after the start of its delivery.
[ref. 4]

conditioning, classical
Pavlovian conditioning
respondent conditioning

Learning in which a behavior comes to be elicited as a reflex response by association with a neutral antecedent *stimulus* through repetition of the stimulus-response pairing.
Note: In classical conditioning, the neutral antecedent stimulus (see *conditioned stimulus*) such as the ringing of a bell is repetitively paired with an *unconditioned stimulus* such as food to elicit a response such as salivation.
[ref. 4]

conditioning, operant

instrumental conditioning

Learning in which appropriate behavior is rewarded, or inappropriate behavior is punished; behavior is modified by learned association with antecedents and consequences.
[ref. 4]
See also *reinforcement*.

cone cell

See *photoreceptor cell.*

conformational epitope

See *epitope, conformational.*

confounding (in data analysis)

1. Situation in which the effects of two processes are not distinguishable from one another.
2. Distortion of the apparent effect of an *exposure* on *risk* brought about by the association of other factors that can influence the outcome.
3. Relationship between the effects of two or more causal factors as observed in a set of data, such that it is not logically possible to separate the contribution that any single causal factor has made to an effect.
4. Situation in which a measure of the effect of an exposure on risk is distorted because of the association of exposure with other factor(s) that influence the outcome under.

[ref. 1]

confounding variable

confounder

Changeable parameter that can cause, modify or prevent the outcome of interest, is not an intermediate in the causal chain of events, and is associated with the factor under investigation.
[After ref. 1]

confusion

Mental state of bewilderment or disorientation in which reactions to environmental stimuli may be inappropriate.
[ref. 4]

congener

1. (in chemistry) One of two or more substances related to each other by origin, structure, or function.
2. (in ecology) One of two or more species within the same genus.
   Note: Congeners in the same ecoregion can compete with one another leading to *adaptations* (microevolution) mitigating pressure on *populations.*
3. (in genetics) One of two or more organisms that have almost identical genomes.
   Note: Recombinant congeneric mice strains are constructed to study various *diseases.*

[ref. 2]

congenic

Differing at a single genetic *locus*.
[ref. 3]

congenital

Present from *birth*, as of a genetic or physical abnormality.
[ref. 5]

congenital adrenal hyperplasia

adrenogenital syndrome

Group of *disorders* caused by *hyperplasia* of the *adrenal* cortex or by *malignant tumors*, resulting in excess secretion of adrenocortical *androgenic hormones*, and characterized by *masculinization* of women, *feminization* of men, or precocious *puberty* in the male.
Note: Congenital adrenal hyperplasia is associated with a decrease in the blood concentration of cortisol and an increase in the level of *androgens* in both sexes, most commonly as a result of *21-hydroxylase* deficiency.
[ref. 5]

congenital malformation

Malformation existing at *birth*, or developing during the first month of life, regardless of the cause.
[ref. 5]
See also *birth defect*.

conjoined twin

One of a pair of *identical twins* fused together with varying degrees of union and of residual duplication of organs.
[After ref. 5]
See also *autosite; parasitic twin*.

conjugate (in biochemistry)

1. *Chemical species* produced in living organisms by covalently linking two chemical moieties from different sources, for example, a conjugate of a *xenobiotic* with some group such as glutathione, sulfate, or glucuronic acid, to make it soluble in water or compartmentalized within the cell.
   See also *phase II reaction*.
2. Material produced by attaching two or more substances together, for example, a conjugate of an *antibody* with a fluorochrome, or an enzyme.

[ref. 5]

conjunctiva

Mucous membrane that covers the eyeball and lines the under-surface of the eyelid.
[ref. 1]

conjunctivitis

Inflammation of the *conjunctiva*.
[ref. 1]

conjunctivitis, allergic

Irritation of the ocular *conjunctiva*, resulting from the activation of conjunctival *mast cells* by airborne *allergens* such as pollens or house *dust*.
[ref. 3]

connective tissue

Extracellular matrix of fibrous proteins and *glycoproteins*, with associated cells such as *fibroblasts*, that fills the spaces between and within organs and tissues.
Note 1: Connective tissue provides the organs and tissues with structural and *metabolic* support.
Note 2: Specialized connective tissues also include bone, *cartilage*, blood components, and adipose tissue.
[ref. 5]

conotoxin

Any of a group of oligopeptide *neurotoxins* produced by marine snails of the genus ***Conus***.
Note: As a group, conotoxins show a variety of neurotoxic symptoms as their individual activities include blockage of several different *ion channels* (including Na^+, K^+, and Ca^{2+} channels) and *acetylcholine receptors*.
[*]

consciousness (n)/conscious (adj)

Aware of and responding to one's surroundings.
[ref. 4]

conservation biology

Science applied to the preservation of *genes, populations, species*, and *ecosystems*.
Note: Conservation biology is concerned with the phenomena that affect the maintenance, loss, and restoration of biological *diversity*.
[ref. 2]

conservation ecology

Science of analyzing and protecting the Earth's biological *diversity*.
Note: Conservation ecology is based on the biological, physical, and social sciences, economics, and the practice of natural-resource management. It concentrates on *population dynamics* issues associated with the small population sizes of rare *species* (*e.g., minimum viable populations*).
[ref. 2]

conservative assessment of risk

Assessment of *risk* that assumes the worst possible case scenario and therefore gives the highest possible value for risk; risk management decisions based on this value will maximize safety.
[ref. 1]

constant (C) domain

See *constant (C) region*.

constant (C) gene

Gene that encodes the *constant (C) region* of *immunoglobulin* chains or *T-cell receptor* chains.
[ref. 3]

constant (C) region

Part of an *immunoglobulin* (Ig) or *T-cell receptor* (TCR) that is relatively constant in amino acid sequence among different Ig or TCR molecules.
Note 1: In an *antibody* molecule the C regions of each chain are composed of up to four C domains.
Note 2: The C region of an antibody determines its general type of interaction.
[ref. 3]
See also *variable (V) region.*

construct validity

Extent to which a measurement is accounted for by theoretical concepts (constructs) concerning the phenomenon under study; for example, if on theoretical grounds, the phenomenon should change with age, a measurement with construct validity would reflect such a change.
[ref. 1]

contact allergen

See *allergen, contact.*

contact dermatitis

See *dermatitis, contact.*

contact hypersensitivity

See *hypersensitivity, contact.*

contact poison

1. *Poison* that injures the target organism through physical contact and skin absorption rather than through ingestion or *inhalation.*
2. *Pesticide (herbicide)* that causes injury to only the plant tissue to which it is applied or which is not appreciably translocated within plants.

[ref. 1]

contact sensitivity

State of immunological *sensitization* in which an *eczematous* epidermal reaction may occur when a *hapten* is applied to the skin of a sensitized individual.
[ref. 3]
See also *contact dermatitis.*

contact urticaria

See *urticaria, contact.*

containment

Process by which possible release, discharge, or spread of a *toxic* substance during normal use or after an accident is prevented by appropriate action.
[ref. 1]

contaminant

1. Minor impurity present in a substance.
2. Extraneous material inadvertently added to a *sample* prior to or during chemical or biological analysis.
3. Unintended component in food that may pose a *hazard* to the consumer.
4. Any undesirable solid, liquid, or gaseous matter occurring, as a result of human activities, in any environmental medium, even without adverse effects being observed.

[ref. 2]
See also *pollutant*.

contamination

1. Presence of a *contaminant*.
2. Process whereby a contaminant reaches the environmental medium or sample affected.

[ref. 2]

content validity

Extent to which a measurement incorporates all aspects of the phenomenon under study.
Example: A measurement of functional *health* status should include such parameters as activities of daily living, occupational and family situations, and social functioning.
[After ref. 1]

continuous effect

Change that can be measured on a continuum, such as growth.
[After ref. 2]
See also *quantal effect*.

continuous epitope

See *linear epitope*.

continuous flow test

See *flow-through test*.

continuous performance test (CPT)

Any of several available neuropsychological procedures that measure a person's sustained attention.
Note 1: An example of a CPT is the computer-administered Conners' test, where, in one version, the test subject is asked to click the spacebar when presented any letter except the letter "X" with 360 presentations over a 14 minute period.
Note 2: CPTs are often used in evaluating children with suspected *attention deficit hyperactivity disorder*.
[ref. 4]

contraceptive

Anything that prevents, or reduces the likelihood of *pregnancy*.
[ref. 5]

contraction

Shortening and tightening of a muscle in response to neural or other electrical stimulation.
[*]

contracture

Chronic condition of shortening and tightening of muscle, tendon, or other tissue, usually *pathological* in nature.
[*]

contraindication

Opposite term: *indication.*

Any condition that renders some particular line of treatment improper or undesirable.
[ref. 1]

contrast medium

Any material (usually opaque to X-rays) employed to delineate or define a structure during a radiological procedure.
[ref. 4]

control

Treatment in a *toxicity* test that duplicates all the conditions of the *exposure* treatments but contains no test material, in order to determine the absence of toxicity under basic test conditions (*e.g.*, health of test organisms, quality of dilution water).
[ref. 2]

control, matched

Control (group, case, or individual) selected to be similar to a study, group, case, or individual in specific characteristics: some commonly used matching variables are age, sex, race, and socioeconomic status.
[ref. 1]

control, negative

Additional sample in an experiment or test that does not contain the agent (*e.g.*, an analyte or toxicant) of interest.
Note: In animal and human studies, the negative control is often a *placebo*. Its use in assays is essential to exclude methodological errors.
[*]

control, positive

Additional sample or group in an experiment or test known to produce the outcome of interest.
[*]

control group

comparison group

Selected subjects of study, identified before a study is done, comprising humans, animals, or other species who do not have the *disease*, intervention, procedure, or other endpoint being evaluated, but in all other respects are as nearly identical to the test group as possible.
[ref. 1]

convection (as applied to air and water motion)

Predominantly vertical motion of air or of water, induced by the expansion of the air or of water heated by the earth's surface, or by human activity, and its resulting buoyancy.
[ref. 1]

conventional dendritic cell

See *dendritic cell, conventional.*

convergent evolution

See *evolution, convergent.*

conversion

See *chemical conversion; biotransformation.*

convertase

Enzyme activity that converts *complement* protein into its reactive form by cleaving it.
Note: Generation of the C3/C5 convertase (EC 3.4.21.43) is the pivotal event in *complement activation.*
[ref. 3]

convulsion

Sudden, violent, irregular movement of the body, caused by involuntary *contraction* of muscles and associated with *brain disorders* such as *epilepsy*, fever in children, or *drug* or alcohol *abuse*.
[ref. 4]

Coombs and Gell classification

See *Gell and Coombs classification.*

Coombs test

Diagnostic test using anti-*immunoglobulin* to agglutinate *antibody*-coated *erythrocytes*.
Note: A Coombs test may be direct or indirect.

- The direct Coombs test, or direct antiglobulin test (DAT) refers to *agglutination* of a blood sample due to antibodies present on the erythrocyte surface.
- In the indirect Coombs test, or indirect antiglobulin test (IAT) antibodies free in the subject's *serum* are tested for their availability to agglutinate erythrocytes of known *antigenicity*.

[ref. 3]

cooxidation

Cometabolism whereby growing microorganisms oxidize a substance without using either carbon or energy derived from the oxidation of that substance.
[ref. 2]

copepod

Minute marine or freshwater crustacean, usually having six pairs of limbs on the *thorax*; some are abundant in plankton and others are parasitic on fish, marine mammals, and macro-invertebrates.
[ref. 2]

coreceptor

Cell surface protein *receptor* that recognizes a substance bound to a primary receptor, and binds to a signaling molecule that thereby enhances the activity of another receptor.

Note 1: Optimal *T-cell activation* in an *immune response* depends on the involvement of relevant coreceptors occurring in a cluster with the *T-cell receptors*. The coreceptors are *CD4* or *CD8* proteins, which lie alongside the T-cell receptor in the *plasma membrane*. Only when both coreceptor and receptor bind the *major histocompatibility complex molecule*-antigen complex simultaneously is the full set of intracellular effector molecules recruited and the signal pathway inside the cell maximally activated.

Note 2: *B-cell receptors* require the contributions of several coreceptors, notably CD19, CD21, and CD81 proteins, for full activation of intracellular signaling pathways.

[ref. 3]

cornu ammonis

Part of the *hippocampus*.

[ref. 4]

coronal

Vertical (longitudinal) plane dividing the body into ventral and dorsal (front and back) sections.

[ref. 4]

coronal suture

Transverse junction in the skull separating the frontal bone from the parietal bones.

[ref. 4]

corpus callosum

Bundle of myelin-enriched neural fibers beneath the *cortex* connecting the two *hemispheres* of the *brain*.

[ref. 4]

corpus cavernosum

Either of the two columns of erectile tissue forming the body of the *clitoris* (corpus cavernosum clitoridis) or penis (corpus cavernosum penis).

[ref. 5]

corpus luteum

Glandular mass of yellowish tissue in the *ovary*, formed by a *Graafian ovarian follicle* that has matured and released its *oocyte*.

Note: The corpus luteum is observed in animal reproductive testing to calculate preimplantation loss.

[ref. 5]

corpus striatum

Striatum together with the *globus pallidus*.

[ref. 4]

corrosion

Process causing a surface-destructive effect on contact; in *toxicology*, this normally means causing visible destruction of the skin, eyes, or the lining of the respiratory tract or the *gastrointestinal tract.*
[ref. 2]

corrosive

1. (n) Substance that causes a surface-destructive effect on contact (see *corrosion*).
2. (adj) Causing *corrosion.*

[After ref. 1]

cortex (in anatomy)

Outer layer of an organ such as the kidney, the cerebellum, or the *adrenal gland.*
[ref. 5]
See also *cortex, cerebral.*

cortex, cerebral

Outer layer of the *cerebrum*, composed of folded *grey matter*, playing an important role in *conscious*ness.
Note: In humans, the cerebral cortex is a 2-3 mm thick covering with gyri and sulci, whereas in rodents, it is smooth.
[ref. 4]
See also *neocortex.*

cortex, motor

Region of the *cerebral cortex*, located primarily in the *frontal lobe,* involved in coordinating *motor activity.*
[ref. 4]

cortex, visual

An area of the *occipital lobe*, part of the cerebral cortex, that receives and processes sensory nerve impulses from the eyes.
[*]

corticosteroid

Any of the family of steroid molecules that are produced in the cortex of the *adrenal gland*, or their synthetic analogs.
Note: Corticosteroids can induce *apoptotic* cell death in *lymphocytes*, especially developing *thymocytes*. Therefore, they are useful anti-inflammatory, anti-*lymphoid* tumor, and *immunosuppressive* agents.
[ref. 3]

cost–benefit analysis (CBA)

Procedure for determining the relationship of the expected benefits of a proposed action to the expected costs in order to decide whether the action provides the best option for the investment of limited resources.
[ref. 2]
Compare *cost–effectiveness analysis.*

cost–effectiveness analysis

Procedure for determining whether the expected beneficial effects of a defined course of action justify the cost when selecting among competing options for the use of limited resources.
Note: Cost–effectiveness analysis is mainly used for comparing the relative value of various clinical and remediation strategies.
[ref. 2]
Compare *cost–benefit analysis.*

costimulation (in immunology)

Delivery of a second signal, in addition to that of *antigen* binding or *antigen presentation*, that is required for *lymphocyte* proliferation.
Note 1: Costimulatory signals are delivered to *T-cells* by the costimulatory molecules, B7.1 and B7.2, related molecules (see *B7 molecule*) that are expressed on the surface of the *antigen-presenting cell*, and that bind the T-cell surface molecule CD28.
Note 2: *B-cells* may receive costimulatory signals from common *pathogen* components such as *lipopolysaccharide*, from *complement* fragments, or from *CD40 ligand* expressed on the surface of an activated antigen-specific *helper T-lymphocyte*.
[ref. 3]

cotolerance

See *cross-resistance.*

cough (in fish)
gill purge

Abrupt, periodic reversal of water flow over the gills that dislodges and eliminates excess mucus from the gills' surfaces.
[ref. 2]

count mean diameter
mean diameter by count

Mean of the diameters of all particles in a population.
[ref. 1]
See also *count median diameter; mass mean diameter.*

count median diameter

Calculated diameter in a population of particles in a gas or liquid phase above which there are as many particles with larger diameters as there are particles below it with smaller diameters.
[ref. 1]
See also *count mean diameter; mass median diameter.*

counter-regulation hypothesis

Hypothesis that all types of infection early in childhood may protect against the development of *atopy* by driving the production of *cytokines* such as *interleukin*-10 and *transforming growth factor-β*, which downregulate both *Th1* and *Th2* responses.
[ref. 3]

"covalent binding" (in toxicology)

Non*enzymatic covalent bond* formation between a reactive metabolite, *e.g.*, that formed in *phase I biotransformation*, and a nearby biomolecule.
Note: Such covalent binding can results in *adverse effects*, such as enzyme inactivation, and DNA *adducts* that can cause *mutagenesis* and *carcinogenesis*.
[*]
See also *hemoglobin adduct; nonenzymatic glycosylation*.

covalent bond

A region of relatively high electron density between nuclei which arises at least partly from sharing of electrons and gives rise to an attractive force and characteristic internuclear distance.
[ref. 8]

Cowper's gland

See *bulbourethral gland.*

crackles

See *crepitations*.

cramp

Painful muscle *spasm* caused by prolonged *tetanic* contraction.
[ref. 4]

cranial nerve

See *nerve, cranial*.

cranial placodes

Thickenings in the surface *ectoderm* of the *embryo* associated with future eye and ear regions.
[ref. 5]

cranial suture

Line where the bony plates of the skull are joined together by fibrous bands of tissue, easily felt in the newborn before closure by *ossification*.
[ref. 5]
See also *fontanelle*.

craniofacial

Pertaining to the *cranium* and the face.
[ref. 5]

craniopharyngioma

Congenital tumor arising from the *pituitary gland* in the *embryonic* tissue between the *brain* and pharynx.
Note: As the specific cells from which a craniopharyngioma arises also contribute to tooth formation, the tumor will often show calcium deposits visible on x-rays.
[ref. 4]

craniorachischisis

Neural tube defect in which both the *cranium* and *vertebral* column remain open.
[ref. 5]

cranioschisis

Developmental failure of the *cranial sutures* to close completely, especially at the *occiput*, usually leading to grossly defective development of the brain.
[ref. 5]

craniosynostosis

Premature closure of the *cranial sutures*.
[ref. 5]

cranium (n)/cranial (adj)

Bony structure surrounding the brain, excluding the bones of the face.
[ref. 5]

cranium bifidum

See *encephalocele*.

Cre/loxP

Bacterial system in which the Cre protein mediates *DNA* recombination between specific DNA sequences known as lox-P sites.
Note: The Cre/loxP system is used in mammalian cells to delete (or invert) a stretch of DNA by flanking it with lox-P sites and then exposing the cell to Cre protein at some predetermined time.
[ref. 4]

crepitation
crepitus

Abnormal crackling sound arising within the body.
Note 1: Crepitations may arise from the grating ends of a fractured bone or within a joint.
Note 2: Crepitations heard on *auscultation* of the chest are produced by movement of air through passages that contain secretion or exudate, or that are constricted by spasm or thickening of their walls. In this case, crepitations are also called crackles or râles (rales).
[*]
See also *rhonchi*.

cretinism

Developmental *disorder* caused by deficiency of *thyroid hormone*, characterized by severe intellectual disability and stunted physical growth, sometimes resulting from maternal iodine deficiency.
[ref. 5]

cri du chat syndrome
Lejeune syndrome
5p– syndrome

Hereditary *congenital syndrome* due to deletion of the short arm of *chromosome* 5.

Note: Cri du chat syndrome is characterized by *hypertelorism, microcephaly*, severe mental deficiency, and a plaintive cat-like cry.
[ref. 5]

crista

One of the inward projections or folds of the inner *membrane* of a mitochondrion.
[ref. 5]

criterion (n)/criteria (pl)

Validated set of data used as a basis for judgment.
[ref. 1]

criterion for effect

See *endpoint.*

criterion validity

Extent to which the measurement correlates with an external *criterion* of the phenomenon under study.
[ref. 1]

critical body residue (CBR)

Whole-body concentration of a chemical that is associated with a given adverse biological response.
Note 1: Stating a CBR assumes each organism is a single compartment, rather than multiple compartments as in reality.
Note 2: CBR has utility as a first approximation of *dose.*
[ref. 2]

critical concentration (for a cell or an organ)

Concentration of a substance at and above which adverse functional changes, reversible or irreversible, occur in a cell or an organ.
[ref. 1]

critical dose

Dose of a substance at and above which adverse functional changes, reversible or irreversible, occur in a cell or an organ.
[ref. 1]

critical effect

For *deterministic effects*, the first *adverse effect* that appears when the *threshold* (*critical*) *concentration* or *dose* is reached in the *critical organ*. Adverse effects with no defined threshold concentration are regarded as critical.
[ref. 1]

critical end-point

Toxic effect used as a basis for a *reference dose.*
[ref. 1]

critical group

Part of a *target population* most in need of protection because it is most *susceptible* to a given *toxicant.*
[ref. 1]

critical life-stage testing

Toxicity testing focused on the *species* life stage thought to be the most sensitive to the *toxicant,* such as newly hatched individuals.
[ref. 2]

critical organ (in toxicology)

First organ that attains the *critical concentration* of a substance and exhibits the *critical effect* under specified circumstances of *exposure* and for a given population.
[ref. 1]

critical organ concentration

Mean *concentration* of a substance in the *critical organ* at the time the substance reaches its *critical concentration* in the most sensitive type of cell in the organ.
[ref. 1]

critical period (in biology)

Specific stage in the development of a biological system (*e.g., organogenesis* in the *fetus*) when it is particularly vulnerable to injury or misdirection of some anatomical, physiological, *metabolic*, or psychological structure or function.
[After ref. 1,5]

critical study

Any study, the outcome of which is essential for future decisions.
Example: Investigation yielding the *no-observed-adverse-effect-level* that is used as the basis of the *reference dose.*
[*]

Crohn disease

Chronic *inflammatory bowel disease* thought to result from an abnormal over-responsiveness to commensal gut flora.
[ref. 3]

cross-matching

1. (n) Test for determining the compatibility between the blood of a donor and that of a recipient before *transfusion*; the clumping of *erythrocytes* indicates incompatibility.
2. (n) Test for determining tissue compatibility between a transplant donor and the recipient before *transplantation*, in which the recipient's *serum* is tested for *antibodies* that may react with the *lymphocytes* or other cells of the donor.
3. (v) Process of performing one of these tests.

[ref. 3]

cross-presentation

cross-priming

Activation of *CD8+ lymphocytes* by the presentation of exogenous *antigens* in association with *major histocompatibility complex class I* molecules.
Note 1: Cross-presentation is in contrast to normal activation of CD8+ lymphocytes (direct-*priming*) that results from presentation of endogenous antigens.
Note 2: The cells that cross-present antigens are the bone marrow-derived *antigen-presenting cells*. The form of antigen they monitor from tissues is predominantly cellular protein, acquired through *phagocytosis* and *macropinocytosis* and presented

through two distinct pathways. In one pathway, antigen is transferred into the cytosol where it is degraded by *proteasomes*, and in the other, the antigen is hydrolyzed in the endocytic compartment.
Note 3: Cross-presentation can lead to different outcomes, *tolerance* or *immunity*.
[ref. 3]

cross-priming

See *cross-presentation.*

cross-product ratio

See *odds ratio.*

cross-reacting antibody

See *antibody, cross-reacting.*

cross-reacting antigen

See *antigen, cross-reacting.*

cross-reactivity

1. Ability of an *antibody* or a *T-cell*, specific for one *antigen*, to react with a second antigen.
2. Measure of relatedness between two *antigenic* substances, and (or) the polyspecificity of the antibody molecule (*e.g.*, some *rheumatoid factors*), or of the *T-cell receptor.*

[ref. 3]

cross-resistance

Condition in which enhanced *tolerance* to one *toxicant* also enhances tolerance to another.
[ref. 2]

cross-sectional study

See *study, cross-sectional.*

cross-sensitivity

State of immunological *hypersensitivity* to one substance that predisposes an individual to *sensitivity* to other substances that are related in chemical structure (*cross-reacting antigens*).
[ref. 3]

cross-tolerance

State of immunological *tolerance* to one substance produced by *priming* an animal with another substance that bears a *cross-reacting antigen.*
[ref. 3]

Crouzon syndrome

branchial arch syndrome

Group of autosomal dominant genetic *diseases* characterized by midfacial *hypoplasia, craniosynostosis, exophthalmos*, and a shortened head.

Note 1: Crouzon syndrome affects the first *branchial arch* (pharyngeal arch), which is the precursor of the maxilla and mandible.
Note 2: Crouzon syndrome is thought to be caused by a *mutation* of the FGFR3 gene, located on *chromosome* 10.
[ref. 5]

cryoglobulin

Immunoglobulin that forms insoluble aggregates at temperatures below body temperature.
Note 1: Cryoglobulins are found in lymphoproliferative (see *lymphoproliferation*) *diseases*, a number of *autoimmune diseases*, as well as chronic infections; many function as *autoantibodies* (*e.g., rheumatoid factor*).
Note 2: Cryoglobulins can cause vasculitic and secondary thrombotic manifestations (*cryoglobulinemic vasculitis, glomerulonephritis*).
[ref. 3]

cryoglobulinemic vasculitis

Cutaneous or *systemic vasculitis* caused by cold-labile proteins (*cryoglobulins*, cryo*fibrinogen*) that leads to increased viscosity, protein precipitation or gelatinification, *complement* activation, and endothelial cell damage, especially in the cold.
Note: Cryoglobulinemic vasculitis is frequently associated with chronic hepatitis C or B infection, but can also be induced by other infections and *malignancies*.
[ref. 3]

cryopyrin

See *NACHT domain-, leucine-rich repeat-, and PYD-containing protein 3*.

crypt (in anatomy)

Small tubular *gland*, pit, or depression.
[ref. 5]
See also *uterine crypt*.

cryptic epitope

See *epitope, cryptic*.

cryptophthalmos

Failure of the eyelids to develop with a fissure between them, usually with defective formation of the eyeballs.
[ref. 5]

cryptorchidism

See *undescended testis*.

cue

Stimulus or associated feature of a stimulus that evokes a response or alerts the subject to a particular behavior.
[ref. 4]

culture (in biotechnology)

1. (n) Stock of healthy cells, freshly prepared *tissue* or *organs*, microorganisms, or plants maintained under well-defined and controlled conditions.
2. (v) Maintain or grow a stock of healthy cells or organisms, plants, or freshly prepared tissue or organs, under well-defined and controlled conditions.

[After ref. 2]

cumulative death rate

See *death rate, cumulative.*

cumulative dose

See *dose, cumulative.*

cumulative effect

See *effect, cumulative.*

cumulative exposure

See *exposure, cumulative.*

cumulative incidence

See *incidence, cumulative.*

cumulative incidence ratio

See *incidence ratio, cumulative.*

cumulative median lethal dose

Estimate of the total administered amount of a substance that causes the death of half a population of animals when the substance is administered repeatedly (cumulatively) in doses that are fractions of the *median lethal dose.*
[ref. 1]

cumulative risk

See *risk, cumulative.*

cumulus oophorus

Mass of *follicular* cells surrounding the *oocyte* in the *Graafian follicle.*
[ref. 5]

cutaneous
dermal

Pertaining to the skin.
[ref. 1]

cutaneous lymphocyte antigen (CLA)

Cell-surface molecule that is involved in *lymphocyte homing* to the skin in humans.
[ref. 3]

cutaneous T-cell lymphoma

See *lymphoma, cutaneous T-cell.*

cyanogenic

Describing any substance able to produce cyanide.
Example: Amygdalin, found in peach and apricot stones.
[ref. 1]

cyanosis

Bluish discoloration of the skin and *mucous membranes* due to excessive concentration of deoxygenated *hemoglobin*, owing to poor circulation or inadequate oxygenation of the blood.
[ref. 5]

cyanotoxin

Toxin produced by ***Cyanobacteria***, sometimes called blue-green algae.
Examples: Microcystin, cylindrospermin.
[ref. 1]

cycad toxin

See *Western Pacific amyotrophic lateral sclerosis and parkinsonism-dementia complex.*

cycle (n)/cyclic (adj)

1. Process that, on completion, returns to its beginning, and may then repeat itself.
2. Components of a cyclic process.

[*]
See also *biogeochemical cycle; cell cycle; estrous cycle; life cycle; menstrual cycle; ovarian cycle; population cycle; reproductive cycle; respiratory cycle; risk cycle; spermatogenic cycle; uterine cycle*

cyclooxygenase-specific inhibitors

Substances, such as aspirin and ibuprofen, that block the activity of cyclooxygenase (COX; prostaglandin-endoperoxide synthase, EC 1.14.99.1), an *enzyme* that is responsible for the formation of prostanoids (including prostaglandins, prostacyclin, and thromboxane).
Note: Inhibition of COX can provide relief from *inflammation* and pain.
[ref. 1]

cyclopia
cyclocephaly
synophthalmia

Rare form of *holoprosencephaly*, a *congenital disorder* characterized by a single orbital *fossa* due to the failure of the *embryonic prosencephalon* to divide the *orbits* of the eye correctly into two cavities.
[ref. 5]

cyst (n)/cystic (adj)

1. In an animal or plant, thin-walled hollow organ or *cavity* containing a liquid secretion.
2. Sac, *vesicle*, or bladder.

[ref. 5]

cytochrome

Protein containing heme as the *prosthetic group* and associated with electron transport and with redox processes.
[ref. 1]

cytochrome P420

Inactive derivative of *cytochrome P450* (EC 1.14.14.1) found in *microsomal* preparations.
[ref. 1]

cytochrome P448

Obsolete term for *cytochrome P450* I (EC 1.14.14.1) polypeptides A1 and A2, one of the major families of the cytochromes P450 hemoproteins.
Note 1: During the monooxygenation of certain substances, often a *detoxification* process, cytochrome P448 iso-enzymes may produce intermediates that can initiate *mutations, cancer, immunotoxic* reactions, and *adverse effects*.
Note 2: "P448" refers to a feature in the visible absorption spectrum (compare Note to *cytochrome P450*).
[ref. 1]

cytochrome P450 (CYP)

Member (EC 1.14.14.1) of a superfamily of heme-containing monooxygenases involved in *xenobiotic metabolism*, cholesterol biosynthesis, and steroidogenesis, in eukaryotic organisms found mainly in the *endoplasmic reticulum* and inner mitochondrial membrane of cells.
Note: "P450" refers to the observation that a preparation of this enzyme exposed to carbon monoxide strongly absorbs light at a wavelength of 450 nm in the difference spectrum recorded against the unexposed enzyme.
[ref. 1]

cytogenetics

Branch of genetics that correlates the structure and number of *chromosomes* and changes in other cell components, seen in isolated cells or tissue sections and associated with variation in *genotype* and *phenotype*.
[*]

cytokine

Any of a group of soluble small proteins released from a variety of cells, and prominently from those of the *immune system*, that affect cell behavior in an *autocrine* or *paracrine* fashion.
Note 1: Cytokines are involved in reproduction, growth, and development; normal homeostatic regulation; response to injury and repair; blood clotting; and host resistance (immunity and tolerance).
Note 2: Cytokines produced by *lymphocytes* are known as *lymphokines*; those produced by *monocytes* are called *monokines*. Other types of cytokines include *chemokines*, *growth factors*, *colony-stimulating factors*, *transforming growth factors*, *interferons*, interleukins, and *tumor necrosis factors*.
[ref. 1,3]

cytokine capture assay

in vivo cytokine capture assay (IVCCA)
Method of detecting *cytokine* release by injecting an animal with a neutralizing biotinylated *antibody* to the cytokine, inhibiting its utilization and allowing its accumulation in the blood. Recovered cytokine-antibody complexes are then measured in an *enzyme-linked immunosorbent assay* with an antibody to a second epitope on the cytokine.
[ref. 3]

cytokine profile

Characteristic pattern of *cytokine* production associated with a defined immunological state.
[ref. 3]

cytokine release assay (CRA)

Method of quantifying *cytokines* released by viable cells, using cytokine-specific *antibodies.*
[ref. 3]

cytokine storm

cytokine cascade
hypercytokinemia

Immunological condition, in which, as a result of a positive feedback loop, white blood cells (*leukocytes*) release large amounts of *cytokines*, which then cause fever, swellings, and additional *allergy*-like symptoms, with a potentially fatal outcome.
[*]

cytolysis, immune

1. Cell lysis caused by a lesion produced by the action of *complement* proteins on the antibody-coated *plasma membrane* of a cell.
2. Cell lysis following plasma membrane reaction with *perforins* released by *natural killer cells.*

[ref. 3]

cytolytic T-cell

See *cytotoxic T-lymphocyte.*

cytomegalovirus (CMV)

visceral disease virus

Any of a group of highly *host*-specific slow growing ***Herpes*** viruses that infect humans, monkeys, pigs, or rodents, with the production of unique enlarged epithelial cells having intranuclear inclusions, and often with a special affinity for the salivary glands.
Note 1: CMV specific for humans causes cytomegalic inclusion *disease*, and it has been associated with a *syndrome* resembling infectious mononucleosis.
Note 2: CMV usually produces very mild symptoms in an infected person but may cause severe neurological damage in people with weakened immune systems and in the newborn.

Note 3: CMV poses the greatest risk to unborn children of women who get CMV for the first time during pregnancy.
[ref. 3,5]

cytopenia

Decrease in the number of one or more types of blood cells.
[ref. 3]
See also *pancytopenia.*

cytoplasm (n)/cytoplasmic (adj)

Fundamental substance or *matrix* of the cell within the *plasma membrane*, surrounding the nucleus, *endoplasmic reticulum, mitochondria*, and other *organelles.*
[ref. 1]

cytoskeleton (n)/cytoskeletal (adj)

Flexible network of structural and contractile components stretching throughout the *cytoplasm* of most *eukaryotic cells.*
Note: The cytoskeleton is composed of actin, *microtubules* and *intermediate filaments*, and functions in both structural support and transport for other cellular components, *e.g.*, proteins, *organelles* such as *mitochondria*, and *vesicles.*
Note: The cytoskeletal transport mechanism involves *dyneins* and *kinesins.*
[*]

cytostasis (n)/cytostatic (adj)

Cessation of cell growth and multiplication, sometimes referring to polymorphonuclear leukocytes.
Note: Many *cancer* chemotherapeutic *drugs* act by a cytostatic mechanism.
[*]

cytotoxicity (n)/cytotoxic (adj)

Causing damage to *cell* structure or function.
[ref. 1]

cytotoxic T-cell

See *cytotoxic T-lymphocyte.*

cytotoxic T-lymphocyte (CTL, Tc)

CD8+ T-cell
cytolytic T-cell
cytotoxic T-cell
killer T-cell

Any of a subset of *T-lymphocytes* bearing the *CD8* surface marker and able to kill *target cells* (infected somatic or tumor cells, recognized by the *antigen receptor* complex) after induction of a specific *immune response* to the *antigens* bound to *major histocompatibility complex class I molecules.*
Note: CD4+ T-lymphocytes may also become cytotoxic.
[ref. 3]

cytotoxic T-lymphocyte antigen 4 (CTLA-4)

CD152

High *affinity* receptor for *B7 molecules* expressed on *T-cells*, binding of which inhibits T-cell *activation*.
Note: Mutations in the gene encoding CTLA-4 have been associated with various *autoimmune diseases*.
[ref. 3]

cytotoxic T-lymphocyte (CTL) assay

Assay based on quantitation of cell death caused by sensitized (see *sensitization*) *lymphocytes* or splenocytes cultured with a fixed number of tumor or other *target cells* that have been prelabeled with ^{51}Cr. The ^{51}Cr is taken up and reversibly binds to cytosolic proteins. When these target cells are incubated with sensitized lymphocytes, the target cells are killed and the ^{51}Cr is released.
[ref. 3]

cytotoxin

cytotoxicant

Substance with a specific *toxic* effect on certain cells.
Note: Major cytotoxins made by *cytotoxic T-lymphocytes* and *natural killer cells* that participate in the destruction of *target cells* include *perforins, granzymes*, and granulolysins.
[ref. 3]

cytotrophoblast

Inner cellular layer of the *trophectoderm* (*trophoblast*); part of the mammalian *placenta*.
[ref. 5]

D gene

See *diversity (D) gene.*

DEC-205

CD205
Surface *antigen* characteristic of *dendritic cells.*
[ref. 3]

DNA

See *deoxyribonucleic acid.*

DNA adduct

See *adduct.*

DNA amplification

See *gene amplification, deoxyribonucleic acid.*

DNA cloning

See *deoxyribonucleic acid cloning.*

DNA, recombinant

See *recombinant DNA.*

DNA, recombinant technology

See *recombinant DNA technology.*

DNA repair

See *deoxyribonucleic acid repair.*

DNA sequencing

See *deoxyribonucleic acid sequencing.*

DNA vaccination

See *vaccination, deoxyribonucleic acid.*

DP, DQ, or DR molecule

Member of the group of *major histocompatibility complex class II molecules* occurring on human *B-lymphocytes* and *antigen-presenting cells.*
[ref. 3]

daily intake, acceptable (ADI)

Estimate by JECFA of the amount of a food additive, expressed on a body weight basis, that can be ingested daily over a lifetime without appreciable health *risk.*

Comprehensive Glossary of Terms Used in Toxicology
By John Duffus, Douglas M. Templeton and Michael Schwenk

Published by the Royal Society of Chemistry, www.rsc.org

Note 1: For calculation of ADI, a standard body mass of 60 kg is used.
Note 2: *Tolerable daily intake* is the analogous term to ADI used for contaminants.
[ref. 1]

daily intake, acceptable, not allocated

See *no-acceptable-daily-intake-allocated.*

damage

See *harm.*

danger hypothesis

Hypothesis that suggests it is not foreignness of a molecule *per se*, but rather its ability to cause cell damage or stress that induces an *immune response*.
Note: This hypothesis is often invoked to explain the causation of *idiosyncratic drug reactions*.
[ref. 3]

Daphnia

Genus of small, mostly planktonic, crustaceans, between 0.2 and 5 mm in length.
Note 1: The genus ***Daphnia*** is a member of the order ***Cladocera***, and is one of several small aquatic crustacean genera commonly called 'water fleas' because of their saltatory swimming style. ***Daphnia*** spp. live in various aquatic environments ranging from acidic swamps to freshwater lakes, ponds, streams, and rivers.
Note 2: *Toxicity* tests on ***Daphnia*** species, usually on ***Daphnia magna***, are required by most regulatory authorities to assess water quality. The results are often interpreted as applicable by extrapolation to the protection of all crustaceans.
[ref. 2]

Daphnia magna reproduction test

Procedure in which young females of the species ***Daphnia magna*** are *exposed* to a substance added to the water and numbers of living offspring and surviving parent organisms are recorded.
[ref. 5]

Darwinian fitness

See *fitness.*

dead-end metabolite

Substance formed by a microbe's metabolism of a substrate (most often during *cometabolism*) that cannot be further metabolized by that organism.
Note: Dead-end metabolites may be further metabolized by coexisting organisms.
[ref. 2]

death (in biology)

Irreversible cessation of all vital functions of an organism.
[ref. 2]

death (in population ecology)

Loss of an *individual*'s ability to reproduce.
[ref. 2]

death domain

Protein-interaction domain originally discovered in proteins involved in the *extrinsic pathway* of *apoptosis*.
[After ref. 3]

death rate

Estimate of the proportion of a population that dies during a specified period, indicating the number of persons dying during the period divided by the size of the population (usually estimated as the mid-year population).
Note 1: The death rate in a population is generally calculated by the formula: [(number of deaths during a specified period)/(number of persons at *risk* of dying during the period)]$\times 10^n$, where n is usually either 3 or 5 giving rates per 1000 or per 100 000 people in the population studied. This rate is an estimate of the person-time death rate, *i.e.*, the death rate per 10^n person-years; if it is low, it is also a good estimate of the *cumulative death rate*.
Note 2: Death rate calculated as in Note 1 is sometimes described as the crude death rate.
[ref. 1]
See also *death rate* (in ecotoxicology); *death rate, per capita*.

death rate (in ecotoxicology)

Number of deaths D in a closed *population* of size N during a specified time interval, Δt. The rate is calculated from the formula

$$D = -\Delta N/\Delta t$$

where ΔN is the change in number of deaths over a specified time period.
[ref. 2]
See also *death rate; death rate, per capita*.

death rate, cumulative

Proportion of a defined group that dies within the specified time period (*e.g.*, month, year).
Note: Cumulative death rate may refer to all deaths or to deaths from a specific cause or causes.
[ref. 1]

death rate, per capita, *m*

Average number of deaths per *population* member per time unit, calculated from death rate, D, and population size, N, as $m = D/N$.
[ref. 2]
See also *population growth rate; per capita rate of increase*.

death rate, specific

Death rate computed for a subpopulation of individual organisms or people having a specified characteristic or attribute, and named accordingly.
Example: Age-specific death rate is calculated as the number of deaths of persons of a specified age during a given period of time, divided by the total number of persons of that age in the population during that time.
[ref. 1]

death receptor

death ligand receptor

Cell-surface *receptor* that, upon binding to extracellular *ligands,* stimulates *apoptosis* in the receptor-bearing cell through the *extrinsic pathway*.
[ref. 3]
See also *tumor necrosis factor*.

decay-accelerating factor (DAF)

CD55

Cell-surface molecule that protects cells from lysis by *complement*.
Note: The decay-accelerating factor binds to C3 *convertases* of both the *alternative pathway* and *classical pathway of complement activation* and, by displacing Bb and C2b respectively, prevents their action. Its absence causes the *disease* paroxysmal nocturnal hemoglobinuria.
[ref. 3]

dechlorinated water

Chlorinated water (*e.g.*, municipal drinking water) that has been treated to remove chlorine and chlorinated compounds from solution.
[ref. 2]

decidua (n)/decidual (adj)

Modified *endometrial* layer that lines the *uterus* during *pregnancy* and is shed with the afterbirth.
[ref. 5]
See also *deciduum*.

decidual cell

Enlarged, ovoid, *connective tissue* cell appearing in the *endometrium* during *pregnancy*.
[ref. 5]
See also *decidua*.

decidual cell response technique

Biological test method in which *pseudopregnant* rats undergo a surgical treatment of the *uterus* to induce uterine *differentiation* and proliferation, resulting in massive tissue growth that mimics the response of the uterus during normal *blastocyst implantation*.
Note: Measurement of *decidual* growth during chemical treatment can be used to assess both *hormonal* status and uterine function. Uterine weight is a sensitive measure of the success of the *decidual cell* response.
[ref. 5]

decidualization

Changes in response to *progesterone* that include the *eosinophil*ic proliferation around arterioles after *ovulation* or progesterone action on *endometrium*.
Note: Decidualization increases *glandular epithelial* secretion, stimulates glycogen accumulation in *stromal cell* cytoplasm, and promotes stromal vascularity (*spiral arterioles*) and *edema*.
[ref. 5]

deciduum

Swelling of a *uterine crypt* produced by its reaction to an *implanted embryo*.
[ref. 5]
See also *decidua*.

decipol

Unit of air quality perceived by a person under standardized conditions against a background of one *olf*.
Note: Air on mountains or by unpolluted sea has a decipol = 0.01; city air with moderate air *pollution* has a decipol = 0.05–0.03; acceptable indoor air quality has decipol = 1.4 (for 80 % satisfaction).
[ref. 1]

decompensation

Explicit *pathological* changes following breakdown of *compensation* for *adverse effects*.
[ref. 1]

decomposer

Organism that breaks down dead matter or wastes of other organisms.
[ref. 2]

decontamination

Process of rendering harmless a region or object, *e.g.*, a natural environment, laboratory area, the workplace, other indoor areas, clothes, food, water, or sewage, by neutralization, *elimination*, or removal of a potentially *toxic substance*.
[ref. 1]

decussate (v)/decussation (n)

Pertaining to two or more things that cross or intersect each other to form an X.
[ref. 5]
See also *chiasma*.

defeminized gonadotropin secretion

Gonadotropin secretion without female sex *hormones*.
[ref. 5]

defensin

Any member of a family of oligopeptides made within the body, notably by *neutrophils* and *macrophages*, and having potent antimicrobial properties.
Note 1: Defensins play important roles against invading microbes. They act against bacteria, fungi, and viruses by binding to their membranes and increasing membrane permeability.
Note 2: Human defensins are classified into the α-defensins and β-defensins on the basis of their sequence homology and their cysteine residues.
[ref. 3]

defoliant

Substance used for removal of leaves by its *toxic* action on living plants.
[ref. 1]

degradation
breakdown
decomposition

Process by which a substance is broken down to simpler structures through biological or *abiotic* mechanisms.
[ref. 2]
See also *biodegradation; mineralization.*

degradation, abiotic

Process in which a substance is converted to simpler products by physical or chemical mechanisms. *Examples: Hydrolysis, photolysis.*
[ref. 1]
See also *abiotic.*

degranulation

Cell reaction that releases antimicrobial *cytotoxic* molecules and other substances (*e.g., histamine*) from secretory vesicles called granules found inside some cells.
Note: Degranulation occurs in several different cells involved in the *immune system*, including *granulocytes* (*neutrophils, basophils*, and *eosinophils*), *mast cells*, and certain *lymphocytes* such as *natural killer cells* and *cytotoxic T-cells.*
[ref. 3]

dehydrogenase

Any *enzyme* that catalyzes oxidation of a compound by removing hydrogen.
[ref. 1]

delayed effect
latent effect

Consequence occurring after a *latent period* following the end of *exposure* to a *toxic* substance or other harmful environmental factor.
[ref. 1]

delayed-type hypersensitivity (DTH)

See *hypersensitivity, delayed-type.*

delayed-type hypersensitivity (DTH) assay

In vivo assay of *cell-mediated immune response*, elicited by *antigen* in the skin and mediated by *CD4+ Th1 cells.*
Note: DTH reactions are often divided into two phases that should be assessed in the assay: the *sensitization* phase, referring to the initial *immunization* with specific antigen, and the efferent or *challenge* phase of the DTH response, which usually follows 6 to 14 days after sensitization.
[ref. 3]

delirium

State of severe *confusion*, characterized by restlessness, *hallucinations* and hyperactivity, during which the person affected may be isolated from normal communication.
Note: Delirium can result from, *e.g., drug* or alcohol toxicity or *withdrawal*, infection, *brain tumor*, head injury, *metabolic* disturbances.
[ref. 4]

demasculinized

Describing a male animal from which the *testes* have been removed.
[ref. 5]
See also *castrated.*

dementia

Serious loss of *brain* function in a previously unimpaired person, affecting memory, thinking, and behavior.
Note: It may be static as a result of brain injury, or progressive with long-term decline due to ongoing *disease.*
[ref. 4]

dementia, presenile

Dementia, often of the *Alzheimer disease* type, developing at or before age 65.
[ref. 4]

dementia, senile

Dementia, often of the *Alzheimer disease* type, developing after the age of 65.
[ref. 4]

de minimis risk

See *risk de minimis.*

demographic stochasticity

Variability in *population* growth rates arising from random differences among individuals in survival and reproduction within a season.
Note: *Demographic stochasticity* is important only in populations that are fairly small.
[ref. 2]

demography (n)/demographic (adj)

Study of *populations*, especially their age structure and growth rates.
[ref. 2]

demyelination (n)/demyelinating (adj)

demyelinization

Destruction of the protective *myelin sheath* that surrounds *nerve* fibres, resulting in diminished function and decreased action potential in those nerves.
[ref. 4]

denaturation

1. Change in molecular structure of proteins so that they cannot function normally, often caused by splitting of hydrogen bonds, salt bridges, hydrophobic interactions, *etc.*, following *exposure* to reactive substances or heat.
2. Addition of methanol, acetone, or other suitable chemical substance(s) to ethanol to make it unfit for drinking.

[ref. 1]

dendrite

Short branched extension of a *nerve cell*, along which impulses received from other cells at *synapses* are transmitted to the cell body.
[ref. 4]
Compare *axon.*

dendritic cell

interdigitating dendritic cell
interdigitating reticular cell

Ameboid cell that is *major histocompatibility complex class II*-positive, *Fc receptor*-negative, and presents processed *antigens* to *T-cells* in the T-cell areas of *secondary lymphoid* tissues.
Note 1: Dendritic cells are potent stimulators of T-cell responses. Nonlymphoid tissues also contain dendritic cells, but these are not able to stimulate T-cell responses until they are activated.
Note 2: There are three major sublasses of dendritic cells, *conventional dendritic cells, Langerhans cells*, and *plasmacytoid dendritic cells*.
Note 3: The dendritic cell referred to in Notes 1 and 2 is a different cell type from the *follicular dendritic cell*, which is *Fc receptor*-positive.
Note 4: Some authors also distinguish myeloid and lymphoid dendritic cells based on lineage.
Note 5: Some confusion in the classification of dendritic cells may arise from systems based on function, morphology, or lineage, and possibly species differences.
[ref. 3]

dendritic cell, conventional

Predominant type of *dendritic cell* active in *antigen* presentation to and *activation* of *naïve T-cells*.
[ref. 3]

dendritic cell, follicular

Major histocompatibility complex class II-negative *Fc receptor*-positive *dendritic cell* that bears *immune complexes* on its surface and is probably involved in the generation of *antibody*-secreting cells and maintenance of *B-cell* memory (see *memory cell*) in *germinal centers*.
[ref. 3]

dendritic cell, plasmacytoid

Dendritic cell of distinct lineage, found in blood and peripheral *lymphoid tissue*, that secretes large amounts of *interferon* upon activation.
[ref. 3]

dendrogram

Tree diagram depicting relationships in a hierarchical cluster.
[*]

denitrification

Reduction of nitrates to nitrites, nitrogen oxides, or dinitrogen catalyzed by facultative *aerobic soil* bacteria under *anaerobic* conditions.
[ref. 1]

density (in ecology)

See *population density*.

density dependence (in population biology)

Variation in characteristics of individuals or of a *population* produced by changes in the *density* of the population.
Note: Density dependence may be seen, *e.g.*, in *mortality rate, birth rate, fitness, sensitivity* to environmental toxicants, transmission of *pathogens*, and parasites.
[ref. 2]

dental fluorosis

Tooth enamel malformations due to excessive fluoride *exposure* during dental development.
[ref. 1]
See also *fluorosis*.

dentate gyrus

Narrow strip of *cerebral cortex* associated with the *hippocampus* that continues forward to the *uncus*.
Note: The dentate gyrus is thought to contribute to the formation of new episodic memories, the spontaneous exploration of novel environments, and other functions.
[ref. 4]

deoxyribonucleic acid (DNA)

Constituent of *chromosome*s that stores the hereditary information of an organism in the form of a sequence of purine and pyrimidine bases.
Note: The hereditary information stored by DNA relates to the synthesis of proteins, and hence it is a determinant of all physical and functional activities of the cell, and consequently of the whole organism.
[ref. 1]

deoxyribonucleic acid (DNA) cloning

Replication of *deoxyribonucleic acid* sequences ligated into a suitable *vector* in an appropriate host organism.
[ref. 1]

deoxyribonucleic acid (DNA) repair

Restoration of the molecular structure of *deoxyribonucleic acid* after it has been damaged by a chemical or physical agent.
Note: DNA repair may involve direct DNA damage reversal, base excision repair, nucleotide excision repair, mismatch repair, or double-strand break repair.
[ref. 1]

deoxyribonucleic acid (DNA) sequencing

Determining the order of base pairs in a *deoxyribonucleic acid* molecule.
[ref. 1]

deoxyribonucleic acid (DNA) synthesis, unscheduled (UDS)

Replication of DNA during nucleotide excision repair of DNA damage.
Note: Assays of UDS with radiolabeled thymidine are used to identify potentially genotoxic substances.
[*]

dependence/dependency

See *addiction; dependence, chemical.*

dependence, chemical

drug addiction
Craving for or addiction to a substance.
[ref. 4]

dependence, physical

See *addiction.*

dependence, psychological

See *addiction.*

depilatory

Substance causing hair loss or device used for that purpose.
[*]

depolarization

Relative reduction in the resting *membrane potential* of an *excitable cell*, transiently making the inside less negative, or even positive with respect to the outside.
[ref. 4]

deposit feeder (n)/deposit feeding (v)

Animal that feeds on particles of matter in the *soil* or *sediment*, usually the topsoil or top sediment where it is filled with organic matter.
Examples: Earthworms, terebellids, fiddler crabs.
Note: Deposit feeding takes place either by ingesting soil or sediment, or by trapping particles as they fall.
[ref. 2]

deposition

1. Process by which a substance settles out of air or an aqueous solution and arrives at a particular organ or tissue site, for example, the "deposition" of particles on the ciliated epithelium of the bronchial airways.
2. Process by which a substance *sediments* out of the atmosphere or water and settles in a certain place.

[ref. 1]
See also *deposition, atmospheric; deposition, dry; deposition, wet.*

deposition, atmospheric

Process that transfers a chemical from the atmosphere to the Earth's surface (land, water, or vegetation) by either dry impingement or by transport in rain or snow.
[ref. 2]
See also *deposition; deposition, dry; deposition, wet.*

deposition, dry

Transfer of chemicals from the atmosphere to the Earth's surface not involving (wet) precipitation, such as rain, snow or hail.
[ref. 2]
See also *deposition; deposition, atmospheric; deposition, wet.*

deposition, immune complex

Precipitation of *immune complexes* in organs and tissues, often causing local *inflammation*.
Note: Immune complex deposition is a prominent feature of *systemic lupus erythematosus, cryoglobulin*emia, *rheumatoid arthritis, scleroderma*, and *Sjögren syndrome*.
[ref. 3]

deposition, wet

Transfer of substances from the atmosphere to the Earth's surface in atmospheric water precipitation (*atmospheric deposition*), *e.g.*, rain, snow, or hail.
Note: Wet deposition is a source of terrestrial *pollutants* that collect in the precipitation, attributed in some models to one of the processes of Brownian capture (random diffusion into the water droplet by Brownian motion), nucleation (of the nascent water droplet around a particulate), dissolution (of pollutant solutes into the water droplet), or impaction (of particulates with the droplet).
[After ref. 2]
See also *deposition; deposition, atmospheric; deposition, dry.*

depression (of the central nervous system)

1. Reduction in the activity of the *central nervous system.*
2. Mental state or *disorder* characterized by feelings of sadness and despair.

[ref. 4]

depuration

Loss of a substance from an organism owing to elimination and *degradation.*
Note: The rate of depuration is expressed by its *half-life* or the time needed to eliminate 50 % of the substance in a clean medium uncontaminated with the substance. This term is often referred to as the depuration time-50 (DT_{50}).
[ref. 2]

derived characteristic

Predicted property of a substance that is dependent upon, or is an approximation to, a fundamental property and the prevailing environmental conditions.
[ref. 2]

dermal

cutaneous

Pertaining to the skin.
[ref. 1]

dermal irritation

Skin reaction resulting from a single or multiple *exposures* to a physical or chemical entity at the same site, characterized by the presence of *inflammation*, that may result in cell death.
[ref. 1]
See also *corrosion.*

dermatitis

Inflammation of the skin showing redness, swelling, infiltration, scaling, and sometimes vesicles and blisters.
[ref. 3]
See also *dermatitis, contact.*

dermatitis, contact

Inflammatory condition of the skin resulting from dermal *exposure* to an *allergen* (sensitizer) or an irritating (corrosive, defatting) substance.
Note: There are three kinds of contact dermatitis, irritant, *allergic*, and *photocontact dermatitis.*
[1,3]

dermatitis, photocontact

Type of *contact dermatitis* arising when substances are transformed into either irritants or *allergens* upon exposure to light.
Note: Aftershave lotions, sunscreens, and certain topical sulfa *drugs* may be changed into allergens causing photocontact dermatitis, while coal tar and certain oils used in manufacturing may become irritants after exposure to sunlight.
[ref. 3]

dermatographism

Condition in which lightly touching or scratching the skin causes raised, reddish marks.
[*]

dermatomyositis

Disease characterized by the presence of *inflammation* of the skin and muscles.
Note: The cause of dermatomyositis is unknown, but it may be associated with a viral infection or an *autoimmune reaction,* and may also present as a paraneoplastic phenomenon (see *paraneoplastic autoimmune syndrome*).
[ref. 3]

dermis (n)/dermal (adj)

Layer of the skin deep under the *epidermis*, consisting of a bed of vascularized *connective tissue*, and containing the nerves and organs of sensation, the hair roots, and sebaceous and sweat *glands*.
[ref. 5]

descriptive epidemiology

See *epidemiology, descriptive*.
[ref. 1]

descriptive study

Study in which a phenomenon is described but no attempt is made to analyze the effects of variables on the phenomenon.
[*]

desensitization

Induction of a generally transient state of specific nonreactivity in a previously sensitized individual, resulting from repeated *antigen* exposures.
[ref. 3]
See also *sensitization*.

desiccant

Drying agent.
[*]

designer drug

Structural or functional analog of a controlled substance that has been designed to mimic the *pharmacological* effects of the original drug, while avoiding classification as illegal and (or) detection in standard drug tests.
[*]

desorption

Opposite term: *adsorption*.

Decrease in the amount of adsorbed substance.
[ref. 1]

despair test

behavioral despair test
See *swimming test; tail suspension test*.

desquamation

Shedding of an outer layer of skin in scales or sheets.
[ref. 1]

desynapsis

Failure of *synapsis* due to separation of *homologous chromosomes* after initial pairing in *meiosis*.
[ref. 5]

detergent

Cleaning or wetting agent that possesses both polar and nonpolar terminals or surfaces allowing interaction with nonpolar molecules and making them miscible with a polar solvent.
[ref. 1]
See also *surfactant*.

determinant, antigenic

Single *antigenic* site (*epitope*) usually exposed on the surface of a complex *antigen*.
[ref. 3]

determinant, biological

Property of living organisms that affects human or environmental health.
Note: Biological determinants may be either endogenous or exogenous. Endogenous biological determinants include genetic characteristics and physiological state. Exogenous biological determinants are other living organisms with which the organisms of concern interact, *e.g.*, beneficial or harmful microorganisms.
[ref. 2]

deterministic (in toxicology)

Term applied to effects, of which the extent varies with the *dose* and for which a threshold is believed to exist.
[ref. 2]
See also *deterministic effect; stochastic*.

deterministic analysis

Detailed study in which all *population* and environmental parameters are assumed to be constant and accurately specified.
[ref. 2]

deterministic effect

deterministic process

Phenomenon of commitment to a particular outcome determined by the laws of physics.
[ref. 1]
See also *stochastic effect.*

deterministic model

Mathematical model that is fully specified and does not include a *stochastic* component.
[ref. 2]

detoxification

detoxication

1. Process(es) of chemical modification that converts a substance into a less *toxic* one.
2. Treatment of patients suffering from *poisoning* in such a way as to remove the poison or to promote physiological processes that reduce the probability or severity of *adverse effects*.

[After ref. 1]

detriment

Opposite term: *benefit.*

Estimated measure of the expected harm or loss associated with an *adverse event*, usually in a manner chosen to facilitate meaningful addition over different events.
Note: Measured detriment is generally the integrated product of arbitrary values of *risk* and *hazard* and is often expressed in terms such as monetary cost, loss in expected years of life or loss in productivity; it is needed for numerical exercises such as cost–benefit analysis.
[ref. 1]

detritus

Organic debris from decomposing plants and animals.
[ref. 2]

detrivore (n)/detrivorous (adj)

Organism that survives by eating *detritus*.
[ref. 2]

developmental biology

Study of biological development from *fertilization* to *adulthood*, usually with an emphasis on the *prenatal* period and regulation of *morphogenesis*, and neural development on through adolescence.
Note: Common model organisms used in developmental biology include ***Caenorhabditis elegans, Xenopus***, ***Drosophila melaogaster***, zebrafish (***Danio rerio***), chick, and mouse.
[ref. 5]

developmental neurotoxicity

Adverse effects of *toxic* substances on the development of the *nervous system.*
[ref. 4]

developmental neurotoxicity study

Procedure in which female rodents are *exposed* to a test substance from the time of *implantation* throughout *lactation.*
Note: Offspring in a developmental neurotoxicity study may be exposed during the preweaning period, either directly or through milk, and are studied with regard to neurological and behavioral abnormalities during the *postnatal* development and until *adulthood.*
[ref. 5]

developmental neurotoxicity testing (DNT)

Any examination that allows detection of substance-induced changes in the structural or functional integrity of the *nervous system* of a developing organism, fetus or child.
[ref. 4]

developmental reference dose (RfDdt)

Reference dose determined for developmental consequences of a single, maternal *exposure* during development.
[ref. 2]

developmental stability

Potential of an organism to develop into a consistent *phenotype* in an environment.
[ref. 2]

developmental susceptibility gene

Any *gene* that encodes a *gene product* that can be altered by environmental agents to cause disturbance of normal development.
[ref. 5]

developmental toxicity

Adverse effects on the developing organism (including structural abnormality, altered growth, functional deficiency, or death) resulting from *exposure* at, or even prior to, the time of *conception*, during *gestation* (including *organogenesis*), and postnatally, up to the time of *sexual maturation* and completion of brain development.
[ref. 1]

developmental toxicology

Study of adverse effects on the developing organism that result from *exposure* of either parent to an agent or substance prior to *conception*, of the mother and *fetus* during *prenatal* development, and of the child from birth until the time development is completed.
Note: Functional brain development continues past the time of *sexual maturation.*
[ref. 5]

dextrocardia

Congenital defect in which the apex of the heart is directed toward the right side of the *thorax* (isolated dextrocardia), or the heart is found in a mirror image position on the right side of the body (dextrocardia *situs inversus*).
[ref. 5]

dextroposition

Displacement of an organ to the right of its normal position, usually applied to position in the *thorax*.
[ref. 5]

diabetes mellitus, insulin-dependent

See *diabetes mellitus type 1*.

diabetes mellitus type 1

insulin-dependent diabetes mellitus (IDDM)
juvenile diabetes
type 1 diabetes

Disease in which the β cells of the pancreatic islets of Langerhans are destroyed with the result that no insulin is produced.
Note: IDDM is believed to result from an *autoimmune* attack on the β cells. It is also known as insulin-dependent diabetes mellitus, as the symptoms can be ameliorated by injections of insulin.
[ref. 3]
See also *diabetes mellitus type 2*.

diabetes mellitus type 2

adult-onset diabetes
type 2 diabetes

Acquired *disease* in which pancreatic insulin secretion is usually increased, but tissue response to insulin is impaired because of down-regulation of insulin *receptors*, leading to insulin resistance.
Note 1: Type 2 diabetes is the leading cause of diabetes mellitus in contemporary society, with obesity and a sedentary life style being major contributing factors.
Note 2: Type 2 diabetes is a risk factor for cardiovascular disease, stroke, and renal disease.
[*]
See also *diabetes mellitus type 1; metabolic syndrome*.

diapedesis

Movement of blood cells, particularly *leukocytes*, from the blood across blood vessel walls into tissues.
[ref. 3]

diaphoresis

hidrosis

Profuse *sweating*.
[ref. 1]

diaphoretic

1. (n) sudorific. Substance inducing *sweating*.
2. (adj) Of a human, sweating heavily.

[ref. 4]

diaphragm

Dome-shaped muscular *membranous* partition separating the *thoracic cavity* from the *abdominal cavity* in mammals.
Note: The diaphragm plays a major role in breathing, as its contraction increases the volume of the *thorax* and so inflates the lungs.
[ref. 5]

diatom

Unicellular member of a major group of *eukaryotic* algae, forming chains or simple colonies, among the most common types of *phytoplankton*.
Note: Diatom cells are encased in a frustule, of widely diverse form, made of silica (hydrated silicon dioxide).
[ref. 2]

diarrheal shellfish poisoning (DSP)

diarrhetic shellfish poisoning (DSP)

Serious illness characterized primarily by diarrhea with rapid onset and resolution after 24 h that is a consequence of consumption of bivalve shellfish (molluscs) such as mussels, oysters, and clams that have ingested, by filter feeding, large quantities of dinoflagellates containing toxins.
Note: DSP toxins include a group of high-molecular-weight structures with multiple ether linkages, such as okadaic acid, dinophysis toxins, pectenotoxins, and yessotoxin.
[ref. 4]

diathesis

Hereditary predisposition to a particular medical condition.
[ref. 5]

diencephalon

Posterior part of the forebrain (*prosencephalon*), containing the *hypothalamus* and other *thalamic* components, and enclosing the third *ventricle*.
[ref. 4]
Compare *telencephalon*.

diethylstilbestrol (DES)

4,4′-[(3*E*)-hex-3-ene-3,4-diyl]diphenol

Synthetic non*steroidal* substance with *estrogen*ic activity.
Note 1: DES was formerly given to reduce the risk of complications and loss of *pregnancy* but was shown to cause a rare *vaginal tumor* in female offspring who had been exposed to this *drug in utero*.
Note 2: DES also has effects on the reproductive organs of male progeny exposed *in utero*.
[ref. 5]

differential (in hematology)

Reported blood count that distinguishes the percentages of the different blood cells present.
[ref. 3]

differential splicing

Utilization and *splicing* of different *exons* from a primary RNA transcript in order to generate different mRNA sequences.
[ref. 3]

differentiated (in biology)

Describing a *cell* or *tissue* in a state resulting from *differentiation*.
[*]

differentiation (n)/**differentiate** (v) (in biology)

Process by which a cell is committed to a lineage and becomes more specialized in structure and function.
[ref. 4]

differentiation antigen

See *antigen, differentiation*.

diffuse source

Opposite term: point source.

Release into the environment from multiple sources covering a wide area as opposed to a single release from a *point source*.
[ref. 2]

diffusion

Spontaneous differential movement of components in a system.
Note 1: In molecular terms, the driving force for diffusion is random thermal motion. In thermodynamic terms, the driving force is a gradient of chemical potential.
Note 2: *Eddy dispersion* (eddy diffusion) in the atmosphere is the process of transport of gases due to turbulent mixing in the presence of a composition gradient. Molecular diffusion is the net transport of molecules that results from their molecular motions alone in the absence of turbulent mixing; it occurs when the concentration gradient of a particular gas, liquid, or solid in a mixture differs locally from its equilibrium value. Eddy diffusion is the most important mixing process in the lower atmosphere, while molecular diffusion becomes significant at the lower pressures of the upper atmosphere.
[ref. 1,2]

diffusion, eddy

See *eddy dispersion*.

diffusion, facilitated

See *transport, facilitated*.

diffusion, exchange

Diffusion across a membrane by means of a carrier molecule that requires no energy and involves the exchange of two ions across the membrane.
[ref. 2]
See also *transport, facilitated.*

diffusion coefficient, D

Proportionality constant D, relating the *flux* (flux density) of amount of entities B, J_n, to their *concentration* gradient

$$J_n = -D\ \nabla(c_{\mathrm{B}})$$

[After ref. 2]

DiGeorge syndrome (DGS)

congenital thymic aplasia
conotruncal anomaly face syndrome
DiGeorge anomaly
Shprintzen syndrome
Strong syndrome
thymic hypoplasia
velocardiofacial syndrome

Condition caused by the deletion of a small piece of *chromosome* 22 near the middle of the chromosome at a location designated 22q11.2.
Note 1: Characteristic signs and symptoms of DGS may include *birth defects* such as *congenital* heart *disease*, defects in the *palate*, most commonly related to neuromuscular problems with closure (*velopharyngeal insufficiency*), learning disabilities, mild deviations in facial features, and recurrent infections.
Note 2: *Immunodeficiency* in DGS is caused by a congenital failure in *thymic* development resulting in a lack of mature functional *T-cells.*
[ref. 3,5]

digit span test

digit span task

Test of memory in which numbers (series of digits) are presented orally or on a computer screen to a test subject who is asked to repeat each number from memory; the numbers increase in length until mistakes are made.
Note: In the backward digit span task the presented numbers must be recalled in reverse order.
[ref. 4]
See also *neurobehavior core test battery.*

digit symbol substitution test (DSST)

digit symbol test

Neuropsychological assessment in which the top two rows of a test sheet function as a key, displaying numbers 1 to 9 (upper row) matched to "non-sense" symbols (lower row). There follow pairs of rows where the numbers 1 to 9 appear in irregular sequence and the test subject must match the correct symbol from the key to each number, as quickly as possible.
Note 1: DSST is used to assess *brain* damage, *dementia* and *depression.*
Note 2: DSST is a subtest in some intelligence tests.
[ref. 4]
See *intelligence quotient; neurobehavior core test battery.*

diluent

Substance used to perform a dilution.
[*]
See also *dilution water.*

dilution "paradigm"

Belief that pollution is alleviated by dilution.
Note: Sometimes the dilution paradigm is stated as "The solution to pollution is dilution".
[ref. 2]

dilution water
diluent

Water used to dilute the test material in an aquatic *toxicity* test in order to prepare either different concentrations of a test chemical or different percentages of an effluent for the various test treatments.
Note: The water control (see *control, negative*) in a test is prepared with dilution water only.
[ref. 2]

dimercaprol

See *British anti-Lewiste.*

diploid

Cell or nucleus containing two complete sets of *chromosomes* (present in homologous pairs), one from each parent, or an organism composed of such cells.
Note: Normal human somatic (nonreproductive) cells are diploid (they have 46 chromosomes), whereas reproductive cells, with 23 chromosomes, are haploid.
[ref. 1,5]
Compare *haploid.*

diplopia
double vision

Simultaneous perception of two images of a single object.
[ref. 4]

direct antiglobulin test (DAT)

See *Coombs test.*

direct Coombs test

See *Coombs test.*

direct ecological effect

Effect where a *stressor, e.g.*, a toxicant, acts immediately on an ecological component of interest and not through the consequences of effects on other components of the *ecosystem.*
[ref. 2]
See also *indirect ecological effect.*

directional asymmetry

See *assymmetry, directional.*

direct photolysis

See *photolysis.*

direct toxicity

See *toxicity, direct.*

disc, embryonic

blastodisc
germinal disc

Bilayer plate of cells in the *blastocyst* from which the mammalian *embryo* develops.
[ref. 5]

disc, intervertebral

spinal disc

Flat circular structure, consisting of a tough, fibrous exterior and a gelatinous core, interposed between adjacent *vertebra*e.
[ref. 4]

discharge

Release of any waste into the environment from a *point source*.
Note: Although the term "discharge" is usually applied to release of liquid waste into water, it may be applied to release of other substances into the natural environment.
[After ref. 2]
See also *effluent; emission.*

discharge standard

discharge release limit
effluent standard
emission standard

Maximum amount of a *pollutant* released from a given source to a specified medium that is acceptable under specified circumstances.
[ref. 1]

discontinuous effect

See *effect, intermittent.*

discontinuous epitope

See *epitope, conformational.*

discrimination ratio

discrimination factor

Ratio (factor) indicating the degree of isotopic selectivity by a biological organism or other environmental compartment, with a ratio of 1 indicating no selectivity.
Note: In the context of discrimination between elements such as cesium and potassium in a trophic exchange, a discrimination factor or ratio is expressed as $[Cs]_{food}/[K]_{food}$ divided by $[Cs]_{body}/[K]_{body}$.
[ref. 2]
See also *isotopic discrimination.*

discordance (genetic)

Opposite term: *concordance*.

Any difference in a characteristic between individuals due to genetic differences such as may occur in dizygotic twins, or between matched pairs in a *case cohort study*.
[ref. 1]

disease

Pathological condition that presents a unique group of symptoms identifying the condition as an abnormal entity different from other normal or pathological body states; literally, dis-ease, lack of ease.
[After ref. 1]

dishevelled

See *WnT*.

disinfectant

Any chemical or physical agent intended to inhibit or destroy *pathogenic* micro-organisms and (or) viruses.
[*]

disintegrin and metalloproteinase domain-containing protein 33 (ADAM33)

Member of the ADAM (**A** **D**isintegrin **A**nd **M**etalloproteinase domain) family of transmembrane proteins, possibly related to *asthma* susceptibility.
[ref. 3]

disorder (in medicine)

Abnormality of biological structure, function, or both.
[*]

disorientation

1. Loss of sense of direction.
2. In clinical assessment, lack of awareness of one's identity, present location, or the current day and time.

[ref. 4]

dispermy

Entrance of two *spermatozoa* into one *egg*.
[ref. 5]
Compare *monospermy; polyspermy.*

dispersant

Substance used to disperse liquid spills, *e.g.*, oil spills in water.
[ref. 2]
See also *surfactant.*

dispersion (in environmental chemistry)

Spreading and resultant dilution of a substance in a fluid medium (*e.g.*, often a *pollutant* in air or water) due to *diffusion* or turbulence.
[ref. 2]

disposition

1. Natural tendency shown by an individual or group of individuals, including any tendency to acquisition of specific *diseases*, often due to hereditary factors.
2. Total of the processes of *absorption* of a chemical into the circulatory systems, *distribution* throughout the body, *biotransformation*, and *excretion*.

[ref. 1]

disruption

Disturbance that interrupts a process or disorganizes a structure.
[ref. 5]

dissipation

Reduction in the amount of a *pesticide* or other compound that has been applied to plants, soil, or another environmental compartment.
Note: The term "dissipation" is used when it is not clear whether this reduction occurs by mineralization, *degradation*, binding, leaching, or some other process.
[ref. 1]

dissolved organic carbon (DOC)

Amount concentration of carbon found dissolved in water samples from aquatic systems, measured as total elemental carbon.
Note 1: The "dissolved" fraction of organic carbon is an operational classification: Operationally, DOC is taken to be the organic matter that is able to pass through a defined filter (filters generally range in size between 0.7 μm and 0.22 μm). Conversely, particulate organic carbon (POC) in water is that carbon that is too large and is filtered out of a sample.
Note 2: The DOC in marine and freshwater systems is part of the greatest *cycled* reservoir of organic matter on Earth and consists mostly of humic substances.
Note 3: DOC is important in the transport and bioavailability of *pollutants* in aquatic systems.
Note 4: Metals may form strong complexes with DOC, increasing metal solubility and concentration in water, while also reducing metal *bioavailability*.
[ref. 2]
See also *dissolved organic matter*.

dissolved organic matter (DOM)

Analogous to *dissolved organic carbon*, but refers to the entire organic pool dissolved in water.
[ref. 2]

dissolved oxygen content (DOC)

Amount concentration of oxygen dissolved in water at a particular temperature and pressure.
Note: Dissolved oxygen content can be a limiting factor on the growth of aquatic *populations*.
[ref. 2]

distal (in anatomy)

Opposite term: *proximal*.

Situated away from the centre of the body or from the point of attachment.
[ref. 5]

distributed source

See *area source.*

distribution

1. Apportionment of a solute between two phases. The terms "partition" or "extraction" may also be used in this sense where appropriate.
2. Dispersal of a substance and its derivatives throughout the natural environment or throughout an organism.
3. Final location(s) of a substance within an organism after dispersal.

[ref. 1]

distribution (in statistics)

Set of numbers and their frequency of occurrence collected from measurements over a statistical *population.*
[ref. 2]

distribution constant

See *partition ratio.*

distribution volume

Theoretical volume of a body *compartment* throughout which a substance is calculated to be distributed.
[ref. 1]

disturbance (in ecology)

Event that introduces, removes, or redistributes organisms, changing the colonization potential of a given environment.
[ref. 2]

diuresis

Production of urine by the kidney, especially in excess.
[ref. 1]

diuretic
micturitic

Agent that increases urine production and elimination.
[ref. 1]

diversity

Quality of consisting of many different entities, forms, kinds, or individuals.
[ref. 2]

diversity (D) gene

Small segment of *immunoglobulin heavy-chain DNA* or *T-cell receptor DNA* between the *variable (V) gene* and *joining (J) gene* segments, coding for the third hypervariable region of the receptors.
[ref. 3]
See also *V(D)J recombination.*

diversity index

Mathematical descriptor of *species* variation within a *community*.
Note: All *diversity* indices are based on the relative *abundance* of a species, *i.e.*, the sum of all individuals of that species divided by the sum of all individuals in the community of interest.
[ref. 2]
See also *Brillouin index; Simpson's diversity index; Shannon–Wiener diversity index.*

diverticulum

Outpouching of a hollow structure in the body, that may be acquired (as in colonic diverticulitis) or be present at *birth.*
Examples: Meckel diverticulum (small intestine), Zenker diverticulum (pharynx).
[After ref. 5]

Dobson unit

Unit describing the ozone content of the Earth's atmosphere over a specified area of the Earth's surface, in increments of the amount of pure ozone at standard temperature and pressure (0 °C, 101 kPa (1 atm)), in a volume having the same area and a thickness of 0.01 mm.
Note 1: Atmospheric ozone content in Dobson units is usually measured by the absorption of UV radiation at the Earth's surface.
Note 2: The Dobson unit is sometimes referred to in terms of numbers of molecules. One square centimeter of pure ozone with a thickness of 0.01 mm (volume 10^{-9} m^3) contains 2.69×10^{16} molecules at standard temperature and pressure.
[ref. 2]

domain (in molecular biology)

Recognized structural element of a biological polymer, *e.g.*, a polypeptide or nucleic acid.
[*]

dominant

Opposite term: *recessive.*

Of a *gene*, determining the *phenotype* even when present only in one copy or inherited from only one parent, *i.e.*, when present in either the homozygous or the heterozygous state.
[ref. 1,5]

dominant half-life

See *half-life, dominant.*

dominant lethal mutation

See *mutation, dominant lethal.*

domoic acid

(2*S*,3*S*,4*S*)-4-[(2*Z*,4*E*,6*R*)-6-carboxyhepta-2,4-dien-2-yl]-3-(carboxymethyl)pyrrolidine-2-carboxylic acid

Neurotoxic kainic acid analog produced by some algal blooms that causes *amnesic shellfish poisoning.*
Note 1: Filter-feeding shellfish become contaminated with domoic acid by trapping and eating these algae.

Note 2: Domoic acid is produced by the red alga called doumoi in Japan (***Chondria armatasome***), diatoms of the genus ***Pseudo-nitzschia***, and by some strains of the diatom species ***Nitzschia navis-varingica***.
[ref. 4]

dopamine (INN)

4-(2-aminoethyl)benzene-1,2-diol

Naturally occurring substance functioning as a *neurotransmitter* in the *sympathetic nervous system*, and a *metabolic* precursor of other substances including *adrenaline*.
Note: Dopamine has an effect on movement and its depletion in the *brain* produces the symptoms of rigidity, *tremors*, and *bradykinesia* that are characteristic of *Parkinson disease*.
[ref. 4]

dopaminergic

Relating to a nerve that releases or responds to *dopamine* as a *neurotransmitter*.
[ref. 4]

dorsal

Opposite term: *ventral*.

On or relating to the upper side or back of an organism.
[ref. 5]

dorsal root

posterior root of spinal nerve

Outgrowth of a spinal *nerve* that carries sensory signals to an appropriate integration centre in the *brain*.
[ref. 4]

dorsal root ganglion

Nodule on a *dorsal root* of the *spine* that consists of *afferent* sensory *neuronal* cell bodies.
[ref. 4]
See also *ganglion*.

dosage

Dose (of substance) divided by product of mass of organism and time of dose.
Note 1: Dosage is often expressed as mg (kg body weight)$^{-1}$ day^{-1}.
Note 2: The word "dose" itself is sometimes used as a synonym for dosage.
[ref. 1]

dose (of radiation)

Energy imparted by any form of radiation to a specified volume of matter during a specified *exposure* time divided by the mass of that volume.
[After ref. 1]
Note: In the SI system, the units are joules per kilogram and designated grays (Gy). In the USA, the CGS unit rad is sometimes used but this is deprecated.
[*]

dose (of substance)

Total amount of a substance administered to, taken up, or absorbed by an organism, organ, or tissue.
[ref. 1]
See also *dosage*.

dose, absorbed (of radiation)

See *dose (of radiation)*.

dose, absorbed (of a substance)
internal dose

Amount of a substance taken up by an organism or into organs or tissues of interest.
[ref. 1]
See also *absorption, systemic*.

dose, benchmark

Statistically calculated lower 95 % confidence limit on the *dose* that produces a defined *response* (called the *benchmark response* or BMR, usually 5 % or 10 %) of an *adverse effect* compared to background, often defined as 0 % or 5 % (respectively).
[ref. 1]
See also *benchmark response*.

dose, cumulative

Total *dose* resulting from repeated *exposures* or continuous exposure to a substance or to radiation over a defined time.
[ref. 2]

dose, effective (ED)

Dose of a substance that causes a defined magnitude of *response* in a given system after a specified *exposure* time; *e.g.*, dose that affects x % of a test *population* after a given time (ED_x).
[ref. 2]
See also *dose, median effective*.

dose, median effective

Statistically derived median *dose* of a chemical substance or physical agent (*e.g.*, radiation) expected to produce a certain effect in 50 % of test organisms in a given *population* or to produce a half-maximal effect in a biological system under a defined set of conditions.
Note: ED_n refers to the median dose that is effective in n % of the test population.
[ref. 1]

dose, reference (RfD)

Estimate, with uncertainty spanning perhaps an order of magnitude, of a daily oral exposure to the human population (including sensitive subgroups) that is likely to be without an appreciable risk of deleterious effects.
Note: RfD also takes into account susceptible populations.
[*]

dose–effect

Relation between *dose* and the magnitude of a measured biological change.
[ref. 1]

dose–effect curve

Graph of the relation between *dose* and the magnitude of the biological change produced measured in appropriate units.
[ref. 1]

dose–effect relationship

Association between *dose* and the resulting magnitude of a change, either in an individual or in a *population*.
[ref. 1]

dose–response curve

Graph of the relation between *dose* and the proportion of individuals in a *population* responding with a defined biological effect.
[ref. 1]

dose–response relationship

Association between *dose* and the *incidence* of a defined biological effect in an *exposed population* usually expressed as percentage.
[ref. 1]

dot plot

Two-dimensional graphical representation of individual data points.
[ref. 3]

double diffusion

See *Ouchterlony technique*.

double-negative cell

Immature T-cell in the *thymus* that lacks expression of the two *coreceptors, CD4* and *CD8*.
Note: Double-negative cells represent about 5 % of *thymocytes* in a normal *thymus*.
[ref. 3]

double-positive cell

Immature T-cell in the *thymus* that is characterized by expression of both *CD4* and *CD8 coreceptor* proteins.
Note: Double-positive cells represent the majority (80 %) of *thymocytes* in a normal *thymus*.
[ref. 3]
See also *pre-T-cell*.

doubling time

Estimated time required for a *population* of living organisms to double its size; it is estimated from the intrinsic rate of increase, r, as $(\ln 2)/r$.
[ref. 2]

Down syndrome

See *trisomy 21*.

drainage basin

Area of land where water from rain, snow melt, or ice drains downhill into a body of water, such as a river, lake, dam, *estuary, wetland*, sea, or ocean.
Note 1: A drainage basin includes the streams and rivers that convey the water as well as the land surfaces from which water drains into those channels, separated from adjacent basins by a drainage divide.
Note 2: A drainage basin acts like a funnel, collecting all the water within the area covered by the basin and channeling it into a waterway. Each drainage basin is separated topographically from adjacent basins by a ridge, hill, or mountain, which is known as a water divide.
Note 3: Terms related to drainage basin include catchment, catchment area, catchment basin, drainage area, river basin, water basin, and watershed.
[ref. 2]

draining lymph node

Lymph node that is downstream of a site of infection and thus receives *antigens* and microbes from the site via the *lymphatic system.*
Note: Draining lymph nodes often enlarge enormously during an *immune response* and can be palpated; they were formerly called "swollen glands".
[ref. 3]

Draize test

1. (ocular) Test for potential to cause irritation to the eye in which the test substance is applied directly to the eye of restrained rabbits.
   Note: The ocular Draize test is widely criticized as unethical. Now it is often replaced with an acute eye irritation test using cadaveric chicken eyes.
2. (dermal) Test for the potential of a material to cause irritation or *corrosion* following local dermal application, generally performed with rabbits.

[ref. 3]

drug
medicine
pharmaceutical

Any substance that, when absorbed into a living organism, may modify one or more of its functions.
Note: The term "*drug*" is generally accepted for a substance taken for a *therapeutic* purpose, but is also commonly used for *abused* substances.
[ref. 1]

drug-induced autoimmunity

See *autoimmunity, drug-induced.*

drug-induced lupus

See *lupus, drug-induced.*

drug-metabolizing enzyme (DME)

Any enzyme that *metabolizes xenobiotics.*
Note: Most if not all *drug*-metabolizing enzymes also metabolize endogenous *substrates.*
[ref. 5]

dry deposition

See *deposition, dry*.

duct

Vessel for transporting fluids such as *lymph*, or *glandular* secretions such as tears or bile.
[ref. 5]

duct, excurrent

See *excurrent*.

ductus arteriosis

Fetal blood vessel connecting the *pulmonary artery* to the *proximal* descending *aorta*.
Note: The ductus arteriosis allows most of the blood from the right *ventricle* to bypass the fetus's fluid-filled nonfunctioning lungs. Upon closure at *birth*, it becomes the *ligamentum arteriosum*.
[ref. 5]
See also *patent ductus arteriosis*.

dung fly test
Dipterian dung fly test

Procedure using dung flies of the order ***Diptera*** where a test substance is mixed with bovine feces to which *eggs* of the fly are added; number, sex, and morphology are determined when the last *adult* has emerged.
[ref. 5]

duodenum

First portion of the small intestine, between the stomach and the *jejunum*, where bile and pancreatic digestive juices enter the intestinal tract.
[ref. 5]

duplicate portion sampling method (of diet/food)
duplicate diet study

Study in which test persons consume their ordinary diet but, for each meal, they prepare for subsequent analysis a duplicate portion of all food as prepared, served, and consumed.
[ref. 1]

duplicate samples

Two *samples* taken under the same or comparable conditions.
[ref. 1]
See also *replicate sampling*.

dura mater

Outermost and most fibrous of the three membranes of the meninges (see *meninx*) covering the *brain* and the *spinal cord*.
[ref. 4]

dust

1. (in air) Sum of particles in the air, originating from many different sources, such as incineration, exhausts, volcanic ash, plant pollen, and other sources.
2. (on surfaces) Particles that have sedimented on to surfaces such as furniture and floors. House dust is usually rich in particles such as textile *filaments* and skin particles.

Note 1: When inhaled, large dust particles sediment in the upper airways and may then be cleared without evidence of harm. Very small dust particles are carried into the deep airways, where they may contribute to lung injury.
Note 2: House dust is a source of exposure by contact or *inhalation*, and from *hand-to-mouth* activity, especially in toddlers.
[*]

dynamic energy budget (DEB) theory

Theory that simple quantitative rules may be applied to define the organization of metabolism of individual organisms.
Note: In DEB theory, "dynamic" refers to changes in energy budgets in relation to the individual *life cycle*. The theory includes stoichiometric constraints and mass balance equations, *allometric* relationships, organizational uncoupling of *metabolic* modules, strong and weak *homeostasis*, and partitionability of reserve kinetics.
[ref. 2]

dynamic stability hypothesis (in ecology)

Hypothesis that long *food chains* are less stable than short ones.
[ref. 2]

dynamically fragile community

Community that is stable for only a very limited range of environmental characteristics, *e.g.*, a stable and predictable environment with respect to *predator*–prey ratios or disturbances caused by humans.
[ref. 2]
See also *dynamically robust community*.

dynamically robust community

Community that is stable within a wide range of conditions, *e.g.*, in very variable and unpredictable environments.
[ref. 2]
See also *dynamically fragile community*.

dynein

Protein associated with motile structures that exhibits adenosine triphosphatase activity; it forms "arms" on the outer microtubules of cilia and flagella and functions as a molecular motor.
Note: Dyneins are involved in *axonal transport* and are targets of various *neurotoxic* substances.
[ref. 4]

dynorphin

Member of a class of *opioid* peptides that arise from the precursor protein prodynorphin.
Note 1: When the dynorphin precursor, prodynorphin, is cleaved during processing by proprotein convertase 2 (PC2; EC 3.4.21.94), multiple active peptides are released: dynorphin A, dynorphin B, and α/β-neo-endorphin.

Note 2: *Depolarization* of a *neuron* containing the dynorphin precursor, prodynorphin, stimulates PC2 processing, which occurs within *synaptic vesicles* in the *presynaptic* terminal.
[ref. 4]

dysaphia

Impairment of the sense of touch.
[ref. 4]

dysarthria

Imperfect articulation of speech owing to disturbances of muscular control resulting from *central* or *peripheral nervous system* damage or emotional stress.
[ref. 4]

dyscrasia

See *blood dyscrasia.*

dysesthesia

1. Condition in which a disagreeable sensation, especially of touch, is produced following damage to peripheral or central sensory pathways.
2. Abnormal sensation experienced in the absence of stimulation.

[ref. 4]

dysfunction

Abnormal, impaired, or incomplete functioning of an organism, organ, tissue, or cell.
[ref. 1]

dysgenesis

Defective or abnormal development of an organ.
[ref. 5]

dysgonesis

Dysgenesis of the *gonads.*
[ref. 5]

dysgraphia

Difficulty in writing.
[ref. 4]

dyskinesia

Difficulty or abnormality in voluntary movement.
[ref. 4]

dyskinesia, tardive

Involuntary, repetitive body movement of slow onset.
Note: Tardive dyskinesia may be induced by *drugs* such as chlorpromazine.
[ref. 4]

dyslexia

Impairment in appreciation of spatial relations, often leading to difficulty in reading.
[ref. 4]

dysmenorrhea

Difficult and painful *menstruation.*
[ref. 5]

dysmorphia (n)/dysmorphic (adj)
dysmorphism

Abnormality of shape of a body part or organ, often referring to a *birth defect.*
[ref. 5]

dysmorphogenesis

Production of *dysmorphia.*
[ref. 5]

dysostosis

Defect in the normal *ossification* of *fetal cartilage.*
[ref. 5]

dysphagia

Difficulty in swallowing.
[ref. 4]

dysphasia

Difficulty in the use of language owing to a *brain* lesion, without mental impairment.
[ref. 4]
See also *aphasia.*

dysplasia

Abnormal development of an organ or tissue identified by *morphological* examination.
[ref. 5]

dyspnea

Difficulty in breathing; shortness of breath.
[ref. 4]

dysreflexia, autonomic (AD)

Over-activity of the *autonomic nervous system* causing an abrupt onset of excessively high blood pressure, *tachycardia*, and constriction of peripheral blood vessels.
[ref. 4]
Compare *hyperreflexia.*

dystonia

State of abnormal (either hypo- or hypertonic) muscle tone resulting in impairment of voluntary movement.
[ref. 4]

early life stage (ELS) test

Toxicity test using an organism in an early life stage such as the *embryo* or *larva*, noting that this stage is often the most sensitive part of the species *life cycle*.
[ref. 5]

earthworm reproduction test

Procedure in which *adult* worms (usually the redworm ***Eisenia fetida***)) are *exposed* to a test substance mixed into the soil; number, weight and behaviour of the adult worms are studied after four weeks and the number of juveniles hatched is counted after a further four weeks.
[ref. 5]

eclampsia

Acute, life-threatening complication of *pregnancy* characterized by tonic-clonic *seizures* (*convulsions*), usually in a woman who has developed *pre-eclampsia*.
[ref. 5]

ecogenetics (n)/ecogenetic (adj)

Study of the influence of hereditary factors on the response of individuals or *populations* to environmental factors.
Note: Examples of ecogenetic phenomena are the effects of *cytochrome P450* polymorphisms on cancer risk, and the mechanisms of development of pesticide resistance in insects and metal tolerance in plants.
[ref. 2]

ecological character

Sum of biological, physical, and chemical components of an *ecosystem* and their interactions that maintain the ecosystem, and its products, functions, and attributes.
[ref. 2]
See also *ecology*.

ecological energetics

Study of the flow of energy within an *ecological* system from the time the energy enters the system until it is irretrievably lost from the system as heat.
Note: Ecological energenetics is also referred to as production ecology, because ecologists use the word "production" to describe the process of energy input and storage in *ecosystems*.
[ref. 2]

ecological epidemiology

See *epidemiology, ecological*.

ecological imbalance

State of instability resulting from a pertubation of any biological, physical, or chemical components of an *ecosystem*, or in their interactions, that results in change in ecological character and its functions and attributes.

Comprehensive Glossary of Terms Used in Toxicology
By John Duffus, Douglas M. Templeton and Michael Schwenk

Published by the Royal Society of Chemistry, www.rsc.org

[After ref. 2]
See also *species imbalance.*

ecological magnification

See *biomagnification.*

ecological mortality

ecological death

Diminution of *fitness* of an individual functioning within an *ecosystem* that is of a magnitude sufficient that its contribution to the ecosystem becomes negligible.
[After ref. 2]

ecological parameter

Measurable variable whose value is a determinant of the characteristics of an *ecosystem*.
[ref. 2]

ecology (n)/ecological (adj)

Branch of biology that studies the interactions between living organisms and all factors (including other organisms) in their environment.
Note: Ecological interactions include those with environmental factors that determine the distributions of living organisms.
[ref. 1]

ecology, human

Interrelationship between humans and the entire environment – physical, biological, socioeconomic, and cultural – including the interrelationships between individual humans, among groups of humans, and among humans and groups of other species.
[ref. 1]
See also *ecology*.

ecology, industrial

Study of the flows of materials and energy in the manufacturing sector, and the effects of these flows on natural *ecosystems.*
[ref. 2]

ecophysiology

Study of physiology and tolerance limits of *species* that enhances understanding of their distribution in relation to abiotic conditions.
[ref. 2]

ecoregion

bioregion

1. Any of a number of regions into which a continent, country, or other geographical region, can be divided according to its distinct environmental conditions and *habitat* types.
2. Large area of land or water with a characteristic, geographically distinct assemblage of natural communities and species comprising a recurring pattern of *ecosystems* associated with characteristic combinations of *soil* and landform.

[ref. 2]

ecosphere

See *biosphere.*

ecosystem

Grouping of organisms (microorganisms, plants, animals) interacting together, with, and through their physical and chemical environments, to form a functional entity within a defined environment.
[ref. 1]

ecosystem, experimental

Manmade construction intended to simulate a natural environment.
[ref. 2]
See also *limnocorral; littoral enclosure; mesocosm; microcosm.*

ecotone

Area of gradual transition between two or more *ecosystems.*
[ref. 2]
See also *edge effect.*

ecotoxicologically relevant concentration (ERC)

environmentally relevant concentration (ERC)
Concentration of a *pesticide* (active ingredient, formulations, and relevant metabolites) that is likely to affect a determinable ecological characteristic of an *exposed* system.
[ref. 1]

ecotoxicology

Study of the *toxic* effects of chemical and physical agents on all living organisms, especially on populations and communities within defined *ecosystems*; it includes transfer pathways of these agents and their interactions with the environment.
[ref. 1]

ectoderm

In an *embryo*, outermost layer that develops into the *epidermis* of the skin and the nervous system.
[ref. 5]
See also *bilaminar embryo; epiblast.*

ectohormone

Hormone secreted into an individual organism's immediate environment to affect the physiology or behavior of other organisms.
[*]
See also *pheromone.*

ectoparasiticide

Substance intended to kill parasites living on the exterior of the host.
[ref. 1]

ectopia (n)/**ectopic** (adj)
ectopy

Abnormal location or malpositioning of an organ, tissue or body part, usually *congenital.*
[ref. 5]

ectopic expression

Expression of a *gene* in a tissue in which it is not normally expressed.
[ref. 5]

ectopic pregnancy

Complication of *pregnancy* in which the *embryo* implants (see *implantation*) and develops outside the *cavity* of the *uterus.*
[ref. 5]

ectotherm (n)/**ectothermal** (adj)/**ectothermic** (adj)

Organism dependent on external sources of heat to maintain their body temperature. Note: Ectotherms, together with *poikilotherms*, are sometimes referred to as "cold-blooded" organisms, although actually their body temperature is determined by the ambient temperature.
[*]
See also *endotherm; heterotherm; homeotherm; poikilotherm.*

ectothermy

Thermal regulation of an organism's body temperature dependent on external sources of heat.
[*]
See also *endothermy; heterothermy; homeothermy; poikilothermy.*

ectrodactyly
lobster-claw deformity
cleft hand
split hand

Congenital absence or deficiency of one or more of the central digits of the hand or foot.
[ref. 5]

ectrosyndactyly

Congenital absence or deficiency of one or more of the central digits of the hand or foot with fusion of the existing ones.
[ref. 5]

eczema
dermatitis

Acute or chronic skin *inflammation* with *erythema*, papules, vesicles, pustules, scales, crusts, or scabs, alone or in combination, of varied or unknown *etiology.*
[ref. 1]

edaphic

Pertaining to the *soil.*
[ref. 2]

eddy diffusion

See *eddy dispersion.*

eddy dispersion

eddy diffusion

1. Process by which substances are mixed in the atmosphere or in any fluid system due to *eddy motion.*
   See also *diffusion, Note 2.*
2. Irregularity in the diffusion of solute molecules that occurs in a porous chromatographic support.

Note: The phenomenon of eddy dispersion is due to the fact that (a) the path lengths of some solute molecules are either shorter or longer than those of most of the molecules, and (b) the rate of solvent flow varies in different regions of the porous support.
[ref. 2]

eddy motion

Movement in a current of water or air, that is contrary to the direction of the main current, especially in a circular motion, leading to irregularity in the motion of molecules.
[ref. 2]

edema

dropsy
oedema

Presence of abnormally large amounts of fluid in body *cavities* and intercellular spaces of *tissues.*
[ref. 5]

edema, hereditary angioneurotic

Clinical name for a genetic deficiency of the *C1 inhibitor* of the *complement system.*
Note: Absence of C1 inhibitor in hereditary angioneurotic edema can result in spontaneous activation of the complement system, causing diffuse fluid leakage from blood vessels, the most serious consequence of which is epiglottal swelling leading to suffocation.
[ref. 3]

edge effect (in ecology)

Influence of the closeness of contrasting environments on an *ecosystem*, seen at boundaries between natural *habitats*, especially forests and disturbed or developed land.
Note 1: Edge effects lead to changes in *species* richness and *population* size at the boundary between two *communities*, most pronounced in smaller habitat fragments.
Note 2: Because of edge effects, *ecotones* often have species assemblages with high *species richness* and high *abundance* of individuals relative to those of the adjacent communities.
[ref. 2]

effect (in toxicology)

Reaction (often adverse) resulting from *exposure* to a substance or agent, whether on the molecular, cellular, tissue, organ, systemic or *population* level.
[*]
See also *response.*

effect, acute

Effect of finite duration occurring rapidly (usually in the first 24 h or up to 14 d) following a single *dose* or short *exposure* to a substance or radiation.
Note: Acute effects may occur continuously following continuous dosing or repeatedly following repeated dosing.
[ref. 1]

effect, additive

Consequence that follows *exposure* to two or more physicochemical agents that act jointly but do not interact: The total effect is the simple sum of the effects of separate exposures to the agents under the same conditions.
[ref. 1]

effect, bystander (in immunology)

Positive or negative effect on the *immune system* seen after exposure to certain *drugs*, radiation, and other agents, induced by nonimmune mechanisms.
[ref. 3]
See also *bystander suppression*.

effect, cumulative

Overall change that occurs after repeated *doses* of a substance or radiation.
[ref. 1]

effect, edge

See *edge effect (in ecology)*.

effect, intermittent (in biology)

discontinuous effect
Biological change that comes and goes at intervals.
[ref. 1]

effect biomarker

See *biomarker of effect*.

effect time (ET)

Time taken for a substance to produce a precisely defined effect.
Note: Effect time is often expressed as ET_{50}, the median time it takes for a *toxicant* to produce a precisely defined effect in 50 % of a *population*.
[ref. 2]

effective concentration (EC)

See *concentration, effective*.

effective dose (ED)

See *dose, effective*.

effective half-life (k_{eff})

See *half-life, effective*.

effector cell

See *cell, effector.*

effects assessment

dose–response assessment
toxicity assessment

Component of *risk assessment* concerned with quantifying the manner in which the frequency and intensity of effects increase with increasing *exposure* to a contaminant or other source of stress.
[ref. 2]

efferent

Opposite term: *afferent.*

Carrying outward; of *nerves*, those that conduct impulses outward from the *central nervous system.*
[ref. 4]

efferent duct

efferent ductule

Seminal duct leading from the *testis* to the head of the *epididymis.*
[ref. 5]

efferocytosis

Engulfment and removal of dying or dead cells by *phagocytic* cells.
Note: Efferocytosis is especially important in the safe removal of *apoptotic* cells by engulfment of intact apoptotic bodies.
[*]

effluent

Fluid, solid, or gas discharged from a given source into the external environment.
[ref. 1]

egg

Female *gamete* after completion of the second *meiotic* division.
Note: The term "egg" is often loosely applied to secondary *oocytes* and early *embryos.*
[ref. 5]
See also *ovum; zygote.*

ejaculation

Expulsion of *semen* from the *genital ducts* and *urethra*, usually resulting from a reflex process during sexual stimulation.
[ref. 5]
Note: In common, nontechnical usage, ejaculation refers to a sudden verbal exclamation.
[*]

ejaculatory duct

Passage formed by the junction of the duct of the *seminal vesicles* and the *ductus deferens* through which *semen* enters the *urethra.*
[ref. 5]

elasticity (community)

Ability of a *community* to return to its prestressed condition.
[ref. 2]

electrocardiogram

Recording of the electrical activity of the heart, or its representation as a visual display or audible signal, using electrodes attached to the skin over the *thorax* and limbs.
[*]

electroconvulsive therapy (ECT)

electroshock therapy

Therapeutic intervention in which *seizure*s are electrically induced in patients with the aim of providing relief from a specific mental illness.
[ref. 4]

electroencephalogram

Test or record of *brain* electrical activity detected by *electroencephalography*.
[ref. 4]

electroencephalography (EEG)

Recording of electrical activity from different parts of the *brain*.
[ref. 4]

electromyography (EMG)

Recording of the electrical activity of muscle, or its representation as a visual display or audible signal, using electrodes attached to the skin or inserted into a muscle.
[ref. 4]

electron transport chain

Molecular assembly that transfers electrons through a series of redox reactions, establishing a proton gradient across a *membrane* that can be dissipated, with the energy being harnessed to synthesize *ATP* or to produce heat.
Note 1: Electron transport chains are found in the *cell membrane* of bacteria, in the inner *mitochondrial* membrane of *eukaryotes*, and in the thylakoid membrane of photosynthetic organisms.
Note 2: *Uncouple*d heat production is an essential, tightly regulated, part of the physiology of warm blooded animals.
[*]
See also *uncoupling*.

electroneurography

Noninvasive method used to examine the integrity and conductivity of a *peripheral nerve*, in which a brief electrical stimulation is given to the nerve at one point, while at the same time the induced electrical activity (compound *action potential*s) is recorded at another point of the nerve's distribution and the interval is displayed on a video monitor.
[ref. 4]

electrophysiology

Study of the electrical properties of cells and tissues.
[ref. 4]

electroporation

Means of introducing molecules into cells by transiently permeabilizing their *membranes* with brief electric field pulses.
[ref. 5]

electroretinogram (ERG)

Recording, with electrodes placed on the cornea or nearby skin, of the electrical activity of *photoreceptors* and other retinal cells in response to standardized, patterned stimuli with light and colour.
[ref. 4]

element (in chemistry)

1. Species of atoms; all atoms with the same number of protons in the atomic nucleus.
2. Pure chemical substance composed of atoms with the same number of protons in the atomic nucleus. Note: Sometimes this concept is called the elementary substance as distinct from the chemical element as defined under 1, but mostly the term chemical element is used for both concepts.

[ref. 8]

element, abundant

Chemical element that is of common occurrence in the Earth's crust.
Note: An abundant element may be so defined in terms of its *abundance* in regions other than the Earth's crust, *e.g.*, oceans.
[ref. 2]

element, essential

See *nutrient, essential.*

element, response (in molecular genetics)

Nucleotide sequence in the promoter region of a *gene* that regulates expression of that *gene* through interaction with a *transcription factor*.
[After ref. 1]

element, trace (in biology)

1. Chemical element required in very small quantities by an organism to maintain health.
   Note: Use of the term trace element in this sense is meaningless unless it is specified which biological organism is referred to.
2. Chemical element present in body fluids or compartments near the detection limits of standard analytical techniques.

[After ref. 2]
See *trace nutrient.*

element, trace (in geology)

Element having an average concentration in a given sample of less than about 100 atoms per million atoms (100 ppm) or less than 100 $\mu g\ g^{-1}$.
[ref. 2]

elevated plus maze

See *maze, elevated plus.*

elicitation (in immunology)

Production of a cell-mediated or *antibody*-mediated *allergic* response by exposure of a sensitized individual to an *allergen.*
[ref. 3]
See also *cell-mediated immune response.*

elimination (in toxicology)

Disappearance of a substance from an organism or a part thereof, by processes of *metabolism, secretion*, or *excretion.*
[ref. 1]
See also *clearance.*

elimination half-life

See *half-life, elimination.*

elimination rate

Differential with respect to time of the *concentration* or amount of a substance in the body, or a part thereof, resulting from *elimination.*
[ref. 1]

eliminator (of a poison)

Substance that contributes to the *elimination* of a *poison* from an organism.
[ref. 1]

elutriate

Aqueous solution obtained after adding water to a solid substance (*e.g., sediment*, tailings, drilling mud, or dredging spoil), shaking the mixture, then separating the solid from the solution.
[After ref. 2]

elutriate test

Test in which a non*benthic* biological *species*, such as ***Daphnia magna***, is *exposed* to an *elutriate* produced by mixing a test *sediment* with water and then separating the solids from the solution.
Note 1: The elutriate test was developed for evaluating the water-soluble constituents potentially released from sediment into open water during dredge disposal operations.
Note 2: When applying an elutriate test in *estuarine* studies, gradients of salinity must be taken into account.
[After ref. 2]

elutriation

Process of separating the lighter particles of a powder from the heavier ones by means of an upward directed stream of fluid (gas or liquid).
[ref. 2]

embolus

Thrombus that detaches from its site of formation to migrate elsewhere in the cardiovascular system, potentially causing occlusion and *infarction.*
[*]
See also *embolism; thromboembolus.*

embolism (n)/embolic (adj)

Occlusion of a blood vessel, *e.g.*, by detachment of a *thrombus* that leaves its site of origin in the vasculature and travels to occlude a vessel elsewhere, by another entity such as an air bubble.
Note: Embolism is associated with *infarction. Brain* embolism is a major cause of *stroke.*
[*]
See also *thromboembolus.*

embryo (n)/embryonic (adj)

1. Stage in the developing mammal at which the characteristic organs and organ systems are being formed: for humans, this involves the stages of development from the second to the eighth week post*conception* (inclusive), or to the end of *organogenesis.*
2. In birds, the stage of development from the *fertilization* of the *ovum* until hatching.
3. In plants, the stage of development within the seed.

[ref. 5]

embryo, bilaminar

bilaminar blastoderm

Early *blastula* having only two of the three primary *germ layers* that it will ultimately have; the two layers present are the cells of the *epiblast* (that will give rise to the *ectoderm*) and those of the *hypoblast* (that will become the *endoderm*) during *gastrulation* - both attached to a *basement membrane* before the *mesoderm* has formed.
[ref. 5]

embryo, trilaminar

trilaminar blastoderm

Disc-like *embryonic* stage in which differentiation into the three *endoderm, mesoderm,* and *ectoderm* layers has occurred.
Note: In the human, the trilaminar embryo occurs in the third week following the onset of *gastrulation.*
[ref. 5]

embryo transfer

Process of *implanting* a *fertilized ovum* into a *uterus.*
[ref. 5]

embryo transport rate analysis

Method to evaluate the potential for early *embryonic* loss in rodents caused by accelerated or retarded arrival of embryos into the *uterus.*
[ref. 5]

embryogenesis

Development and growth of an *embryo* in the period from formation of the *bilaminar embryo* to the beginning of the *fetal* period (in humans, the second through the eighth week after *conception*).
[ref. 5]

embryoid body

Structure resembling an *embryo* that is formed by *embryonic stem cells* or *teratocarcinoma* cells when they are removed from a growth-promoting medium.
[ref. 5]

embryology

Study of the origin and development of the organism from *fertilization* of the *oocyte* to the beginning of *fetal* life (in humans, the end of the eighth week).
Note: In common usage this term "embryology" includes all the stages of *prenatal* life.
[ref. 5]

embryonic induction

Process whereby the development of one group of cells, called the competent region, is altered by an inducing factor from another group, called a signaling center or organizer.
[ref. 5]

embryonic period

Period from *fertilization* to the end of major *organogenesis*.
[ref. 5]
See also *embryo; embryogenesis*.

embryonic stem (ES) cell

Undifferentiated, *pluripotent* cell from an early stage of the pre*implantation embryo* (inner cell mass of the *blastocyst*).
Note 1: ES cells have the potential to proliferate and differentiate into various cell types of the body.
Note 2: ES cells can be genetically manipulated in tissue culture and then inserted into mouse blastocysts to generate mutant lines of mice; often genes are deleted in ES cells by homologous recombination and the mutant ES cells are then used to generate gene *knockout mice*.
Note 3: ES cells may also be used to *clone* organisms.
[3,5]

embryotoxicity (n)/embryotoxic (adj)

1. Production by a substance of *toxic* effects in the *embryo*.
2. Any *toxic* effect on the *conceptus* as a result of *exposure* during the embryonic stages of development.

Note: Embryotoxic effects may include malformations and variations, malfunctions, altered growth, prenatal death, and altered postnatal function.
[ref. 1]

embryotropic effect

Change in the *embryo* and the regulation of its development.
[ref. 1]

emergent properties

New properties that appear with upward steps in hierarchical systems, such as ecological *communities* or *ecosystems*, and that cannot be predicted solely from our limited understanding of the system's parts or components.
Note: Emergent properties arise during the self-organization of complex systems and are the product of the evolution of these systems.
[ref. 2]

emesis

Vomiting.
[ref. 1]

emetic

1. (n) Substance that produces vomiting.
2. (adj) Producing vomiting.

[ref. 4]

emission

discharge
effluent
release

Release of a substance from a source, including a discharge into the wider environment.
[ref. 1]

emission and exposure control

Technical and administrative procedures and specifications applied for the monitoring, reduction, or *elimination* of *emissions* from a source or *exposure* to a target.
[ref. 1]

emission standard

Quantitative limit on the *emission* or discharge of a substance from a source, usually expressed in terms of a time-weighted average *concentration* or a *ceiling value*.
[ref. 1]

emphysema

Lung *disease*, usually chronic, characterized by a widening of the lower airways, fusion of the alveoli, and progressively decreasing *pulmonary* gas exchange.
[*]

emulsifier

Chemical substance that aids the fine mixing (in the form of small droplets) of an otherwise hydrophobic substance with water.
[ref. 2]
See also *dispersant*.

encephalitis

Inflammation of the *brain*.
[ref. 4]

encephalocele

See *meningoencephalocele.*

encephalopathy

Any *disorder* of the *brain* that affects its functioning.
Note: Common causes of encephalopathy include trauma, infection, liver failure, anoxia, kidney failure, or exposure to a *neurotoxin.*
[ref. 4]

endemic

Present in a community or among a group of people; said of a *disease* prevailing continually in a region.
[ref. 1]

endemism

Ecological state of being restricted to a place.
Note: There are two subcategories of endemism—paleoendemism and neoendemism.

- Paleoendemism refers to a species that was formerly widespread but is now confined to a smaller area.
- Neoendemism refers to a species that has recently arisen, *e.g.*, by hybridization (see *hybrid*) and is now classified as a separate species. This is a common process in plants, especially those that exhibit *polyploidy*.

[ref. 2]

endocardial cushion
atrioventricular canal cushion

Subset of cells in the primordial tube-like heart that is essential to the development of the *ventricular septum* and the *atrioventricular* valves of the heart.
Note: Endocardial cushion defects may cause various types of heart *malformation.*
[ref. 5]

endocardium

Endothelial lining of the heart chambers, also containing small blood vessels and a few bundles of smooth muscle, continuous with the endothelium of the great blood vessels.
[ref. 5]

endochondral ossification

Formation and growth of bone tissue (especially of the long bones) during *fetal* development of the mammalian skeletal system, and in repair of bone fractures, that takes place in the presence of *cartilage.*
Note: Endochondral ossification is one of two mechanisms for bone formation, the other being *intramembranous ossification.*
[ref. 5]

endocon

Portion of a *conjugated* metabolite that is derived from a natural product (such as a sugar, amino acid, or other organic acid) of the metabolizing organism.
[ref. 1]
See also *exocon; phase II reaction.*

endocrine

Pertaining to *hormones* or to the glands that secrete hormones directly into the bloodstream.
[ref. 1]

endocrine disrupter

endocrine modifier

Exogenous substance that, at some dose, alters function(s) of the *endocrine* system and consequently causes adverse health effects in an intact organism, its progeny, or (sub)populations.
[ref. 5]

endocrine modifier

See *endocrine disrupter.*

endocytosis

Opposite term: *exocytosis.*

Cellular ingestion of macromolecules, often *receptor*-bound ("receptor-mediated endocytosis") by invagination of *plasma membrane* to produce an intracellular vesicle that encloses the ingested material.
[After ref. 3]
See also *phagocytosis; pinocytosis.*

endogenous

Opposite term: *exogenous.*

Produced within or caused by factors within a biological organism.
[ref. 1]

endometrium

Inner lining of the *uterus* that is shed during *menstruation.*
[ref. 5]

endonuclease

Enzyme that cleaves the phosphodiester bond of a polynucleotide such as *DNA.*
[*]
See also *restriction endonuclease.*

endoplasmic reticulum (ER)

Intracellular complex of membranes in which proteins and lipids, as well as molecules for export, are synthesized and in which the *biotransformation* reactions of the monooxygenase enzyme systems occur.
Note 1: Based on its appearance under the electron microscope, the endoplasmic reticulum is divided into rough ER and smooth ER. Rough ER is studded with *ribosomes* that, along with those free in the cytoplasm, are the site of protein synthesis in the cell. Smooth ER lacks ribosomes and carries out other metabolic functions such as synthesis of lipids, phospholipids and *steroids.*
Note 2: Endoplasmic reticulum may be isolated as *microsomes* following cell fractionation procedures.
[ref. 1]

endoplasmic reticulum stress

ER stress

unfolded protein response (UPR)

Highly conserved cellular stress response resulting from a disturbance of normal endoplasmic reticulum (ER) physiology, due the presence of misfolded protein in the ER *lumen* that triggers cellular repair mechanisms, or, alternatively, *apoptosis*.

Note: Misfolding in the process of protein synthesis and modification occurs continually at a slow rate, but can be increased during ER stress by factors such as hypoxia and hyperoxia, loss of Ca^{2+} *homeostasis*, and excess lipid accumulation.

[*]

endorphin

Portmanteau formed from endogenous morphine-like substance, referring to one of several peptides (including the *enkephalins*) that activate the body's *opiate receptors*, causing an *analgesic* effect.

[ref. 4]

See also *enkephalin.*

endosome

Intracellular smooth surfaced vesicle in which endocytosed (see *endocytosis*) material passes on its way to the *lysosomes*.

[ref. 3]

endothelium (n)/endothelial (adj)

Layer of flat cells that line the blood vessels, lymphatic vessels, and the chambers of the heart.

[ref. 5]

endotherm (n)/endothermal (adj)/endothermic (adj) (in biology)

Organism that regulates its body temperature to be almost constant.

Note: Sometimes endotherms are referred to as "warm-blooded".

[After ref. 2]

See also *ectotherm; heterotherm; homeotherm; poikilotherm.*

endothermy

Thermal regulation of an organism that maintains almost constant body temperature by appropriate control of metabolism in relation to heat loss to, or heat gain from, the surrounding environment.

[*]

See also *ectothermy; heterothermy; homeothermy; poikilothermy.*

endotoxin

Pathogenic lipopolysaccharide that forms an integral part of the cell wall of certain Gram-negative bacteria and is released only upon breakdown of the bacterial cell.

Note: Endotoxins elicit fever and an immune response and do not form *toxoids*.

[*]

See also *exotoxin.*

endpoint (of toxicity)

Objective of measurement of a *toxicity* test.
Note: Endpoints of toxicity vary with the level of biological organization being examined and may include changes in biochemical markers or enzyme activities, mortality or survival, growth, reproduction, primary production, and changes in structure, *abundance*, and function in a community.
[ref. 2]

endpoint assessment

Quantitative or quantifiable expression of the parameter considered to be at *risk* in a *risk analysis*.
[After ref. 2]

enhancement (in immunology)

See *immune enhancement*.

enhancing antibody

See *antibody, enhancing*.

enkephalin

Either of two endogenous pentapeptides with *opiate*-like *effects* that are especially involved in modulating *pain* responses in the *central nervous system*.
[ref. 4]
See also *endorphin*.

enrichment factor (EFcrust)

anthropogenic enrichment factor

Measure of natural or *anthropogenic* enrichment in defined *environmental* samples of an *element* above natural levels in the Earth's crust.
Note 1: EF_{crust}, denoted more correctly as $E_{f\ (crust)}$, is an element's concentration ($C_{element}$) measured in a sample divided by the its concentration expected in the Earth's crust. For example, in the equation $E_{f\ (crust)} = [C_{element}/C_{aluminium}]_{sample}/[C_{element}/C_{aluminium}]_{crust}$, both sample and crustal concentrations are normalized with respect to aluminium concentrations.
Note 2: Alternatively, normalization with respect to iron may be used in the EF_{crust} calculation. Recent studies have shown that iron may be a better predictor than aluminium for background *trace element* levels.
[ref. 2]

enteritis

Intestinal *inflammation*.
[ref. 1]

enterohepatic circulation

Cyclical process involving intestinal re*absorption* of a substance that has been excreted through the bile, followed by transfer back to the liver, making it available for biliary *excretion* again.
[ref. 1]

enterotoxin

Toxin affecting intestinal cells and thus causing food poisoning.
Note: Enterotoxins stimulate many types of *T-cells* by binding to *major histocompatibility complex class II molecules* and the Vb domain [see *variable (V) domain*] of certain *T-cell receptors*. Enterotoxins have thus been referred to as *superantigens*.
[ref. 3]

environment (n)/environmental (adj)

Aggregate, at a given moment, of all external conditions and influences to which a system under study is subjected.
[ref. 1]

environmental assessment (EA)

Short, preliminary assessment of potential environmental harm used to determine if a full *environmental impact statement* is required.
[ref. 2]

environmental availability

See *availability, environmental.*

environmental bioavailability

See *bioavailability, environmental.*

environmental damage

Adverse effects to the natural environment.
[ref. 1]

environmental epidemiology

See *epidemiology, environmental.*

environmental exposure level (EEL)

Level (*concentration* or amount or a time integral of either) of a substance to which an organism or other component of the environment is *exposed* in its natural surroundings.
[ref. 1]

environmental factor

Physical, chemical, or biological agent or condition in the environment that has the potential to affect development and health of an organism, either in a positive or a negative manner.
[ref. 5]

environmental fate

Destiny of a chemical or biological *pollutant* after release into the natural environment.
[ref. 1]

environmental health

Human welfare and its influence by the environment, including technical and administrative measures for improving the human environment from the point of view of *health.*
[ref. 1]

environmental health impact assessment

Estimate of the *risks* or *adverse effects* to *health* likely to follow from a proposed or expected environmental change or development.
[ref. 1]
See also *environmental impact assessment.*

Environmental Health Criteria document

Any one of the critical publications of the International Program on Chemical Safety (IPCS) containing reviews of methodologies and existing knowledge - expressed, if possible, in quantitative terms - of selected substances (or groups of substances) on identifiable, immediate, and long-term effects on human *health* and welfare.
[ref. 1]

environmental hygiene
environmental sanitation

Practical control measures used to improve the basic environmental conditions affecting human *health*, for example, clean water supply, human and animal *waste* disposal, protection of food from biological contamination, and housing conditions, all of which are concerned with the quality of the human environment.
[ref. 1]

environmental impact assessment (EIA)

Appraisal of the possible environmental consequences of a past, ongoing, or planned action, resulting in the production of an environmental impact statement or *finding of no significant impact.*
[ref. 1]
See also *environmental health impact assessment.*

environmental impact statement (EIS)

Report resulting from an *environmental impact assessment.*
[ref. 1]

environmental medicine

Specialty devoted to the prevention and management of environmentally induced injury, illness, and disability, and the promotion of the health of individuals, families, and communities by ensuring a healthy environment.
[ref. 1]

environmental monitoring

Continuous or repeated measurement of agents, and (or) *biological indicators*, and (or) *biomarkers* in the environment to evaluate environmental *exposure* and possible damage by comparison with appropriate reference values based on knowledge of the probable relationship between *ambient* exposure and resultant adverse effects.
[ref. 2]

environmental protection

1. Actions taken to prevent or minimize *adverse effects* to the natural environment.
2. Complex of measures designed to protect the evironment, including monitoring of environmental *pollution*, development and practice of environmental protection principles (legal, technical, and hygienic), as well as *risk assessment, risk management*, and *risk communication.*

[ref. 1]

environmental quality objective (EQO)

Overall state to be aimed for in a particular aspect of the natural environment, for example, "water in an estuary such that shellfish populations survive in good *health*". Note: Unlike an *environmental quality standard*, the EQO is usually expressed in qualitative and not quantitative terms.
[ref. 1]

environmental quality standard (EQS)

ambient standard

Amount *concentration* or mass concentration of a substance that should not be exceeded in an environment, often expressed as a *time-weighted average* measurement over a defined period.
[ref. 1]
See also *limit value*.

environmental risk analysis

See *risk analysis, environmental.*

environmental risk assessment

See *risk assessment, environmental.*

environmental sanitation

See *environmental hygiene.*

environmental security

United Nations concept of global environmental well-being, threatened by relative instability of Earth's natural *ecosystems* as a consequence of human activity, most notably i) global climate change caused by human release of greenhouse gas; ii) deforestation caused by so-called "clearing" of lands; or iii) *soil* depletion and desertification caused by intensive monoculture techniques.
[*]

environmental tobacco smoke (ETS)

See *sidestream smoke.*

environmental transformation

See *transformation, environmental.*

environmentally relevant concentration

See *ecotoxicologically relevant concentration.*

environmental transport

See *transport, environmental.*

enzootic

Present in a *community* or among a group of animals; term applied to a *disease* prevailing continually in a region.
[ref. 2]

enzymatic

Referring to a process or reaction that is catalyzed by an *enzyme*.
[*]

enzyme

Protein, nucleic acid, or a *conjugate* of a protein with another compound (coenzyme), that acts as a biological catalyst.
[ref. 1]

enzyme induction

Process whereby an *enzyme*'s expression is increased in response to a specific substance or to other agents.
Examples: Induction of *ctochrome p450* by phenobarbital, induction of stress response genes by *oxidative stress*, induction of *heat shock proteins*.
[After ref. 1]

enzyme-linked immunosorbent assay (ELISA)

Procedure for detection or quantitation of an *antibody* or *antigen* using a *ligand* (*e.g.*, an anti*immunoglobulin*) *conjugated* to an enzyme that changes the color of a substrate.
Note: There are two kinds of ELISAs:

- In a "competitive" ELISA performed with a fixed amount of immobilized antigen, the amount of labeled antibody bound decreases as the concentration of unlabeled antigen is increased, allowing quantification of unlabeled antigen.
- In a "sandwich" ELISA performed with a fixed amount of one immobilized antibody, the binding of a second, labeled antibody increases as the concentration of antigen increases, allowing quantification of antigen.

[ref. 3]
See also *enzyme-linked immunospot assay; immunosorbent.*

enzyme-linked immunospot (ELISPOT) assay

Adaptation of the *enzyme-linked immunosorbent assay* in which cells are placed over *antibodies* or *antigens* attached to a plastic surface.
Note: In ELISPOT, the immobilized antigen or antibody traps the cells' secreted products, which can then be detected using an enzyme-coupled antibody that cleaves a colorless substrate to make a localized colored spot, allowing quantitation of the number of cells producing a given product such as a *cytokine*.
[ref. 3]

eosinophil

Circulating granular *leukocyte* (*granulocyte*) having prominent granules that stain specifically by eosin and containing numerous *lysosomes*.
Note 1: Eosinophils are important effector cells in immune reactions to *antigens* that induce high levels of *immunoglobulin E antibodies* (*e.g.*, parasites).
Note 2: Eosinophils are also abundant at sites of *immediate-type hypersensitivity* reactions.
[ref. 3]

eosinophil chemotactic factor of anaphylaxis (ECF-A)

Cytokine that facilitates *anaphylaxis* and attracts *eosinophils* during substrate release by *mast cells*.
[ref. 3]

eotaxin
CCL11

CC chemokine that acts predominantly on *eosinophils*.
[ref. 3]

epaxial

Located above or on the *dorsal* side of an axis.
[ref. 5]

ependymal tissue

Glial cells that line the cavities within the *brain*'s *ventricle*s.
[ref. 4]

ependymoma

Growth in the *brain* or *spinal cord* arising from *ependymal tissue*.
Note: Because *cerebrospinal fluid* normally flows through the ependymal tissue-lined *ventricle*s, blockage due to an ependymoma can cause build up of fluid, increased *intracranial pressure*, and *hydrocephalus*.
[ref. 4]

epibenthic

Living on the bed of an aquatic system, normally on *sediment*.
[ref. 2]
See also *benthic; epifaunal; infaunal; nektonic*.

epiblast

Primitive *ectoderm* of the early *embryo*.
[ref. 5]

epicardium
visceral pericardium

Inner layer of the *pericardium*, a sac of fibrous tissue that surrounds and lies upon the heart and the base of the great vessels.
[ref. 5]

epidemiology (n)/epidemiological (adj)

Study of the distribution and determinants of *health* and *disease* states or events in specified populations, and the application of this study to the prevention and management of health-related problems.
[ref. 1]

epidemiology, descriptive

Study of the occurrence of *disease* or other *health*-related characteristics in populations, including general observations concerning the relationship of disease to basic characteristics such as age, sex, race, occupation, and social class; and is also concerned with geographical location and time trends.
[ref. 1]

epidemiology, ecological

Application of *epidemiological* methods to determine the cause, incidence, prevalence, and distribution of adverse effects in nonhuman *species* inhabiting contaminated sites.
Note: Ecological epidemiology is frequently associated with retrospective ecological *risk assessment*.
[ref. 2]
See also *risk assessment, retrospective*.

epidemiology, environmental

Subdiscipline of human epidemiology concerned with *diseases* caused by chemical, physical or biological agents in the environment.
[ref. 2]

epidemiology, genetic

Study of the correlations between phenotypic trends and genetic variation across population groups, and the application of the results to control and management of human health.
[After ref. 1]

epidemiology, molecular

Use in *epidemiological* studies of techniques of molecular biology such as DNA profiling and genetic analysis, with the aim of detecting genetic patterns characteristic of susceptible populations or of groups at risk of *disease*.
[ref. 5]

epidermis (n)/epidermal (adj)

In *vertebrates*, protective outer stratified squamous layer of the skin consisting mainly of keratinocytes.
[ref. 5]

epidermolysis bullosa

Group of inherited skin *diseases* characterized by the development of blisters following minimal pressure to the skin.
Note: Very rarely, epidermolysis bullosa can be life-threatening.
[*]
See also *Stevens-Johnson syndrome; toxic epidermal necrolysis*.

epididymis (n)/epididymal (adj)

Tightly-coiled, thin-walled tube that conducts *sperm* from the *testis* to the *vas deferens*.
[ref. 5]

epididymal appendix
appendix epididymidis

Cystic structure sometimes found on the head of the *epididymis*.
Note: The epididymal appendix represents a remnant of the *mesonephric duct*.
[ref. 5]

epidural

extradural

Immediately outside the *dura mater*.
[ref. 4]

epifauna (n)/epifaunal (adj)

Animals that live on the surface of *soil* or of the bed of an aquatic system, normally on *sediment*.
[ref. 2]
Compare *benthic, epibenthic*.
See also *infauna*.

epigastric

Pertaining to the upper-middle region of the abdomen.
[ref. 5]

epigenesis (n)/epigenetic (adj) (in biology)

Phenotypic change in an organism brought about by alteration in the *expression* of genetic information without any change in the *DNA genomic* sequence itself.
Note: Common examples of epigenesis include changes in nucleotide base methylation and changes in histone acetylation. Changes of this type may become heritable.
[ref. 1]

epigenetic (in geology)

Describing a deposit of later origin than the rocks among which it occurs.
[ref. 2]

epilepsy

Chronic neurological *disorder* marked by sudden recurrent episodes of sensory disturbance, loss of *conscious*ness, or *convulsions*, associated with abnormal electrical activity in the *brain*.
[ref. 4]

epileptiform

Occurring in severe or sudden spasms, as in *convulsion* or *epilepsy*.
[ref. 1]

epinephrine

See *adrenaline*.

epiphyseal plate

The disk of *hyaline cartilage* between the metaphysis and the epiphysis of an immature long bone that permits the bone to grow longer.
[ref. 5]

episodic

Discontinuous.
[ref. 1]

epispadias

Malformation in which the *urethra* does not develop to full length, opening typically on the dorsum of the penis (and rarely, in females, between the *clitoris* and labia); frequently associated with *exstrophy* of the bladder.
[ref. 5]

epistasis

Situation in which the *phenotypic expression* of one *gene* obscures the phenotypic effects of another gene.
[ref. 5]

epithalamus

Dorsal part of the *diencephalon*, including the *pineal gland* and adjacent structures in the roof of the third *ventricle*.
[ref. 4]

epithelial-to-mesenchymal transition (EMT)

Sequence of events, where *epithelial* cells detach, migrate and become *mesenchymal stem cells* that can differentiate.
Note: The EMT plays a role in *embryogenesis*, wound healing and *cancer*.
[ref. 5]
See also *mesenchymal-to-epithelial transition.*

epithelioma

Any tumor derived from *epithelium.*
[ref. 1]

epithelium (n)/epithelial, epithelioid (adj)

Sheet of one or more layers of cells covering the internal and external surfaces of the body and hollow organs.
[ref. 1]

epitope

Part of a molecule recognized by an *antibody antigen receptors* on *T-cells* or *B-cells* (T-cell epitopes or B-cell epitopes).
Note: A macromolecule can contain many different epitopes, each capable of stimulating production of a different specific *antibody*.
[ref. 3]
See also *antigenic determinant.*

epitope, conformational

discontinuous epitope

Epitope on a protein *antigen* formed from several separate regions in the primary sequence of a protein brought together by protein folding.
[ref. 3]
See also *epitope, linear.*

epitope, cryptic

Epitope that cannot be recognized by a *lymphocyte receptor* until the *antigen* has been broken down and processed or modified by *hapten* binding.
[ref. 3]

epitope, immunodominant

Epitope in an *antigen* that is preferentially recognized by *T-cells*, which then come to dominate the *immune response*.
[ref. 3]

epitope, linear

continuous epitope

Antigenic determinant that is contiguous in the amino acid sequence of a protein and therefore does not require the protein to be folded into its native conformation for *antibody* to bind.
[ref. 3]
See also *epitope, conformational*.

epitope retrieval

antigen retrieval

Treatment of denatured *antigen* with heat or other agents in order to regenerate (unmask) lost *antibody* binding capacity.
[ref. 3]

epitope spreading

Increase in the number of *epitopes* targeted by *autoantibodies* and/or *T cells*. The epitopes may be on the same *autoantigen* (intramolecular epitope spreading) and/or on other autoantigens (intermolecular epitope spreading).
Note: Epitope spreading is a characteristic sign of progression of *autoimmune disease* from initial activation to a chronic state.
[ref. 3]

epizootic

Outbreak of disease in a nonhuman *population* or in a large number of individuals of a *species*.
[After ref. 2]
See also *zoonosis*.

epoxide hydrolase

epoxide hydratase

Detoxification enzyme (EC 3.3.2.9), located mainly in the endoplasmic reticulum, that hydrolyzes epoxides, converting them to metabolites that can be more rapidly excreted.
[ref. 5]

Epstein–Barr virus (EBV)

Virus responsible for infectious mononucleosis and Burkitt lymphoma.
Note: The Epstein-Barr virus is used to immortalize human *B-lymphocytes* in vitro.
[ref. 3]

equilibrium/equilibria (pl)

State of a system in which the defining variables (temperature, pressure, chemical potential) have constant values in time.
Note: In a chemical reaction at equilibrium, the rates of forward and backward reactions are equal and the sum of the chemical potentials of the reactants and products is zero, *i.e.*, $\Delta G_r = \Delta G_r^0 - RT\ln K = 0$.
[*]

equilibrium partitioning (EqP)

Tendency for a substance to achieve the same chemical activity (fugacity) in different compartments of a complex system.
[ref. 2]

equilibrium partitioning (EqP) approach

Approach to estimating the fate of chemicals in the aquatic environment that is based on *equilibrium partitioning*.
Note: In practical application of the EqP approach to predict the partitioning of a substance of interest between sediment and aquatic organisms, the activities of the substance are approximated as its concentrations, normalized to organic carbon content of the sediment and to the lipid content of the aquatic organisms. These normalized *biota-sediment accumulation factor* values are considered to be independent of particular sediments and species.
[After ref. 2]

equivalence (in immunology)

Ratio of *antibody* to *antigen* at which *immunoprecipitation* of the reactants is virtually complete.
[ref. 3]

equivalence zone (in immunology)

Range of concentrations of *antigen* and *antibody* in which neither is in significant excess in a *precipitin* reaction.
[ref. 3]

equivalent diameter (of a particle)

Diameter of a spherical particle of the same density as a particle under investigation that, relative to a given phenomenon or property, would behave in the same way as the particle under investigation.
[ref. 1]

erectile dysfunction

Inability of a male to have or to maintain an erection.
[ref. 5]

ergotism

St Anthony's fire
ignis infernalis
ignis sacer

Poisoning produced by eating food contaminated by ergotamine alkaloids (ergot) produced by the fungus ***Claviceps purpurea*** growing on rye and wheat.
Note: Ergotism typically results in *hallucinations*, *headache*, vomiting, diarrhea, a painful burning sensation in the limbs and extremities, and gangrene of the fingers and toes.
[ref. 4]

erythema

Redness of the skin produced by congestion of the capillaries.
[ref. 1]

erythroblast

See *normoblast.*

erythroblastosis

Abnormal presence of *normoblasts* in the blood.
[*]

erythroblastosis fetalis

See *hemolytic disease of the newborn.*

erythrocyte

Red blood cell.
[ref. 3]

erythropoiesis

Erythrocyte production.
[ref. 3]

erythropoietin

Glycoprotein hormone that stimulates the production of *erythrocytes* from *stem cells* in *bone marrow.*
Note: Erythropoietin is produced mainly by the kidneys and is released in response to decreased levels of dioxygen in body tissue.
[ref. 3]

eschar

Slough or dry scab on an area of skin that has been burnt.
[ref. 1]

essential element

See *nutrient, essential.*

essential metal

See *nutrient, essential.*

essential nutrient

See *nutrient, essential.*

estimated daily intake (EDI)

Prediction of the daily *intake* of a potentially harmful substance based on the most realistic estimation of its *concentration* in food, and the best available food consumption data for a specific population.
Note: In deriving an EDI, substance concentrations are estimated taking into account known uses of the substance, the range of contaminated commodities, the proportion of a commodity likely to contain the substance, and the quantity of home-grown or imported commodities; and are often expressed in mg of a substance for a person.
[After ref. 1]

estimated environmental concentration (EEC)

expected environmental concentration (EEC)
predicted environmental concentration (PEC)

Predicted *concentration* of a substance, typically a *pesticide*, within an environmental *compartment* based on estimates of quantities released, discharge patterns, and inherent *disposition* of the substance (fate and distribution), as well as the nature of the specific receiving *ecosystems*.
[ref. 1]

estimated exposure concentration (EEC)

predicted exposure concentration (PEC)

Measured or calculated amount or mass *concentration* of a substance to which an organism is likely to be *exposed*, considering *exposure* by all sources and routes.
[ref. 1]

estimated exposure dose (EED)

Measured or calculated *dose* of a substance to which an organism is likely to be *exposed*, considering *exposure* by all sources and routes.
[ref. 1]

estimated maximum daily intake (EMDI)

See *maximum daily intake, estimated.*

estradiol

17β-estradiol

Steroid sex *hormone*, involved in many regulatory processes, but most prominently in the development of female sex organs, the *menstrual cycle*, and *pregnancy*.
[ref. 5]

estriol

Hormonally active metabolite of *estradiol*, eliminated in urine, especially during *pregnancy*.
[ref. 5]

estrogen

Any substance, natural or synthetic, that exerts the *hormonal* effects of the natural *estrogen, estradiol*, usually by interaction with the estrogen *receptor*.
Note: Phytoestrogens are substances that occur in plants and have estrogenic activity.
[ref. 5]
See also *endocrine disruptor*.

estrogen activity assay, in vitro

1. Test using estrogen-sensitive cells to evaluate estrogenic activity of a substance or environmental sample.
2. Procedure in which a *tumor* cell line is *exposed* to a test substance and activation of the *estrogen receptor* is studied by a reporter molecule in order to assess the estrogen-*sensitivity* of the tumor.

[ref. 5]
Compare *uterotrophic assay*.

estrogen-mimetic

Behaving like an *estrogen*.
[ref. 5]

estrogenic

Exhibiting *hormonal* activity similar to that of an *estrogen*.
[ref. 5]

estrogenism

See *clover disease*.

estrous cycle

Sequence of recurring (*cyclic*) physiological *uterine, ovarian*, and other changes, induced by reproductive *hormones* in female higher animals, resulting in readiness for *insemination*.
Note 1: The estrous cycle starts in *adulthood* (at *menarche*), transiently discontinues during *pregnancy*, and disappears at the *menopause*.
Note 2: Not to be confused with *estrus*.
[ref. 5]

estrus

oestrus
heat

Recurrent period of sexual receptivity and arousal in the female of most mammals except the higher primates, during which *conception* is possible.
Note: Not to be confused with *estrous cycle*.
[ref. 5]

estrus syndrome

Persistent *estrus* caused by elevated *estrogenic* activity, either due to endogenous estrogens (*e.g.*, in *polycystic ovary syndrome*) or due to exogenous substances.
Note: Estrus syndrome is associated with *infertility*.
[ref. 5]

estuary (n)/estuarine (adj)

1. Tidal mouth of a great river, where the tide meets the current of freshwater.
2. Tidal opening, inlet, or creek through which the tide enters; arm of the sea indenting the land. Rare in modern use.

Note 1: An estuary is often associated with sedimentation of material from terrestrial runoff.
Note 2: An estuary is often associated with a high rate of biological productivity.
[ref. 2]

etiologic(al) agent

Factor contributing to the cause of a *disease*.
[ref. 2]

etiology

aetiology

1. In individuals, the cause or origin of *disease*.
2. Science dealing with the cause or origin of disease.

[ref. 1]

euglobulin

Member of a class of proteins insoluble in water but soluble in saline solutions.
[ref. 3]

eukaryote (n)/eukaryotic (adj)

Cell or organism with well-developed cell organelles, having its genetic material enclosed in a membrane-bounded, structurally discrete nucleus, and in mitochondria or chloroplasts when present.
Note: The term "eukaryote" includes all organisms except archaebacteria, eubacteria, and cyanobacteria (until recently classified as ***Cyanophyta*** or blue-green algae).
[ref. 1]
See also *prokaryote*.

Euler–Lotka equation

Equation used to estimate the intrinsic rate of population growth from life-table data.
[ref. 2]

euphoria (n)/euphoric (adj)

Characterised by or feeling intense excitement and happiness.
[ref. 4]

euploid

Referring to a cell or organism with *chromosome*s present in an integral multiple of the *haploid* number.
Note: A human cell with the normal number of 46 chromosomes, an integral multiple of the monoploid number, 23, is thus euploid. However, a human with abnormal, but integral, multiples of this full set (*e.g.*, 69 chromosomes) would also be considered as euploid.
[ref. 5]
See also *diploid; haploid; polyploid*.

eutherian

Subclass of mammals having a *placenta* through which the *fetus* is nourished.
[ref. 5]

eutrophic

Describing an environment having a high concentration of nutrients.
Note: Eutrophic is usually used to describe nutrient-rich bodies of water or soil having a high or excessive rate of biological production.
[After ref. 2]
See also *eutrophication; oligotrophic*.

eutrophication

Adverse change in the chemical and biological status of a body of water following depletion of the dioxygen content caused by decay of organic matter, resulting in and from high primary production as a result of enhanced input of nutrients.
[ref. 1]
See also *eutrophic*.

eutrophy

1. State of being *eutrophic*.
2. (in medicine) Good nutrition.

[ref. 2]
See also *oligotrophy*.

eventration

herniation of intestines

Protrusion of *omentum* and/or intestine through a defect or weakness in the abdominal wall while the skin remains intact.
[ref. 5]
See also *omphalocele.*

evocation

Specific *induction* of a tissue within a developing *embryo* that results from the action of a single *hormone* or other chemical (the evocator).
[ref. 5]

evoked potential

Electrical potential that is triggered by presentation of a stimulus (somatosensory, auditory, visual) and measured with electrodes near the *nerve* or near the *brain* region in which the signal is processed.
Note: Speed, amplitude and location of the evoked potential provide information about the intactness of the response.
[ref. 4]

evoked response

Electrical potential recorded from the *nervous system* following exposure to a stimulus, as distinct from spontaneous potentials detected by *electroencephalography, electromyography*, or other *electrophysiological* recording methods.
[ref. 4]

evolution (n)/evolutionary (adj) (in biology)

Theory that all living organisms have arisen by diversification from simpler life forms during the Earth's history, especially by a process of *natural selection* of inherited and adaptive genetic traits.
[*]
See also *neo-Darwinism.*

evolution, convergent

Independent evolution of similarity between molecules or between biological *species.*
[ref. 3]

evolutionary adaptation

See *genetic adaptation.*

evolutionary tree

See *cladogram.*

excess lifetime risk

Additional or excess *risk* incurred over the lifetime of an individual by *exposure* to a *toxic* substance.
[ref. 1]

excess rate

See *rate difference.*

exhalation

Process in which the *pulmonary* airways contract, thus removing from the lungs residual air that is enriched in CO_2 and depleted of dioxygen.
Note: Exhalation is an excretory pathway not only for endogenously produced CO_2, but also for volatile *xenobiotics* (*e.g.*, solvents, *narcotics*) and volatile substances formed in the organism (*e.g.*, products of lipid peroxidation).
[*]

exchange diffusion

See *diffusion, exchange.*

exchange transfusion

Method of active *elimination* of a *toxic* substance by replacement of blood of the patient with donor blood or blood components.
[After ref. 1]

excipient

Any largely inert substance added to a *drug* to give suitable consistency or form to the drug.
[ref. 1]

excitable cell

Cell that can respond to stimuli, often by creating an electric current: muscle fibres and nerve cells are in this category.
[After ref. 4]
See also *excitation.*

excitation

State of enhanced activity of a cell, organism, or tissue that results from stimulation.
[ref. 4]
See also *excitable cell.*

excitatory post-synaptic potential (EPSP)

Referring to a more positive *membrane potential* at the *postsynaptic* side of the *synaptic cleft* that makes the postsynaptic *neuron* more likely to generate an *action potential.*
Note 1: EPSP's are commonly produced by excitatory *neurotransmitter*s such as *glutamate.*
Note 2: Postsynaptic electrical activity is in part a function of the balance of EPSP's and *inhibitory post-synaptic potential*s.
[ref. 4]

excitotoxicity (n)/excitotoxic (adj)

Pathological process by which *neurons* are damaged and killed by the overactivation of *receptors*, such as the *N-methyl-D-aspartate* (NMDA) and *2-amino-3-hydroxy-5-methyl-4-isoxazole propionate receptors,* for the excitatory *neurotransmitter glutamate*.
Note: Excitotoxins like NMDA and *kainic acid* bind to *glutamate receptors*, and can cause excitotoxicity by allowing high levels of calcium ions to enter cells, activating *enzymes* such as phospholipases, *endonucleases*, and *proteases* such as calpain which damage cell structures, including the *cytoskeleton*, membranes, and *DNA*.
[ref. 1,4]

excretion

Discharge or *elimination* of an absorbed or *endogenous* substance, or of a *waste* product, and (or) its *metabolites*, through some tissue of the body; and its appearance in urine, feces, or other products normally leaving the body.
Note 1: Excretion does not include the passing of a substance through the intestines without *absorption*.
Note 2: Excretion is sometimes misused to describe the elimination of a substance from a cell. The proper term here is *secretion*.
[ref. 1]
See also *clearance; elimination.*

excretion rate

Amount of substance and (or) its *metabolite*s that is excreted divided by a time period of *excretion*.
[ref. 1]

excurrent

Pertaining to a vessel (or opening) conveying fluid outwards.
Note: The male excurrent *ducts* are those involved in the transport, enrichment and *ejaculation* of *semen*.
[ref. 5]

exencephaly
exencephalus

Exposed *brain* resulting from failure of the neural tube to close and absence of the top of the skull.
Note: In humans, exencephaly is followed by degeneration of the brain, resulting in *anencephaly*.
[ref. 5]

exfoliation (n)/exfoliative (adj)
desquamation

Detachment and shedding of superficial cells of an *epithelium* or tissue surface, especially of the horny layer of the *epidermis*.
[ref. 5]

exocon

Portion of a *conjugated* metabolite that is derived from the parent molecule.
[ref. 1]
See also *endocon*.

exocrine

Relating to or denoting *glands* that secrete through *ducts* opening on to superficial *epithelium* (*e.g.*, the intestinal tract) rather than into the blood.
[ref. 5]

exocytosis
Opposite term: *endocytosis*.

Release of the content of an intracellular *vesicle* to the exterior of the cell.
Note: In exocytosis, the vesicles make their way to the *plasma membrane*, with which they fuse to permit the contents to be released to the external environment.
[ref. 3]

exogenous

Opposite term: *endogenous.*

Resulting from causes or derived from materials external to an organism.
[ref. 1]

exogenous substance

Substance arising outside the body.
[ref. 1]
See also *xenobiotic.*

exomphalos

See *omphalocele.*

exon

Coding section of a *gene* that is separated from other coding sequences of the same gene by intervening noncoding sequences (*introns*).
[ref. 1]

exophthalmia

exophthalmos

Marked protrusion of the eyeballs, usually resulting from an increased volume of the *orbital* contents.
[ref. 5]

exothelium

Layer of flattened epithelial cells external to an organ or tissue.
[ref. 1]

exotherm

See *poikilotherm.*

exotoxin

Toxin secreted by, or released upon lysis of, a bacterium.
[*]
See also *endotoxin.*

expected environmental concentration (EEC)

See *estimated environmental concentration.*

expected exposure concentration (EEC)

See *estimated environmental concentration.*

expected life span

Average length of time an organism can be expected to survive, or a substance can be expected to persist.
[ref. 2]

experimental allergic encephalomyelitis (EAE)

See *encephalomyelitis, experimental allergic.*

experimental ecosystem

See *ecosystem, experimental.*

explant

Living tissue removed from its normal environment and transferred to an artificial medium for growth.
[ref. 1]

exploitation competition

Interspecies competition in which *species* compete for some limiting resource such as food.
[ref. 2]

exponential decay

Decrease in the amount of an entity according to the equation

$$A = A_0 e^{-\lambda t}$$

where A and A_0 are the values of the entity being considered at time t and zero, respectively, and λ is an appropriate constant ($\lambda = \ln 2/t$ when $t = t_{1/2}$).
[ref. 1]

exponential growth

See *growth, exponenetial.*

exposed

Opposite term: unexposed.

Subject to a factor or agent (*e.g., toxic*, nutritional, therapeutic, *hazardous, infectious* or psychological) in the *environment.*
[ref. 1]

exposed group (in epidemiology)

Set of biological organisms that has been subjected to a substance or agent of interest.
[*]

exposome

Totality of human *environmental* (*i.e.*, nongenetic) exposures from *conception* onwards.
[*]

exposure

1. Condition, in which a substance becomes available for contact and *absorption* by the *target population*, organism, *organ, tissue*, or *cell*, by any route.
2. Amount, or intensity of a particular physical or chemical agent that reaches a *target population*, organism, *organ, tissue*, or *cell*, usually expressed in numerical terms of *concentration*, duration, and frequency (for chemical agents and microorganisms) or intensity (for physical agents).

[After ref. 1]
See also *exposure, external; exposure, internal.*

exposure, accidental

Unintended contact with a substance or change in the physical environment (including, *e.g.*, radiation).
[ref. 1]

exposure, acute

Opposite term: *chronic exposure.*

Exposure of short duration.
[ref. 1]
See also *acute.*

exposure, bystander

Liability of members of the general public to come in contact with substances arising from activities of other individuals in their vicinity.
[ref. 1]

exposure, cumulative

Total *exposure* resulting from repeated and continuous exposure to a substance or to radiation over a defined time.
[ref. 2]

exposure, external

1. *Concentration*, amount, or intensity of a particular physical or chemical agent or environmental agent that reaches the *target population*, organism, organ, tissue, or cell, usually expressed in numerical terms of concentration, duration, and frequency (for chemical agents and microorganisms) or intensity (for physical agents).
2. Process by which a substance becomes available for *absorption* by the target population, organism, organ, tissue, or cell, by any route.

[After ref. 1]

exposure, internal

Fraction of the *external exposure* dose that is absorbed by an organism and spread throughout the organism by systemic circulation, *i.e.*, the internal dose.
[*]

exposure assessment

Process of estimating and (or) measuring the amount, frequency and duration of *exposure* to an agent, of people or other organisms at risk, taking into account the sources and routes of exposure, the nature of the population exposed, and the numbers of people or organisms likely to be affected.
[*]
See also *exposome.*

exposure biomarker

See *biomarker of exposure.*

exposure characterization (in ecological risk assessment)

Description of the presence and characteristics of contact between a *contaminant* and an *ecological* entity of concern, and a summary of this information in an *exposure* profile.
[ref. 2]

exposure control

See *emission and exposure control.*

exposure–effect curve

See *concentration–effect curve.*

exposure limit

Regulatory term defining a substance *concentration* or intensity of *exposure* that should not be exceeded.
[ref. 1]

exposure pathway

Route by which an individual is exposed to a substance, including the source and point of contact.
[ref. 2]

exposure profile

Outline of the magnitude and spatio-temporal pattern of *exposure* developed during the process of *risk assessment*.
[ref. 2]

exposure ratio

In a *case control study*, value obtained by dividing the rate at which persons in the case group are *exposed* to a *risk* factor (or to a protective factor) by the *rate* at which persons in the control group are exposed to the risk factor (or to the protective factor) of interest.
[ref. 1]

exposure–response relationship

See *concentration–response relationship, dose–response relationship.*

exposure scenario

See *scenario, exposure*.

exposure surface

Surface on a *target* organism where a substance (*e.g.*, a *pesticide*) is present.
Note 1: Examples of outer *exposure* surfaces include the exterior of an eyeball, the skin surface, and a conceptual surface over the nose and open mouth in mammals.
Note 2: Examples of inner exposure surfaces include the *gastrointestinal tract*, the respiratory tract, and the lining of the urinary tract.
[ref. 1]

exposure test

1. Determination of the level, *concentration*, or *uptake* of a potentially *toxic* compound and (or) its *metabolite*(s) in biological samples (*e.g.*, blood, urine, hair) from an organism, and the interpretation of the results to estimate the absorbed *dose* or degree of environmental *pollution*.
2. Measurement of biochemical effects, usually not direct *adverse effect*s of the substance, and assessment of their relation to the quantity of substance absorbed, or to its concentration in the environment.

[ref. 1]

expressed sequence tag (EST)

Partial or full complementary *DNA* sequence that can serve as a marker for a region of the *genome* that encodes an expressed product.
[ref. 1]

expression, gene

1. Transcriptional activation of a *gene* so that its corresponding *RNA* and functional protein product are produced.
   [ref. 1]
2. Process through which a specific genotype produces its characteristic phenotype.
   [*]

exstrophy

Congenital malformation in which a hollow organ has its interior exposed through eversion; most commonly observed in the urinary bladder (ectopia vesicae).
[ref. 5]

external genitalia

Genitalia visible outside the body.
[ref. 5]

external validity

Generalizability of the results of a particular study, beyond the limits of the population actually studied.
[ref. 1]

extinction probability

Likelihood that a population will become extinct within a specified interval of time, or eventually.
Note: Very small populations have a high extinction probability; they are likely to go extinct just by chance due to *demographic stochasticity.*
[After ref. 2]

extra risk

See *risk, extra.*

extracellular matrix (ECM)

Mesh of molecules, secreted by cells into the surrounding *extracellular space.*
Note: Cells may adhere to the extracellular matrix and this can provide them with structural and biochemical support.
[ref. 5]

extracellular space
interstitial space

Volume within a tissue, outside cells, and excluding *vascular* and *lymphatic* space.
[ref. 1]
See also *interstitial fluid.*

extracellular volume

Volume of fluid outside the cells but within the outer surface of an organism.
[ref. 1]

extraction ratio

Amount of substance extracted from a source divided by the total contained within the source.
[ref. 1]

extraembryonic membrane

One of the *membranes* that surrounds the *embryo*, including the *yolk sac, allantois, amnion,* and *chorion.*
[ref. 5]

extraembryonic mesoderm

Cells outside the *embryo* that, although derived from the *zygote*, are not part of the embryo proper, and contribute to the *fetal* membranes (*yolk sac, allantois, amnion,* and *chorion*).
[ref. 5]

extraneous residue limit (ERL)

Term referring to a *pesticide* residue or contaminant arising from environmental sources (including former agricultural uses) other than the use of a pesticide or contaminant substance directly or indirectly on the commodity.
Note 1: The ERL is the maximum *concentration* of a pesticide residue or contaminant that is recommended by the *Codex Alimentarius Commission* to be legally permitted or recognized as acceptable in or on food, agricultural commodity, or animal feed.
Note 2: The mass content ERL is expressed in milligrams of pesticide residue or contaminant per kilogram of commodity.
[ref. 1]

extrapolation (in ecotoxicology)

Calculation, based on quantitative observations in *exposed* test *species* or in vitro test systems, of predicted *dose–effect* and *dose–response relationships* for a substance in the same species at other doses or in humans and other species at similar doses.
Note 1: The term "extrapolation" may be applied to predictions of such relationships in susceptible groups from knowledge of a group used for testing.
Note 2: The term "extrapolation" may also be used for qualitative information applied to species or conditions that are different from the ones in which the original investigations were carried out.
[ref. 2]

extrapolation factor

Quantity used in effect and *exposure* assessments to adjust estimated exposures or *concentrations/doses* for uncertainties, to make corrections in the data, or to improve safety.
[ref. 2]

extrapyramidal movement disorder

Frequent involuntary movements mediated by signaling through neurons of the *extrapyramidal system*, often describing side effects of psychiatric medications.
[After ref. 1]

extrapyramidal system

See *motor system.*

extravasation

Movement of cells or fluid from within blood vessels to the surrounding tissues.
[ref. 3]

extrinsic allergic alveolitis

See *pneumonitis, hypersensitivity*.

extrinsic pathway (of apoptosis)

Apoptotic pathway of cell death initiated upon occupancy of so-called death *receptors* at the cell surface with their ligands such as Fas/CD95 and tumor necrosis factor-α, and involving activation of *caspase* 8.
Note: The extrinsic pathway converges with the *intrinsic pathway* at the level of cleavage of procaspase 3 to caspase 3 (EC 3.4.22.56) by either caspase 8 (EC 4.4.22.61; extrinsic pathway) or caspase 9 (EC 3.4.22,62; intrinsic pathway).
[ref. 5]

exudate

Extravascular fluid containing proteins and cellular debris that accumulates during *inflammation*.
[ref. 3]

F1 generation

Indicating 'first filial' generation, denoting offspring from genotypically (see *genotype*) distinct parents.
Note: F2 generation denotes offspring resulting from mating (inbreeding) of individuals from the F1 generation. The term may be extended to F3 and beyond.
[ref. 5]

F2 generation

See *F1 generation*.

Fab fragment

Monovalent *antigen*-binding ('ab') fragment obtained following papain digestion of *immunoglobulin*.
Note: It consists of an intact *light chain* and the N-terminal VH and C H1 domains of the *heavy chain*.
[ref. 3]

F(ab′)2 fragment

Bivalent *antigen*-binding fragment obtained following pepsin digestion of *immunoglobulin*; consists of both *light chains* and the N-terminal part of both *heavy chains* linked by disulfide bonds.
Note: Because it lacks the *Fc fragment* it does not bind the *Fc-receptor, e.g.*, in flow cytometry.
[ref. 3]

Fas

CD95

Member of the *tumor necrosis factor receptor* gene family. Engagement of Fas on the surface of the cell by the Fas *ligand* (CD178) present on *cytotoxic* cells can trigger *apoptosis* in the Fas-bearing *target cell*.
[ref. 3]

Fc fragment

Crystallizable, non*antigen*-binding fragment of an *immunoglobulin* molecule obtained following papain digestion, consisting of the C-terminal portion of both *heavy chains*, and responsible for binding to *Fc receptors* and *complement* factor C1q.
[ref. 3]

Fc receptor

Receptor expressed on a wide range of cells, interacting with the Fc portion (see *Fc fragment*) of *immunoglobulins* belonging to various *isotypes*.
Note: *Membrane*-bound Fc receptors mediate different effector functions (*e.g., endocytosis, antibody-dependent-cellular cytotoxicity*) and induce mediator release. Both the membrane-bound and soluble forms of Fc receptors regulate *antibody* production by *B-lymphocytes*.
[ref. 3]

Comprehensive Glossary of Terms Used in Toxicology
By John Duffus, Douglas M. Templeton and Michael Schwenk

Published by the Royal Society of Chemistry, www.rsc.org

Fc region

See *Fc fragment.*

Fd fragment

Heavy chain portion of an *immunoglobulin* N-terminal to the papain hydrolysis site, after reduction and separation of the *light chain* portion.
[ref. 3]
See also *Fab fragment.*

FETAX

Assay for *teratogenicity* using *embryos* of the frog, ***Xenopus laevis***.
Note: The term "FETAX" is derived from the first letters of the words "frog embryo teratogenesis assay ***Xenopus***".
[ref. 5]

fMLP peptide

Formyl-methionyl-leucyl-phenylalanine, a chemoattractant (see *chemotactic factor; chemotaxis*) derived from *degradation* of bacterial or mitochondrial proteins that causes *neutrophil activation.*
[ref. 3]

Foxp3

Transcription repressor that is specifically expressed in *CD4+CD25+T-cells.*
Note: Mutations in the FOXP3 gene may lead to an *autoimmune* syndrome called IPEX (*immunodysregulation–polyendocrinopathy–enteropathy, X-linked*).
[ref. 3]

FUS

See *fused in sarcoma.*

Fv fragment

Variable (V) region fragment of an *antibody heavy chain* or *light chain.*
[ref. 3]

facial cleft

Congenital anomaly resulting from the failure of facial structures in the *embryo* to fuse properly.
[ref. 5]
See also *orofacial cleft.*

facies

In medicine, facial expression of an individual that is typical of a particular *syndrome, disease*, or condition.
[ref. 5]

facilitated diffusion

See *transport, facilitated.*

facilitated transport

See *transport, facilitated.*

facilitation

1. Neural facilitation: Increase in *postsynaptic excitation* as a result of very rapid firing of *action potentials* by a *presynaptic neuron.*
2. Presynaptic facilitation: Increase of *prepsynaptic* excitation when an excited *neuron* receives additional excitatory impulses from other neurons.

[ref. 4]

Fallopian tube

oviduct
uterine tube
salpinx

One of a pair of tubes, on either side of the upper or outer extremity of the *ovary* that provides a path by which an *ovum* travels from the ovary to the *fundus* of the *uterus.*
Note: Each Fallopian tube is largely enveloped by its expanded *infundibulum*, where, if the ovum is fertilized in the tube, it will implant (see *implantation*) as a *zygote.*
[ref. 5]

false negative

Type of experimental finding where the true result would indicate a positive effect of an agent, but the experimental outcome wrongly classifies the observed result as a "no effect" or negative result.
Note: Such a finding can be due to problems with the experimental method, or caused by statistical error.
[*]
See also *false positive.*

false positive

Type of experimental finding where the true result would show no effect of an agent, but the experimental outcome wrongly classifies the observed result as an effect.
[*]
See also *false negative.*

falx

falx cerebri

Continuation of *dura mater* between the right and left *hemispheres* of the *brain.*
[ref. 4]

familial cold autoinflammatory syndrome (FCAS)

Episodic *autoinflammatory disease*, induced by exposure to cold, and caused by mutations in the gene CSA1, encoding *cryopyrin.*
[ref. 3]

familial hemophagocytic lymphohistiocytosis (FHL)

Progressive and potentially lethal inflammatory *disease* caused by an inherited deficiency of *perforin.*
Note: In FHL, large numbers of *polyclonal CD8+ T-cells* accumulate in *lymphoid tissue* and other organs, and this is associated with activated *macrophages* that *phagocytose* blood cells, including *erythrocytes* and *leukocytes.*
[ref. 3]

farmer's lung

Hypersensitivity disease caused by the interaction of *immunoglobulin G antibodies* with large amounts of an inhaled *allergen,* such as hay *dust* or mold spores, in the alveolar wall of the lung, causing alveolar wall *inflammation* and compromising gas exchange.
[After ref. 3]

Farnsworth D-15 dichotomous test

Test for color blindness in which 15 distinct color chips have to be arranged in a correct order.
[*]
See also *Lanthony D-15 color test.*

fasciculation

Involuntary contractions, or twitchings, of groups (fasciculi) of muscle fibers.
Note: Fasiculation is a coarser form of repetitive muscular contraction than *fibrillation.*
[ref. 4]

fate (in ecology)

Disposition of a material in various environmental *compartments* (*e.g., soil* or *sediment*, water, air, biota) as a result of transport, partitioning, *transformation*, and *degradation.*
[ref. 2]

fatigue

Mental state characterized by weakness, sleepiness and reduced performance, often a consequence of physical exhaustion, *disease*, or chemotherapy.
Note: "Chronic fatigue *syndrome*" is a poorly defined term for a long lasting state of perceived fatigue without an identifiable cause of exhaustion or a defined underlying disease.
[ref. 4]

fatty liver
fatty liver disease (FLD)

Reversible accumulation of triglycerides in *vacuoles* in the *hepatocytes*, causing a yellowish discoloration of the liver.
Note 1: *Chronic* alcohol *abuse* is a common cause of fatty liver.
Note 2: Nonalcoholic fatty liver *disease* (NAFLD) may be associated with *metabolic syndrome* and obesity, and may be caused by certain *hepatotoxic drugs.*
[*]

feasibility study (FS)

Part of a remedial investigation that compares the various options available for *remediation* and identifies those that are practicable.
[ref. 2]

fecundation
impregnation

Process of *fertilization.*
[ref. 5]

fecundity

1. Ability to produce offspring within a given period of time.
2. Quantity of reproductive output.

Note 1: In assessing fecundity, the potential reproductive capacity of an organism or *population* may be measured by the number of *gametes* (*eggs*), number in the seed set, or number of entities of asexual propogation (*propagules*).
Note 2: Fecundity is controlled by both genetic and environmental factors, and is the major determinant of *fitness*.
[ref. 2]

fecundity selection

Component of the *life cycle* of an individual in which *natural selection* can occur, involving the production of more offspring by matings of certain *genotype* pairs than by others.
[ref. 2]

feminization

Development of female characteristics as part of normal female maturation, or, in a male, pathologically as a result of endocrine imbalance.
[ref. 5]

Fenton reaction

Fenton catalysis
Iron-catalyzed decomposition of hydrogen peroxide to generate hydroxyl, a component of the *Haber-Weiss reaction*.
Note: The Haber-Weiss and Fenton reactions are an important source of *reactive oxygen species* in cells and tissues experiencing *oxidative stress*.
[*]

feromone

See *pheromone*.

fertility

Ability of a female to conceive and to produce live offspring, and of a male to induce *conception*.
Note 1: For litter-bearing species, the number of offspring per litter is used as a measure of fertility.
Note 2: Reduced fertility is sometimes referred to as subfertility; *sperm* count and *motility* are important contributing factors to subfertility in the male.
[ref. 1,5]
See also *infertility*.

fertility toxicant

Substance that produces abnormalities of male or female reproductive functions or impairs reproductive capacity.
[ref. 1]

fertilization (n)/**fertilize** (v) (in reproductive biology)

Union of male and female *gametes* to form a *zygote* from which an *embryo* can develop.
[ref. 5]
See also *conception*.

fertilization effect

Enhanced growth of plants as a result of *exposure* to low levels of *pollutants* such as nitrogen and sulfur oxides in acid precipitation.
[ref. 2]

fertilizer

Substance applied to *soil* or hydroponic systems for improving the root nutrition of plants with the aim of increasing crop yields and (or) controlling production.
[ref. 1]

fetal alcohol syndrome (FAS)

fetal alcohol spectrum disorder (FASD)
Condition developing in the *fetus* and resulting in *congenital* abnormalities, caused by alcohol intake by the mother during pregnancy, typically characterized by decreased cognitive development, stunted growth and a characteristic *facies*.
Note: FAS is the most serious form of fetal alcohol spectrum *disorder*, but a range of milder forms exists that may show reduced skills in learning, social development, memory, and control of emotions.
[ref. 5]

fetal antigen

See *antigen, fetal.*

fetal period

See *fetus.*

fetal tolerance

Lack of *rejection* of a fetal *allograft* carrying paternal *major histocompatibility complex* and *minor histocompatibility antigens* that differ from those of the mother.
[ref. 3]

α-fetoprotein (AFP)

Serum protein coded by the AFP gene, related to serum albumin in evolution, produced by and abundant in *fetal* tissues, and reoccurring in the serum of patients with liver cancer.
Note 1: AFP has various *immunomodulating* and *immunosuppressive* effects.
Note 2: An abnormally high amount of AFP in the *amniotic fluid* or maternal serum may indicate a *neural tube defect*, or some other loss of structural integrity in the fetus.
[ref. 3,5]

fetoscopy

Procedure in which a *fetus* may be directly observed *in utero*, using a fiber-optic endoscope (fetoscope) introduced under local anesthesia through a small incision in the abdomen.
Note: Fetoscopy allows photographs to be taken, and *amniotic fluid,* fetal cells, or blood to be sampled for prenatal diagnosis of many *congenital* anomalies or genetic defects.
[ref. 5]

fetotoxicity

Toxicity to the *fetus.*
[ref. 1]

fetus (n)/fetal (adj)

Young mammal within the *uterus* of the mother, from the visible completion of characteristic *organogenesis* until *birth.*
Note: In humans, the fetal period is usually defined as from the third month after *fertilization* until birth; prior to this the young mammal is referred to as an *embryo.*
[ref. 5]

fibrillation

Rapid contractions or twitching of muscle fibrils, but not of the muscle as a whole.
Note: The term "fibrillation" is commonly used for atrial fibrillation, where the muscles of the cardiac *atrium* show the phenomenon, leading to loss of normal rhythmic contraction, and also for loss of synchronized contraction of the *ventricles, i.e.*, ventricular fibrillation.
[ref. 4]
Compare *fasciculation.*

fibrillation, ventricular

Life threatening *arrhythmia* characterized by uncoordinated contractions of the cardiac *ventricles*, leading to failure to pump blood.
[*]

fibrin

Insoluble protein formed from *fibrinogen* during the *clotting* of *blood*, forming a fibrous mesh.
[*]

fibrinogen

Soluble protein present in *blood plasma*, from which *fibrin* is produced by the action of the *enzyme* thrombin (EC 3.4.21.5).
[*]

fibrinolysis

Enzymatic lysis of a *fibrin* clot.
[ref. 3]

fibrinolytic

Pertaining to, characterized by, or causing the breakdown of *fibrin* (*fibrinolysis*), usually by the action of plasmin; also referring to a *drug* administered for that purpose.
[After ref. 3]

fibroblast
fibrocyte
desmocyte

Flat fibrous tissue or connective tissue cell, with stellate or spindle shape, associated with the formation of collagen fibers and other components of the *extracellular matrix.*

Note 1: Fibroblasts may develop into a number of precursor cells, such as collagenoblasts, *osteoblasts*, or *chondroblasts*.
Note 2: Fibroblasts play an important part in wound healing.
[3,5]

fibroblast growth factor (FGF)

Any member of a family of more than twenty protein *growth factors* involved in *angiogenesis*, wound healing and, in early *embryonic* development, induction of *mesoderm*, patterning and *morphogenesis*, and development of the limbs and *brain.*
[ref. 5]
See also *sonic hedgehog*.

fibrosis

Abnormal formation of fibrous tissue.
[ref. 1]

fiducial limit

Form of confidence limit given as a stated probability, for example, $P = 0.95$.
Note: In toxicology, the terms "fiducial limits" and "confidence limits" are generally considered to be synonymous.
[ref. 1]

filament (n)/**filamentous** (adj) (in biology)

Thread-like structure.
Note: Several different types of filament are distinguished.

- Protein filament: Chain of protein subunits found in hair, muscle (myofilament), and flagella.
  See also *cytoskeleton; intermediate filament; paired helical filament.*
- Cell filament: Chain of cells connected end to end.
- Plant filament: Natural fiber, root hair or other hair-like growth.

[*]

filter feeder

See *suspension feeder*.

final acute value (FAV)

Estimate of the concentration of a substance corresponding to a cumulative probability of 0.05 in the acute *toxicity* values for all *genera* for which acceptable acute tests have been conducted on the substance.
[ref. 2]

final chronic value (FCV)

Estimate of the concentration of a substance corresponding to a cumulative probability of 0.05 in the chronic *toxicity* values for all *genera* for which acceptable chronic tests have been conducted on the substance.
Note: The FCV can also be calculated by dividing the *final acute value* by the final *acute-to-chronic toxicity ratio*.
[ref. 2]

finding of no significant impact (FONSI)

Statement prepared and issued to the public when the results of an environmental impact assessment identify no harmful effects of concern.
[ref. 1]
See also *environmental impact assessment.*

finger tapping test

Procedure in which a test subject is asked to tap a finger at maximal rate on a surface; relatively high rates of tapping indicate better neuromuscular function.
[ref. 4]

finite rate of increase

Rate of increase of *population* size measured over set intervals, such as between age classes of a life table or generations of a population with nonoverlapping generations, *e.g.*, that of an annual plant.
[ref. 2]

first line of defence

Surface tissues, notably the skin, respiratory tract, and *gastrointestinal tract.*
Note 1: Surface tissues are rich in *immunocompetent* cells that form a first line of defense by recognizing *pathogens*, destroying them with secretory *antibodies*, or preventing their intrusion into the organism.
Note 2: Internal organs may also have a first line of defense, *e.g.*, the *microglia* have been considered as a first line of defense against *brain infections*.
[ref. 3]

first-order chemical reaction

first-order reaction

1. Chemical reaction where the initial rate is directly proportional to the *concentration* of one of the reactants.
2. Any process in which a variable decreases with time at a constant fractional amount.

[ref. 1]

first-pass effect

1. (hepatic) *Biotransformation* and, in some cases, biliary *elimination* of a substance in the liver after *absorption* from the intestine and before it reaches the *systemic* circulation.
2. (intestinal) Biotransformation of an ingested substance in intestinal *epithelial* cells; the metabolites are then either absorbed and moved via the portal blood to the liver, or eliminated into the intestine (presystemic elimination).

[*]

first-pass metabolism

See *first-pass effect.*
[ref. 1]

fish acute toxicity syndrome (FATS)

Behavioral, physiological, and biochemical response of fish used to classify substances by mode of action.
[ref. 2]

fish embryo test (FET)

Fish embryo acute toxicity test
Procedure in which fish (often zebrafish, ***Danio rerio***) *eggs* and *embryos* are exposed to a test chemical and subsequent development or death of the animals is studied.
[ref. 5]

fish reproduction assay

Procedure in which sexually mature male and spawning female fish are exposed to a test substance and multiple endpoints, including *egg* production, *endocrine* activity, *vitellogenin*, and *gonadal histopathology*, are measured.
[ref. 5]

fish sexual development test

Procedure in which fish are exposed from the time of *fertilization* of the *egg* until sexual differentiation is completed and markers of possible *endocrine disruptor* activity are studied, including *vitellogenin* concentration, *gonadal histopathology*, sex ratios, and the occurrence of *intersex*.
[ref. 5]

fistula

Permanent abnormal passage from an internal organ to the body surface or between two internal organs or structures.
[ref. 5]

fitness (in ecology)

Ability of an individual to survive and reproduce successfully, *i.e.*, to transfer genes to the next generation.
Note 1: If differences in individual *genotypes* affect fitness, then the frequencies of the genotypes increasing fitness will increase over generations due to *natural selection*.
Note 2: Several types of fitness are distinguished:

- Darwinian fitness is the lifetime reproductive success of an organism or genotype, indexed by the average number of offspring that it produces, relative to other organisms or genotypes, and hence the relative number of copies of its genes that it passes on to future generations.
- Absolute fitness (W_{abs}) of a genotype is the number of individuals with that genotype after selection divided by those before selection, calculated for a single generation from absolute numbers or from frequencies, $W_{abs} = N_{after}/N_{before}$. If $W_{abs} > 1.0$, the genotype frequency increases. If $W_{abs} < 1.0$, its frequency decreases.
- Relative fitness is the fitness of individuals with a genotype (a) relative to fitness of individuals with competing genotypes (b, c, . . .),

$$W_{rel}(a) = W_{abs}(a)/(W_{abs}(b) + W_{abs}(c) + \ldots).$$

  Relative fitness can therefore take any nonnegative value including 0.
- Inclusive fitness is the degree of *adaptation* of an organism to its environment, estimated from the number of genes belonging to its genotype that are passed on to the next generation, relative to those of other genotypes, counting both genes that it passes on directly and those that it shares with close relatives and passed on by them.

[ref. 2, 5]

fitness advantage

Increased *relative fitness* of a resistant *genotype* in a polluted environment compared to a nonresistant genotype.
[ref. 2]

fitness cost

Reduced relative *fitness* of a resistant *genotype* in an unpolluted environment compared to a nonresistant genotype.
[ref. 2]

fixed dose procedure

Acute *toxicity* test in which a substance is tested initially at a small number (3 or 4) predefined *dose*s to identify which produces evident toxicity without lethality.
Note: The fixed dose procedure may be repeated at one or more higher or lower defined discriminating doses to satisfy the criteria.
[ref. 1]

flaccid

Relaxed, flabby, or without tone.
Note 1: Flaccid *paralysis* is a condition where one or more muscles are without tone. It is often caused by the lack of motor nerve impulses due to *nerve* trauma, *disease* or specific pharmaceuticals.
Note 2: Curare causes flaccid paralysis by binding to *acetylcholine receptor*s and inhibiting their action.
[ref. 4]

flexure, hepatic
right colic flexure

Bend between the ascending colon and the transverse colon.
[ref. 5]

flocculation

Formation of a light, loose precipitate (*i.e.*, a floc) from a solution.
[ref. 2]

Flory–Huggins theory

Theory in which the thermodynamic quantities of a polymer solution are derived from entropy of mixing and a reduced Gibbs energy parameter, c.
Note: In environmental toxicology, Flory–Huggins theory predicts nonideal behavior resulting in a nonlinear relationship between K_{ow} and lipophilicity for very lipophilic compounds. This explains the nonlinear relationship between K_{ow} and *bioconcentration factor*.
[ref. 2]

flow cytometry

Measurement of physical and biochemical characteristics of cells suspended in a fluid as they pass through the path of one or more laser beams.
Note: In flow cytometry, cell components are fluorescently labeled and excitation by each laser causes them to emit light at a characteristic wavelength.
[*]
See also *fluorescence-activated (-assisted) cell sorting*.

flow-through system

Exposure system for aquatic *toxicity* tests in which test solutions and clean water flow into and out of test chambers on a once-through basis, either intermittently or continuously.
[ref. 2]

flow-through test

Aquatic *toxicity* test performed in a *flow-through system.*
[ref. 2]

fluctuating asymmetry

See *asymmetry, fluctuating.*
See also *antisymmetry; asymmetry, directional.*

fluid feeder

Organism that feeds on the fluids of other animals or of plants.
Examples: aphids, ticks, mosquitoes, leeches, and hummingbirds.
[ref. 2]

fluorescein isothiocyanate (FITC)

Green fluorescent dye used to 'tag' *antibodies* for use in *immunofluorescence.*
[ref. 3]

fluorescence-activated (-assisted) cell sorting (FACS)

Specialized type of *flow cytometry* that sorts a heterogeneous mixture of biological cells into two or more containers, one cell at a time, based upon specific light scattering and fluorescent characteristics of each cell.
[*]

fluorescent antibody

See *antibody, fluorescent.*

fluoridosis

See *fluorosis.*

fluorosis

fluoridosis

Adverse effects of fluoride, as in *dental fluorosis* or *skeletal fluorosis.*
[ref. 1]

flux (of a quantity)

Flow rate of an entity through a cross-section perpendicular to the flow divided by the cross-sectional area.
[ref. 1]

fly ash

Combustion residue that escapes sedimentation and filtration in the combustion unit, is emitted into ambient air, and consists of a *mixture* of organic and inorganic particles.
[*]

focus/foci (pl) **of neoplasia**

Small group of cells distinguishable, in appearance or histochemically, from the surrounding tissue.
Note: Foci are indicative of an early stage of a lesion that may lead to the formation of a *neoplastic* nodule.
[ref. 1]

foetus

Alternative spelling of *fetus* found in British English usage.
Note: This usage reflects incorrect etymology and should be deprecated.
[After ref. 5]

fold

plica

1. Ridge or margin apparently formed by the doubling back of a lamina.
   Note: In anatomy, used as a common identifier, as, for example, in nail f., neural f., tail f., transverse f., and *urogenital* f.
2. In the *embryo*, a transient elevation or reduplication of tissue in the form of a lamina.

[ref. 5]

folic acid

Water-soluble B vitamin involved in breakdown of carbohydrates, releasing energy and promoting biosynthesis.
Note 1: Folic acid deficiency may lead to a range of serious abnormalities of the developing *fetus*, including *neural tube defects* and to reduced production of red blood cells in the adult.
Note 2: Alcohol intake is associated with acquired folic acid deficiency.
[After ref. 5]

follicle (n)/**follicular** (adj)

1. Small, secretory sac, such as the dental follicles that enclose the teeth before eruption or the hair follicles within the *epidermis*.
2. Fluid- or colloid-filled ball of cells in some *glands* such as the *thyroid gland* and the *ovaries*.

[ref. 5]

follicle-stimulating hormone (FSH)

Hormone secreted by the anterior *pituitary* that stimulates the *Graafian follicles* of the *ovary* and subsequent *follicular* maturation, and in the male contributes to inducing *spermatogenesis*.
[ref. 5]

follicle-stimulating hormone-releasing hormone (FSH-RH)

gonadoliberin

Hormone, released by the *hypothalamus*, inducing the secretion of *follicle-stimulating hormone* and *luteinizing hormone* by the *pituitary gland*.
[ref. 5]

follicular

See *follicle*.

follicular atresia

Degeneration and resorption of an *ovarian follicle* before it reaches maturity and ruptures.
[ref. 5]

follicular dendritic cell

See *dendritic cell, follicular*.

follicular phase

First half of the human *menstrual cycle*, during which one or more *follicles* in the *ovary* may mature, culminating in *ovulation*.
[ref. 5]

follow-up study

See *study, follow-up*.
[ref. 1]

fontanelle

Any of several soft spots in specific locations on the skull of the newborn where the bones have not yet fused and the *brain* is covered by skin and a tough *membrane*.
[ref. 5]
See also *cranial suture*.

food additive

Any substance, whether or not it has nutritive value, that is added intentionally to food for a technological (including *organoleptic*) purpose in the manufacture, processing, preparation, treatment, packing, packaging, transport, or holding of the food. Addition results, or may be reasonably expected to result (directly or indirectly), in the substance or its byproducts becoming a component of, or otherwise affecting, the characteristics of the food to which it is added.
Note: The term "food additive" does not include *contaminants*, or substances (food supplements) added to food for maintaining or improving nutritional qualities.
[ref. 1]

food allergy

Hypersensitivity reaction to substances in the diet to which an individual has previously been sensitized.
[ref. 1]

food chain

Sequence of transfer of matter and energy in the form of food from organism to organism in ascending or descending *trophic levels*.
Note 1: Commonly a food chain will be in a hierarchical sequence from prey organism to *predator* organism.
Note 2: Interconnected food chains combine to form a *food web* in which most organisms consume or are consumed by more than one other type of organism.
[After ref. 1, 2]

food intolerance

Physiologically-based reproducible, nonallergic *sensitivity* of an individual to *adverse reaction* to a specific food or food ingredient.
Note: Food intolerance must be distinguished from *allergy* (*hypersensitivity*) that is immunologically based.
Example: Lactose intolerance.
[After ref. 1]

food-mass feeder

Animal that feeds on the body parts of other animals.
Note: Examples of food-mass feeders are avivores (feed on birds), carnivores (feed on meat), piscivores (feed on fish), insectivores (feed on insects), and ophiophagous species (feed on snakes).
[After ref. 2]

food web

Network of *food chains*.
[ref. 1]

footpad test

Test for *allergic contact dermatitis* in which the test substance is injected into the front footpad of a guinea pig and *challenge* is performed seven days later.
[ref. 3]

foramen/foramina (pl)

Opening, hole.
Note 1: The skull has several foramina that act as passageways for structures, notably *nerve*s and blood vessels.
See also *foramen magnum*.
Note 2: The *vertebral column* is perforated by the vertebral foramina through which nerves from the *spinal cord* exit to the periphery.
[ref. 4]

foramen magnum

Large *foramen* in the base of the skull, through which the *spinal cord* passes.
[ref. 4]

foramen ovale

1. In the *fetal* heart, opening that allows shunting of blood between the right and left *atria* and normally closes at birth.
2. One of the larger *foramina* in the base of the skull.

[ref. 5]

forced diuresis

Method of stimulating diuresis based on performing hydrational therapy, sometimes with parallel introduction of *diuretics*, with the aim of achieving increased clearance of a *toxic* substance in urine.
[ref. 1]

forebrain

See *prosencephalon.*

foreskin

See *prepuce.*

foreign substance

See *xenobiotic.*

Forssman antigen

See *antigen, Forssman.*

forward genetics

See *genetics, forward.*

fossa

In anatomy, a depression or hollow, often in a bone.
[ref. 5]

fossa ovalis

Oval depression *(fossa)* in the heart, on the lower part of the *septum* of the right *atrium.*
Note: The fossa ovalis is a remnant of the *foramen ovale.*
[ref. 5]

fossil

Mineralized or otherwise preserved remnant or trace (such as a footprint) of an animal, plant, or other organism.
[ref. 2]

founder effect

Changes in *allelic* frequencies that occur when a small group is separated from a large *population* and establishes a colony in a new location.
[ref. 1]

fractionation

Process of classification of an analyte or a group of analytes from a *sample* according to physical properties, *e.g.*, size or solubility, or chemical properties, *e.g.*, bonding or reactivity.
[ref. 1]

frame-shift mutation

Point *mutation* involving either the deletion or insertion of one or two nucleotides in a *gene.*
Note: As a result of a frame shift mutation, the normal reading frame used when decoding nucleotide triplets in the gene is altered.
[ref. 1]

framework region

One of several relatively conserved amino acid sequences that flank the *hypervariable regions* in *immunoglobulin* and *T-cell receptor variable (V) regions,* and maintain a common overall structure for all V region domains.
[ref. 3]

free ion activity model (FIAM)

Model for acute metal *toxicity* to aquatic organisms based on the idea that toxicity occurs when the concentration of the free metal cation in solution reaches a certain level.
Note: The FIAM has been developed into the *biotic ligand model.*
[ref. 2]

Freund's adjuvant

Complete Freund's *adjuvant* is an emulsion of aqueous *antigen* in mineral oil that contains heat-killed ***Mycobacteria.***
Note 1: Incomplete Freund's adjuvant lacks the Mycobacteria.
Note 2: Freund's adjuvant can cause painful local *inflammation* and should be used with care.
[After ref. 3]

Freundlich adsorption isotherm

Empirical equation that describes the adsorption of a *contaminant* to *soil.* The equation is

$$x/m = (K_f\ C_e)\ \exp(1/n)$$

where x/m is the mass ratio of concentrations of adsorbed substance at equilibrium divided by the concentration of the contaminant in soil, C_e is the contaminant concentration in the aqueous phase at equilibrium, K_f is the equilibrium constant (the Freundlich adsorption constant), and $1/n$ is a contaminant-specific exponent.
[ref. 2]

frontal lobe

See *lobe, frontal.*

frontonasal dysplasia (FND)

frontonasal dysostosis
frontonasal malformation
median cleft face syndrome

Tessier cleft numbers 0/14 (See *Tessier classification*)
Congenital malformation of the midface in which the nose has a flat, wide appearance, the eyes may be wide-set, and there is a groove of varying size, running down the middle of the face across the nose.
[ref. 5]

frontotemporal dementia (FTD)

frontotemporal lobular degeneration (FTLD)

Neurodegenerative disease characterized by progressive *neuron*al defects in the *frontal* and *temporal lobe*s of the *brain*, leading to *dementia*
[ref. 4]

fugacity, *f*, *p*

1. Of a substance B, f_B or p_B in a gaseous *mixture* is defined by

$$f_B = \lambda_B \lim_{p \to 0} p_B / \lambda_B$$

   where p_B is the partial pressure of B and λ_B its absolute activity.
2. Tendency for a substance to transfer from one environmental medium to another.

Note: In this sense, fugacity is analogous to chemical potential as it pertains to the tendency of a chemical to escape from a phase (*e.g.*, from water).
[After ref. 2]

fulvic acid

Humic substance that is soluble at all pHs, consisting of networks of highly oxidized aromatic and aliphatic components
Note: Most of the humic substance in natural water is fulvic acid.
[ref. 2]

fumigant

Substance that is vaporized in order to kill or repel *pests*.
[ref. 1]

functional domain

In the *brain*, referring to the concept that discrete regions are involved in specific aspects of *cognitive function*, thus giving rise to modularity.
Note: An alternative to the functional domain theory, distributive processing, holds that *cognition* involves more interaction of *brain* regions.
[ref. 4]

functional genomics

Development and implementation of technologies to characterize the mechanisms through which *genes* and their products function and interact with each other and with the environment.
[ref. 1]

functional observational battery

Structured set of tests to examine changes in neuromuscular, arousal, autonomic and sensory functions that assesses the presence, absence or severity of specific neurological signs.
Note: Usually performed in rodents after exposing them to potentially *neurotoxic* substances.
[ref. 4]

functional redundancy

Presence of a number of *taxonomically* distinct species that all exhibit similar ecological functions.
Note: The functioning of *ecosystems* with high functional redundancy will be more affected by the removal of a function than of a species.
[*]

functional response

Change in some *predator* function, such as prey consumption rate, in response to changes in prey density.
[ref. 2]

fundamental niche

See *niche, fundamental.*

fundus

Part of a hollow organ (*e.g.*, the *uterus*) that is furthest from its opening.
[ref. 5]

fungicide

Substance intended to kill fungi.
[ref. 1]

fused in sarcoma transcription factor (FUS)

Nuclear DNA- and RNA-binding protein involved in transcription, splicing, and RNA-transport.
Note: Mutation in the FUS gene is believed to have a role in several *neurodegenerative diseases*.
[ref. 4]

G protein

Any member of a family of guanine nucleotide-binding proteins that binds GTP, converts it to GDP, and thus mediates a signal from a so-called *G protein-coupled receptor* in the process of cell *signal transduction*.
Note: There are two kinds of G protein, the heterotrimeric (α, β, γ) receptor-associated G proteins, and the small G proteins, such as Ras and Raf, that act downstream of many transmembrane signaling events.
[ref. 3]

G-protein-coupled receptor (GPCR)

See *receptor, G-protein coupled.*

GABA

See *γ-aminobutyric acid.*

GABA receptor

See *γ-aminobutyric acid receptor.*

GABAergic

Pertaining to the action of *γ-aminobutyric acid* or to neural or *metabolic* pathways in which it functions as a *neurotransmitter*.
[ref. 4]

gp120

Viral *glycoprotein*, noncovalently associated with gp41 in the viral envelope of *human immunodeficiency virus*.
Note: The gp120 portion of the glycoprotein complex binds with high *affinity* to the cell-surface molecule *CD4*. Before fusion and entry of the virus, gp120 must bind to a *coreceptor* in the membrane of the host cell, for instance *chemokine receptors* (mainly CCR5).
[ref. 3]

Gaia hypothesis

Hypothesis proposed by James Lovelock that the Earth's temperature, *albedo*, and surface chemistry are homeostatically regulated by the sum of all the biota of the Earth.
[ref. 2]

gall bladder

Pear-shaped muscular sac underneath the liver that stores *bile* secreted by the liver before its release into the *duodenum*.
[ref. 5]

gamete

Reproductive cell (either *sperm* or *egg*) containing a *haploid* set of *chromosomes*.
[ref. 1]

Comprehensive Glossary of Terms Used in Toxicology
By John Duffus, Douglas M. Templeton and Michael Schwenk

Published by the Royal Society of Chemistry, www.rsc.org

gamete intrafallopian transfer (GIFT)

Technique of assisted reproduction by placing *eggs* and *sperm* into a woman's *Fallopian tubes* in order that *fertilization* may occur there.
Note: After GIFT, the *embryo* is expected to travel through the Fallopian tube and *implant* in the *uterus* as it would have done had natural fertilization occurred.
[ref. 5]

gametic selection

Natural selection resulting from differential success of *gametes* produced by *heterozygotes*.
[ref. 1]

gametocide

Substance intended to kill *gametes*.
[ref. 1]

gametogenesis

Development of male or female *gametes* to maturity.
[ref. 5]

gametophyte

Of seed plants and *algae, haploid* multicellular organism that develops from a haploid *spore* having one set of *chromosomes*, and then develops sex organs that produce *gametes* - haploid sex cells that participate in fertilization to form a *diploid zygote*.
Note 1: Gametophytes that produce *egg* and *sperm* on separate plants are termed "dioecious".
Note 2: Because the two gametophytes differ in form and function, they are described as "*heteromorphic*".
[*]
See also *megagametocyte; microgametocyte*.

gammaglobulin

See *γ-globulin*.

gamma-interferon

See *γ-interferon*.

ganglion/ganglia (pl)

1. Cluster of *nerve cell* bodies located outside the *brain* and *spinal cord, i.e.*, in the *peripheral nervous system*.
   Note: Ganglia interconnect to form a complex network known as a *plexus* and serve as relay stations where different neurons can modulate each other's signals.
   Compare *basal ganglion*.
2. Fibrous cyst usually attached to a tendon sheath.

[ref. 4]

ganglion cell

Neuron located in a *ganglion*.
Note: Included are cells in the ganglion cell layer of the *retina*, cells of the *sympathetic nervous system* in the adrenal medulla, cells in *sympathetic* and

parasympathetic ganglia, and cells in the spiral (cochlear) ganglion involved in hearing.
[ref. 4]

ganglioside

Glycosphingolipid chemically similar to *cerebrosides* but containing one or more sialic (*N*-acetylneuraminic or *N*-glycolylneuraminic) acid residues, expressed at high densities in peripheral nervous tissues, but also in spleen and thymus.
Note 1: Accumulation of gangliosides can be associated with *disease*. Ganglioside GM1 accumulates in generalized gangliosidosis; GM2 accumulates in Tay-Sachs disease.
Note 2: Gangliosides are targets of *autoantibodies* in *autoimmune* peripheral neuropathies (*e.g.* anti-GM1, -GQ1b, -GD1b).
Note 3: *Natural autoantibodies* induced by *infection* may cross-react with gangliosides and become *pathogenic* after *affinity maturation* and *class switching*.
After [3, 4]

ganglioside, tetanus toxin-binding

Ganglioside that binds *tetanus toxin*, facilitating its internalization at the *presynaptic neuronal membrane*.
[ref. 4]

gasotransmitter

Gaseous molecule that is either synthesised in an organism, *tissue* or *cell* – or is received by the organism, tissue or cell from outside – and that transmits a signal inducing specific physiological or biochemical changes.
Note: Common gasotransmitters include CO, NO, H_2S, and the plant hormone ethylene.
[*]

gastritis, autoimmune

Autoimmune-mediated destruction of the gastric *mucosa* that may result in the development of *pernicious anemia*.
Note: Autoimmune gastritis is associated with *autoantibodies* to H^+/K^+-ATPase of gastric *parietal* cells as well as *autoantibodies* to the intrinsic factor produced by these cells.
[ref. 3]

gastroenteritis

Inflammation of the stomach and intestine.
[ref. 1]

gastrointestinal

Pertaining to, or communicating with, the stomach and intestine.
[ref. 1]
See also *gastrointestinal excretion; gastrointestinal tract*.

gastrointestinal excretion

Excretion through the intestinal mucosa by active or passive processes.
Note 1: Gastrointestinal excretion may involve loss of cell-bound substances by normal cell sloughing of the intestinal wall.

Note 2: Some chemical *species* of metallic elements such as cadmium and mercury can undergo significant levels of gastrointestinal excretion.
Note 3: Intestinal *epithelial* cells possess *membrane transporters* for export of organic molecules into the intestinal *lumen*, thus participating in gastrointestinal excretion.
[After ref. 2]

gastrointestinal tract (GIT)

alimentary canal
Tubular *organ* system extending from the oral *cavity* to the *anus*, involved in the intake of food and its digestion, nutrient *absorption*, and processing and excretion of waste.
Note: The GIT serves *endocrine* and *exocrine* functions, acts as a physical and *immunological* barrier for entry into the body, is an incubator for *microbiota*, and plays a role in *drug metabolism* and *detoxification*.
[*]

gastroschisis

Congenital defect characterized by a fissure in the anterior abdominal wall through which the small and (or) large intestine protrude.
[ref. 5]

gastrula

Embryonic stage that develops from two to three *germ layers* during *gastrulation*.
[ref. 5]

gastrulation

Stage of *embryo* development in which the two-layered *blastula* transforms into the *gastrula* by developing *ectoderm* and *endoderm*, and a third layer (*mesoderm*) through the movement of specific cells.
[ref. 5]

gavage

Administration of materials directly into the stomach by esophageal intubation.
[ref. 1]

Gell and Coombs classification

Classification of immune mechanisms of tissue injury into four types: type I, *immediate-type hypersensitivity* reactions, mediated by interaction of *immunoglobulin E antibody* and *antigen* causing the release of *histamine* and other mediators; type II, antibody-mediated *hypersensitivity* reactions, due to antibody–antigen interactions on cell surfaces; type III, *immune complex*-mediated local or general inflammatory responses due to formation of circulating immune complexes and their deposition in tissues; and type IV cell-mediated hypersensitivity reactions, initiated by sensitized *T-lymphocytes* either via release of *lymphokines* or by T-cell-mediated cytotoxicity.
[ref. 3]
See also *cytotoxic T-lymphocyte*.

gene

Length of *DNA* or *RNA* (in viruses) that encodes a functional product, which may be a polypeptide or a ribonucleic acid.
Note: A gene is the fundamental unit of heredity.
[ref. 1]

gene, Mendelian

Gene located in a *chromosome* that obeys the laws of *Mendelian inheritance*.
[ref. 5]

gene, recessive

Allele that, in the heterozygous state, is expected to have no effect on the *phenotype* of the organism that carries it.
[ref. 1]

gene, recombination activating (RAG)

Gene whose products are involved in *V(D)J recombination* in *B-cells* and *T-cells*.
Note: Two recombination-activating genes having been identified as RAG-1 and RAG-2.
[ref. 3]

gene, tumor suppressor

Gene that protects cells from entering a cancerous state.
Note: According to Knudson's "two-hit" hypothesis, both alleles of a particular *tumor* suppressor gene must acquire a mutation before the cell will enter a transformed state.
[ref. 1]

gene amplification

Occurrence of extra copies of a *gene*; with respect to a *plasmid*, an increase in the number of plasmid copies per cell, which may be induced by a specific treatment.
Note: Spontaneous gene amplification frequently occurs in tumor cells.
[ref. 1]

gene expression

See *expression, gene*.

gene knockout

Method of disabling a specific gene by homologous recombination with an introduced DNA construct designed for that purpose.
[ref. 3]
See also *gene targeting; knockout; knockout mouse*.

gene map

Map showing the positions in the *genome* of *gene*s or other genetic markers, either relative to each other or as a physical map of absolute distances.
[ref. 1]

gene product

Both the *messenger RNA* resulting from transcription of a *gene* and the polypeptides translated from that mRNA.
[ref. 5]

gene rearrangement

Structural alteration in a *chromosome* that changes the order of its genetic loci, occurring by *DNA recombination*, *e.g.*, during development or in some *cancer*s.

Note: In *immunology*, gene rearrangement refers to recombination of gene segments in *immunoglobulin* and *T-cell receptor* loci to produce a functional *variable (V) region* sequence.
[ref. 3]

gene silencing

Prevention of the expression of a specific *gene*.
Note: Gene silencing may occur by natural genetic or *epigenetic* processes, or by experimental intervention, as in *gene targeting knockout mutation*, or *RNA interference*.
[ref. 5]

gene targeting

Use of *homologous recombination* to change a *gene, e.g.*, to delete a gene, remove exons, add a gene, or introduce point *mutations*.
[ref. 5]
See also *gene knockout*.

gene therapy

Introduction of genetic material into an individual, or the modification of the individual's genetic material, in order to achieve a *therapeutic* or prophylactic objective.
[ref. 1]

general adaptation syndrome (GAS)

Specific *syndrome* associated with *Selyean stress* composed of three phases: the alarm reaction, *adaptation* or resistance, and exhaustion; adaptation in all phases of the GAS results in restoration of *homeostasis* or reduced deviation from homeostasis.
[ref. 2]

generally regarded as safe (GRAS)

Phrase used to describe the legal philosophy that justifies approval of *food additives* that may not meet the usual test criteria for *safety* but have been used extensively and have not demonstrated that they cause any harm to consumers.
[After ref. 1]

generation time

Average length of time between the birth of parents and the birth of offspring.
[ref. 2]

genetic

Of, or relating to, *genes*, heredity, and the science of *genetics*.
[*]

genetic adaptation

See *adaptation, genetic*.

genetic drift

Evolutionary process of change in the *allele* frequencies in a *population* due to random changes in the frequency by which different alleles are transferred to the next generation.
Note: In small populations, genetic drift may result in extinction of some alleles leading to evolutionary change over time.
[ref. 2]

genetic engineering

Molecular methodology that permits manipulation of genetic material to alter the nature of organisms.
Note: The applications of genetic engineering include scientific research, health benefits, agricultural improvement, and biological warfare.
[*]

genetic epidemiology

See *epidemiology, genetic.*

genetic equilibrium

See *Hardy–Weinberg equilibrium.*

genetic hitchhiking

1. Condition in which a given *allele* changes in frequency as a result of linkage or gametic phase disequilibrium with another selected locus.
2. Situation in *ecotoxicology* in which a scored *locus* is acting only as a marker for a closely linked *gene* that is actually responsible for the difference in tolerance among *genotypes.*

[ref. 2]

genetic polymorphism

See *polymorphism, genetic.*

genetic risk

See *risk, genetic.*

genetic susceptibility

Predisposition to a particular *disease* or *sensitivity* to a substance due to the presence of a specific *allele* or combination of alleles in an individual's *genome.*
[ref. 1]

genetic toxicology

Study of chemically or physically induced changes to the structure of *DNA*, including *epigenetic* phenomena or *mutations* that may or may not be heritable.
[ref. 1]

genetically modified food

Foodstuff, such as an agricultural cash crop, produced by a *genetically modified organism.*
[*]

genetically modified organism (GMO)

Individual life form whose genetic material has been deliberately altered using techniques of *genetic engineering.*
[*]

genetics

Scientific study of heredity in its widest sense, with the objective of relating reproductive behaviour and processes to *genotype*s, resultant *phenotype*s, and the factors

that influence them, including environment and related processes of selection, including those used by ***Homo sapiens***.
[*]

genetics, forward

Approach to genetic investigation, in which the aim is to identify the *gene* that governs a particular function.
Note: Mutant *phenotypes* indicate the responsible gene, and co-inherited genetic markers indicate the region of the *genome* where it occurs.
[ref. 5]
See also *genetics, reverse*.

genetics, reverse

Approach to elucidating the function of a *gene* by studying the effects on *phenotype* of expressed variations in a known *DNA* sequence.
Note: The term is intended to indicate the reverse of the approach (starting from a phenotype and working back to identify the gene) of *forward genetics*.
[ref. 5]

genital

1. Of or relating to human or animal reproduction.
2. Of or relating to the *genital organs*.
3. Of or relating to the final stage of psychosexual maturation.
4. *Genital organ*.

[ref. 5]

genital fold
genital ridge
genitourinary ridge
labioscrotal swelling
urogenital ridge

Embryonic structure that will develop into the penis and *scrotum* in males or the labia in females.
[ref. 5]
See also *fold*.

genital organ

Organ of reproduction or generation, both external and internal to the body.
[ref. 5]

genital tract
reproductive tract
genital duct

Genital passages of the *urogenital* apparatus.
Note: In females, the genital tract runs from the *ovaries* to the *vulva*, in males from the *testicles* to the external *urethral* orifice of the penis.
[ref. 5]

genital tubercle

Primordium of the penis or *clitoris*.
[ref. 5]

genitalia

1. Plural of *genital*.
2. Externally visible sex organs.

[ref. 5]
See also *external genitalia*.

genitourinary

See *urogenital.*

genome (n)/genomic (adj)

Complete set of *chromosomal* and extrachromosomal *genes* of an organism, a cell, an organelle (*e.g.*, mitochondria or chloroplasts), or a virus, *i.e.*, the complete *DNA* component of an organism (or the complete *RNA* component of an RNA virus).
[ref. 5]

genomics

Science of using *DNA*- and *RNA*-based technologies to study the *genome* and demonstrate effects on *gene expression.*
[After ref. 1]
See also *toxicogenomics*.

genotoxic

Capable of causing a change to the structure of the *genome.*
[ref. 1]

genotype (n)

1. Genetic constitution of an organism, especially as distinguished from its *phenotype*.
2. All of the *genes* present in an organism or *species*.
3. Specific *alleles* present at a given *locus*.
4. Type-species of a genus.

[ref. 2]

genotype (v)

Establish the *genotype* of an organism.
[ref. 2]

genus/genera (pl)

Low-level *taxonomic* rank, above *species* and below family, used in the biological classification of living and fossil organisms.
Note 1: A genus includes one or more similar species.
Note 2: In Latinized binomial nomenclature, the italicized genus name precedes the species name and is capitalized, *e.g., **Homo sapiens***.
[*]

geographic information system (GIS)

Computerized system to handle spatial data and mapped information.

Note: Most geographical information systems allow one to archive, organize, integrate, statistically analyze, and display many kinds of spatial information, such as emission sources, using a common coordinate system.
[ref. 2]

germ

1. Describing a reproductive cell.
2. Reproductive seed or spore
3. *Pathogenic* microorganism.
4. Nucleation center for growth and development.

[*]

germ cell

See *germ line cell.*

germ cell gene mutation assay

Procedure in which *mutations* induced by an agent are studied in *germ line cells* or *somatic stem cells* from a *transgenic* animal (rodent), containing reporter *genes* for detection of various *mutations.*
[ref. 5]

germ-free

Descriptor applied to an environment that has been sterilized and is free from microorganisms, notably from *pathogens.*
[*]

germ-free animal

axenic animal

Animal grown under sterile conditions in the period of postnatal development: Such animals are usually obtained by Caesarean operation and kept in special sterile boxes in which there are no viable intestinal or other microorganisms (sterile air, food, and water are supplied).
Note: Germ-free animals have depleted *immune systems*, but they can respond normally to any specific *antigen*, provided it is mixed with a strong *adjuvant.*
[ref. 1,3]
See also *gnotobiote.*

germ line (in immunology)

Refering to genes in their unrearranged state rather than those rearranged for production of *immunoglobulin* or *T-cell receptor* molecules.
[ref. 3]

germ-line cell

germ cell

Gamete, or *haploid* or *embryonic* cell that can develop into a gamete.
Note: In animals, the germ-line cells are the *sperm* or *egg* (synonym *gamete*); in plants, the *pollen* cell or the *ovum.*
[After ref. 1,5]

germ layer

Any of three distinct layers of cells (*endoderm, ectoderm*, and *mesoderm*) that become recognizable as the *embryo* develops.
[ref. 5]

germ warfare

See *biological warfare.*
[ref. 1]

germinal aplasia

Complete failure of gonad development.
[ref. 1]

germinal center

Discrete area within *lymph nodes* and *spleen* where *B-cell maturation* and immunologic *memory* development occur.
[ref. 3]

gestation

pregnancy

Period between *conception* and *birth* during which an *embryo* or *fetus* is carried in the *uterus* of a female mammal.
[ref. 5]

gestation period

Time from *conception* to *birth,* during which a *fetus* develops.
[ref. 5]

giant axon

squid giant axon

Very large *axon* (typically 0.5 mm in diameter) that functions in the propulsion system of the squid.
Note: The large size of the axon has facilitated studies on the mechanism of the *action potential.*
[ref. 4]

giant axonal neuropathy

Rare human genetic neurological *disorder* in which the *neurofilaments* become disordered, resulting in abnormal size and shape of neurons.
[ref. 4]

giant cell

Large multinucleate cell derived from fused *macrophages* and often present in *granulomas.*
[ref. 3]

gigantism

Condition of abnormal size or overgrowth of the entire body or of any of its parts.
Note: Gigantism is often caused by increased levels of *growth hormone.*
[ref. 5]
See also *acromegaly.*

gill purge

See *cough.*

gland (n)/**glandular** (adj)

Organized aggregation of cells functioning as a secretory or excretory organ.
[ref. 5]

glans

Any small rounded mass or *gland*-like body.
[ref. 5]

glans clitoridis

Rounded mass of sensitive erectile tissue that forms the head of the *clitoris.*
[ref. 5]

glans penis

Rounded mass of sensitive erectile tissue at the distal end (head) of the *penis*, analogous to the *glans clitoridis.*
[ref. 5]

glaucoma

Disease of the eye characterized by increased intraocular pressure, resulting in *atrophy* of the optic nerve.
[After ref. 5].

glia (n)/**glial** (adj)

neuroglia

Non*neuronal* cellular elements of the *central* and *peripheral nervous system* having metabolic and support functions.
Note: In the central nervous system, the glia include *oligodendroglia, astrocyte*s, *ependymal* cells, and *microglia* cells. In the peripheral nervous system they include *ganglion* satellite cells and *Schwann cell*s.
[ref. 4]

glial cell

Cellular component of the *glia*, including *oligodendroglial cell*s, *astrocyte*s, *ependymal cells* and *microglial cell*s.
[ref. 4]

glial-derived neurotrophic factor (GDNF)

Protein that promotes and guides the growth of *neuron*s and facilitates the survival of mature neurons by suppressing cell death.
[ref. 4]

glial fibrillary acidic protein (GFAP)

Cytoskeletal intermediate *filament* protein found in mature fibrillary *astrocyte*s and in neural progenitor cells.
Note 1: Stains for GFAP are frequently used in the differential diagnosis of neurologic lesions.
Note 2: GFAP staining does not reveal the full distal *arborization* of the cell.
[ref. 4]

glioblastoma

glioblastoma multiforme

Glioma consisting chiefly of undifferentiated anaplastic cells of *astrocytic* origin.
Note: Glioblastomas grow rapidly, invade extensively, and occur most frequently in the *cerebrum* of adults.
[ref. 4]

glioma

Neoplasm originating from any of the *glia cells* in the *brain* and *spinal cord*.
Note: Glioma is the predominant form of malignant brain tumor.
[ref. 4]

gliosis, reactive

Damage-induced proliferation, enlargement and overgrowth of *glial cells*, often *astrocytes* in the *central nervous system*, resulting in an *astrocytic scar*.
[ref. 4]

global distillation

Process by which persistent and relatively *volatile organic compounds* (*e.g.*, organochlorines) are distilled from warmer regions of use, finally condensing in cooler regions of the globe.
[After ref. 2]

global fractionation

Process by which some *persistent organic pollutants* (POPs) move more rapidly than others toward the polar regions.
Note: Global fractionation occurs because POPs differ in their individual rates of *degradation*, vapor pressure, and lipophilicity. The net result is a redistribution of the different POPs from the equator or site of origin toward the cold polar regions of the Earth.
[ref. 2]

Globally Harmonized System (GHS)

Internationally agreed system for regulation of classification and labeling of chemicals, created by the United Nations beginning in 1992, and gradually implemented in many countries.
Note: GHS was designed to replace the various classification and labeling standards used in different countries with consistent criteria on a global level. It supersedes earlier systems used in the European Union and in the United States.
[*]

global warming

Heating of the Earth's climate thought to result from the increased atmospheric carbon dioxide (CO_2) concentrations from fossil fuel burning, release of other greenhouse gases, and the worldwide destruction of forests.
[ref. 2]
See also *greenhouse effect*.

globoside

Glycosphingolipid, specifically a *ceramide* tetrasaccharide (tetraglycosylceramide), isolated from kidney and erythrocytes.
Note: Globoside accumulates in people with Sandhoff *disease*.
[ref. 3]

γ-globulin

One of a group of *serum* proteins, mostly *immunoglobulins*, that have the greatest mobility towards the cathode during serum protein electrophoresis.
[ref. 3]

glomerular

Pertaining to a tuft or cluster, as of a plexus of capillary blood vessels or nerve fibers, especially referring to the capillaries of the *glomerulus* of the kidney.
[ref. 1]

glomerular filtration

Formation of an ultrafiltrate of the blood occurring in the capillaries of the *glomerulus* of the kidney.
Note: The resulting filtrate is concentrated in the renal tubules.
[ref. 1]

glomerular filtration rate (GFR)

Volume of ultrafiltrate formed in the kidney tubules from the blood passing through the glomerular capillaries divided by time of filtration.
[ref. 1]

glomerulonephritis

Any of a group of kidney *diseases* involving *inflammation* of the renal *glomeruli*, often as a result of *antibody-antigen* complexes that localize in the kidney.
Note: Glomerulonephritis, in common with other acute *nephritides,* is usually characterized by blood in the urine.
[After ref. 3]

glomerulonephropathy

glomerulopathy

Disease of the renal *glomeruli* that may show either thickening of the glomerular basement membrane due to the accretion of proteins, or to a minimal change disease in which there is functional damage but little structural change observable by light microscopy.
[ref. 3]

glomerulus/glomeruli (pl)

Tuft or a cluster, as of a plexus of capillary blood vessels or nerve fibers (*e.g.*, capillaries of the filtration apparatus of the kidney).
[ref. 1]

glucocorticoid

Any member of the group of steroid hormones, such as cortisone, produced by the *adrenal cortex,* that inhibit inflammation and mediate a response to stress that alters protein, fat, and carbohydrate metabolism.
Note: Glucocorticoids also play an important role in the normal regulation of the *immune system* and act as physiological *immunosuppressants* involved in the control of immune and inflammatory hyperactivity.
[ref. 3,5]

glucuronosyltransferase
UDP-glucuronosyltransferase

Any of a group of enzymes (EC 2.4.1.17) that uses uridine-5′-diphosphoglucuronic acid to transfer glucuronic acid residues to substrates.
Note: Transfer of glucuronic acid to xenobiotic molecules by UDP-glucuronosyl transferase is a major *phase II biotransformation* reaction.
[*]

glue-sniffing

Inhalation of solvent vapor from plastic cements or other adhesives, in order to become intoxicated.
[ref. 1]
See also *solvent abuse*.

glutamate

Salt of glutamic acid (2-aminopentanedioic acid).
Note 1: Glutamate is a major excitatory neurotransmitter in the vertebrate nervous system.
[ref. 4]
Note 2: Glutamate activates the umami taste *receptors* and monosodium glutamate (MSG) is commonly used in the food industry as a flavour enhancer, but at high doses MSG has been reported to give rise to feelings of *headache* and discomfort.
[*]

glutamate-induced excitotoxicity

Form of *excitotoxicity* where excess *glutamate* release in *synapses* (glutamatergic storm) leads to overstimulation, followed by excess cellular calcium uptake, cytotoxicity and apoptosis.
Note 1: *N-methyl-D-aspartatic acid, kainic acid*, and other ligands of the glutamate *receptor* induce an effect similar to glutamate-induced excitotoxicity.
Note 2: Excitotoxicity may occur after acute *neuronal ischemia* and damage. It is believed to be a factor in chronic *diseases* of the *nervous system*, and in some *withdrawal* phenomena.
[ref. 4]

glutamatergic storm

See *glutamate-induced excitotoxicity*.

glutamic acid decarboxylase (GAD)

Enzyme (EC 4.1.1.15) that catalyzes the decarboxylation of *glutamate* to *γ-aminobutyric acid*.
Note 1: GAD is an *autoantigen* targeted in *diabetes mellitus type 1* and stiff-person *syndrome* (a neurological *autoimmune disease*).
Note 2: GAD is localized in pancreatic β cells and γ-aminobutyric acid-responsive (GABAergic) neurons.
[After ref. 3]

glutathione
γ-L-glutamyl-L-cysteinylglycine

Tripeptide that serves as a major cellular defense against oxidative damage and particularly thiol oxidation, is *conjugated* to *xenobiotics* in *phase II*

biotransformations, and acts as a redox sensor modulating protein function through glutathionylation.
[*]

glutathione peroxidase

Family of enzymes (EC 1.11.1.19) that uses reduced glutathione (GSH) to reduce peroxides to water and the corresponding alcohol, with production of oxidized glutathione (GSSG).
Note: The product of glutathione peroxidase (GSSG) is reduced back to GSH by glutathione reductase (EC 1.8.1.7) at the expense of NADPH.
[*]

glutathione reductase

See Note to *glutathione peroxidase.*
[*]

glutathione-S-transferase

Family of enzymes (EC 2.5.1.18) acting in *phase II biotransformations* to transfer *glutathione* to a substrate.
Note: Following subsequent cleavage of the glutamate and glycine residues from the glutathione *conjugate*, the resulting mercapturic acid is excreted, mainly via the kidneys.
[*]

gluten

1. Any of the prolamins found in cereal grains, especially the prolamins in wheat, rye, barley, and possibly oats, which cause digestive *disorders*, notably *celiac disease.*
2. Mixture of water-insoluble proteins found in wheat, including gliadins, that give wheat dough its elastic texture.

[ref. 3]

gluten enteropathy

See *celiac disease.*

gluten intolerance

See *celiac disease.*

glycobiology

See *glycomics.*

glycolysis

Biochemical breakdown of glucose into pyruvic acid with the production of ATP.
Note: If the pyruvate resulting from glycolysis is not used efficiently in aerobic metabolism, it may then be converted to ethanol (fermentation) or lactic acid (anaerobic glycolysis).
[ref. 5]

glycome

Description of the complete set of carbohydrates and their functions in a living organism.
[ref. 1]

glycomics
glycobiology

Global study of the structure and function of carbohydrates, especially oligosaccharides (short chains of sugars) in a living organism.
[ref. 1]

glycoprotein

Any protein that has carbohydrate groups *covalently* attached to the polypeptide chain.
[*]

glycosphingolipid

Any representative of a group of glycolipids where a carbohydrate is connected with *sphingosine* (see also *sphingolipid*).
Note 1: Important glycosphingolipids are *cerebrosides*, *gangliosides* and *globosides*.
Note 2: Glycosphingolipids are components of cell membranes, notably *nerve cell* membranes.
[ref. 4]

glycosylation (n)/glycosylate (v)

Enzymatic or nonenzymatic modification of an organic molecule, especially a protein, by *covalent* addition of a sugar molecule.
[*]
See also *glycoprotein; nonenzymatic glycosylation.*

gnotobiont

See *gnotobiote.*

gnotobiota

Specifically and entirely known microfauna and microflora of a specially reared laboratory animal.
[ref. 1]
See also *gnotobiote.*

gnotobiote (n)/gnotobiotic (adj)
gnotobiont

Laboratory animal specially reared under aseptic conditions, whose microflora and microfauna are known in their entirety.
[After ref. 1]

goiter

Noncancerous enlargement of the thyroid gland, visible as a swelling at the front of the neck, that is often associated with iodine deficiency.
[ref. 1]

goitrogen

Any substance (*e.g.,* thiouracil) that induces the formation of a goiter.
[ref. 1]

Golgi apparatus
Golgi body

Complex structure of folded *membranes* and *vesicles* found in the *cytoplasm* of most *eukaryotic cells*.
Note 1: The Golgi apparatus facilitates intracellular transport and secretion, and is a site of post-translational modification and *glycosylation* of proteins.
Note 2: The Golgi apparatus consists of cis-, medial-, and trans-Golgi components, progressing from the *endoplasmic reticulum* towards the *plasma membrane*.
[*]

Golgi staining
Golgi's method

Method of *silver staining* of histological sections of tissue from the *nervous system*, in which a limited number of *neurons* stain in their entirety upon formation of micro-crystals of silver chromate, thus allowing visualization in the light microscope of some individual neurons in densely packed tissue.
[ref. 4]

gonad (n)/**gonadal** (adj)

Organ in animals that produces *gametes, i.e.*, the *testis* or the *ovary*.
[ref. 5]

gonadotropic

Pertaining to effects on sex glands and on the systems that regulate them.
[ref. 1]

gonadotropin
gonadotrophin

Glycopeptide hormone, produced by the *fetal placenta*, that maintains the function of the *corpus luteum* during the first few weeks of *pregnancy*.
[ref. 5]

gonadotropin-releasing hormone (GnRH, GRH)
gonadoliberin

luteinizing hormone-releasing hormone (LHRH)
Any factor from the *hypothalamus* that stimulates the anterior *pituitary* to release both *follicle-stimulating hormone* and *luteinizing hormone*.
[ref. 5]

good agricultural practice (GAP) (in the use of pesticides)

Nationally authorized safe uses of *pesticides* under actual conditions necessary for effective and reliable pest control.
Note: GAP encompasses a range of levels of pesticide applications up to the highest authorized use, applied in a manner that leaves a residue that is the smallest amount practicable. Authorized safe uses include nationally registered or recommended uses, which take into account public and occupational *health* and environmental safety considerations. Actual conditions include any stage in the production, storage, transport, distribution, and processing of food commodities and animal feed.
[ref. 1]

good laboratory practice (GLP) principles

Fundamental rules incorporated in Organization for Economic Cooperation and Development (OECD) guidelines and national regulations concerned with the process of effective organization and the conditions under which laboratory studies are properly planned, performed, monitored, recorded, and reported.
[ref. 1]

good manufacturing practice (GMP) principles

Fundamental rules incorporated in national regulations concerned with the process of effective organization of production and ensuring standards of defined quality at all stages of production, distribution, and marketing.
Note: Minimization of *waste* and its proper disposal are part of this process.
[ref. 1]

Goodpasture syndrome

Goodpasture disease

Autoimmune disease of humans in which *glomerulonephritis* and *pulmonary* hemorrhage are produced by *complement*-mediated tissue damage caused by *antibodies* directed against the renal glomerular and alveolar basement membranes.
[ref. 3]

Graafian follicle

vesicular ovarian follicle

Mature *ovarian follicle* within which an *oocyte* attains full size and which ruptures during *ovulation* to release the *ovum*.
[ref. 5]

graded effect

Opposite term: *all-or-none effect.*

Consequence that can be measured on a graded scale of intensity or severity and its magnitude related directly to the *dose* or *concentration* of the substance producing it.
[ref. 1]
See also *quantal effect; stochastic effect.*

graft

Tissue *transplant*ed into a *host* or surgically moved from one site to another within an individual.
[ref. 3]
See also *allograft; autograft; isograft; xenograft.*

graft rejection

See *rejection, graft.*

graft-versus-host disease (GVHD)

Disease that occurs following *bone marrow transplantation* between genetically non-identical people and in which mature *T-cells* in the transplanted bone marrow attack and destroy the recipients's tissues.
[ref. 3]
See also *graft-versus-host reaction.*

graft-versus-host (GVH) reaction

Reaction occurring when *T-lymphocytes* present in a *graft* recognize and attack *host* cells.
[ref. 3]

graminicide

Pesticide (herbicide) intended to kill weedy grasses (***Gramineae***).
[ref. 1]

granule cell

One of several types of *neurons* with small cell bodies, involved in *neural networks* in several regions of the *brain, including the cerebellum, hippocampus*, and *cerebral cortex.*
Note 1: Granule cells give rise to the name granular layer within these regions.
Note 2: Granule cells should not be confused with granular cells of the kidney.
[ref. 4]

granulocyte

White blood cell, distinct from a lymphocyte, containing cytoplasmic granules (*i.e.*, granulocytes are *neutrophils, eosinophils*, and *basophils*).
[ref. 5]

granulocyte colony-stimulating factor (G-CSF)

Hematopoietic (see *hematopoiesis*) factor augmenting the production of *neutrophils* in the *bone marrow.*
[ref. 3]

granulocyte–macrophage colony-stimulating factor (GM-CSF)

Cytokine that stimulates production of *granulocytes* and *monocytes* from *stem cells.*
[ref. 3]

granulocytopenia

Deficiency of circulating *granulocytes,* especially *agranulocytosis.*
[After ref. 3]

granuloma (n)/granulomatous (adj)

Mass or nodule of granulation tissue, with actively growing *fibroblasts* and capillary buds, characterized by the presence of aggregates of modified *macrophages* resembling epithelial cells (epithelioid histiocytes), and *lymphocytes*, surrounded by a rim of giant multinucleate cells, either of the *Langerhans* or foreign body type.
Note: Granuloma is due to a chronic inflammatory process associated with infectious *disease*, such as tuberculosis, syphilis, *sarcoidosis*, leprosy, and lymphogranuloma, or with invasion by a foreign body.
[ref. 3]

granulosa

Pertaining to cells of the *cumulus oophorus*, surrounding the oocyte.
[ref. 5]

granzyme

Member of a family of serine esterases present in the granules of *cytotoxic T-lymphocytes* and *natural killer cells.*
Note: Granzymes induce *apoptosis* in the *target cell* that they enter through *perforin* channels inserted into the target cell membrane by the cytotoxic lymphocyte.
[ref. 3]

grass pea poisoning

See *lathyrism.*

grasshopper effect

Global distillation of *persistent organic pollutants* involving seasonal cycling of temperatures such that movement toward the higher latitudes occurs in annual pulses.
[ref. 2]

Graves disease

Hyperthyroidism associated with diffuse hyperplastic goitre resulting from production of a *thyroid stimulating hormone receptor*-binding *autoantibody.*
[ref. 3]

green chemistry

Development and adoption of chemical processes and their products that minimizes any harmful impact upon living organisms and the environment.
[*]

greenhouse effect

Net warming of the Earth resulting from increasing atmospheric concentrations of carbon dioxide (CO_2), water vapor, and other *greenhouse gases.*
Note: Gases and vapors implicated in the greenhouse effect, such as CO_2 and water vapor, are relatively transparent to light but absorb long-wave, infrared radiation radiating from the Earth's surface. The net balance for sunlight influx, infrared radiation absorption by greenhouse gases, and infrared efflux from the Earth's surface determines the steady-state temperature of the Earth.
[ref. 2]

greenhouse gas

Atmospheric gas that is relatively transparent to sunlight entering the atmosphere but absorbs infrared radiation generated at the Earth's surface.
Note: Greenhouse gases include water vapor, carbon dioxide (CO_2), methane, dinitrogen oxide (nitrous oxide), chlorofluorocarbons, chloroethane (methylchloroform), carbon tetrachloride, and the fire retardant, halon. Ozone in the troposphere can also act as a greenhouse gas.
[ref. 2]

grey matter

Regions of the *brain* and *spinal cord* that are made up primarily of the cell bodies and *dendrite*s of *nerve cell*s rather than of *myelin*ated *axon*s.
[ref. 4]
Compare *white matter.*

gross pathology

See *macroscopic pathology*.

ground treatment of plants

Dusting or spraying of plants with *pesticides* by hand, by special machines, or by apparatus fixed to tractors or driven by them.
[ref. 1]

groundwater

Water that is enclosed beneath the earth's surface.
Note: Groundwater is often derived from surface water that has seeped down through the earth, and may be contaminated with pesticides, substances solubilized from landfill waste, or fertilizers (*e.g.*, nitrates).
[*]

growth

Increase in size and (or) number.
[ref. 2]
See also *growth, exponential; growth, intrinsic rate of; growth, logistic.*

growth, exponential

Growth of cells, organisms, or *populations* in which the number or mass increases exponentially and growth at any time is proportional to the number or mass present.
Note: The mathematical form for exponential growth is of the same as that for *exponential decay.*
[ref. 2]

growth, intrinsic rate of (r)

Rate of population *growth* if no density-dependent factors operate, and thus $r =$ (birth rate + immigration) – (death rate + emigration)
[ref. 2]
See also *growth; growth, exponential; growth, logistic.*

growth, logistic

Growth of a *population* under environmental constraints that set a maximum population size, giving an S-shaped curve.
[ref. 2]
See also *carrying capacity; growth.*

growth dilution

Decrease in *contaminant* concentration in a growing organism because the amount of tissue in which the contaminant is distributed is increasing.
Example: Growth dilution happens in young children when the load of *persistent organic pollutants*, which they have ingested as babies with their mothers' milk, are diluted in a growing body (fat) volume.
[ref. 2]

growth factor

Naturally occurring or genetically engineered protein or *steroid hormone* that binds to a *receptor* to regulate cell *growth*, proliferation or differentiation.
[ref. 5]

growth hormone (GH)
somatotropin
somatotropic hormone (STH)

Peptide *hormone* secreted by the anterior *pituitary* that stimulates growth, energy *metabolism*, and cell proliferation.
Note: Human growth hormone (hGH) isolated from cadavers or produced by recombinant technology is used clinically to treat deficiency of the hormone and other growth *disorders*, and inappropriately to enhance athletic performance.
[ref. 5]

growth hormone releasing factor (GHRF)
growth hormone releasing hormone (GHRH)

Peptide produced in the *hypothalamus* that regulates release of *growth hormone* by the anterior *pituitary*.
[ref. 5]

gubernaculum

Fetal mesenchyme ligament that passes through the anterior abdominal wall and connects the lower pole of each developing *gonad* with the developing *scrotum* in men, and with the developing labia majora in women.
Note: In men, the gubernaculum guides descent of the *testes* into the scrotum.
[ref. 5]

guide to air quality

Set of atmospheric *concentrations* and *exposure* times that is associated with specific effects of varying degrees of *pollution* on humans, animals, vegetation, and the environment in general.
[ref. 1]

guide to environmental quality

Set of *concentrations*, numbers and *exposure* times that is associated with the specific effects of factors in environmental media on humans, animals, vegetation, and the environment in general.
[ref. 1]

guideline for exposure limits
guideline value

Scientifically judged quantitative value (a *concentration* or number) of an environmental constituent that ensures aesthetically pleasing air, water, or food and from which no *adverse effect* is expected concerning noncarcinogenic endpoints; or that gives an acceptably low estimate of lifetime *cancer risk* from those substances that are proven human *carcinogens,* or that show at least *limited evidence* of human *carcinogenicity*.
[ref. 1]

guild (in ecology)

Group of functionally similar *species* whose members interact strongly with one another but weakly with the remainder of the community.
[ref. 2]

Guillain-Barré syndrome (GBS)

Type of idiopathic *polyneuritis* in which autoimmunity to *peripheral nerve myelin* leads to a condition characterized by chronic *demyelination* of the spinal roots (see *spinal cord*), *peripheral nerves*, and *cranial nerves*.
Note: Guillain-Barré *syndrome* is often preceded by a respiratory or *gastrointestinal infection* and shows gradual but complete recovery in most cases.
[ref. 4]

guinea pig maximization test (GPMT)

Skin sensitization test for *allergic contact dermatitis* in which shaved guinea pig skin is exposed to intradermal injections of a test agent together with complete *Freund's adjuvant*, followed by an occlusive patch for boosting (see *booster*) for 48 h beginning on day 7, and *challenged* on day 21.
[ref. 3]

gut-associated lymphoid tissue (GALT)

Lymphoid cells and tissues lining the *mucosa* that seem to serve as the first point of *antigen* contact via this route, including *Peyer's patches*, the *appendix, tonsils*, adenoids, and mesenteric *lymph nodes*.
Note: Large aggregates of GALT have distinct B-cell follicles and T-cell areas. Antigen-presenting accessory cells are also present.
[ref. 3]

H-2

Region of mouse chromosome 17 coding the *major histocompability complex.*
[ref. 3]

H-2 complex

Mouse *major histocompatibility complex (MHC)* coded by *H-2*.
[ref. 3]

H-chain

See *heavy chain.*

Haber-Weiss reaction

Reaction of hydrogen peroxide and superoxide to generate hydroxyl according to

Reaction 1. $H_2O_2 + O_2^{-\bullet} \rightarrow O_2 + HO^- + HO^\bullet$

Note 1: Hydroxyl can react further with peroxide to produce additional superoxide, according to

Reaction 2. $H_2O_2 + HO^\bullet \rightarrow H_2O + O_2^{-\bullet} + H^+$

Note 2: The reaction of H_2O_2 with $O_2^{-\bullet}$ is slow, but it can be catalyzed by a transition metal ion, such as $Fe^{II/III}$ or Cu^{II}/Cu^{I}, *e.g.*, according to

Reaction 3. $Fe^{3+} + O_2^{-\bullet} \rightarrow Fe^{2+} + O_2$

This is catalytic because the Fe^{3+} is then regenerated by

Reaction 4. $Fe^{2+} + H_2O_2 \rightarrow Fe^{3+} + HO^- + HO^\bullet$

Reaction 1 is the Haber-Weiss reaction and reaction 4 is the *Fenton reaction*. Taken together, reactions 3 + 4 can be called the Fenton catalytic *cycle*, and they sum to reaction 1.
Note 3: The Haber-Weiss and Fenton reactions are an important source of *reactive oxygen species* in cells and tissues experiencing *oxidative stress.*
[*]

habitat

1. Spatial area (geographical area) where a particular *species population* lives, large enough to comprise a breeding population.
   Note: A microhabitat or microenvironment is the immediate surroundings and other physical factors of an individual plant or animal within its *habitat.*
2. Physical conditions that surround a species, or species population, or assemblage of species, or community.

[ref. 2]

habituation

Decrease or cessation of a response to a stimulus after its repeated presentation.
[ref. 4]

Comprehensive Glossary of Terms Used in Toxicology
By John Duffus, Douglas M. Templeton and Michael Schwenk

Published by the Royal Society of Chemistry, www.rsc.org

haem

See *heme.*

hairy cell leukemia

See *leukemia, hairy cell.*

half-life ($t_{1/2}$) (in chemistry)

half-time

Time required for the *concentration* of a reactant in a given reaction to reach a value that is the arithmetic mean of its initial and final (equilibrium) values. For a reactant that is entirely consumed, it is the time taken for the reactant concentration to fall to one-half of its initial value.
Note: The half-life of a reaction has meaning only in special cases:

1. For a first-order reaction, the half-life of the reactant may be called the half-life of the reaction.
2. For a reaction involving more than one reactant, with the *concentration*s of the reactants in their stoichiometric ratios, the half-life of each reactant is the same, and may be called the half-life of the reaction.
3. If the concentrations of reactants are not in their stoichiometric ratios represented in the product, there are different half-lives for different reactants, and one cannot speak of the half-life of the reaction.

[ref. 1]
See also *half-life, biological; half-life, elimination.*

half-life, biological ($t_{1/2}$)

For a substance, the time required for the amount of that substance in a biological system to be decreased to one-half of its value by biological processes, assuming the rate of removal is exponential.
[ref. 1]

half-life, dominant

Half-life of a fraction of a substance in a specific organ or *compartment* if it defines approximately the overall *clearance* rate for that substance at a specific time point.
[ref. 1]

half-life, effective (k_{eff})

Estimated *half-life* in a *compartment model* that has numerous elimination mechanisms, each with an associated k, such that $k_{eff} = (\ln 2)/\Sigma k_i$.
[ref. 2]

half-life, elimination

elimination half-time

Period taken for the *plasma concentration* of a substance to decrease by half.
Note: the term "elimination half-life" may also be applied to body compartments other than plasma, such as blood, specific organs, or tissues.
[ref. 1]

half-time, $t_{1/2}$

See *half-life.*

hallucination (n)/**hallucinate** (v)

The apparent, often strong, subjective perception of an external object or event when no such stimulus or situation is present.
Note: Hallucinations may be visual, auditory, olfactory, gustatory, or tactile.
[ref. 4]

hand-to-mouth activity

See *mouthing behaviour.*

haploid

monoploid

State in which a cell contains only one set of *chromosomes*.
[ref. 1]

haplotype

1. Contraction of "haploid genotype", thus genetic constitution of an individual with respect to one member of a pair of allelic *genes*.
2. Note: Haplotype can refer to only one *locus* or to an entire *genome*. A genome-wide haplotype would comprise half of a diploid genome, including one *allele* from each allelic gene pair.
3. Set of *single nucleotide polymorphisms* found to be statistically associated on a single chromatid, or more generally of *allelic* variants present at a given genetic region.

[ref. 1,3]

hapten (n)/**haptenic** (adj)

Low-molecular-mass *species* which is not itself antigenic unless complexed with a *carrier*, such as a protein.
Note: Once bound to its carrier, the hapten presents an *epitope* that can cause the *sensitization* of *lymphocytes*.
[ref. 1]

hard acid

Lewis acid with an acceptor center of low polarizability.
Note: Other things being approximately equal, complexes of hard acids and bases or *soft acids* and bases have an added stabilization (sometimes called the 'HSAB' rule). For example, the hard O- (or N-) bases are preferred to their soft S- (or P-) analogs by hard acids. Conversely, a soft acid possesses an acceptor center of high polarizability and exhibits the reverse preference for coordination of a soft base.
[ref. 2]
See also *class 'a' metal ion; class 'b' metal ion.*

hard water

Water that contains mineral salts of divalent cations, commonly Ca^{2+} and Mg^{2+} and sometimes Fe^{2+} ions, principally as hydrogen carbonates, chlorides, and sulfates.
Note: *Hardness* caused by calcium hydrogen carbonate is known as temporary, because boiling converts the hydrogencarbonate to calcium carbonate ($CaCO_3$), which has a very low solubility; hardness from the other salts is called permanent.
[ref. 2]

hardness (water)

Concentration of all metallic cations, except those of the alkali metals, present in water.
Note: In general, the concentration of calcium and magnesium ions in water, frequently expressed as mg L^{-1} calcium carbonate or equivalent, is used as a measure of hardness.
[ref. 2]
See also *hard water.*

Hardy–Weinberg equilibrium (genetic equilibrium)

State of a *population* if the frequencies of different *alleles* of all genes in the genome remain constant between generations.
Note 1: The Hardy–Weinberg equilibrium requires the following conditions: (1) the population is large ("infinite"), (2) mating is random, (3) there is no selection, (4) the net mutation rate is zero, and (5) there is no migration.
Note 2: The Hardy–Weinberg equilibrium is a very rare situation in natural populations. Deviation from the Hardy–Weinberg equilibrium is the basis for *microevolution.*
[ref. 2]

harelip

See *cleft lip.*

harm (n)/**harmful** (adj)
adverse effect

Damage or *adverse effect* to a population, species, individual organism, organ, tissue, or cell.
[ref. 1]

harmful occupational factor

Component of the work environment, the effect of which on a worker under certain conditions leads to ill *health* or reduction of working ability.
[ref. 1]

harmful substance
noxious substance

Substance that, following contact with an organism, can cause ill *health* or *adverse effects* either at the time of *exposure* or later in the life of the present and future generations.
[ref. 1]

Hashimoto thyroiditis
chronic lymphocytic thyroiditis

Autoimmune disease where the body's own *antibodies* attack the cells of the thyroid.
[ref. 3]

hay fever
pollenosis

Allergic condition affecting the mucous membranes of the upper respiratory tract and the eyes, characterized by nasal discharge (see *rhinitis*), sneezing, and itchy, watery eyes; and usually caused by an abnormal *sensitivity* to airborne pollen.
[ref. 3]

hazard (n)/**hazardous** (adj)

Set of inherent properties of a substance, *mixture* of substances, or a process involving substances that, under production, transport, usage, or disposal conditions, make it capable of causing *adverse effects* to organisms or the environment, depending on the degree of *exposure*; in other words, it is a source of danger.
[ref. 1]
See also *risk*.

hazard assessment

Determination of factors controlling the likely effects of a *hazard* such as the *dose–effect* and *dose–response relationships*, variations in *target susceptibility, bioaccumulation* potential, *persistence*, and mechanism of *toxicity*.
[ref. 1]

hazard characterization

Second step in the process of *hazard assessment*, consisting of the qualitative and, wherever possible, quantitative description of the nature of the hazard associated with the agent of concern.
Note: Hazard characterization may cover various aspects of the hazard such as the mechanisms of action of the agent, the biological extrapolation of these mechanisms to physiological consequences, and *dose–effect* and *dose–response relationships*, among other properties that may be relevant to the specific circumstances under consideration.
[*]

hazard communication standard

U.S. OSHA standard requiring all employers to inform employees of the *hazard* of substances in the workplace and the steps necessary to avoid harm, now covered by the *Globally Harmonized System*.
[After ref. 1]

hazard evaluation

Establishment of a qualitative or quantitative relationship between *hazard* and benefit of a substance, involving the complex process of determining the significance of the identified hazard and balancing this against identifiable *benefit*.
Note 1: Hazard evaluation should include consideration of the whole *life cycle* of the substance from production through use, transport and final disposal.
Note 2: Hazard evaluation may subsequently be developed into *risk evaluation*.
[After ref. 1]

hazard identification

Determination of substances of concern, their *adverse effects*, *target* populations, and conditions of *exposure*, taking into account *toxicity* data and knowledge of effects on human *health*, other organisms, and their environment.
[ref. 1]

hazard index (HI)

Sum of the *hazard quotients* for substances that affect the same target organ or organ system.
Note 1: Ideally, hazard quotients should be combined for pollutants that cause *adverse effects* by the same mechanism in calculating the HI.

Note 2: Aggregate exposures below a HI of 1.0 are unlikely to result in adverse health effects over a lifetime of *exposure*. A hazard index greater than 1.0 does not necessarily suggest a likelihood of adverse effects.
Note 3: The HI cannot be translated to a probability that adverse effects will occur, and is not likely to be proportional to risk.
[*]

hazard pictogram

Any of a set of icons used for classification and labeling of chemicals that indicate the nature of hazardous properties.
Note: Hazard pictograms should have the advantage over text that they are intelligible to illiterate persons and independent of language. However, interpretation of pictograms may be confused by cultural differences.
[*]

hazard quotient (HQ)

Toxicant exposure (estimated or measured) divided by a reference value regarded as corresponding to an exposure value identified as the threshold of *toxicity*.
Note 1: In the natural environment, the *hazard* quotient is usually determined as the *predicted environmental concentration* divided by the *predicted no-effect concentration*, HQ = PEC/PNEC.
Note 2: If the HQ exceeds unity, the toxicant may produce an adverse effect, but normally this will require an HQ of several times unity; an HQ of less than one indicates that no adverse effects are likely over a lifetime of *exposure*.
[After ref. 2]

hazardous concentration (HC_p, HCS)

Concentration of a substance producing a defined effect on p % (usually 5 %) of *species* of concern, derived by means of a statistical extrapolation procedure.
[ref. 2]
See also *species sensitivity distribution*.

hazardous production factor
hazard at work
hazardous occupational factor

Aspect of production that may, under certain conditions, result in injury or impairment of *health* for a worker involved
[After ref. 1]

headache

Pain in one or more parts of the *cranium*, not confined to the area of distribution of any *nerve*.
[ref. 4]

headache, rebound

Headache caused by stopping *analgesics* following their overuse to relieve headaches.
[ref. 4]

headache, tension

Headache associated with anxiety or other states of distress, often with chronic contraction of the scalp muscles.
[ref. 4]

health

1. According to the World Health Organization, "State of complete physical, mental, and social well-being, and not merely the absence of *disease* or infirmity".
2. State of dynamic balance in which an individual's or a group's capacity to cope with circumstances is at an optimal level.

Note: Taken together, these definitions of health imply a state of well-being characterized by anatomical, physiological, and psychological integrity; the ability to deal with and perform under conditions of physical, biological, psychological, and social stress; and a justified feeling of well-being and freedom from the *risk* of disease and untimely death.

3. In *ecology*, a sustainable steady state in which humans, other living organisms, and their offspring can coexist indefinitely.

[*]

health advisory level (HAL)

In the United States, nonregulatory *health*-based reference level of chemical traces in drinking water (usually implying in the mg L^{-1} range) at which there are no adverse health *risks* when ingested over various periods of time.
Note: Such levels are established for 1 day, 10 days, long-term and life-time *exposure* periods. They allow for a wide *margin of safety*.
[ref. 1]

health-based exposure limit

Maximum *concentration* or intensity of *exposure* that can be tolerated without significant effect, based only on scientific evidence concerning exposure levels associated *health* effects, and ignoring economic considerations.
[After ref. 1]

health hazard

Any *scenario*, factor, or *exposure* that may adversely affect *health*.
[ref. 1]

health surveillance

Periodic medico-physiological examinations of populations or *exposed* workers, with the objective of protecting *health* and preventing occupationally related *disease*.
[ref. 1]

healthy worker effect

Epidemiological phenomenon that workers usually exhibit lower overall *disease* and death rates than the general population, because the old, severely ill, and disabled are ordinarily not working.
Note: Because of this healthy worker effect, disease rates or death rates in the general population may be misleading if this effect is not taken into account.
[After ref. 1]

heat shock protein

Member of an evolutionarily conserved group of proteins whose synthesis is increased by greater transcription of the corresponding genes, to assist in the survival of cells when they are exposed to elevated temperatures.

Note 1: Production of high levels of heat shock proteins can also be triggered by *exposure* to different kinds of environmental stress conditions, for example, *infection, inflammation*, exposure of the cell to chemicals (such as ethanol, arsenicals, or certain metal species), ultraviolet light, starvation, hypoxia (oxygen deprivation), nitrogen deficiency (in plants), or water deprivation. Hence, the alternative name, stress proteins. Their upregulation is sometimes described more generally as part of the stress response.
Note 2: Heat shock proteins often act as *chaperones* of misfolded proteins or in a protective role against *oxidative stress*.
[*]
See also *stress protein*.

heavy chain

H-chain

Larger of the two types of polypeptide chain found in *immunoglobulin* molecules.
Note: Each H-chain is linked by disulfide bonds to a light chain and to another, identical heavy chain. Each heavy chain consists of an *Fc fragment* and an *Fd fragment*. Heavy chains carry the *antigenic determinants* that differentiate the various immunoglobulin classes.
[ref. 3]

heavy metal

Term used commonly in the environmental and biological literature, but having no generally agreed meaning, and sometimes even applied to nonmetals; therefore a source of confusion, to be avoided.
Note: When "heavy metal" is used, the term "metal" alone is often adequate without the qualifying adjective, but this can be misleading as it may imply the elemental form when the intended reference is to a toxic *chemical species*.
[ref. 1]
See also *toxic substance*.

helminthagogue

See *anthelmint(h)ic*.

helminthic

See *anthelmint(h)ic*.

helper cell

See *helper T-lymphocyte (Th)*.

helper T-lymphocyte (Th)

helper cell
helper T-cell
T-helper cell

Member of a subclass of *T-lymphocytes* that provides help (in the form of *cytokines* and/or cognate interactions) necessary for the expression of effector function by other cells in the *immune system*.
Note: Helper T-lymphocytes recognize *antigen* in association with *major histocompatibility complex (MHC) class II* gene products. Depending on their capacity to produce various cytokines, one can functionally differentiate *Th1* (*interleukin*-2- and *IFN*-γ-producing) and *Th2* (interleukins IL-3-, IL-4-, and IL-6-producing) cells.
[ref. 3]

hemagglutination

Agglutination of *erythrocytes*.
[ref. 3]

hemagglutination, passive

Method of measuring *antibody titer*, in which *antigen*-coated *erythrocytes* are agglutinated (see *agglutination*) by adding antibody specific for the antigen.
[ref. 3]

hemagglutinin

Any molecule that *agglutinates erythrocytes*.
[ref. 3]

hemal

1. Pertaining to blood or blood vessels.
2. Situated, in common with the heart and major blood vessels, on the *ventral* side of the body with respect to the *vertebral* column or its *embryonic* precursors.

[ref. 5]

hemangioma

Benign *tumor* formed by a vascular *malformation* present at birth or developing during life, in which proliferation of blood vessels leads to a vascular tangle.
Note 1: Hemangiomas can occur anywhere in the body but are most frequently noticed in the skin and subcutaneous tissues; most hemangiomas present at birth undergo spontaneous regression.
Note 2: Hemangioma in the *brain* (*central nervous system* cavernous hemangioma) can be accompanied with multiple neurological symptoms, ranging from *headache* to *seizures*.
[ref. 5]

hematemesis

Vomiting of blood.
[ref. 1]

hematoma

Region of bleeding into a tissue or organ.
Note 1: Hematoma is often a result of trauma, defective blood clotting or *drugs* that suppress blood clotting.
Note 2: Hematoma of the *brain* is a common cause of *stroke* and is accompanied by potentially lethal increase of *intracranial pressure* and *neuron*al damage.
[ref. 4]

hematopoiesis

hemopoiesis

Development of each of the types of blood cell (*erythrocytes, leukocytes*, and *platelets)* from common precursor cells, located mainly in the bone marrow.
[ref. 5]

hematopoietic stem cell

See *stem cell, hematopoietic*.

hematotoxicity

Adverse changes to the blood caused by *exposure* to chemicals.
[ref. 1]

hematuria

Presence of blood in the urine.
[ref. 1]

heme

haem

Complex consisting of an iron ion coordinated to a *porphyrin* ring acting as a tetradentate ligand, with one or two axial ligands.
Note 1: Heme is a constituent of *hemoglobin* and *cytochromes*.
Note 2: Carbon monoxide has a high affinity to heme and can displace dioxygen from hemoglobin, forming carbonmonoxyhemoglobin (*carboxyhemoglobin*) and interfering with the dioxygen-delivery function of blood.
Note 3: Cyanide has a high affinity to the oxidized (Fe^{III}) state of heme, thus *poisoning* various enzymes, including cytochrome c oxidase (EC 1.9.3.1) in the respiratory electron transport chain.
[*]

heme oxygenase (HOX)

Enzyme (EC 1.14.99.3) activity that catalyzes ring opening of heme to produce biliverdin or its globin *conjugate*, verdoglobin, with release of CO and Fe^{2+}.
Note: Heme oxygenase occurs in three isoforms. HOX-1 is induced by oxidative and hypoxic stress, some metals, and certain *cytokines*. HOX-2 is expressed constitutively. HOX-3 is catalytically inactive but may play a role in O_2-sensing.
[*]

hemimelia

Congenital partial absence of all or part of the *distal* half of a limb.
[ref. 5]

hemiplegia

Paralysis of one side of the body, including the arm, trunk and leg.
[ref. 4]

hemisphere, cerebral

Right or left half of the *brain* in *sagittal* section.
[ref. 4]

hemisphere, dominant

Cerebral hemisphere containing the representation of speech and controlling arm and leg preference in skilled movements.
Note: In most people, the left hemisphere is the dominant hemisphere.
[ref. 4]

hemivertebra

Congenital defect of the *vertebral* column in which one side of a vertebra fails to develop completely due to failure of the *chondrification* center to form on that side.

Note: The resulting wedge-shaped hemivertebra can cause an angle in the spine leading to *kyphosis*, *scoliosis*, or *lordosis*.
[After ref. 5]

hemochromatosis

Inherited *disorder* affecting iron *metabolism*, in which excessive amounts of iron are absorbed in the gut and accumulate in some body tissues.
Note: Because iron deposition is prominent in liver, heart, pancreas and the pituitary gland, common complications of *hemochromatosis* are liver dysfunction and *cirrhosis*, cardiomyopathy, *diabetes mellitus*, and *impotence*. As well, a bronze pigmentation of the skin may be seen.
[ref. 1]

hemodialysis

Use of an artificial kidney in patients with end-stage *renal disease*, designed to remove *toxic* metabolic wastes from the blood by passing it through a tube of semipermeable membrane.
Note: The hemodialysis tubing is bathed in a dialyzing solution to restore the normal chemical composition of the blood while permitting diffusion of toxic substances from the blood.
[ref. 1]

hemoglobin

Heme-containing protein in *erythrocytes*, serving the important function of transporting dioxygen from the lungs to body tissues.
[ref. 1]
See also *heme*.

hemoglobin adduct

Adduct of *hemoglobin*, typically arising from environmental exposure to a harmful substance (*e.g.*, acrylamide, aromatic amines) or excess of an endogenous nutrient or metabolite (*e.g.*, glucose).
Note: Hemoglobin adducts are useful in *biomonitoring* for the respective environmental exposure, and in medical evaluation, as in the use of the glucose adduct HbA1c used to assess long-term glycemic control in *diabetes mellitus*.
[*]

hemoglobinuria

Presence of free *hemoglobin* in the urine.
[ref. 1]

hemolysin

Toxin, usually protein or lipid in nature, produced by a *pathogenic* organism and capable of damaging the membrane of erythrocytes *in vitro*, thus causing the release of *hemoglobin*.
[*]

hemolysis

Rupture (lysis) of the erythrocyte membrane releasing cellular contents, notably *hemoglobin*, giving the blood plasma a red discoloration.
Note: Hemolysis may occur in connection with *disease*, but may also occur *in vitro* upon storage.
[*]

hemolytic anemia

Anemia resulting from the lysis of *erythrocytes*.
[ref. 3]

hemolytic disease of the newborn

erythroblastosis fetalis

Two severe, potentially fatal *anemias* occurring in a *fetus* or newborn infant: *Rhesus (Rh) factor* incompatibility *disease* and *ABO blood group* incompatibility disease.
Note: Hemolytic disease of the newborn is caused by incompatibility between a mother's blood and her unborn baby's blood, causing the mother's *immune system* to launch an *immune response* against the baby's *erythrocytes*.
[ref. 3]

hemolytic plaque assay

See *antibody-forming cell assay*.

hemoperfusion

Passing blood through a column of charcoal or other adsorbent resin, usually for the removal of *drug*s or other *toxic substances*.
[ref. 1]

hemorrhage

Copious escape of blood from a disrupted blood vessel.
Note: When hemorrhage occurs in the *brain*, this is called a hemorrhagic *stroke*.
[ref. 4]

hemosiderin

Insoluble iron(III) hydroxide-based pigment deposited in cells in conditions of iron overload.
[ref. 1]

hen test

Procedure using birds to study acute and delayed *neurotoxic*ity, notably of *organophosphate*s.
Note: After the birds in the hen test are exposured to the test substance, they are observed for *motor activity*, gait changes, *motor coordination*, and related parameters.
[ref. 4]

Henderson–Hasselbalch equation

Equation of the form $pH = pK_a - \log([HA]/[A^-])$, used for the calculation of the pH of solutions where the ratio $[HA]/[A^-]$ is known: HA and A^- are the hydronated and dehydronated forms of an acid, respectively, and pK_a is the acid dissociation constant.
[ref. 1]

Henry's law

Statement that *fugacity* (f_B) of a *solute* (B) in a *solution* at pressure p^θ is directly proportional to the activity (a_B) of the solute, thus

$$f_B = a_{x,B}\, p^\theta / K_{x,B} = \gamma_{x,B} x_B k_{H,B}$$

where $K_{x,\mathrm{B}}$ is the solubility coefficient for infinite dilution (*i.e.*, for pure *solvent*), $\gamma_{x,\mathrm{B}}$ is the activity coefficient of B on a mole fraction basis, x_{B} is the equilibrium mole fraction of dissolved gas, and $k_{\mathrm{H,B}}$ is the *Henry's law constant*. That is, in an ideal solution, the vapor pressure of a dissolved substance is proportional to its mole fraction.
Note 1: The above equation can be taken as a definition of the *Henry's law constant*.
Note 2: Henry's law is often used as a limiting law for converting solubility data from the experimental pressure to standard partial pressure, and this is adequate provided the mole fraction of the gas in the liquid is small and the difference in pressures is small.
[*]

Henry's law constant

Henry coefficient
Henry's law coefficient
Henry constant

At constant temperature and pressure, the ratio of the partial pressure of a gas above a liquid divided by its solubility in the liquid: it is therefore a measure for that gas of its partition between the gas phase and the solute phase.
Note 1: In calculating the Henry's law constant, the solubility may be expressed in any convenient units, such as amount fraction, molality, or substance concentration, but the units must always be given.
Note 2: The Henry's law constant is the limiting value of the solubility of the gas at zero partial pressure.
[After ref. 1]
See also *Henry's law*.

heparin-induced thrombocytopenia (HIT)

Most frequent *antibody*-mediated *drug*-induced *thrombocytopenia*, which occurs in 1–2 % of patients treated with heparin intravenously for longer than four days.
Note: HIT is mediated by antibodies to complexes formed between heparin and the endogenous *platelet* factor 4.
[ref. 3]

hepatic

Pertaining to the liver.
[ref. 1]

hepatic coma

Coma occurring in patients with reduced liver function because of a decreased capacity to *detoxify* neurotoxic substances, formed by the intestinal *microbiota*, that then accumulate in the blood.
Note: Hepatic coma is an example for an endogenous intoxication.
[*]

hepatocyte

Parenchymal cell of the *liver*.
Note 1: The hepatocyte plays a central role in energy *metabolism*.
Note 2: The hepatocyte is the leading cell type for detoxification by *biotransformation* of *xenobiotics*, including *drugs* and ethanol, and is also an excretory organ, as it transports amphiphilic substances into *bile*.

Note 3: Other cell types in the liver serve different functions, *e.g.*, hepatic *Kupffer cells* are phagocytosing cells of the immune system and hepatic stellate cells are fat- and vitamin A-storing cells that become involved in the etiology of liver fibrosis.
[*]

hepatosplenomegaly

Enlargement of the liver and spleen.
[ref. 5]

hepatotoxicity (n)/hepatotoxic (adj)

Toxicity to the liver.
Note 1: Hepatotoxicity is often a consequence of *reactive intermediate* formation (*e.g.*, from carbon tetrachloride, nitrosamines, aflatoxins) during *phase I biotransformation*, which causes *acute hepatocyte necrosis*, and chronically predisposes to liver cirrhosis or liver cancer.
Note 2: Some substances (*e.g.*, paracetamol) exert their hepatotoxicity by *phase II* conjugation to gluathione, thus depleting the hepatocyte of protection against *oxidative stress* by glutathione.
Note 3: Hepatotoxicity can also be attributed to the presence of *ABC-transporters* that cause accumulation of organic molecules (*e.g.*, phalloidin) in liver cells.
[*]

herbicide

Substance intended to kill plants.
[ref. 1]

herbivore (n)/herbivorous (adj)

Feeding on plants.
[*]

hereditary angioneurotic edema

See *edema, hereditary angioneurotic*.

hermaphrodite

Person or other animal having the reproductive organs and many of the *secondary sex characteristics* of both sexes.
[ref. 5]
See also *pseudohermaphrodite*.

hermaphroditism

State of being *hermaphrodite*.
[ref. 5]
See also *pseudohermaphrodite*.

hernia (n)/herniation (n)/herniate (v)/herniated (adj)

Protrusion of an organ or structure through an abnormal opening in *connective tissue* or in the muscle wall of the *cavity* in which it is normally enclosed.
[ref. 5]

hernia, hiatal
hiatus hernia

Upward protrusion of a part of the stomach through a rupture of the *diaphragm* at the esophageal opening.
[ref. 5]

herniation, supratentorial

Abnormal protrusion of *brain* structures into compartments above the *tentorium*, or over the edge of the *tentorium*, due to increased *intracranial pressure*.
[ref. 4]

herniation, transtentorial

Bulging of *brain* tissue from the *cerebrum* through the notch of the *tentorium*, caused by increased *intracranial pressure*.
[ref. 4]

hepatosplenomegaly

Simultaneous enlargement of both the liver (hepatomegaly) and the spleen (splenomegaly).
[*]

herpes

Family of viruses including herpes simplex types 1 and 2, and herpes zoster (also called varicella zoster).
Note: Herpes viruses cause several *infections*, all characterized by blisters and ulcers, including chickenpox, shingles, genital herpes, and cold sores or fever blisters.
[ref. 5]

Hershberger bioassay

Short-term in vivo procedure in which the *androgenic* or antiandrogenic effects of a test substance are studied in castrated, peripubertal male rodents, as indicated by changes in the weights of androgen-dependent tissues.
[ref. 5]

heteroantigen
heterogenetic antigen

Identical or similar *cross-reacting antigen* shared by several species, *e.g., Forssman antigen.*
Note: *Antibodies* produced against a heteroantigen will also react with the other antigens of the set even though these are derived from a different species; such antibodies are also called *heterophile antibodies.*
[ref. 3]

heterologous antibody

See *antibody, heterologous.*

heterologous antigen

See *antigen, heterologous.*

heteromorphic

Occurring in two or more different forms, especially at different stages in the *life cycle*.
[*]

heterophagy

Digestion of exogenous material taken up by a cell by *phagocytosis* or *pinocytosis*, following fusion of the phagocytic or pinocytic vacuole with a *lysosome*.
[ref. 3]

heterophile antibody

See *antibody, heterophile*.

heterophile antigen

See *antigen, heterophile*.

heterosis

See *heterozygote advantage*.

heterotherm (n)/heterothermal (adj)/heterothermic (adj)

Animal that partially regulates its body temperature, sometimes maintaining its temperature at a certain level, *e.g.*, when active, but at other times allowing it to fluctuate with the environment.
Note: Heterothermic organisms can switch between *poikilothermy* and *homeothermy*.
[ref. 2]

heterothermy

Thermal regulation of an organism that can switch between *poikilothermy* and *homeothermy*.
[*]

heterotroph

Organism that cannot utilize inorganic sources of carbon such as carbon oxides and is dependent upon organic carbon for growth.
Note 1: A heterotroph obtains organic food by consuming other organisms or their excreta.
Note 2: Animals, fungi, and most bacteria are heterotrophs.
[*]
See also *autotroph, auxotroph*.

heterotrophy (n)/heterotrophic (adj)

Requirement of an organism for organic carbon derived from other living organisms to support growth.
[*]
See also *autotrophy; auxotrophy*.

heterotrophic succession

See *succession, heterotrophic*.

heterozygote

Organism that has different allelic forms of a specified *gene* on each of a pair of homologous *chromosomes* or describing the *genome* of that organism.
[ref. 1]

heterozygote advantage

heterosis

Greater *Darwinian fitness* (reproductive output) from heterozygous than from homozygous individuals of a species.
Note: Heterozygote advantage tends to preserve variation in the *population* gene pool.
[ref. 2]

heterozygous

Possessing different *alleles* at a given locus on the two homologous chromosomes.
[ref. 3]

hexosaminidase A

See β-*N-acetylhexosaminidase*.

hidromeiosis

Reduced *sweat*ing due to blocking of sweat glands.
[*]

hidrosis

See *diaphoresis*.
[*]

high endothelial venule (HEV)

Specialized venule in *lymphoid* tissues that has walls permeable to migrating *lymphocytes*, allowing them to move from blood into the lymphoid tissues.
[ref. 3]

high-mobility group box (HMGB) protein

Any of a group of universal sensors of nucleic acids, required for the induction of transmembrane and *cytoplasmic* receptor-mediated *innate immune responses*.
[ref. 3]

highly active antiretroviral therapy (HAART)

Approach to the treatment of *acquired immune deficiency syndrome* patients involving a combination of nucleoside analogs, which prevent reverse transcription, with *drugs* that inhibit responses to the virus.
[ref. 3]

Hill plot

Graphical method for analyzing binding of a molecule A to a macromolecule P with n binding sites.
Note: A Hill plot of $\log[\theta/(1-\theta)]$ vs. $\log[A]$ has a slope of 1 if binding is noncooperative and >1 for cooperative binding, where $\theta = [A]_{bound}/n[P]_{total}$ is the fraction of sites occupied.
[ref. 1]

hinge region

Amino acids between the F_{ab} and F_c regions of *immunoglobulin* that permit flexibility of the molecule.
[ref. 3]

hippocampal slice culture

Maintenance *in vitro* of freshly prepared slices of the *hippocampus*.
Note 1: Vital hippocampal slice cultures can be kept for weeks and maintain structure and *neuronal* functions ("organotypic").
Note 2: Hippocampal slice cultures are useful for many types of *brain* research including electrophysiological, biochemical and morphological measurements in studies of *neurotoxicity*.
[ref. 4]
See also *brain slice*.

hippocampus (n)/hippocampal (adj)

Structural component of the *limbic system* of the *vertebrate brain* involved in short-term and long-term memory and spatial navigation.
[ref. 4]
See also *CA pyramidal cell; dentate gyrus; granule cell*.

Hirschsprung syndrome
aganglionic megacolon

Absence of nerve *ganglia* throughout all or part of the *gastrointestinal tract*, causing dysregulation of intestinal motility.
[ref. 5]

hirsutism

Presence of excessive bodily and facial hair.
[ref. 5]

histamine
2-(1*H*-imidazol-4-yl)ethan-1-amine

Bioactive metabolite produced in living organisms by deamination of the amino acid histidine.
Note: Histamine acts as a *neurotransmitter* in the *brain*. It also serves as a mediator in the regulation of various body functions such as gastric secretion, bronchial constriction, *vasorelaxation*, and local *inflammation*.
[ref. 4]
See also *Scombroid poisoning*.

histaminergic

Pertaining to the action of *histamine* or to *neural* pathways in which it functions as a *neurotransmitter*.
[ref. 4]

histaminosis

Histamine intolerance, which may contribute to food intolerance as part of a *pseudoallergic reaction*.
[ref. 3]

histocompatibility

Relationship between a tissue or organ donor and a recipient who have sufficient similarity in *major histocompatibility complex antigens* to avoid *rejection* of a *graft*.
[ref. 3]
See also *histoincompatability*.

histogenic origin

Germ cell layer of the *embryo* from which a given adult tissue develops.
[ref. 1]

histoincompatibility

Relationship between a tissue or organ donor and a recipient who have sufficient differences in *major histocompatibility complex antigens* to cause *rejection* of a *graft*.
[ref. 3]

histology

Study (usually microscopic) of the anatomy of tissues and their cellular and subcellular structure.
[ref. 1]

histopathology

Microscopic study of the anatomy and cell structure of tissues in *disease* to reveal abnormal or adverse structural changes.
[ref. 1]

hit-and-run effect

Toxicity that follows a single *exposure* to a substance.
[ref. 1]

hives

nettle rash
urticaria

Vascular reaction pattern of the skin marked by the transient appearance of smooth, slightly elevated patches (*wheals*) that are either more red or more pale than the surrounding skin and are accompanied by severe itching.
Note: Hives are usually, but not always, caused by an *allergic* reaction to food or to a *drug*, but can also be induced by physical stimuli such as cold or exercise.
[ref. 3]

Hodgkin disease

Hodgkin lymphoma

Immune system tumor characterized by large cells called *Reed–Sternberg cells* that derive from mutated B-lineage cells.
Note: Hodgkin *disease* exists in at least two forms, Hodgkin lymphoma and nodular sclerosis.
[ref. 3]

holoprosencephaly

(formerly arhinencephaly)

Birth defect in which the *embryonic forebrain* fails to divide completely to form the *cerebral hemispheres*.

Note: Holoprosencephaly results in varying degrees of mental impairment and abnormal development of eye, nose, and lip.
[ref. 5]

homeobox

Any of a class of closely similar DNA sequences, occurring in various *genes* and involved in regulating pattern formation, segmentation and *morphogenesis* during *embryonic* development in many species.
[ref. 5]
See also *homeosis*.

homeobox gene

Gene containing a *homeobox* sequence.
[ref. 5]

homeosis (n)/homeotic (adj)

Replacement of part of one segment of an insect or other segmented animal by a structure characteristic of a different segment, especially through *mutation*.
[ref. 5]

homeostasis (n)/homeostatic (adj)

1. Totality of processes occurring in either an open or a closed system, especially a living organism, enabling it to regulate its internal environment to maintain stable, constant conditions.
2. Outcome of processes maintaining stable, constant conditions in a living organism.

[After ref. 2]

homeotherm (n)/homeothermal (adj)/homeothermic (adj)

Organism that maintains a stable internal body temperature though the ambient temperature varies.
Note 1: Homeothermic regulation may be achieved by behavioural mechanisms alone.
Note 2: Homeotherms are not necessarily *endotherms*.
[*]
See also *ectotherm; endotherm; heterotherm*; *poikilotherm*.

homeothermy

Thermal regulation of an organism that provides a stable internal body temperature in spite of variation in ambient temperature.
[*]
See also *ectothermy; endothermy; heterothermy; poikilothermy*.

homing

Movement of *leukocytes* to specific locations in the body.
[ref. 3]

homing receptor

See *receptor, homing*.

homocytotropic antibody

See *antibody, homocytotropic.*

homologous

1. Having the same relationship, relative position, or structure.
2. (of organs) Similar in position, structure, and evolutionary origin but not necessarily in function.
3. (of *chromosomes*) Pairing at *meiosis* and having the same structural features and pattern of *genes.*
4. (of a series of chemical compounds) Having the same functional group(s) but differing in structure by a fixed group of atoms.

[ref. 5]

homologous recombination

See *recombination, homologous.*

homology (in biology)

1. Similarity of anatomical structures in different species because of shared ancestry.
2. Unspecified degree of similarity of *DNA* or *RNA* nucleotide sequences, or of protein amino-acid sequences, supporting the hypothesis that they share a common ancestor.
   Note: Homology among DNA or RNA nucleotide sequences, or among protein amino-acid sequences, is often concluded on the basis of sequence similarity. In general, if there are almost identical sequences, it is likely that they are homologous. However, it is possible that highly similar sequences were not derived from a common ancestor, *i.e.*, they are similar but not homologous.

[ref. 1]

homozygote

Organism that has the same allelic form of a specified *gene* on each of a pair of homologous chromosomes or describing the genome of that organism.
[ref. 1]

homozygous

Possessing the same *allele* at a given locus on the two homologous chromosomes.
[ref. 3]

honey bee larval toxicity test

Procedure in which larvae of honey bee (***Apis mellifera***) are exposed to a test chemical in the diet and subsequent mortality is recorded daily up to the 72-h LD_{50}.
[ref. 5]

hormesis (n)/hormetic (adj)

Apparent beneficial effect of exposure to a low dose of a substance or physical agent that is generally considered to be harmful, identified by an atypical dose response curve.
[After ref. 1]

hormone (n)/**hormonal** (adj)

Substance formed in one organ or part of the body and carried in the blood to another organ or part where it selectively alters functional activity.
[ref. 5]

horror autotoxicus

Term (Latin: dread of self-poisoning) to describe the body's innate aversion to immunological self-destruction.
Note: The term horror autotoxicus was introduced by Paul Ehrlich (1902).
[ref. 3]

host (in immunology)

Recipient of foreign cells or tissue, or of an infectious agent.
[ref. 3]

host defense

Ability of an individual to resist invasion by *opportunistic* agents and production of *disease* associated with exposure to microorganisms, foreign tissue, and particulates, as well as certain types of *neoplasia*.
Note 1: Host defense may be either nonspecific (*innate* or *natural immunity*) or specific (*adaptive* or *acquired immunity*) in nature.
Note 2: Immunological host defense may involve *chemotaxis, phagocytosis*, reaction with *immunoglobulins* and (or) with *complement*, and *T-cell cytotoxicity*.
[ref. 3]

host-resistance assay

Evaluation of *host resistance* in rodents to *in vivo challenge* with an infectious organism under normal conditions and after pharmacological and nutritional alterations of the *immune system*.
[ref. 3]

human chorionic gonadotropin (HCG)

See *chorionic gonadotropin.*

human ecology

See *ecology, human.*

human equivalent dose

Dose of an substance given to a human that is believed to induce the same magnitude of a *toxic* effect that a known dose has induced in an animal.
[ref. 1]

human exposure threshold (of toxicological concern)

Generic value of *exposure* to a substance, or a group of substances falling within a defined structural class, below which there is expected to be no appreciable risk to human *health*.
[ref. 1]

Human Genome Project (HGP)

International research project that started in 1990 with the goal of determining the base-pair sequence of the human *genome*. The project was declared complete in 2003.
Note 1: The HGP also involved studying the genome of a number of organisms other than humans, including insects, fish, plants, and other mammals.
Note 2: The HGP found that there are between 20,000 and 25,000 genes in the human genome, not 100,000 or more as had previously been believed.
[After ref. 5]

human immunodeficiency virus (HIV)

Causative agent of *acquired immune deficiency syndrome*.
Note 1: HIV is a retrovirus of the lentivirus family that selectively infects *macrophages* and *CD4+ T-cells*, leading to their slow depletion, eventually resulting in *immunodeficiency*.
Note 2: There are two major strains of HIV, HIV-1 and HIV-2, of which HIV-1 causes most HIV infections worldwide. HIV-2 is endemic to West Africa but is spreading.
[ref. 3]

human leukocyte antigen (HLA)

Antigen coded by genes of the human *major histocompatibility complex (MHC)*.
Note 1: Human HLA-A, -B and -C (resembling mouse H-2K, D and L) are *MHC class I* molecules, whereas HLA-DP, -DQ and -DR (resembling mouse I-A and I-E) are *MHC class II* molecules.
Note 2: The genes for HLAs are situated on chromosome 6.
[ref. 3]

human leukocyte antigen (HLA) polymorphism

Discontinuous genetic variation in the *major histocompatibility complex* that results in the occurrence of several different forms of MHC molecules among people.
Note: Specific HLA polymorphisms are associated with a number of *diseases, e.g.*, HLA-B27 is associated with ankylosing spondylitis, psoriatic arthritis, *rheumatoid arthritis (RA), etc.*, and some chemical sensitivities.
[ref. 3]

human leukocyte antigen (HLA) type I

Molecules that enable the body to recognize infected cells and tumor cells and destroy them with *cytotoxic T-lymphocytes*.
Note: HLA type I molecules are made by all nucleated cells in the body, possess a deep groove (the *peptide-binding groove*) that can bind peptide *epitopes*, typically 8–11 amino acids long, from endogenous *antigens*; and present HLA type I/peptide complexes to *CD8+ lymphocytes* that have a complementary shaped *T-cell receptor*.
[ref. 3]

human leukocyte antigen (HLA) type II

Molecules that enable *CD4+ lymphocytes* to recognize *epitopes* of exogenous *antigens* and discriminate self from *nonself*.
Note: HLA type II molecules are made by *antigen-presenting cells*, such as *dendritic cells, macrophages*, and *B-lymphocytes*, possess a deep groove (the *peptide-binding groove*) that can bind peptide *epitopes*, typically 10–30 amino acids long but with an optimum length of 12–16 amino acids, from exogenous antigens; and present HLA type II/peptide complexes to CD4+ lymphocytes that have a complementary shaped *T-cell receptor*.
[ref. 3]

humanized antibody

See *antibody, humanized.*

humic substance

Group of nonvolatile organic anionic polyelectrolytes, of biological origin, in the molecular mass range 500–5000, which have complex structures and some variability in composition.
Note 1: Humic substances occur naturally as deposits on *sediment* and *soil* particles and constitute (30–50) % of the *dissolved organic carbon* in natural waters.
Note 2: Humic substances are classified according to solubility and may contain humic acid, *fulvic acid*, and humin.
[ref. 2]

humoral

Pertaining to extracellular fluid such as *plasma* and *lymph*.
[ref. 3]
See also *humoral immunity*.

humoral immune response

Immune response in which specific *antibodies* induce the effector functions (such as *phagocytosis* and activation of the *complement system*).
[ref. 3]

humoral immunity

Specific *immune response* that is mediated primarily by *humoral* factors circulating in solution in the *blood plasma* and *lymph* (*i.e., antibodies* and *complement*).
Note: The induction of the *humoral immune response* generally requires the cooperation of cellular immune mechanisms.
[ref. 3]

humorally mediated immunity (HMI)

See *humoral immunity*.

Huntington disease

Genetic autosomal dominant *neurodegenerative disease* resulting from a mutation in the Huntingtin gene and resulting notably in decline of *cognitive function* and a characteristic *chorea*.
[ref. 4]

Hutchinsonian niche

See *niche, Hutchinsonian.*

hyalin (n)/hyalinized (adj)

Translucent, horny, proteinaceous substance deposited during *collagenous* scar formation, tissue degeneration or amyloid deposition.
Note: Hyaline is an alternate spelling of hyalin, but may also refer to hyaline cartilage, a bluish, translucent, collagen-rich substance found on joint surfaces.
[*]

hyaline

See *hyalin*.

hybrid

1. Result of interbreeding between two animals or plants of different *taxa*.
   Note: Hybrids between different *species* within the same *genus* are sometimes known as interspecific hybrids or crosses. Hybrids between different subspecies within a species are known as intra-specific hybrids. Hybrids between different *genera* are sometimes known as intergeneric hybrids.
2. Cross-breed between *populations*, breeds, or cultivars within a single species.
   Note: Production of hybrids is often used in plant and animal breeding to obtain desirable characteristics not found or inconsistently present in the parent individuals or populations.

[ref. 2]
See also *hybridization*.

hybridization (in genetics)

Process of combining different varieties or *species* of organisms to create a *hybrid*.
[ref. 2]

hybridoma

Hybrid cell line obtained by fusing a lymphoid tumor cell with a *lymphocyte*.
Note: The resultant cell line has both the immortality of the tumor cell and the effector function (*e.g.*, *monoclonal antibody* secretion) of the lymphocyte.
[ref. 3]

hydatidiform mole

Vesicular or *polycystic* mass resulting from the proliferation of the *trophoblast*, with *hydropic* degeneration and *avascularity* of the *chorionic villi*.
Note: The abnormal tissue of a hydatidiform mole typically results from *gene expression* from paternally derived *chromosomes* and a loss of maternal chromosomes.
[ref. 5]

hydranencephaly

Rare condition in which the *brain*'s *cerebral hemispheres* are replaced by sacs filled with *cerebrospinal fluid*.
[ref. 5]

hydrocele

Accumulation of *serous* fluid in a sacculated *cavity*; specifically, such an accumulation in the space of the *tunica vaginalis testis*, or in a separate pocket along the *spermatic cord*.
[ref. 5]

hydrocephalus

Accumulation of excess *cerebrospinal fluid* within the *ventricles* of the *brain*.
Note: Hydrocephalus is associated with raised *intracranial pressure* that may damage the brain and lead to an enlargement of the skull.
[ref. 5]

hydrocephalus, communicating

Hydrocephalus where flow of *cerebrospinal fluid* is not blocked but there is a failure of its reabsorption.
[ref. 3]

hydrocephalus, obstructive

Hydrocephalus where flow of the *cerebrospinal fluid* is blocked.
[ref. 3]

hydrolysis (n)/hydrolytic (adj)

Reaction of a substance with water, usually resulting in the breaking of an ionic (salt hydrolysis) or covalent bond.
[*]

hydromicrocephaly

Microcephaly with excess *cerebrospinal fluid.*
[ref. 5]

hydromyelia

Pathological dilation of the *spinal cord* due to expansion of the *cerebrospinal fluid*-filled central canal of the cord.
[ref. 3]

hydronephrosis

Swelling of the funnel-shaped part of the kidney, where urine is collected to enter the ureter.
Note: Hydronephrosis may be a *congenital* deformity or the consequence of an obstruction in the ureter.
[ref. 5]

hydrophilic (adj)/hydrophilicity (n)

lipophobic/lipophobicity
Opposite term: *hydrophobic/hydrophobicity*.

Describing the character of a substance, material, or molecule that has an affinity for water.
[ref. 1]

hydrophobic (adj)/hydrophobicity (n)

lipophilic/lipophilicty
Opposite term: *hydrophilic/hydrophilicity*.

Describing the character of a substance, material, or molecule that has poor solubility in water, or resists wetting or hydration.
Note 1: Hydrophobicity also suggests that an organic substance with poor water-solubility tends to have a high affinity for nonpolar *solvents* or surfaces.
Note 2: Hydrophobicity is a physicochemical property that describes a partitioning equilibrium of solute molecules between water and an immiscible organic solvent, favoring the latter.
Note 3: Increasing hydrophobicity correlates with *bioaccumulation* but extreme hydrophobicity may prevent passage through the phospholipid bilayer of the cell *membrane* into the internal aqueous phase of the *cytoplasm*.
[After ref. 1]

hydrops (n)/**hydropic** (adj)

Gross *edema* of the entire body, with severe *anemia*, occurring in *hemolytic disease of the newborn.*
[ref. 5]

hydrosphere

Water above, on, or in the Earth's crust, including oceans, seas, lakes, groundwater, and atmospheric moisture.
[ref. 2]

hydroureter
ureterectasia

Dilation of a ureter with fluid.
[ref. 5]

21-hydroxylase

See *steroid 21-monooxygenase.*

4-hydroxynonenal (4-HNE)
4-hydroxy-2-nonenal

Major harmful end product of *lipid peroxidation.*
Note 1: Low concentrations of 4-HNE may have a *hormetic effect* by initiating *signal transduction*, cell proliferation, and increasing antioxidant defenses, while higher concentrations may induce *apoptosis* and *necrosis.*
Note 2: 4-HNE is a potent *inhibitor* of *glutathione-S-transferase* and is shuttled out of cells bound to *glutathione.*
[*]

5-hydroxytryptamine (5-HT)

See *serotonin.*

hygiene

Science of *health* and its preservation.
Note: Hygienic measures are aimed at avoiding unhealthy exposures, notably in the living and working environments.
[After ref. 1]

hygiene hypothesis

See *counter-regulation hypothesis.*

hygroma (n)/**hygromous** (adj)
hydroma

Accumulation of fluid in a sac, *cyst*, or *bursa.*
[ref. 5]

hymen

Thin, *membranous* fold of highly variable appearance that, before its rupture, partly occludes the opening of the *vagina.*
[ref. 5]

hyoid arch

Second *pharyngeal* or *branchial* arch of the developing *embryo*, from which different tissues around the neck, ear and face will develop.
[ref. 5]

hypaxial

Ventral to the long axis of the body.
[ref. 5]

hyper-

Opposite term: *hypo-*.

Prefix meaning above or excessive.
[ref. 1]

hyperalimentation

Ingestion or administration of nutrients in excess of optimal amounts.
[ref. 1]

hyperbilirubinemia

Excessive *concentration* of bilirubin in the blood.
[ref. 1]

hypercalcemia

Excessive *concentration* of calcium in the blood.
[ref. 1]

hypercapnia

Abnormally increased carbon dioxide concentration in the blood resulting in an increased rate and depth of breathing.
Note: Hypercapnia may result either from insufficient *pulmonary* respiration or from increased levels of carbon dioxide in the ambient air.
[ref. 4]

hyperesthesia

Excessive *sensitivity* to touch, pain, or other sensory stimuli.
[ref. 4]

hyperextension

Extension of a limb or part of a limb beyond the normal limit.
[ref. 5]

hyperflexion

Flexion of a limb or part of a limb beyond the normal limit.
[ref. 5]

hypergammaglobulinemia

Increase of *gammaglobulins* in the blood by paraproteinemia or increased production of *immunoglobulins*.
[ref. 3]

hyperglycemia

Excessive *concentration* of glucose in the blood.
Note: Hyperglycemia may be an indicator of *diabetes mellitus*.
[After ref. 1]

hyperhidrosis

Excessive *sweat*.
Note 1: Focal hyperhidrosis is excessive sweat in specific regions of the body.
Note 2: Secondary hyperhidrosis is excessive sweat, secondary to another *disease* condition, usually involving the whole body.
[*]

hyperimmunoglobulin E syndrome

Job syndrome
Rare *primary immunodeficiency syndrome* characterized by recurrent severe staphylococcal skin abscesses (hence Job syndrome), lung infections, and markedly elevated *serum immunoglobulin E* levels.
[ref. 3]

hyperimmunoglobulin M syndrome (HIGM)

Primary *T-cell* defect due to mutations in the *CD40 ligand*, characterized by recurrent (*opportunistic*) infections and very low levels of *immunoglobulin G* and *immunoglobulin A*.
Note: *Autoimmune* manifestations (*e.g.*, *cytopenia*, *arthritis*, sclerosing cholangitis) are often seen in HIGM *syndrome*.
[ref. 3]

hyperkalemia

Excessive *concentration* of potassium in the blood.
Note: Hyperkalemia produces cardiac arrhythmias.
[After ref. 1]

hypermutation

See *somatic hypermutation*.

hypernatremia

Excessive *concentration* of sodium in the blood.
[ref. 1]

hyperparathyroidism

Abnormally increased activity of the parathyroid glands that affects, and is affected by, *plasma* calcium *concentration*.
[ref. 1]

hyperplasia

Abnormal multiplication or increase in the number of normal cells in a tissue or organ.
[ref. 1]

hyperpolarization
Opposite term: *depolarization.*

Transient increase in *membrane polarization* of *nerve cells* or muscle cells.
[ref. 4]

hyperreactivity

Abnormally increased response to a stimulus.
[ref. 3]

hyperreflexia

Increased or exaggerated *reflex* response.
[ref. 4]

hypersensitivity

State in which an individual reacts with *allergic* effects following exposure to a certain substance (*allergen*) after having been exposed previously to the same substance; sometimes used loosely for any increased response.
Note: Four types of hypersensitivity are recognized. Most common chemically induced allergies are type I (*immunoglobulin E*-mediated) and type IV (cell-mediated) hypersensitivity.
[ref. 3]
See also *allergy; Gell and Coombs classification.*

hypersensitivity, cell-mediated

See *hypersensitivity, delayed-type.*

hypersensitivity, contact

Immune response following skin contact with an *antigen.*
[ref. 3]

hypersensitivity, delayed-type (DTH)
cell-mediated hypersensitivity
Gell and Coombs Type IV reaction
type IV hypersensitivity

Form of *T-cell*-mediated *immunity* in which the ultimate effector cell is the activated mononuclear *phagocyte* (*macrophage*).
Note 1: The DTH response to *antigen* appears fully over 24 to 48 h after exposure, and a previous exposure to the antigen is required.
Note 2: Examples of DTH include response to ***Mycobacterium tuberculosis*** (*tuberculin test*) and *contact dermatitis.*
[ref. 3]

hypersensitivity, immediate-type
immediate-type allergy
type I hypersensitivity

Reaction provoked by re-exposure to an *antigen* (*allergen*) that causes *plasma cells* to secrete *immunoglobulin E (IgE)* that binds to *Fc receptors* on the surface of tissue *mast cells* and blood *basophils*, sensitizing them, so that later exposure to the same allergen cross-links the bound IgE, leading to *degranulation* and the secretion of pharmacologically active mediators such as *histamine, leukotriene*, and *prostaglandin* that act immediately on the surrounding tissues.

Note: The principal effects of the products of immediate-type hypersensitivity are vasodilation and smooth-muscle contraction. The reaction may be either local or *systemic*. Symptoms vary from mild irritation to sudden death from *anaphylactic shock*.
[ref. 3]

hypersensitivity, immunoglobulin E (IgE)-mediated

State in which an individual reacts with allergic effects caused fundamentally by the reaction of *antigen*-specific *immunoglobulin E* following *exposure* to a certain substance (*allergen*) after having been *exposed* previously to the same substance.
Note: IgE-mediated hypersensitivity is called "type I allergy", involves release of *histamine* from *mast cells*, and in a severe form may cause *anaphylactic shock*.
[ref. 1]
See also: *hypersensitivity; immunoglobulin E-binding Fc receptors*.

hypersensitivity, type I

See *Gell and Coombs classification; hypersensitivity, immediate-type*.

hypersensitivity, type II

See *Gell and Coombs classification*.

hypersensitivity, type III

See *Gell and Coombs classification*.

hypersensitivity, type IV

See *Gell and Coombs classification; hypersensitivity, delayed-type*.

hypersensitivity pneumonitis (HPS)

See *pneumonitis, hypersensitivity*.

hypersensitization

Development of excessive *immune* reactivity to an *antigen*.
[ref. 3]

hypersusceptibility

Adverse *immunological effects* in an individual occurring under conditions of *exposure* to an *allergen* that result in no effects in the great majority of the *population*, or an individual exhibiting exaggerated effects in comparison with the great majority of those showing some *adverse effects*.
[ref. 3]

hypertelorism

Abnormally wide space between two organs, especially referring to the eyes.
[ref. 5]

hypertension

Persistently high blood pressure in the arteries (systemic hypertension), or in an arterial circuit (*e.g.*, *pulmonary* hypertension or hepatic portal hypertension).
[After ref. 1]

hypertonia

Extreme tension of muscles or arteries.
Note: Hypertonia is often a result of an *upper motor neuron* lesion in the *brain*, and is accompanied by decreased *synaptic inhibition* and increased excitability of muscle.
[ref. 5]

hypertrichosis

See *hirsutism*.

hypertrophy

Excessive growth in bulk of a tissue or organ through increase in size, but not in number, of the constituent cells.
[ref. 1]

hypervariable region

Amino acid sequence within the *immunoglobulin* and *T-cell receptor variable regions* that shows the greatest variability and contributes most to the *antigen-* or peptide-*major histocompatibility complex molecule* binding site.
[ref. 3]

hypervitaminosis

Adverse condition resulting from the ingestion of an excess of one or more vitamins.
[After ref. 1]

hypnotic

Agent that may reduce anxiety and induces sleep.
[ref. 4]
See also *soporific*.

hypo-

Opposite term: *hyper-*.

Prefix meaning under or deficient.
[ref. 1]

hypoblast

Innermost of the three primary *germ layers*, adjacent to the *blastocyst cavity*: the hypoblast develops subsequently into the *endoderm*.
[ref. 5]

hypocalcemia

Abnormally low calcium *concentration* in the blood.
[ref. 1]

hypocapnia

Abnormally decreased carbon dioxide concentration in the blood.
Note: An increased respiratory rate during normal metabolic activity may cause hypocapnia that may be associated with *spasms*.
[ref. 4]

hypogammaglobulinemia

Immunodeficiency state marked by abnormally low levels of all classes of *immunoglobulins*, associated with increased susceptibility to infectious *diseases*.
Note: Hypogammaglobulinemia may be primary (inherited), or secondary (acquired), or it may occur physiologically in normal *neonates*.
[ref. 3]

hypogonadism

Inadequate functioning of the *testes* or *ovaries* as manifested by deficiencies in *gametogenesis* or in secretion of *gonadal hormones*.
Note: Primary hypogonadism refers to a defect that is inherent in the gonad while secondary hypogonadism refers to a defect lying outside the gonad, often an *endocrine* effect.
[ref. 5]

hypohidrosis

Abnormally low excretion of *sweat*.
[*]

hypokalemia

Abnormally low potassium *concentration* in the blood.
Note: Hypokalemia carries a risk of cardiac arrhythmias.
[After ref. 1]

hypomagnesemia

Abnormally low magnesium *concentration* in the blood.
[ref. 1]

hyponatremia

Abnormally low sodium *concentration* in the blood.
[ref. 1]

hypophysectomy

Surgical removal of the *pituitary gland* (*hypophysis*).
[ref. 4]

hypophysis

See *pituitary*.

hypoplasia

Underdevelopment or *atrophy* of a tissue or organ.
[ref. 5]

hyporeflexia

Diminished *reflex* response.
[ref. 4]

hyposensitization therapy

Dermal application of a selected *allergen* to an *allergic* person in stepwise increasing dosage, with the aim of reducing the *immune system's* tendency for the corresponding *allergic reaction*.
[ref. 3]

hypospadias

Birth defect in which the *urethra* opens on the underside of the penis, or into the *vagina*.
[ref. 5]

hypotension

1. Subnormal arterial blood pressure.
   Note: Hypotension can be a cause of dizziness, weakness and fainting.
2. Lower than normal pressure or tension of any kind (used less commonly).

[ref. 4]

hypothalamus

Region at the base of the *brain* containing specialized *nerve cell*s that help activate, control, and integrate peripheral *autonomic* mechanisms, endocrine activities, and some somatic functions such as body temperature, sleep, and appetite.
[ref. 4]

hypotonia

1. Condition in which there is a diminution or loss of muscle tone.
2. Relaxation of the arteries.
3. Lower than normal tension in any part, as in intraocular pressure of the eyeball.

[ref. 4]

hypovolemic

Pertaining to an abnormally decreased volume of circulating fluid (*plasma*) in the body.
[ref. 1]

hypoxemia

Deficient oxygenation of the blood.
[ref. 1]

hypoxia (n)/hypoxic (adj)

1. Abnormally low dioxygen content or tension.
   Note: Even short periods of hypoxia may result in irreversible *brain* damage.
2. Deficiency of dioxygen in the inspired air, in blood, or in tissues, short of anoxia.

[After ref. 4]

hypoxic

Deficient of dioxygen.
[ref. 1]

Ia antigen

See *antigen, Ia.*

IPEX syndrome

See *immunodysregulation–polyendocrinopathy–enteropathy, X-linked.*

IQ test

See *intelligence quotient.*

ir genes

See *immune response genes.*

iatrogenic

Any adverse condition resulting from medical treatment.
[ref. 1]

ichthyosis (n)/**ichthyotic** (adj)

fish-skin disease
fish-scale disease
xeroderma

Congenital disorder of *keratinization*, characterized by dryness and scaling of the skin, often associated with other defects and with abnormalities of lipid *metabolism.*
[ref. 5]

icterus (n)/**icteric** (adj)

jaundice
hyperbilirubinemia

Pathological condition characterized by deposition of bilirubin in the skin and mucous membranes, including the conjunctival membranes, giving them a yellowish discolouration.
Note 1: The most common cause of icterus is liver dysfunction.
Note 2: Neonatal jaundice is a result of the immaturity of the fetal liver. A certain degree of icterus may be normal in the neonate, but it requires treatment with phototherapy in premature infants who are especially at risk for *kernicterus.*
[*]

ictus

Sudden attack, *stroke* or *seizure.*
[ref. 4]

identical twin

monozygotic twin

One of a pair of twins resulting from one *zygote* that, at an early stage of *embryonic* development, separated into two independently growing cell aggregations giving rise to two individuals of the same sex and identical genetic constitution.
[ref. 5]

Comprehensive Glossary of Terms Used in Toxicology
By John Duffus, Douglas M. Templeton and Michael Schwenk

Published by the Royal Society of Chemistry, www.rsc.org

idiopathic

Term that describes a primary symptom or *disease* in which no underlying cause or associated *disorder* can be found.
Note: In many cases of idiopathic disease, *autoimmune* processes are involved in the *pathogenesis* (*e.g.*, idiopathic *Addison disease,* idiopathic *thrombocytopenic purpura*).
[ref. 3]

idiopathic environmental intolerance

See *multiple chemical sensitivity.*

idiopathic thrombocytopenic purpura (ITP)

Thrombocytopenia of unknown cause, probably related to the production of anti-*platelet* antibodies, and leading to bruising (*purpura*).
[ref. 3]

idiosyncrasy (n)/idiosyncratic (adj) (in toxicology)

Genetically based unusually high *sensitivity* of an organism to the effect of certain substances.
[ref. 1]
See also *idiosyncratic drug reaction.*

idiosyncratic drug reaction (IDR)

Rare and unpredictable *adverse drug reaction* occurring only in susceptible individuals.
Note: A dose–response relationship in IDRs may not be apparent within the dose range used clinically.
[ref. 3]

idiotope

Epitope made up of amino acids within the *variable region* of an *antibody* or *T-cell receptor* that reacts with an anti-idiotope *antibody*.
Note: The anti-idiotopic region of the anti-idiotope antibody may mimic the epitope-binding characteristics of the *antigen* without sharing any sequence homology.
[ref. 3]
See also *antibody, anti-idiotypic; idiotype.*

idiotype (n)/idiotypic (adj)

The combined *antigenic determinants* (*idiotopes*) expressed in the *variable region* of *immunoglobulins* of an individual that determine *antibody* specificity to a particular *antigen*.
[ref. 3]
See also *antibody, anti-idiotypic.*

idiotypic network

idiotype network

Regulatory network based on interactions of *anti-idiotypic antibodies* and *idiotypes* present on *antibodies* and *T-cell receptors*, resulting in feedback inhibition of ongoing *B-cell* or *T-cell* responses.
[ref. 3]

ileocecal

Relating to the *ileum* and the *cecum*.
[ref. 5]

ileum

Third portion of the small intestine, between the *jejunum* and the *cecum*.
[ref. 5]

iliac artery
hypogastric artery

Main artery of the pelvis.
[ref. 5]

immature (in immunology)

Describing cells that are not fully developed and unable to participate immediately in an *immune response*.
Note: Immature *B-cells* and *T-cells* migrate from their *primary lymphoid* sites (*bone marrow* and *thymus*) through the vascular and *lymphatic systems* to *secondary lymphoid* sites. These sites include the *spleen, lymph nodes, tonsils*, and *Peyer's patches* in the intestine and *appendix*. The immature B cells and T cells mature only after they encounter an *antigen*.
[ref. 3]

immediately-dangerous-to-life-or-health-concentration (IDLHC)

According to the U.S. NIOSH, the maximum *exposure concentration* from which one could escape within 30 min without any escape-impairing symptoms or any irreversible *health* effects.
[ref. 1]

immediate-type hypersensitivity

See *hypersensitivity, immediate-type*.

immission

Environmental *concentration* of a *pollutant* resulting from a combination of *emissions* and dispersals (often synonymous with *exposure*).
[ref. 1]

immune

Possessing *immunity*.
[*]

immune adherence

Attachment of a particulate *antigen* coated with the complement component C3b to cells expressing C3b *receptors*, resulting in enhanced *phagocytosis* of bacteria by *macrophages*.
[ref. 3]

immune complex

Product of an *antigen–antibody* reaction that may also contain components of the *complement* system.
[ref. 3]

immune complex disease

Illness resulting from deposition of *antigen-antibody* complexes in tissues.
[ref. 3]

immune deviation

Regulatory mechanism of the preferential activation of one aspect (cellular or humoral) of the *adaptive immune system* at the expense of the other.
Note: Although not a form of true *tolerance*, immune deviation may be involved in the induction and maintenance of *self-tolerance*.
[ref. 3]

immune elimination

Removal of *pathogens* or tumor cells by the immune system; the first step of *immunoediting* of tumors.
[ref. 3]

immune enhancement

Therapeutic stimulation of the *immune response*, especially in tumor therapy.
[ref. 3]

immune equilibrium

State in carcinogenesis where there is an equilibrium between elimination of tumor cells by the *immune system* and growth of non*immunogenic* tumor cells; the second step in *immunoediting*.
[ref. 3]

immune escape

Biological feature of an infectious agent or of a tumor cell that prevents its elimination by the *immune system*.
Note 1: Immune escape can be acquired by a selection process.
Note 2: Immune escape is the third step in *immunoediting* of tumors.
[ref. 3]

immune evasion

Property of a *pathogen* that results in avoidance of attack by the *immune system, e.g.*, because of reduced *phagocytosis*, lack of recognition by the *innate immune system*, or *suppression* of the *immune response*.
[ref. 3]

immune modulation

immunomodulation

Alteration of the *immune response* to alleviate harmful effects of the *immune system* or to promote its activity by changes in regulatory factors; often part of deliberate *therapeutic* intervention.
[ref. 3]

immune regulation

immunoregulation

Capacity of the *immune system* to regulate itself so that an *immune response* does not become excessive and cause tissue damage, an *autoimmune* reaction, or an *allergic reaction*.
[ref. 3]

immune reserve hypothesis

Hypothesis that the *immune response* involves multiple redundancies capable of compensating for acute reductions in certain immune functions.
Note: The hypothesized immune reserve might prevent a serious reduction in *host resistance* after temporary *immunosuppression* of selected parameters (*e.g., natural killer cell* function).
[ref. 3]

immune response

Selective reaction of the body to substances that are foreign to it, or that the *immune system* identifies as foreign, shown by the production of antibodies and *antibody*-bearing cells or by a *cell-mediated hypersensitivity* reaction.
[ref. 1]

immune response, adaptive

Immune response based on the principle of clonal recognition, such that upon first exposure to an *antigen*, primed *lymphocytes* either differentiate into immune effector cells or form an expanded pool of *memory cells* that respond to secondary exposure to the same antigen by mounting an amplified and more rapid response.
Note: The response may be classified as cellular (*T-cell*-mediated) or *humoral* (*antibody*-dependent).
[ref. 3]
Compare *innate immunity*.

immune response, cell-mediated

Specific *immune response* in which *T-lymphocytes* mediate the effects, either through the release of *cytokines* or through *cytotoxicity*.
[ref. 3]

immune response, secondary

Qualitatively and quantitatively improved *immune response* that occurs upon the second encounter of *primed lymphocytes* with a given *antigen*.
[ref. 3]

immune response-associated (Ia) protein

Protein found in *antigen-presenting cells* and *B-lymphocytes* in mice.
[ref. 3]
Compare *Ia antigen*.

immune response genes

Genes, including those within the *major histocompatibility complex*, that together determine the overall level of *immune response* to a given *antigen*.
[ref. 3]

immune surveillance
immunosurveillance

Recognition, and in some cases elimination, of tumor cells by the *immune system* before they become clinically detectable.
[ref. 3]

immune system

Integrated network of organs, glands, and tissues that has evolved to protect the body from foreign substances, including bacteria, viruses, and other infection-causing parasites and *pathogens*.
Note 1: The immune system may produce *hypersensitivity* reactions that, in the extreme, can be fatal.
Note 2: If the immune system misidentifies normal body components as foreign, this leads to *autoimmune disorders*, such as *systemic lupus erythematosus*, in which the body destroys its own constituents.
[ref. 1]

immune thrombocytopenic purpura

See *thrombocytopenic purpura, idiopathic (ITP)*.

immunity

Inherited, acquired, or induced *resistance* to infection by a specific *pathogen*.
[ref. 3]

immunity, acquired

State of protection against *pathogen*-induced injury, with rapid *immune elimination* of pathogenic invaders owing to previous *immunization* or *vaccination*.
[ref. 3]

immunity, innate

Immunity that is not intrinsically affected by prior contact with *antigen, i.e.*, all aspects of immunity not directly mediated by *lymphocytes*.
[ref. 3]

immunity, natural

Repertoire of host defense mechanisms that do not require prior exposure to *antigen*.
Note: Natural immunity may involve the actions of *macrophages* and *natural killer cells*, mucocutaneous or integumental barriers, the action of cilia or microvilli, or physiological processes, *e.g.*, urinary outflow, vascular perfusion of tissues, or the presence of native flora, which "outcompete" *pathogens*.
[ref. 3]

immunization

Making an organism immune to a specific agent, such as an *allergen, pathogen*, or *cancer* cell.
[ref. 3]
See also *immunization, active; immunization, passive; vaccination*.

immunization, active

Immunization with *antigen*, as distinct from the transfer of *antibody* to an unimmunized individual, which is called *passive immunization*.
[ref. 3]

immunization, passive

Immunization of an individual by the transfer of *antibody* synthesized in another individual.
[ref. 3]

immunization, primary

First introduction of a *vaccine* into the body for the purpose of inducing *immunity*.
[ref. 3]
See also *primary immune response*.

immunoactivation

Activation of the *immune system* as a whole to react more rapidly to *antigens*.
[ref. 3]

immunoactivator

Agent that activates the *immune system* as a whole to react more rapidly to *antigens*.
[ref. 3]

immunoadsorption

Method for removal of *antibody* or *antigen* by allowing it to bind to a corresponding antigen or antibody immobilized in the solid phase.
[ref. 3]

immunoassay

Ligand-binding assay that uses a specific *antigen* or *antibody*, capable of binding to the analyte, to identify and quantify substances.
Note: The antibody in an immunoassay can be linked to a radioisotope (*radioimmunoassay, RIA*) or to an enzyme that catalyzes an easily monitored reaction (*enzyme-linked immunosorbent assay, ELISA*), or to a highly fluorescent compound by which the location of an antigen can be visualized (*immunofluorescence*).
[ref. 3]

immunoblot

Supporting substrate (often a nitrocellulose, nylon, or poly(1,1-difluoroethylene) [obsolete: poly(vinylidene fluoride), PVDF] membrane) onto which proteins that have been separated by gel electrophoresis are transferred and then identified by the binding of specific *antibodies*.
[ref. 3]
See also *immunoblotting*.

immunoblotting
western blotting

Technique for the detection, isolation, and quantitative measurement of specific immunoreactive polypeptides, separated into bands by polyacrylamide gel electrophoresis, after which the bands are transferred from the gel to a membrane (*immunoblot*), followed by immunological detection of the immobilized *antigen* by the binding of specific *antibodies* typically labeled with peroxidase or radioactivity.
[ref. 3]

immunochemistry

Study of biochemical and molecular aspects of *immunology*, especially the nature of *antibodies, antigens*, and their interactions.
[ref. 1]

immunocompetence (n)/immunocompetent (adj)

Having the ability to exhibit an *immune response*.
[ref. 3]

immunocompromised

Unable to mount a full or effective *immune response.*
[ref. 3]

immunoconjugate

antibody conjugate

Antibody or antibody fragment to which a functional molecule, such as a *drug*, has been chemically linked.
[ref. 3]
See also *immunocytokine.*

immunocytochemistry

See *immunohistochemistry.*

immunocytokine

Antibody or antibody fragment to which a *cytokine* has been chemically linked.
Note: An immunocytokine construct may be used to direct a cytokine to the antibody's target cell.
[ref. 3]

immunodeficiency (n)/immunodeficient (adj)

Inability to produce a normal repertoire of *antibodies* or immunologically sensitized *T-lymphocytes*, especially in response to specific *antigens.*
Note 1: Immunodeficiencies arise from effects in one or more components of the immune system result in the inability to eliminate or neutralize antigens.
Note 2: Congenital or primary immunodeficiencies are genetic or due to developmental *disorders*, such as congenital *thymic* aplasia (see also *thymic atrophy*).
Note 3: Acquired or secondary immunodeficiencies develop as a consequence of malnutrition, malignancies, *immunosuppressive* compounds, radiation or infection of *immunocompetent* T-lymphocytes with *human immunodeficiency virus.*
Note 4: Defects in *natural immunity* may also result in immunodeficiency.
[ref. 3]

immunodeficiency, acquired

See *acquired immunodeficiency syndrome.*

immunodeficiency syndrome

See *acquired immunodeficiency syndrome.*

immunodeficiency, X-linked severe combined

Sex-linked trait of *severe combined immunodeficiency syndrome* carried on the X-chromosome, resulting from nonfunctional *B-lymphocytes* and lack of *T-lymphocytes* and *natural killer lymphocytes*, and leading to recurrent, persistent, and severe infections.
[ref. 3]

immunodominant epitope

See *epitope, immunodominant.*

immunodysregulation–polyendocrinopathy–enteropathy, X-linked
IPEX syndrome

X-linked *syndrome* characterized by immunodysregulation, polyendocrinopathy (*diabetes mellitus type 1, thyroiditis*), *hemolytic anemia, thrombocytopenia, dermatitis*, and enteropathy, caused by mutations in the gene encoding *Foxp3*.
[ref. 3]

immunoediting

Process of continuing *immunosuppression* of *immunogen*ic tumor cells, which may finally result in the selection of nonimmunogenic tumor cells.
Note: Immunoediting consists of the steps *immune elimination, immune equilibrium*, and *immune escape*.
[ref. 3]

immunofluorescence

Technique for detection of cell- or tissue-associated *antigens* by the use of a fluorescently tagged *ligand* (*e.g.*, an anti-*immunoglobulin conjugated* to *fluorescein isothiocyanate*).
[ref. 3]

immunogen (n)/immunogenic (adj)

Any substance that elicits an *immune response*.
Note: Whilst all *immunogens* are *antigens*, not all antigens are immunogens.
[ref. 3]
See also *hapten*.

immunogenicity

1. Property of being an *immunogen*.
2. Extent to which a substance elicits an *immune response*.

[*]

immunoglobulin (Ig)

Member of a *glycoprotein* family to which *antibodies* and *B-cell receptors* belong.
Note 1: Immunoglobulins bind to substances in the body that are recognized as foreign *antigens* (often proteins on the surface of bacteria and viruses).
Note 2: Immunoglobulins play a central role in *allergies* when they bind to antigens that are not otherwise a threat to health and provoke an inflammatory reaction.
[ref. 3]
See also specific *immunoglobulins A, D, E, G*, and *M*.

immunoglobulin A (IgA)

Class of *immunoglobulin (Ig)* characterized by α *heavy chains*.
Note: IgA antibodies are secreted mainly by *mucosal lymphoid* tissues, and in the dimeric form are present in mucosal secretions. IgA in the monomeric form is present in blood.
[ref. 3]
See also *secretory immunoglobulin A*.

immunoglobulin D (IgD)

Class of *immunoglobulin (Ig)* characterized by δ *heavy chains*.
Note: IgD appears as a surface immunoglobulin on mature native *B-cells* (see *native lymphocyte*) but its function is unknown.
[ref. 3]

immunoglobulin E (IgE)

Class of *immunoglobulin (Ig)* characterized by ε *heavy chains.*
Note: IgE is involved in the defense against parasite infections and in *allergic reactions.*
[ref. 3]

immunoglobulin E (IgE)-binding Fc receptors

High-*affinity* IgE-binding *Fc-ε-R* type I *receptors* are expressed on *mast cells* and *basophils* and interact with IgE *antibodies* with high affinity.
Note 1: The cross-linking of IgE-binding Fc receptors, induced by allergen binding, results in release of mediators such as *histamine.*
Note 2: The IgE-binding Fc receptors are composed of α, β, and γ chains; the α chain contains the IgE binding site, while the γ chain is responsible for *signal transduction.*
Note 3: The low-affinity IgE binding *Fc receptor* (*CD23*) is expressed on *B-cells*, and its soluble (truncated) form is generated by proteolytic cleavage and regulates IgE production by B-cells.
[ref. 3]

immunoglobulin E (IgE)-mediated hypersensitivity

See *hypersenitivity, immunoglobulin E (IgE)-mediated.*

immunoglobulin G (IgG)

Class of *immunoglobulin* characterized by γ *heavy chains.*
Note: Immunoglobulin G is the most abundant class of immunoglobulin found in the *plasma.*
[ref. 3]

immunoglobulin (Ig) gene superfamily

Genes encoding proteins containing one or more *immunoglobulin domains* (homology units) that are homologous to either Ig *variable region* or *constant region* domains.
Note: Cell surface and soluble molecules mediating recognition, adhesion, or binding functions in and outside the *immune system*, derived from the same precursor, belong to the Ig gene superfamily of molecules.
Examples: Immunoglobulin, *T-cell receptor, major histocompatibility complex class I* and *class II molecules, CD4, CD8*, FcγR.
[ref. 3]
See also *immunoglobulin superfamily.*

immunoglobulin M (IgM)

Class of *immunoglobulin* characterized by μ *heavy chains.*
Note 1: IgM is the first class of immunoglobulin to appear during sensitization to an allergen on the surface of *B-cells* and the first to be secreted.
Note 2: Unlike other immunoglobulins that exist in the monomeric (*immunoglobulins A, D, E,* and *G*) or dimeric (*immunoglobulin A*) state, IgM is found in the blood as a pentamer.
[ref. 3]

immunoglobulin (Ig) superfamily

Large family of proteins characterized by possession of "immunoglobulin-type" domains of approximately 110 amino acids folded into two β-pleated sheets. Members

include *immunoglobulins A, E, G,* and *M; T-cell receptors*; and *human leukocyte antigen major histocompatibility complex molecules.*
[ref. 3]
See also *immunoglobulin gene superfamily.*

immunoglobulin Y (IgY)

Immunoglobulin found in chickens.
[ref. 3]

immunohistochemistry

Detection of cell-associated molecules in the microscope with *antibodies* labeled with enzymes that change a substrate into a colored precipitate.
[ref. 3]

immunological ignorance

Absence of a *pathogenic autoimmune* response in spite of the concomitant presence in the *host* of the *autoantigen* and *T-cells* bearing the specific *autoreactive T-cell receptor.*
[ref. 3]

immunological incompetence

Inability of the *immune system* to function in a normal fashion.
[ref. 3]

immunologically privileged site

Any of various sites in the body where foreign tissue *grafts* do not induce an immune reaction.
Note: Immunologically privileged sites include the eye, *brain*, testis, and unborn fetus. Although *antigens* do migrate from these privileged sites, they either induce *immunological tolerance* or a nondestructive response.
[ref. 3]

immunological memory
immunological anamnesis

Ability of the *immune system* to respond faster and more effectively to subsequent exposures to an *antigen* following a *primary immune response* to the same antigen.
Note: Typically for immunological memory, *memory T-cells* appear five days following initial immunization, whereas *memory B-cells* may take about a month to reach maximum levels. Populations of such cells may persist for the lifetime of the individual.
[ref. 3]

immunological synapse

See *synapse, immunological.*

immunological tolerance

See *tolerance, immunological.*

immunology (n)/immunological (adj)

Science that deals with the *immune system* including *cell-mediated immunity* and *humoral* aspects of *immunity* and *immune responses.*
[ref. 3]

immunology, reverse

High-throughput procedure where information on potential *immunogenic tumor* proteins is gained from the amino acid sequences of *gene products* specifically expressed by the tumor, followed by predicted fitting of putative *antigenic* peptides to a *peptide-binding groove*, and finally experimental verification.
[ref. 3]

immunomagnetic separation

Method of separating specific cell types or macromolecules with the aid of cell-specific *antibodies* coupled to paramagnetic beads.
[ref. 3]

immunomodulation (n)/immunomodulating (adj)

Modification of the functioning of the *immune system* by the action of a substance that increases or reduces the ability to produce an *immune response*.
[ref. 3]

immunopathology

1. Study of *diseases* of the *immune system*.
2. The occurrence of such diseases.

[ref. 3]

immunopathy

Any *disease* of the *immune system*.
[ref. 3]
See also *immunopathology*.

immunopharmacology

1. Study of the *immune system* using *drugs* as diagnostic tools.
2. Use of *pharmaceutical* molecules to support and stimulate the immune system in patients with *immunodeficiency*, or to suppress or specifically influence the reactivity of the immune system in order to control a pathological immune reaction or *disease*.

[ref. 3]

immunophenotyping

Use of a panel of *antibodies* to determine a subset of proteins expressed on the surface of a cell or heterogeneous group of cells, often for diagnostic purposes, *e.g.*, identifying the presence of *leukemia* cells in a population of *lymphocytes*.
[ref. 3]

immunophilin

Any of a group of *cytoplasmic* proteins in *T-cells* that are targets of the *immunosuppressant drugs* cyclosporin A, tacrolimus (fujimycin), rapamycin, and related compounds.
[ref. 3]

immunopotentiation

Enhancement of the capacity of the *immune system* to produce an effective response.
[ref. 1]

immunoprecipitate

Precipitate formed in an *antigen–antibody* reaction.
[ref. 3]

immunoprecipitation

Process of precipitating something by reaction with a specific *antibody* or *antigen*.
[ref. 3]

immunoreceptor tyrosine-based activation motif (ITAM)

Consensus sequence for src-family *tyrosine kinases*, found in the cytoplasmic domains of several signaling molecules including the *signal transduction* units of *lymphocyte antigen receptors* and of *Fc receptors*.
[ref. 3]
See also *killer cell activatory receptor; killer cell immunoglobulin-like receptor*.

immunoreceptor tyrosine-based inhibitory motif (ITIM)

Consensus sequence, present in the cytoplasmic domains of certain cell surface molecules (*e.g.*, Fc γ RIIB, *killer cell inhibitory receptors*), that mediates inhibitory signals.
[ref. 3]
See also *killer cell immunoglobulin-like receptor*.

immunosensitivity

Reactivity to *antigens*.
[ref. 3]

immunosensitizer

Substance that makes the *immune system* more reactive to *antigens*.
[ref. 3]

immunosorbent

Solid *matrix* on to which a specific *antibody* or *antigen* is adsorbed and used to capture the corresponding antigen or antibody from solution.
[ref. 3]

immunostimulating complex (ISCOM)

Immunological *adjuvant* composed of saponin, cholesterol, phospholipid, and an *immunogen*, usually protein.
Note: ISCOM was originally designed to form a *vaccine* delivery system that combined certain aspects of virus particles such as their size and orientation of surface proteins, with the powerful *immunostimulatory* activity of saponins.
[ref. 3]

immunostimulation (n)/immunostimulatory (adj)

Increase in immune function, *e.g.*, by use of *bacille Calmette–Guérin vaccine* or *drugs*.
Note: Immunostimulation may be beneficial (*e.g.*, restoration of a depressed *immune response*) or detrimental (*e.g.*, induction by drugs of *allergy, hypersensitivity*, or *autoimmunity*).
[ref. 3]

immunosuppressant

Substance that depresses the function of the *immune system.*
[ref. 3]

immunosuppression

Depression of the normal functioning of the *immune system.*
Note: Immunosuppression may be due to 1. inhibition of the normal response of the immune system to an *antigen*, or 2. prevention, by chemical or biological means, of the production of an *antibody* to an antigen by inhibition of the processes of transcription, translation, or formation of tertiary structure.
[ref. 3]

immunosuppressive

Causing depression of the normal function of the *immune system.*
[ref. 3]

immunosurveillance

Mechanisms by which the *immune system* is able to recognize and destroy *malignant* cells before the formation of an overt *tumor.*
[ref. 1]

immunotherapy

Treatment or prevention of a *disease* using agents that can modify the *immune response*.
Note 1: Immunotherapy is applied most widely in the treatment of leukemias, melanoma, and hypernephroma.
Note 2: Immunotherapy may involve *active* or *passive immunization, immunopotentiation* or *immunosuppression, hyposensitization, bone marrow transplantation*, or *thymus* implantation.
[ref. 3]

immunotoxic

Harmful to the *immune system.*
[ref. 1]

immunotoxicant

Substance that is harmful to the *immune system.*
[ref. 3]

immunotoxicology

Discipline applying cardinal principals of both *immunology* and toxicology to study the ability of certain substances to alter the *immune response.*
[ref. 3]

immunotoxin

Biochemical *conjugate*, or recombinant fusion protein, consisting of an immune targeting molecule such as an *antibody* or antibody fragment together with a *cytotoxic* molecule.
[ref. 3]
Compare *toxin.*

imperforate anus
anal atresia

Congenital absence of an *anal* opening due to the persistence of the *epithelial* plug (persistence of the anal membrane) or to complete absence of the *anal canal.*
[ref. 5]

impermeable

Of a *membrane*, not allowing a given substance to pass through.
Note: When applied to nonbiological membranes without a qualifier, impermeable normally refers to impermeability to water.
[ref. 1]

implantation
nidation

Embedding of the early *embryo* in the lining of the *uterus.*
[ref. 5]

imposex

Pseudohermaphrodite condition in female gastropods (snails) manifested by the development (imposition) of male characteristics such as a penis or vas deferens.
Note: Quantitation of imposex in the dog whelk (***Nucella lapillus***) has been used to monitor *pollution* by the antifouling agent tributyl tin oxide in marine environments.
[ref. 2]

imposition

See *imposex.*

impotence (in physiology)

Inability of a man to achieve an erection sufficient to sustain sexual intercourse (impotentia coeundi) or to produce viable semen (impotentia generandi).
Note 1: Some *toxic substances* that interfere with *vasorelaxation* of the *corpora cavernosa* (*e.g.*, ethanol) can contribute to insufficient erection.
Note 2: Treatment of insufficient erection can involve *drugs* that increase the *concentration* of *nitric oxide* in the *blood, e.g.* by inhibition of the *enzyme* cGMP-specific phosphodiesterase type 5 (EC 3.1.4.17).
Note 3: The term is sometimes applied to failure to *ejaculate* in spite of an adequate erection.
[*]
See also *sexual dysfunction.*

imprinting (in genetics)

Differential *expression* of a *gene*, depending on whether it was transmitted through the *sperm* or the *egg.*
Note: Imprinting is an *epigenetic* modulation of gene expression, thought to be regulated by attachment of methyl groups to the DNA, and by chromatin structure.
[ref. 5]

imprinting, metabolic

Process by which the *metabolism* of the developing *fetus* may be programmed during *gestation, e.g.*, giving rise to a predisposition to diabetes in the the *offspring* when the *pregnant* mother suffers from *diabetes mellitus type 2.*
[*]

in silico

Phrase applied to data generated and analyzed using computer modeling and information technology.
[ref. 1]

in utero

See *intrauterine*.

in vitro

Opposite term: *in vivo.*

In glass, referring to a study in the laboratory usually involving isolated organ, tissue, cell, or biochemical systems.
[ref. 1]

in vitro fertilization (IVF)

Fertilization outside the body, used as a treatment for *infertility*.
[ref. 5]

in vivo

Opposite term: *in vitro.*

In the living body, referring to a study performed on a living organism.
[ref. 1]

inactivated vaccine

See *vaccine, inactivated*.

inbred strain

Strain of an animal that has been inbred by brother-sister matings for more than 20 generations, and consequently all the individuals of the strain are more than 98% genetically identical.
[ref. 5]

incidence

Number of occurrences of a defined effect (*e.g.*, a specific illness), or number of organisms showing the defined effect, during a given period in a specific *population*, usually expressed as a rate.
Note: When incidence is expressed as a rate, it is the number of affected organisms divided by the average number of organisms in the specified population during a defined period, or alternatively divided by the estimated number of organisms at the midpoint of that period.
[After ref. 2]

incidence, cumulative

incidence proportion

Number or proportion of individuals in a group who experience the onset of a *health*-related event during a specified time interval.
Note: The study interval for cumulative incidence is the same for all members of the group, in contrast to lifetime *incidence*, which varies depending on the lifetime of each individual.
[ref. 1]

incidence density

Average *person-time incidence rate.*
[*]

incidence rate (in epidemiology)

cumulative incidence rate

Measure of the frequency at which new events occur in a population.
Note: The incidence rate is the value obtained by dividing the number of new events that occur in a defined period by the number of individuals in the population at *risk* of experiencing the event during this period, sometimes expressed as person-time.
[ref. 1]

incidence ratio, cumulative

Value obtained by dividing the *cumulative incidence* in an *exposed* group by the cumulative incidence in an unexposed group.
[*]

incidence study

See *study, incidence.*

incipient LC_{50}

Concentration of a chemical that is *lethal* to 50 % of the test organisms as a result of *exposure* for periods long enough for acute lethal action to cease; in other words, the concentration below which 50 % of individuals will have a normal lifespan despite the previous exposure to a *toxicant.*
[ref. 2]
See also *median lethal concentration.*

inclusion body

Particle in a cell, detectable under the light microscope.
Note: Inclusion bodies often consist of aggregates of *misfolded proteins* and are often found in *neurodegenerative diseases*, such as the *β-amyloid plaques* in *Alzheimer disease.*
[ref. 4]

inclusive fitness

See *fitness.*

incremental unit risk estimate

For an air *pollutant*, additional lifetime *cancer* risk occurring in a hypothetical *population* in which all individuals are *exposed* continuously from birth throughout their lifetimes to a concentration of 1 $\mu g\ m^{-3}$ of the pollutant in the air they breathe.
[ref. 2]

independent joint action

Production of an effect by each *toxicant* in a given *exposure* that is independent of the others and occurs by a different mode of action.
[ref. 2]

index/indices (pl)

Numerical record or measure for comparing values of things that change according to each other or relative to a fixed standard.
[*]

index, biological integrity

Composite *index* combining 12 qualities of fish communities of warm-water, low-gradient streams to determine the level of stream *degradation*; widely used in the United States.
[ref. 2]

index, biotic

One of several ranking systems calculated from the presence or *abundance* of sensitive species relative to tolerant species.
Note: Biotic indices measure decreased environmental quality from effects on especially sensitive species and should not be compared to *diversity indices*, which measure *community structure*.
[ref. 2]

index, Brillouin (H_B)

Quantitative value for community *species* diversity calculated as

$$H_B = (\ln N! - \Sigma \ln n_i!)/N$$

where N is the total number of individuals and n_i is the number of individuals in the ith species.
Note 1: Evenness, E, for the Brillouin *index* is estimated as

$$E = H_B/H_{Bmax}$$

where H_{Bmax} is the maximum possible Brillouin diversity that occurs when all species are equally abundant.
Note 2: When a subsample is taken from a given area, the Brillouin index provides a better estimate of diversity than the *Shannon–Wiener index* for samples of the same size. It also corresponds to situations of sampling without replacement, whereas the Shannon–Wiener index is appropriate for sampling with replacement.
[ref. 2]
See also *diversity index.*

index, female fertility

In rodents, number of *pregnant* females divided by the number of females mated, multiplied by 100.
Note: The female fertility *index* measures the female's ability to become pregnant and may be used as a general indicator of *fertility*.
[ref. 5]

index, gestation

In rodents, number of females with live born *offspring* divided by number of females with evidence of *pregnancy*, multiplied by 100.
[ref. 5]

index, male fertility

In rodents, number of males impregnating females divided by number of males mated, multiplied by 100.
Note: The male fertility *index* measures the male's ability to produce *sperm* that are capable of impregnating a female, assuming all mated females are *fertile*.
[ref. 5]

index, saprobic

Means of classifying the *saprobic* state of running waters, covering the full range from unpolluted to extremely *polluted* waters.
[ref. 2]

index, salt tolerance

See *tolerance index, salt.*

index, Shannon–Wiener diversity *(H)*

Shannon index

Quantity of biodiversity, derived from the mathematical relationship

$$H = -\sum_{i=1}^{S} p_i \log p_i$$

where p_i is the fraction of individuals belonging to the i'th *species* and S is the number of species, based on the assumptions that all species are represented in a study sample and that the sample was obtained randomly,
Note 1: The Shannon *index* is affected by both the number of species and their equitability, or evenness. A greater number of species and a more even distribution will both increase diversity as measured by H.
Note 2: The most important source of error in this index is failure of sampling to include all species from the *community* of interest.
[ref. 2]
See also *diversity index.*

index, Simpson's diversity *(D)*

Quantity describing dominance, weighted toward the *abundance* of the most common *species* in a *community*, giving the probability of any two individuals drawn at random from an infinitely large community belonging to different species. The bias corrected mathematical form of Simpson's *index* is

$$D = \sum_{i=1}^{S} p_i^2$$

where p_i is the fraction of all organisms that belong to the i'th *species* and S is the number of species.
Note: Since D and diversity are negatively related, Simpson's index is usually expressed as either a reciprocal or a complementary form ($1/D$ or $1\text{-}D$) so that, as the index goes up, so does the measure of *diversity*.
[ref. 2]
See also *diversity index.*

index, species richness *(S)*

Total number of *species* in an ecosystem.
Note: The species richness *index* makes no use of relative species *abundances*.
[ref. 2]
See also *biodiversity*.

index, tubular fertility

Percentage of *seminiferous tubules* containing identifiable *spermatogonia*.
[ref. 5]

indication

1. Quantity value provided by a measuring instrument or a measuring system.
   [ref. 1]
2. (in medicine) Evidence-based reason to apply a specific diagnostic or *therapeutic* procedure.
   [*]

indicator

1. (in biology) Organism, *species*, or *community* whose presence shows the presence of defined environmental conditions.
   Examples: Abundance, yield, and age/weight ratios are indicators of *population* production. A low cholinesterase activity is an indicator of *exposure* to cholinesterase-inhibiting pesticides.
   See also *indicator species*.
2. (in chemistry) Substance that shows a visible change, usually of color, at a defined point in a chemical reaction.
3. Device that indicates the result of a measurement, *e.g.*, a pressure gauge or a moveable scale.
   [ref. 2]
4. (in medicine) Diagnostic parameter that is characteristic for a *disease* or *adverse effect*.

[*]

indicator species

Species whose presence shows the occurrence of defined environmental conditions.
[ref. 2]

indigenous

Native to a given region or *ecosystem*.
Note: The term "indigenous" is applied to a native *species* to distinguish it from species introduced as a result of human activity.
[After ref. 2]
Compare *endemic*.

indirect antiglobulin test (IAT)

See *Coombs test*.

indirect Coombs test

See *Coombs test*.

indirect ecological effect

1. Effect resulting from imposed *biotic* or *abiotic* factors that alter *ecosystem* properties and consequently favor or disfavor an ecological component of

importance (*e.g.*, a *species*) and thus indirectly lead to improved or reduced *fitness* of that species.
2. Result of imposed biotic or abiotic factors allowing *indigenous* or new species to dominate, thereby affecting ecosystem composition.

[ref. 2]

indirect exposure

1. *Exposure* to a substance in a medium or vehicle other than the one originally receiving the substance.
2. Exposure of people to a substance by contact with a person directly *exposed*.

[ref. 1]

indirect immunofluorescence

Method of visualizing an *antigen* in which it is first reacted with an unlabeled *antibody* directed against it, and then is detected by staining with a second fluorescently tagged *immunoglobulin G* directed against the first antibody.
[ref. 3]

indirect photolysis

Degradation of a *contaminant* through interaction with other molecules in solution that have absorbed light energy; this can occur either through energy transfer or by chemical reaction with short-lived reactive species.
Note: Dissolved *humic* and *fulvic acids* are good examples of photoactive compounds that can increase the degradation of contaminants through indirect photolysis.
[ref. 2]

indirect toxicity

See *toxicity, indirect.*

individual

One whole organism.
Note: Individuals have size, shape, *health* status and condition; they grow, reproduce, and die over time.
[ref. 2]

individual effective dose (IED)

Concept that there is a basal limit to the dose required to produce a defined effect in any individual organism: this concept is implicit in *dose–response* models applied to the production of toxic effects.
[After ref. 2]

individual monitor

See *personal sampler.*

individual protective device (IPD)

personal protective device (PPD)
personal protective equipment (PPE)

Piece of equipment designed for protection of individual workers against hazardous and harmful factors in their workplace, including protection of the eyes, respiratory tract, skin, and whole body.
[After ref. 1]

individual risk

See *risk, individual.*

indoleamine-2,3-dioxygenase (IDO)

Enzyme (EC 1.13.11.52) catalyzing the initial rate-limiting step of *tryptophan degradation.*
Note: Tryptophan is required for *T-cell* proliferation, and local degradation of tryptophan by IDO thus modulates T-cell activity.
[ref. 3]

induced pluripotent stem (iPS) cell

See *stem cell, induced pluripotent.*

inducer

Substance that causes *induction.*
[ref. 1]

inducible co-stimulatory protein (ICOS)

Highly specific *receptor* for the protein B7H/B7RP-1 that is expressed on the surface of *B-cells* and *macrophages*, and also appears on the surface of *T-cells* during the process of T-cell *activation.*
Note: Stimulation of the B-cell and subsequent *antibody* production takes place after the ICOS receptor attaches to its partner B7RP-1 molecule. Thus, the co-stimulatory molecules, ICOS and B7H/B7RP-1, provide specificity for the *immune system* activation process.
[ref. 3]

induction

1. Process of stimulating and determining *morphogenetic* differentiation in a developing *embryo* through the action of chemical substances transmitted from one *embryonic* part to another.
   See also *evocation.*
2. Mechanism increasing the expression of a protein or set of proteins, especially an enzyme or enzymes, triggered by an endogenous mediator, a *xenobiotic*, or a change in environmental conditions.
   [After ref. 5]
   See also *enzyme induction.*
3. Initiation (see *initiator*) of a cancer.
4. Pharmacological or mechanical stimulation of the onset of labor and childbirth.

[*]

induction period

latent period
latency period

Time from the onset of *exposure* to a causative agent and the appearance of signs of its effects or of a resultant *disease.*
[After ref. 1]

industrial ecology

See *ecology, industrial.*

industrial hygiene

See *occupational hygiene.*

industrial melanism

See *melanism, industrial.*

inert chemical

Substance that is not chemically reactive.
[After ref. 1]

inert ingredient

Any ingredient intentionally added to a *mixture* that does not contribute to a desired biological effect,
Note: Inert ingredients do not include impurities and this definition does not imply that the inert ingredient has no biological effects.
[ref. 1]
Compare *active ingredient.*

inertia (of a community)

Ability of a *community* to resist change.
[ref. 1]

infarction

Macroscopic area of *tissue necrosis* following disruption of the *blood* supply, and hence cessation of delivery of dioxygen, to an *organ.*
[*]
Compare *ischemia.*

infauna (n)/infaunal (adj)

Animals living in the sediment of an aquatic system but not on its surface.
[ref. 2]
See also *epifauna.*

infection (n)/infected (adj)

Invasion of a biological organism by a *pathogenic* microorganism that can multiply, causing tissue injury and *disease.*
[*]

infectious

Describing a *disease*, or a disease-causing organism or material contaminated with such an organism, liable to be passed on amongst individuals.
[*]

infectious tolerance

See *tolerance, infectious.*

infectiousness

1. Pathological state resulting from having been *infected.*
2. Property of a *pathogenic* organism capable of causing and spreading *infection.*

[*]

infecundity

See *infertility.*

inferior cerebellar peduncle

Part of the *cerebellum* that is important for a number of motor functions, including balance, position sensing and *motor coordination*.
[ref. 4]

infertility

barrenness
infecundity
sterility

Persistent inability of either a male or a female to achieve *conception* or to produce offspring.
[ref. 5]

infertility, autoimmune

Infertility caused by sperm *antibodies, autoimmune* ovarian *inflammation* (oophoritis), or autoimmune orchitis.
Note: Autoimmune infertility may be part of a polyendocrinopathy.
[ref. 3]

inflammasome

High-molecular-weight complex that activates inflammatory *caspases* and the *cytokines interleukin*-1β (IL-1β) and IL-18.
Note: There appear to be at least three types of inflammasomes. Those identified initially were the NALP1 inflammasome, the *NALP3* (*cryopyrin*) inflammasome, and the *interleukin*-1β converting enzyme protease-activating factor (IPAF) inflammasome.
[ref. 3]
See also *inflammation*.

inflammation (n)/inflammatory (adj)

Reaction of the body to injury or to infectious, *allergic*, or chemical irritation; characterized by redness, swelling, heat, and pain resulting from dilation of the blood vessels accompanied by leakage of *plasma* and *leucocytes* into the tissues.
Note: Inflammation differs in the *brain* (see *neuroinflammation*), where lymphocytic invasion requires compromise of the *blood-brain barrier*, although T-cells can enter the brain for surveillance.
[ref. 3,4]

inflammatory bowel disease (IBD)

Group of chronic inflammatory conditions resulting in the inappropriate and persistent activation of the *mucosal immune system* of the bowel.
Note 1: *Idiopathic* IBD is a set of chronic conditions probably driven by the presence of normal intestinal flora.
Note 2: *Autoantibodies* against proteins of *neutrophil granulocytes*, pancreatic acinus, intestinal goblet, and colonic epithelial cells are detectable in IBD.
Note 3: *Crohn disease* and ulcerative colitis are two variants of IBD with overlapping clinical manifestations and probable *autoimmune* origins. Crohn disease is characterized immunologically by antibody to ***Saccharomyces cerevisiae*** and *Th1 cell*-dominated responses.
[ref. 3]

inflammatory response

See *inflammation*.

informosome

Complex, formed by combination of *messenger RNA* with protein, that permits transfer of messenger RNA from the cell nucleus to ribosomes in the cytoplasm.
[*]

infratentorial

Below the *tentorium*.
[ref. 4]

infundibulum

Anatomical funnel-shaped opening, often referring to the hollow stalk that connects the *hypothalamus* and the posterior *pituitary* gland, or to the portion of the *Fallopian tube* that receives the *ovum*.
[ref. 5]

infusion (in physiology)

Therapeutic introduction of a solution (usually saline) into a vein.
[ref. 1]

ingestion

1. Process of taking food and drink into the body by mouth.
2. Process of taking in particles by a *phagocytic* cell.

[ref. 1]

inguinal canal

Passage in the lower anterior abdominal wall, through which passes the *spermatic cord* in men and the round ligament of the *uterus* in women.
[ref. 5]

inhalation (n)/**inhale** (v)

Act of drawing in gas (often referring to air) or vapor, or any suspended *particulates*, into the lung.
[ref. 1]

inherently biodegradable

Describing substances for which there is unequivocal evidence of *biodegradation* (primary or ultimate) in any appropriate test of biodegradability.
[After ref. 1]

inhibin

Any of a group of peptide *hormones* secreted by the *follicular granulosa cells* of the *ovary* and the *Sertoli cells* of the *testis*, inhibiting *follicle stimulating hormone* secretion by the anterior *pituitary*.
[ref. 5]

inhibition (n)/**inhibit** (v) (in physiology and biochemistry)

1. Slowing down or preventing a process occurring in a living organism
2. Reduction in the activity of an *enzyme* or other biologically active substance.

[*]
See also *inhibition, enzyme*.

inhibition, enzyme

Inhibition of an *enzyme.*
Note: Enzyme inhibition is often classified as competitive, noncompetitive, mixed, and uncompetitive.

- Competitive inhibition refers to a situation where the *inhibitor* binds directly to the active (catalytic or substrate binding) site and competes directly with the substrate for binding.
- Noncompetitive inhibition refers to a situation where the inhibitor binds to the enzyme at a site other than the substrate-binding site (*e.g.*, the active site or an allosteric site), regardless of the presence of bound substrate. The inhibitor does not compete with the substrate for binding, but decreases enzyme activity through conformational (allosteric) effects.
- Mixed inhibition is similar to noncompetitive inhibition except that the inhibitor has a different affinity for the bound and unbound states of the enzyme.
- Uncompetitive inhibition refers to a situation where the inhibitor binds only to the enzyme-substrate complex, inhibiting the formation or release of product, thus decreasing the rate of reaction by effectively lowering the concentration of productive enzyme-substrate complex.

[*]

inhibitor, enzyme

Substance that binds to or otherwise interacts with an *enzyme* and *inhibits* its activity.
[*]
See also *inhibition, enzyme*.

inhibitor, receptor

See *antagonist*.

inhibitory concentration (IC)

Concentration of a substance that causes a defined inhibition of a given reaction or process.
Note: IC_{50} denotes the median concentration that causes 50 % *inhibition.*
[After ref. 1]
See also *inhibitory dose*.

inhibitory dose (ID)

Dose of a substance that causes a defined inhibition of a given biological system or process.
Note: ID_{50} denotes the median dose that causes a 50 % *inhibition.*
[After ref. 1]
See also *inhibitory concentration*.

inhibitory post-synaptic potential (IPSP)

Referring to a more negative *membrane potential* at the *postsynaptic* side of the *synaptic cleft* that renders the postsynaptic *neuron* less likely to generate an *action potential.*
Note 1: IPSP's are commonly produced by inhibitory *neurotransmitter*s such as *γ-aminobutyric acid* and glycine.
Note 2: Postsynaptic electrical activity is in part a function of the balance of IPSP's and *excitatory post-synaptic potentials*.
[ref. 4]

inhibitory time (IT)

See *median inhibitory time.*

iniencephaly

Malformation producing a cranial defect at the *occiput*, with the *brain* exposed, often combined with a cervical *rachischisis* and retroflexion.
[ref. 5]

iniopagus

Twins conjoined at the *occiput.*
[ref. 5]

initiating event

Specific action that results in a *risk* being incurred.
[ref. 2]

initiation (of cancer)

Occurrence of genetic changes that lead to the induction of *tumors*, often only after exposure to a second agent, called a *promoter.*
[*]
See also *induction; initiator.*

initiator

1. Agent that induces a change in a *chromosome* or *gene* that leads to the induction of *tumors*, often only after exposure to a second agent, called a *promoter.*
   See also *inducer.*
2. Substance that starts a chain reaction
   Note: An initiator is consumed in a chain reaction, in contrast to a catalyst.

[ref. 1]

innate immunity

See *immunity, innate.*

inotropic

Able to modify the force or speed of muscular contraction.
[*]

insecticide

Substance intended to kill insects.
Note: Insecticides commonly target the *nervous system* of insects.
[ref. 4]

insemination

Delivery of *sperm* into the female reproductive system for the purpose or with the result of causing *pregnancy.*
[ref. 5]

insomnia

Inability to sleep during the period and in conditions when sleep should normally occur.
[ref. 4]

insulin-dependent diabetes mellitus (IDDM)

See *diabetes mellitus type 1.*

intake

Amount of a substance that is taken into the body, regardless of whether or not it is absorbed.
Note: Intake is often expressed as total *daily intake*, the sum of the intake by an individual during a day from food, drinking-water, inhaled air, and other sources.
[ref. 1]

integral indicator of toxic effect

Parameter (such as body weight or temperature) characterizing the overall changes in the general state of the organism *exposed* to a *toxic* substance.
[ref. 1]

integrated risk information system (IRIS)

USEPA database containing *reference doses, slope factors*, and drinking-water health advisories (one-day, ten-day, longer-term, and lifetime advisories), and associated information.
[ref. 2]

integrin

Member of a family of cell membrane heterodimeric *glycoproteins* that mediate cell-to-cell and cell-to-*extracellular matrix* interactions.
[ref. 5]

intelligence quotient (IQ)

Numeric measure of a person's cognitive function based on one of several standardized tests of a problem-solving nature.
Note 1: IQ is expressed as a ratio of the individual's score to the median raw score of a sufficiently large reference population, the latter score taken as 100.
Note 2: The tests and numeric value of IQ are age-specific.
Note 3: Historically, IQ test results have been prone to misuse in drawing invalid conclusions about differences in intelligence based on genetic background, gender or race, ignoring potentially confounding factors such as education, socioeconomic status and other environmental influences on test performance.
[ref. 4]

intention tremor

See *tremor.*

interactome

Large-scale protein–protein interaction map.
[ref. 1]

intercellular adhesion molecule (ICAM)

Member of the *immunoglobulin superfamily* that interacts with *integrins* and is found on the surface of several cell types, including *antigen-presenting cells* and *T-cells.*
[ref. 3]

interclonal competition

Process that favors survival of foreign-specific *lymphocytes* at the expense of self-specific lymphocytes.
Note: Interclonal competition is a secondary mechanism involved in the induction and maintenance of *self-tolerance*.
[ref. 3]

interdigitating dendritic cell

See *dendritic cell*.

interfacial layer

Inhomogeneous region of space comprising and adjoining the boundary between two different phases (gas, liquid or solid) or immiscible fluids, within which properties of matter have values significantly different from their corresponding values in either of the adjoining bulk phases.
[After ref. 1]

interference competition

Interspecies competition in which one *species* interferes with another, as might occur with territoriality or aggressive behavior.
[ref. 2]

interferon (IFN)

Any *glycoprotein* produced by cells in response to stimuli, such as exposure to a virus, bacterium, parasite, or other *antigen*, that prevents viral replication in newly infected cells and, in some cases, modulates specific cellular functions.
Note 1: There are three classes of interferon: α, β, and γ. Alpha interferon (IFN-α) is made by *lymphocytes* and *macrophages*. Beta interferon (IFN-β) is synthesized by *fibroblasts* and epithelial cells. Alpha and β interferons were once called type 1 interferon. Gamma interferon [see *γ-interferon (IFN-γ)*], also called type 2 interferon, is synthesized by lymphocytes.
Note 2: All three interferon classes can be induced during viral infection. They have antiviral and antiproliferative effects, and all induce expression of *major histocompatibility complex class I molecules*.
[ref. 3]

γ-interferon (IFN-γ)

Member of a group of *cytokines*, the *interferons*, that has as its primary action the activation of *macrophages* and that can induce cells to resist viral replication.
Note: γ-Interferon is a product of *CD4+ Th1* cells, *CD8+ T-cells*, and *natural killer cells*.
[ref. 3]

interleukin (IL)

Member of a group of immunoregulatory *glycoproteins*, also called *lymphokines, monokines*, or *cytokines*.
Note 1: General features of interleukins are low molecular mass (about 80 kDa) and frequent *glycosylation*; regulation of immune cell function and *inflammation* by binding to specific cell surface *receptors*; transient and local production; action in *paracrine, autocrine*, or endocrine manner, with stimulatory or blocking effect on growth/differentiation; very potent, function at picomolar concentrations.

Note 2: Interleukins represent an extensive series of mediators with a wide range of overlapping functions. Other mediators in this series are c-kit *ligand, interferons, tumor necrosis factor, transforming growth factor* β, and a family of low relative molecular mass mediators, called *chemokines*.
[ref. 3]

intermediate filament (IF)

Any of a group of fibrous proteins (including *keratin* fibres, *neurofilament*s, desmin, and *vimentin*) that make up part of the *cytoskeleton* of most eukaryotic cells; so named because, at about 10 nm diameter, they are intermediate in thickness between actin *filament*s and microtubules.
Note: Most types of intermediate filaments are cytoplasmic, but one type, the lamins, is nuclear.
[ref. 5]

intermittent effect (in biology)

See *effect, intermittent*

internal dose (of a substance)

See *dose, absorbed.*

internal image

Epitope on an anti-*idiotype* that binds in a way that structurally and functionally mimics the *antigen*.
[ref. 3]

internal validity

Selection and comparison of index and *comparison groups* in such a manner that, apart from *sampling error*, the observed differences between these groups with respect to dependent variables under study may be attributed only to the hypothesized effect under investigation.
[ref. 1]

interphase
resting phase

Stage of progress between successive *mitotic* divisions of a *cell*, or between the first and second divisions of *meiosis*.
[*]

interpolation

Estimation of a value between two known data points, based on an assumption about the shape of the function between the points.
[ref. 1]

interpretation (of data or findings)

Evaluation of the observations from an investigation, study or diagnostic test in order to determine their significance for human *health*, for the environment, or for both.
[ref. 1]

intersexuality
intersex

Condition of having both male and female characteristics: thus, the state of being intermediate between the sexes.
[ref. 5]

interspecies competition

Interference with or inhibition of one *species* by another.
[ref. 2]

interspecies dose conversion

Process of extrapolating from the doses of one animal species to another, *e.g.*, from a rodent dose to its human equivalent.
[ref. 1]

interspecific competition

Competition by different species for the same limited resource(s).
[ref. 2]

interspecific interaction

Relations between different *species* in a *community*.
[ref. 2]

interstitial fluid

Aqueous solution filling the narrow spaces between cells.
[ref. 1]
Compare *interstitial water*.

interstitial pneumonia

Chronic form of pneumonia involving increase of the interstitial *tissue* volume at the expense of functional lung tissue.
[After ref. 1]

interstitial water

Water in *sediment* or *soil* that surrounds the solid particles.
Note: The percent amount of interstitial water is calculated from the mass of water in the sediment divided by the mass of the wet *sediment*.
[ref. 2]
Compare *interstitial fluid*.

intervention study

See *study, intervention*.

intestinal reabsorption

Absorption further down the intestinal tract of a substance that has been absorbed previously and subsequently excreted into the intestinal tract, usually through the *bile*.
[ref. 1]

intolerance (in immunology)

Extreme sensitivity or *allergy* to a *drug*, food, or other substance.
[ref. 3]

intoxication

1. *Poisoning*: pathological process with clinical *signs* and *symptoms* caused by a substance of *exogenous* or *endogenous* origin.
2. Drunkenness following consumption of beverages containing ethanol or other substances affecting the *central nervous system*.

[ref. 1]

intracranial pressure (ICP)

Pressure within the *cranial cavity*.
Note 1: Increased ICP may result from increased volume of the *cerebrospinal fluid*.
Note 2: Even minor increases in ICP, *e.g.*, due to intracranial bleeding, may cause serious damage to the *brain*.
[ref. 4]

intracytoplasmic sperm injection (ICSI)

Infertility treatment in which the *sperm* is injected through the *membrane* of the *egg* into its *cytoplasm*.
[ref. 5]

intradermal test

Diagnostic test for a possible cause of *hypersensitivity* in an individual in which a small drop of *antigen* is placed on a scarified skin surface or injected intradermally.
Note: Production of an *immune response* in the treated skin is a positive intra*dermal* test result.
[ref. 3]

intra-epithelial lymphocyte (IEL)

Lymphocyte found in the epithelial layer of mammalian *mucosal* linings, such as those of the *gastrointestinal* and reproductive tracts.
[ref. 3]

intramembrous ossification

Creation of bone tissue during *fetal* development of jawed *vertebrates*, and in the healing of bone fractures; the tissue forms from *mesenchymal stem cells* residing in an *extracellular matrix* devoid of collagen.
Note: Intramembrous ossification is one of two mechanisms of bone formation, the other being *endochondral ossification*.
[ref. 5]

intraspecific competition

Competition by individuals of the same *species* (population) for the same (limited) resources.
[ref. 2]

intrauterine growth restriction (IUGR)
intrauterine growth retardation

Subnormal, poor growth of the *fetus*.
Note: IUGR can be due to maternal or fetal causes, as well as to malnutrition and *toxic* exposures.
[ref. 5]

intrathecal

Within a sheath, as within either the *subarachnoid* or the *subdural* space.
[ref. 4]

intrinsic activity

Ability of a substance to produce a maximal stimulatory effect in relation to that of a given reference compound, *i.e.*, a full *agonist* has an intrinsic activity of 1.
[After ref. 1]

intrinsic clearance

Volume of *plasma* or *blood* from which a substance is completely removed per unit of time by an excreting organ, *e.g.*, the liver, when there is no restriction of blood flow or of other physiological limitation.
[ref. 1]

intrinsic factor (in biochemistry)

Protein, secreted by cells in the gastric *glands* of the stomach, required for the *transporter*-mediated absorption of vitamin B12 in the distal small intestine (*ileum*).
[After ref. 1]

intrinsic pathway

Apoptotic pathway of cell death initiated from within the cell by signals initiated by mitochondrial damage and (or) DNA damage, a defective *cell cycle*, detachment from the *extracellular matrix*, hypoxia, loss of cell survival factors, or other types of severe cell stress; characterized by the activation of *caspase* 9.
Note 1: The intrinsic pathway involves the release of pro-apoptotic proteins from the mitochondria.
Note 2: The intrinsic and extrinsic pathways converge with cleavage of procaspase 3 by either caspase 8 (extrinsic pathway) or caspase 9 (intrinsic pathway).
[ref. 5]

intrinsic rate of growth

See *growth, intrinsic rate of.*

intrinsic (Malthusian) rate of increase

Rate of increase in the size of a *population* growing under no constraints.
[ref. 2]
See also *Malthusian theory*.

introitus

See *ostium*.

intron

Noncoding sequence within *genes* that separates the *exons* (coding regions).
Note: Introns are spliced out of the *mRNA* molecule created from a gene after *transcription* and prior to *translation*.
[ref. 1]

invariant chain

CD74

Protein (31 kDa) of the *endoplasmic reticulum lumen* that binds to newly formed *major histocompatibility complex* heterodimeric proteins, preventing binding of endogenous peptides to their groove.
Note: The invariant chain protein acts as a *chaperone* for these molecules until they leave the *Golgi apparatus* and enter the *endosome* pathway. It is degraded proteolytically but leaves a fragment (called CLIP) bound within the groove of the *major histocompatibility complex class III molecules*. In acid vesicles, after leaving the Golgi apparatus, CLIP exchanges with peptides derived from exogenous *antigens*.
[ref. 3]

inverse agonist

See *agonist, inverse*.

inversion, chromosomal

Rearrangement of a *chromosome* in which, after breakage at two points, a segment is reversed, resulting in a change in sequence of nucleotides.
[ref. 5]

ion channel

Pore-forming transmembrane protein that can gate the transmembrane flux of small ions.
Note 1: Ion channels are generally involved in regulation of the electrical *membrane potential* and cell volume.
Note 2: Both *voltage-gated* and *ligand-gated* ion channels promote electrical signals in *neurons* and muscle cells.
Note 3: Many of the known ion channels are susceptible to inhibition by specific *neurotoxins*.
[ref. 4]

ion channelopathy

Neuromuscular *disease* resulting from a *genetic* defect in an *ion channel*.
Note: Documented ion channelopathies include those arising from mutations in channels for Na^+, K^+, Cl^-, and Ca^{2+}.
[ref. 4]

ionized calcium-binding adapter molecule 1 (Iba-1)

allograft inflammatory factor 1 (AIF-1)

Protein that is expressed in several tissues, but in *brain* is a specific immunomarker for *microglia*.
Note: The expression of Iba-1 is up-regulated upon activation of *microglial cells*, thus allowing identification of areas of brain injury or *inflammation*.
[ref. 4]

ionizing radiation

Any radiation consisting of ionizing particles, or of photons with energies higher than those of ultraviolet light, or a mixture of both such particles and photons.
[ref. 1]

ionotropic

Able to open ion channels that permit specific ions to move into or out of a *cell*.
[*]

irreversible alteration

Change from normal structure or function that persists or progresses after cessation of *exposure* of the organism.
[ref. 1]

irritant

1. (n) Substance that causes *inflammation* following immediate, prolonged, or repeated contact with skin, *mucous membrane*, or other biological material.
   Note: A substance capable of causing inflammation on first contact is called a primary irritant.
2. (adj) Causing inflammation following immediate, prolonged, or repeated contact with skin, mucous membrane, or other *tissues*.

[ref. 1]

Irwin battery

Set of neurobehavioral tests, including observations of behavior in novel environments, of reactions, and of motor functions; used in various modifications and resembling the *functional observational battery*.
[ref. 4]

ischemia (n)/ischemic (adj)

Local deficiency of *blood* supply, and hence of dioxygen, to an *organ* or *tissue*, caused by constriction or obstruction of the blood vessels.
Note 1: Ischemic cerebrovascular insult (see *stroke*) is due to decreased *cerebral* blood flow or dioxygen supply, due to vascular occlusion or intracranial bleeding.
Note 2: Prolonged ischemia can lead to *infarction*.
[ref. 4,5]

ischemia-reperfusion injury

Progression of *tissue* injury following reestablishment of *blood* flow to an *organ* where it has been interrupted by a period of *ischemia*, typically seen in the heart following acute myocardial *infarction*.
Note: Multiple mechanisms contribute to ischemia-reperfusion injury, including generation of *reactive oxygen species*, cellular calcium overload, and restoration of the *apoptotic* program upon resumption of *oxidative phosphorylation* and *ATP* repletion.
[*]
See also *reperfusion*.

islet cell antibody (ICA)

See *antibody, islet cell*.

isoantigen

See *alloantigen*.

isobole

Line on a graph (isobologram) joining points of equal activity.
[*]
See also *isobole analysis*.

isobole analysis

Method of evaluating the interaction of two biologically active substances such as *drugs* or *toxicants* that both produce a defined *effect* of interest.
Note 1: In an isobole analysis, a third graph is derived from the *dose-effect curve* of each substance by plotting dose pairs that are expected to yield the specified effect at some constant magnitude (often 50% of the maximum effect). This third curve is the additive *isobole*. The graph of the concentration or dose of one substance against that of the other is a decreasing curve that may be nonlinear. Points on the curve (*e.g.*, drug or toxicant dose pairs) are expected to produce quantitatively the same specified effect and lie on the linear isobole. If they do not, experimental points found to be below the isobole mean that less than additive quantities are needed to produce the effect, indicating a *synergistic* interaction. An experimental point on the graph that plots above the isobole indicates a sub-additive interaction.
Note 2: In biochemistry, isobole analysis is based on a plot (isobologram) of varying concentrations of inhibitor and substrate that give a constant *enzyme* activity.
[*]

isoenzyme

See *isoform*.

isoform

1. (of a protein) Any one of two or more proteins with similar function (*e.g.*, the same *enzymatic* activity) and a similar, but not identical, amino acid sequence.
   Note 1: Protein isoforms usually arise from differential splicing, single-nucleotide polymorphisms, post-translational modifications, or in some cases coding by distinct genes.
   Note 2: Isoforms of proteins with enzymatic activity are called isoenzymes. Isoenzymes will have the same *substrate* specificity and reaction mechanism, but may differ in their kinetic parameters.
2. (of a gene transcript) Any of two or more *mRNAs* coded from the same gene *locus* but differing, *e.g.*, in *transcription* start sites or untranslated regions.

[*]

isograft

syngraft

Tissue *transplant*ed between two *genetically* identical individuals.
[ref. 3]
See also *graft*.

isohemagglutinin

Naturally occurring *imunoglobulin M antibody* specific for the *erythrocyte antigens* of the *ABO blood groups*, thought to result from *immunization* by bacteria in the *gastrointestinal* and respiratory tracts.
[ref. 3]

isotretinoin (INN)

13-*cis*-retinoic acid
(2*Z*,4*E*,6*E*,8*E*)-3,7-dimethyl-9-(2,6,6-trimethylcyclohex-1-enyl)nona-2,4,6,8-tetraenoic acid

Vitamin A-like medication used, amongst other things, for acne treatment.
Note: Intake of isoretinoin during *pregnancy* has a high *teratogenic* risk.
[ref. 5]

isotonic

Denoting a liquid exerting the same *osmotic* pressure, or having the same chemical potential of water, as another liquid with which it is being compared.
Note: In medical usage, isotonic refers to a fluid that has the same osmotic pressure as *blood plasma*.
[After ref. 1]
See also *water potential*.

isotope effect

Difference in the *equilibrium* or *rate constant* of two chemical reactions that differ only in the isotopic composition of one or more of their otherwise chemically identical components.
Note: An isotope effect on the rate of a reaction is a kinetic isotope effect, and there is a distinction between a primary kinetic isotope effect (where a bond to the isotope is made or broken) and a secondary isotope effect (where no bond to the isotope is directly involved in the reaction). When the effect is observed on the equilibrium constant of a reaction, this is called a thermodynamic (or equilibrium) isotope effect.
[After ref. 2]

isotopic discrimination

Differential behavior in the rate or extent of participation of two stable isotopes of the same element in a biological or chemical process.
Note: Isotopic discrimination depends strongly on the masses of the isotopes.
[ref. 2]
See also *isotope effect*.

isotype

Class of *antibody* that differs from others in the *constant region* of the *heavy chain* (*Fc* portion).
[ref. 3]

isotype control

Antibody exhibiting the nonspecific characteristics of the antibody-*isotype* but lacking any specificity for the *antigen* in question; used as a negative *control* in antibody-antigen detection assays, notably in *flow cytometry*.
[ref. 3]

isotype switch

Process by which a *B-cell* switches from making *antibody* of one *isotype* to another without altering the specificity of the antibody, producing an isotype with the same *variable regions* but a different *heavy chain constant region*.
[ref. 3]

itai-itai disease

Illness (renal osteomalacia) observed in the Toyama prefecture of Japan in the early-to-mid 20th Century, resulting from the ingestion of cadmium-contaminated rice.
Note: In itai-itai *disease*, damage occurred to the kidneys, bones and joints of affected individuals, and the resultant bone pain was severe ("itai" means "ouch" or "it hurts" in Japanese).
[After ref. 1]

iteroparous species

Species whose members reproduce more than once during their lifetime.
[ref. 2]

J chain

See *joining (J) chain.*

J gene

See *joining (J) gene.*

JAK/STAT signaling pathway

Mechanism that transmits information from chemical signals outside the *cell* to gene *promoters* on the *DNA* in the cell nucleus, activated by the binding of *Janus-family tyrosine kinase (JAK)* to the nonpolypeptide portion of occupied *receptors* for some *interleukins*.
Note 1: JAK phosphorylates signal transducer and activator of transcription (STAT) proteins apart from STAT 5a and 5b.
Note 2: JAK2 is activated after it binds occupied *receptors* for *somatotropin*, several *cytokines*, and leptin. It then phosphorylates STAT proteins that dimerize and enter the nucleus to activate *transcription* of specific *genes*.
[ref. 3]

JAM test

Method to estimate *cell-mediated cytotoxicity* or *apoptosis* by assessing *DNA* fragmentation after preincubating cells with radiolabeled nucleotides.
Note: The name JAM derives from "**J**ust **A**nother **M**ethod".)
[ref. 3]

Janus-family tyrosine kinase (JAK)

Tyrosine kinase activated by *cytokines* binding to cell *receptors*.
Note: The name JAK is derived from Janus, the Roman god who had two faces, and refers to the two similar phosphate-interacting domains, one with kinase activity and one with regulatory activity.
[ref. 3]
See also *JAK/STAT signaling pathway*.

jaundice

See *icterus*.

jejunum

Second part of the small intestine between the *duodenum* and *ileum*.
[ref. 5]

Jerne plaque assay

See *antibody-forming cell (AFC) assay*.

joining (J) chain

Polypeptide that forms part of the polymeric structure of pentameric *immunoglobulin M* and dimeric *immunoglobulin A*.
[ref. 3]

Comprehensive Glossary of Terms Used in Toxicology
By John Duffus, Douglas M. Templeton and Michael Schwenk

Published by the Royal Society of Chemistry, www.rsc.org

joining (J) gene

Gene coding for a joining segment that connects *variable regions* and *constant regions* of *immunoglobulin (Ig)* or *T-cell receptor (TCR)* chains that, upon gene rearrangement, encodes part of the third *hypervariable region* of the *antigen receptors*.
Note: In Ig *light chains* and TCR, a *variable gene* segment rearranges to a *joining gene* segment; in Ig *heavy chains* and TCR, a *diversity gene* segment rearranges to a *joining gene* segment.
[ref. 3]
See also *V(D)J recombination*.

joint effect

Simultaneous or successive effect of factors of diverse types (chemical, physical, biological) on an organism.
[ref. 1]

junctional diversity

Diversity of the splice junctions in the recombined *variable gene, diversity gene* (for *immunoglobulin heavy chains*, and for *T-cell receptor* β and δ chains), and *joining gene* segments of *antibody* and *T-cell receptor* genes.
[ref. 3]
See also *D gene* and *V gene*.

K cell

See *killer cell.*

K-strategist

Organism that has stable populations and produces relatively low numbers of *offspring*.
Note: Species of K-strategists are characterized by long *gestation periods*, slow maturation and long life spans. They are usually found in stable biological *communities*.
[*]
Compare *r-strategist.*

K-strategy

Parental investment in a lower number of *offspring*, each with a higher degree of competitiveness in their *niche* and a greater chance of survival.
[*]
Compare *r-strategy*.
See also *Verhulst equation*.

kainic acid

(2*S*,3*S*,4*S*)-3-(carboxymethyl)-4-(prop-1-en-2-yl)pyrrolidine-2-carboxylic acid

Natural amino acid produced by some seaweeds that activates a subclass of *glutamate receptor*s ("kainate receptors") to produce *excitotoxicity*.
Note: Kainic acid is used experimentally to induce focal *seizure*s to model *epilepsy*.
[ref. 4]

kairomone

Semiochemical produced by one organism that induces a response in an organism of another species, that response being unfavorable to the emitter.
[ref. 1]
See also *allomone*; *pheromone*; *synomone*.

kallikrein

Any of a group of *enzymes* found in the *blood* and body fluids that acts on certain *plasma globulins* to produce *bradykinins*.
[ref. 3]

Kamofsky's law

Assertion that any agent will be *teratogenic* if it is present at concentrations or intensities producing *cell toxicity*.
[ref. 2]

Kaplan–Meier method

See *product-limit method*.

Comprehensive Glossary of Terms Used in Toxicology
By John Duffus, Douglas M. Templeton and Michael Schwenk

Published by the Royal Society of Chemistry, www.rsc.org

Kaposi sarcoma (KS)

Form of skin *cancer* that can involve internal *organs*. It is most often found in patients with *acquired immunodeficiency syndrome* and can be fatal.
[ref. 3]

kappa (κ)-light chain

Smaller of the two types of *light chain* found in human *immunoglobulins*, the other type being a *lambda (λ)-light chain*.
[ref. 3]
See also *Bence-Jones protein*.

karyolysis

Dissolution of a *cell nucleus*, especially during *mitosis* and *meiosis* but also following *necrosis*.
[ref. 5]
See also *karyorrhexis*.

karyorrhexis

Irreversible fragmentation of the nucleus of a dying *cell* following *karyolysis*, whereby its *chromatin* is distributed irregularly throughout the *cytoplasm*.
[ref. 5]

karyotype

1. (v) Characterize the number, form, and size of the *chromosomes* of an individual or a species.
2. (n) Photomicrograph of an individual's chromosomes, arranged according to a standard classification for the species.

[ref. 5]

keratin

Fibrous protein forming the main structural constituent of hair, feathers, hoofs, claws, and horns.
[ref. 5]

keratinization

cornification

Replacement of the outer *epithelial* layer of cells, especially in skin, with *keratin*-rich structures.
[ref. 5]

keratinocyte

Epidermal cell that produces *keratin*.
[ref. 3]

kernicterus

Neurotoxicity due to *bilirubin*.
Note: Premature infants with *icterus* are especially at risk for kernicterus, and may require phototherapy to reduce circulating bilirubin levels.
[*]

ketoacidosis

Acidosis, as in *diabetes*, *pregnancy*, or starvation, accompanied by the accumulation of *ketone bodies* in body tissues and fluids.
[ref. 5]

ketone body

Intermediate product of the breakdown of fats in the body; any of three compounds, acetoacetic acid, acetone, and (or) β-hydroxybutanoic acid [3-hydroxybutanoic acid], found in excess in *blood* and urine of persons with metabolic *disorders*.
Note 1: β-Hydroxybutanoic acid is not itself a ketone, but is called a ketone body because, like the other compounds, it is derived from ketones.
Note 2: Ketone bodies tend to accumulate in the blood and urine of individuals affected by starvation or uncontrolled *diabetes mellitus*.
[ref. 5]

ketosis

Pathological increase in the production of *ketone bodies*, *e.g.*, following blockage or failure of carbohydrate *metabolism*.
[ref. 1]

key event (in an adverse outcome pathway)

Empirically observable precursor step that is a necessary component of an *adverse outcome pathway* or is a biologically based marker for such a component.
[*]

keystone habitat

High-quality *habitat* patch essential to maintaining the vitality of the *metapopulation*.
[ref. 2]

keystone species

Species, usually a top *predator*, that influences the *ecological community* by its activity or role, not its numerical dominance.
[ref. 2]

killer activatory receptor (KAR)

killer activation receptor

Subclass of *killer cell immunoglobulin-like receptor* expressed on the surface of *natural killer (NK) cells*, and some *γ:δ* and *α:β T-cells*, that recognizes *major histocompatibility complex class I molecules* and activates NK cells.
Note: *Immunoreceptor tyrosine-based activation motif (ITAM)* sequences present in the KAR *cytoplasmic* domain are involved in NK cell activation.
[*]
See also *killer cell immunoglobulin-like receptor*; *killer cell inhibitory receptor*.

killer cell

Cell that displays *cell-mediated cytotoxicity*, including *cytotoxic lymphocytes*, *natural killer* cells, and *natural killer T-cells*. Some also consider activated *macrophages*, *monocytes*, and *interferon*-activated *neutrophils* to be killer cells.
[ref. 3]

killer cell immunoglobulin-like receptor

Receptor expressed on the surface of *natural killer cells* that binds to *major histocompatibility complex (MHC) class I* molecules on *target cells*; binding MHC class I allows receptors of this type to identify MHC self-variants and those associated with viral infection or *cell transformation.*
Note 1: Killer cell immunoglobulin-like receptors come in two subclasses: Most (*killer cell inhibitory receptors*) are inhibitory and suppress the *cytoxicity* of the *NK cell* against self, but some (*killer activatory receptors*) activate the killing response upon MHC class I recognition.
Note 2: If *immunoreceptor tyrosine-based inhibitory motif (ITIM)* sequences are present in the killer cell immunoglobulin-like receptor *cytoplasmic* domain, MHC class I molecule binding is inhibitory to the *killer cell.* Killer cell immunoglobulin-like receptors lacking ITIMs can associate with *immunoreceptor tyrosine-based activation motif (ITAM)*-containing adaptor molecules, in which case binding of MHC class I molecules can activate the killer cell.
Note 3: The killer cell immunoglobulin-like receptor is sometimes known by the acronym KIR, but this is also used for the killer cell inhibitory receptor subclass, and its use for the unspecified receptor should be avoided.
[*]
See also *C-type lectin*; *killer lectin-like receptor.*

killer cell inhibitory receptor (KIR)

Subclass of *killer cell immunoglobulin-like receptor* expressed on the surface of *natural killer cells* that recognize *major histocompatibility complex (MHC) class I molecules* and inhibit signaling that would otherwise arise from *NK cell binding and* lead to target cell killing.
Note 1: KIRs interact with, and inactivate, *killer activatory receptors.*
Note 2: *Immunoreceptor tyrosine-based inhibitory motif (ITIM)* sequences present in the KIR cytoplasmic domain are involved in inhibitory signaling.
[*]
See also *killer cell immunoglobulin-like receptor.*

killer lectin-like receptor (KLR)

Killer cell receptor that binds to *major histocompatibility complex class I molecules* and, like the *C-type lectin* receptors also found on these cells, can either inhibit or activate the killer cells.
[ref. 3]

killer T-cell

See *cytotoxic T-lymphocyte.*
[ref. 3]

kinase

Enzyme that catalyzes transfer of a phosphate group from a donor (almost always *ATP*) to a biomolecule acceptor.
[*]
See also *carbohydrate kinase; lipid kinase; protein kinase.*

kindling

Increase of epileptogenic (see *epilepsy*) activities as a result of repeated, longer-lasting subthreshold *brain* stimulation, *e.g.*, with electrical stimuli.

Note: Kindling is used in experimental models to study the development of *seizures* and epilepsy, and also for studying *withdrawal* phenomena.
[ref. 4]

kinesin

Motor protein occurring in *eukaryotic cells*.
Note: Kinesins are ATPases that move along *microtubule filaments*, powered by ATP hydrolysis.
[*]

kinetics (in chemistry)

Branch of chemistry concerned with measuring and studying rates of chemical reactions.
[ref. 1]

kinetics (in toxicology)

See *toxicokinetics.*
[ref. 1]

kinin

Any of a family of polypeptides that is released during *inflammatory* responses and increases *vascular* permeability and smooth muscle contraction.
[After ref. 3]

Klimisch score

Classification of the reliability of toxicological reports for regulatory purposes according to four categories: reliable without restriction, reliable with restriction, not reliable, and reliability not assignable.
[*]

Klinefelter syndrome

Syndrome in males resulting from a *genetic* defect in which an extra female *X chromosome* (thus an XXY *genotype*) is present in a male, characterized by small *testes*, long legs, enlarged breasts, reduced *sperm* production, and intellectual disability.
[ref. 5]

knock-down

Technique used to decrease the *expression* of a particular *gene* in a *cell* or living organism.
[ref. 1]
See also *knock-out*.

knock-in

Technique used to express an *exogenous gene* or to overexpress an *endogenous* gene in a living organism.
Note: In mammalian *toxicology*, this technique is most readily applied to the mouse.
[ref. 1]
See also *knock-out*.

knock-out

Technique used to inactivate a particular *gene* in a living organism, often in order to define its function.
Note 1: Knock-out involves use of *homologous recombination* in embryonic *stem cells* to replace a functional gene with a defective copy of the gene.
Note 2: In mammalian *toxicology*, the knock-out technique is most readily applied to the mouse. The resultant animals can be bred to *homozygosity*, thus allowing the generation of a null *phenotype* for that *gene product.*
[1,3]
See also *knock-out mouse.*

knock-out mouse

Mouse produced from *embryonic cells* containing *DNA* that has been genetically engineered (see *genetic engineering*) so that it does not express a particular *gene* or group of genes.
[ref. 3]
See also *knock-out.*

knock-out mutation

null mutation
Mutation that leads to the loss of function of a particular *gene.*
[ref. 5]
See also *knock-out.*

Kupffer cell

Fixed tissue *macrophage* found lining the *blood sinuses* in the liver.
[ref. 3]
See also *macrophage, resident(ial).*

Kviem reaction

Test for *sarcoidosis*, eliciting a *granuloma* at the site of intradermal injection of a *lymph node* extract from a person with active *disease.*
Note: The Kviem reaction is generally considered nonspecific for sarcoidosis.
[ref. 3]

kyphosis
hunchback

Rearward curvature or convexity of the *spine* in excess of normal, resulting in a protuberant upper back.
[ref. 5]

L-selectin

Any of a group of *leukocyte* surface *adhesion molecules*; they are classed as CD62 in the *cluster of differentiation antigen* marker system. All have *lectin* family carbohydrate binding domains and epidermal growth factor (EGF) repeats.
Note: L-selectins are expressed on the surfaces of *platelets* and endothelial cells as well as leukocytes.
[ref. 3]

LOD score

logarithm (base 10) of odds

Ratio of the likelihood of two or more *loci* remaining together (true linkage) when *chromosomes* recombine (see *recombination, genetic*) to the likelihood of this occurring by chance alone.
Note: A LOD score of 3 or greater is considered indicative of *genetic* linkage with odds greater than 1000:1.
[ref. 5]
See also *linkage analysis*.

l*x* life table/schedule

Tabular summary of *mortality* data for a *population*.
Note: "l*x*" is the number of individuals in a *cohort* alive at an age or a life stage class, *x*.
[After ref. 2]

l*x*m*x* life table

Tabular summary of both mortality and natality data for a *population*.
Note 1: "l*x*" in "l*x*m*x*" is the actual number or the proportion (as a decimal or percentage) of survivors at the beginning of age interval *x*. Since several samples are often averaged together, the l*x* values may not always be whole numbers.
Note 2: "m*x*" in "l*x*m*x*" is the number of female births to each age group of "mothers". Because, for most organisms, one male can fertilize a number of females, the size of the population is more dependent on the number of females present, and the calculations for the table usually use only the number of females. In a species with a 1:1 sex ratio, the number of females is m*x*/2 where m*x* = total *eggs* or young produced per female at age *x*.
[After ref. 2]

Ly-6

Family of multi-*gene*-encoded, small, generally glycosylphosphatidyl inositol-anchored *membrane* proteins thought to be involved in *cell* adhesion and signaling, and in *antigen*-independent *activation* of *lymphocytes*.
[ref. 3]
See also *protectin*.

lab-on-a-chip (LOC)

Miniaturized device, typically about (5×10) cm and few mm thick, that has integrated channels (microfluidic systems), pumps and reaction chambers that allow rapid

Comprehensive Glossary of Terms Used in Toxicology
By John Duffus, Douglas M. Templeton and Michael Schwenk

Published by the Royal Society of Chemistry, www.rsc.org

performance of a set of (bio)chemical reactions on small samples under automated, standardized conditions.
Note: Applications of LOC include screening in forensic analysis, environmental monitoring, medical diagnostics, *genomics*, and other related studies.
[*]

labor (in biology)

Physical efforts of expulsion of the *fetus* and the *placenta* from the *uterus* during *birth.*
[ref. 5]

lachrymation

See *lacrimation.*

lachrymator

See *lacrimator.*

lacrimation

Secretion and discharge of tears.
[ref. 1]

lacrimator

Substance that irritates the eyes (see *irritant*) and causes the production of tears or increases the flow of tears.
[ref. 5]

lactation

Secretion of milk from the *mammary gland*, usually to feed the infant during the *neonatal* period.
[ref. 5]

lactation period

Time following *pregnancy* during which the *mammary glands* secrete milk.
[ref. 5]

Lamarckianism

See *Weismannism.*

Lambert–Eaton myasthenic syndrome (LEMS)

Paraneoplastic (see *paraneoplastic autoimmune syndrome*) neurological *disorder* associated with small cell lung *cancer* and caused by *autoantibodies* against *voltage-gated* calcium *ion channels.*
[ref. 3]

lambda (λ)-light chain

One of the two types of *light chain* of human *immunoglobulins*, the other type being the *kappa* (κ)*-light chain.*
[ref. 3]

lamin

Fibrous *intermediate filament* protein functioning as a nuclear structural component and in the regulation of *transcription*.
Note 1: Lamins combine with nuclear membrane-associated proteins to form the nuclear lamina on the interior of the *nuclear envelope*.
Note 2: Lamins take part in the disassembling and reforming of the nuclear envelope during *mitosis* and are also involved in positioning nuclear pores.
Note 3: Not to be confused with the *extracellular matrix* protein laminin.
[*]

lamina propria

Layer of *connective tissue*, underlying the *epithelium* of a *mucus membrane*, containing capillaries and *lymphatic* vessels as well as *fibroblasts* and cells of the *immune system*.
[ref. 5]

Langerhans cell

Immature, phagocytic *dendritic cell* of the mammalian skin, characterized by the presence of *Fc receptors, major histocompatibility class II molecules*, and *epidermal* dendritic cell marker *CD1*.
Note: It contains a cytoplasmic organelle called the Birbeck granule.
[ref. 3]

Lanthony D-15 color test

Lanthony D-15 desaturated hue panel

Test of color vision using 15 distinct color chips with low color saturation that have to be arranged in a correct order.
Note: The low color saturation makes the Lanthony D-15 color test more difficult than the *Farnsworth D-15 dichotomous test* and thus it can detect more subtle color vision deficiencies.
[ref. 4]

large granular lymphocyte (LGL)

Lymphocyte of greater than normal size that contains *cytoplasmic* granules and functions as a *natural killer cell* or *killer cell*.
Note: Activated *CD8+ cytotoxic T-lymphocytes* also assume an LGL morphology.
[After ref. 3]

larva

Recently hatched insect, fish, or other organism that has physical characteristics different from those seen in the adult, requiring *metamorphosis* to reach the adult body structure.
[ref. 2]

larvicide

Substance intended to kill larvae.
[ref. 1]

laryngospasm

Reflex spasmodic closure of the sphincter of the *larynx*, particularly the glottic sphincter.
[ref. 1]

larynx (n)/**laryngeal** (adj)

Part of the respiratory tract between the *pharynx* and the *trachea*, having walls of *cartilage* and muscle and containing the vocal cords.
[ref. 5]

lassitude

A state of lethargy or fatigue.
Note: Partial synonyms of lassitude include exhaustion, listlessness and tiredness.
[*]

late phase reaction
type I reaction

Immunoglobulin E-mediated immune response occurring 5 h to 8 h after exposure to *antigen*, after the "*wheal* and flare" reaction of immediate *hypersensitivity* has diminished, with *inflammation* peaking around 24 h, and then subsiding.
Note: The latent phase reaction type I is not to be confused with a delayed type IV allergic reaction (see *hypersensitivty, delayed-type*).
[After ref. 3]

latency

See *latent period.*

latent

Not yet manifest; dormant but potentially discernible.
[ref. 4]

latent effect

See *delayed effect.*

latent period

1. Delay between *exposure* to a harmful substance and the manifestations of a *disease* or other *adverse effect.*
2. Period from disease initiation to disease detection.

[ref. 1]
See also *latent.*

lateral flow immunochromatographic assay
lateral flow test

Type of *immunoassay* performed on a minituarized device, where the analyte fluid (*e.g.*, urine) flows through a porous *matrix* into a region in which *antigen* reacts with an integrated *antibody*, and then flows further to a detection system.
Note: The lateral flow immunochromatographic assay can be useful for point-of-care testing (*e.g., drug* testing, *pregnancy* testing), where results can be gained quickly by nonprofessionals.
[*]

latex agglutination test
latex fixation test

Use of latex beads coated with *antibodies* to detect *antigen* in biological samples.
[ref. 3]

latex allergen

See *allergen, latex.*

lathyrism (n)/lathyritic (adj)

grass pea poisoning

Disease characterised by *spastic paralysis* of the legs and lower part of the body, pain, *hyperesthesia*, and *paresthesia.*
Note: Lathyrism is due to excessive ingestion of seeds of plants of the genus ***Lathyrus***, which includes many kinds of pea, including ***Lathyrus sativa*** (grass pea). These seeds contain the *glutamate* analog and *neurotoxicant* oxalyldiaminopropionic acid (3-[(carboxycarbonyl)amino]alanine)).
[ref. 4]

lavage

Irrigation or washing out of a hollow *organ* or *cavity* such as the stomach, intestines, or lungs.
[ref. 1]

law of frequence

Proposal that there are comparatively many rare (low *abundance*) biological *species*, and possibly comparatively many common (high abundance) species, but relatively few in the middle (of medium abundance).
Note: According to the law of frequence, if one collects data on species presence/absence in a set of quadrants, one tends to find a U-shaped pattern in the distribution of species frequencies.
[ref. 2]

laxative

cathartic
purgative

Substance that causes evacuation of the intestinal contents.
[ref. 1]

leach (in environmental science)

leaching

1. With reference to water–soluble substances, the action of percolating water in dissolution and drainage from *soil*, ash, or similar material.
   Modified from [ref. 2]
2. Loss of mineral and organic solutes due to percolation from soil.

[*]

leachate (in the natural environment)

Water that has percolated through a column of *soil*, ash, or similar material, carrying with it substances dissolved from that material.
[After ref. 2]

lead colic

painters' colic

Chronic intestinal pains and constipation caused by lead *poisoning*.
[ref. 1]

lectin

Member of a family of proteins that binds specific sugars on *glycoproteins* and glycolipids.
Note: Some plant lectins are *mitogenic*, *e.g.*, *phytohemagglutinin* and *concanavalin A*.
[After ref. 3]

lentic

lenitic

Inhabiting or occurring in standing water in *riparian*-wetland areas such as lakes, ponds, seeps, bogs, and meadows.
[After ref. 2]

lentic water

Nonflowing or still inland water; *e.g.*, lakes, ponds.
[ref. 2]

leprosy

Disease caused by infection with the bacterium ***Mycobacterium leprae***, often affecting the skin and nerves and causing body parts to become deformed.
Note: *Thalidomide* is used as a *therapeutic drug* for leprosy and thalidomide-associated *embryo*pathy occurs in regions where leprosy is endemic.
[ref. 5]

leptocephaly

Malformation characterized by an abnormally tall, narrow *cranium*.
[ref. 5]

leptodactyly

Abnormally slender digits.
[ref. 5]

lesion

1. Region of pathologically altered tissue, *e.g.*, an infected patch of skin.
2. Injury or wound.

[After ref. 1]

Leslie matrix

Leslie model

Square matrix used in *population* biology to predict population growth. The top row of the matrix is the fecundity (f_1, f_2, … f_i) for each age class x of mothers, and a subdiagonal is constructed from the number of individuals surviving (s_1, s_2, … s_{i-1}) from age class x to $x + 1$.
Note: Multiplying the Leslie matrix by the population vector of the number of female *offspring* in each age class x at time t ($[n_1, n_2, \ldots n_i]_t$) allows prediction of the age distribution of the population at the next time step $t+1$ ($[n_1, n_2, \ldots n_i]_{t+1}$), corresponding to the age class interval $x + 1$.
[After ref. 2]

lethal
deadly
fatal

Causing death.
[ref. 1]

lethal body burden (LBB)

Total body uptake of a substance that is associated with *mortality* in short-term *exposures*.
[ref. 2]

lethal concentration (LC)

Concentration of a substance in an environmental medium that causes death following a certain period of *exposure*.
Note: LC_{50} is the median concentration that causes death in 50 % of the test *population*.
[ref. 2]

lethal concentration, absolute (LC_{100})

Lowest *concentration* of a substance in an environmental medium that kills 100 % of test organisms or *species* under defined conditions.
[ref. 1]

lethal dose (LD)

Amount of a substance or physical agent (*e.g.*, radiation) that causes death when taken into the body.
Note: LD_{50} is the median *dose* that causes death in 50 % of the test *population*.
[ref. 1]

lethal dose, absolute (LD_{100})

Lowest amount of a substance that kills 100 % of test animals under defined conditions.
[ref. 1]

lethal synthesis
suicide metabolism

Metabolic formation of a highly *toxic* compound from one that is relatively nontoxic (*bioactivation*), often leading to death of affected *cells*.
[After ref. 1]

lethal time (LT)

Time taken for a defined percentage, usually 50 %, of a test *population* to die.
Note: The median lethal time (MLT) for 50 % of the test population is referred to as the MLT_{50}.
[ref. 2]
See also *effect time; median inhibitory time.*

lethality

Ability to cause death.
[ref. 2]

lethargy

Relatively mild impairment of *consciousness* resulting in reduced alertness and awareness.
Note: Lethargy has many causes but reflects a generalized suppression of *brain* activity.
[ref. 4]

leucism

Lack of pigmentation in the skin, hair, or feathers as a result of a failure of pigment cells to develop, or to migrate to those locations from their origin in the *neural crest*, in the *embryo*.
Note: Unlike *albinism*, where the defect is in the production of melanin pigment only, animals with leucism usually have pigment in the eye, as *retinal* pigment cells do not derive from the neural crest.
[ref. 5]

leukemia

Progressive, *malignant disease* of the *blood*-forming organs, characterized by distorted proliferation and development of *leucocytes* and their precursors in the *bone marrow* and blood.
[ref. 1]

leukemia, acute lymphoblastic (lymphocytic) (ALL)

Highly aggressive, undifferentiated form of *lymphoid malignancy* derived from a progenitor cell that is thought to be able to give rise to both *T*- and *B-cell* lineages.
Note: Most ALLs show partial differentiation toward the B-cell lineage (so-called B-ALL) whereas a minority show features of T-cells (T-ALL).
[ref. 3]
See also *leukemia*.

leukemia, acute myelogenous (AML)

Cancer characterized by rapid growth of abnormal *granulocytes* that accumulate in the *bone marrow*.
[ref. 3]
See also *leukemia*.

leukemia, chronic lymphocytic (CLL)

B-cell tumor found in the blood.
Note: The great majority of CLL tumors express *CD5* and unmutated *variable (V) genes* and are therefore thought to arise from *B1 cells*.
[ref. 3]
See also *leukemia*.

leukemia, chronic myelogenous (CML)

Cancer characterized by overgrowth of the *bone marrow* with *malignant* white *blood cells*, usually exhibiting a *chromosomal* abnormality (*Philadelphia chromosome*), which causes uncontrolled proliferation of cells that are released into peripheral blood.
[ref. 3]
See also *leukemia*.

leukemia, hairy cell

B-cell neoplasm, usually occurring during middle age, constituting about 2 % of all *leukemias* and responding well to chemotherapy. The neoplastic cells have fine, hairlike surfaces.
[ref. 3]

leukocyte

White *blood cell.*
Note: There are different types of leukocytes including *neutrophils, basophils, eosinophils, lymphocytes*, and *monocytes.*
[After ref. 3]

leukocyte, peripheral blood (PBL)

Leukocyte derived from the peripheral circulatory system.
[ref. 3]

leukocyte, polymorphonuclear

Mature *leukocyte* with granular cytoplasm and a segmented and irregularly shaped nucleus.
Note 1: The polymorphonuclear leukocyte is the predominant leukocyte in the *blood* and is found in *tissues* during acute inflammatory processes, and in the superficial surfaces of lesions during *subacute* or *chronic inflammation.*
Note 2: There are three major types of polymorphonuclear leukocytes - *neutrophils, eosinophils*, and *basophils.*
[ref. 3]

leukocyte common antigen (LCA)

Antigen common to both *T-lymphocytes* and *B-lymphocytes.*
[ref. 3]

leukocyte functional antigen (LFA)

Any of a group of cell-surface *antigens* involved in intercellular adhesion.
[ref. 3]

leukocytopenia

Amount of *leukocytes* below normal values that is a characteristic feature of *systemic autoimmune diseases* (*e.g.*, Felty *syndrome, systemic lupus erythematosus, Sjögren syndrome, mixed connective tissue disease*).
[ref. 3]

leukocytosis

Abnormal increase in the number of *leukocytes.*
[ref. 3]

leukopenia

See *leukocytopenia.*

leukotriene

Metabolic product of arachidonic acid that promotes *inflammatory* processes (*e.g., chemotaxis*, increased vascular permeability) and is produced by a variety of cell types including *mast cells, basophils*, and *macrophages*.
[ref. 3]

levocardia

Normal position of the heart in the left hemi-*thorax* with the apex pointed to the left, and transposition of other *viscera*.
[ref. 5]
See also *dextrocardia; situs inversus*.

Leydig cell

Cell in the *testis* that produces *androgens*, mainly *testosterone*, in the presence of *luteinizing hormone*.
[ref. 5]

libido

Conscious or *unconscious* sexual desire; passionate interest in life force.
[ref. 4]

library (in bioscience)

1. (in bioinformatics) Collection of sequences (*e.g.*, of *DNA* or proteins) in a searchable electronic form.
2. (in molecular biology) Collection of *genomic* or *complementary DNA* sequences that have been *cloned* in a *vector* and grown in an appropriate host organism (*e.g.*, bacteria, yeast).

[After ref. 1]

Liebig's law of the minimum

Observation that a *population*'s size (number of individuals or biomass) is limited by some essential factor in the *environment* that is scarce relative to the amount of other essential factors, *e.g.*, phosphorus-limited *algal* growth in a lake.
[ref. 2]

life cycle (n)/**life-cycle** or **lifecycle** (adj)

Series of stages, from a given point in one generation to the same point in the next generation, *e.g., egg* to *larva* to adult and back to egg.
[ref. 2]
See also *cycle; life-cycle study; life history*.

life-cycle study

Comprehensive study to determine the impact of a substance or *mixture* on the survival, growth, *reproduction*, development, or other important qualities at all stages of the *life cycle* of a *species*.
[ref. 2]

life history

Description of *life-cycle* events through which an organism passes, with particular reference to those events that influence survival and *reproduction*.
[ref. 2]

life-long exposure

Subjection to a potentially *toxic* substance during the whole lifetime.
[ref. 1]

life table

1. (in ecology) Summarizing method used to describe the pattern of *mortality* and survival in *populations*.
   Note 1: Survival data in the life table are time-specific, cumulative probabilities of survival of a group of individuals, assuming, throughout life, the appropriate *age-specific death rates*.
   Note 2: Life tables can be used to study any defined *health* endpoint such as onset of *disease* or occurrence of consequences of disease.
   Note 3: For life tables in *ecology, fertility* for each *age class* is normally included in the tables of consequences of disease.
   [*]
2. (in actuarial science) Statistical table that follows a hypothetical *cohort* of 100 000 persons born at the same time as they progress through successive ages, with the cohort reduced from one age to the next according to a set of *death rates* by age until all persons eventually die.
   Note: The life table is used mainly to indicate expectation of life at various ages. However, it also provides information on numbers of individuals who survive to various ages, median age at death, *age-specific death rates*, and the probability of dying at certain ages.
   [After ref. 2]

life-table response experiment (LTRE)

Retrospective comparison of two or more *populations* in which the response variable is a *life table* or a complete set of stage-specific survival rates.
[ref. 2]

ligamentum arteriosum

Fibrous remnant of the *ductus arteriosus* linking the *aortic arch* with the top of the left *pulmonary artery*.
[ref. 5]

ligand

Ion, molecule, or molecular group that binds to another chemical entity to form a larger complex.
Note: A ligand may bind specifically to a *receptor* and trigger a response such as activation of a *signal transduction* pathway.
[ref. 3]

ligand-gated ion channel

Ion channel that opens upon binding an activating *ligand*.
[ref. 4]
Compare *voltage-gated ion channel*.

ligand of inducible co-stimulatory protein (ICOSL, LICOS)

Protein involved, after binding to *inducible co-stimulatory protein (ICOS)*, in several harmful *immune responses*, such as *autoimmunity, allergy*, or *graft-versus-host reaction*.

Note: Prolonged ICOS and ICOSL expression at *chronic inflammatory* sites seems to give rise to *pathology*.
[ref. 3]

light chain

Small polypeptide subunit of an *antibody* (*immunoglobulin*).
Note: A typical antibody is composed of two immunoglobulin *heavy chains* and two light chains.
[ref. 3]

limacide

Substance intended to kill molluscs, including the gastropod mollusc, ***Limax***.
[ref. 1]

limbic system

Collection of interconnected *neurons* lying underneath the *cerebrum* on either side of the *thalamus*, related more by anatomical location than as a single functional entity.
Note 1: Various structures of the limbic system, including the cingulate gyrus, the isthmus, the *hippocampus*, the *uncus*, and the *amygdala* are associated with various emotions and feelings such as anger, fear, sexual arousal, pleasure, and sadness.
Note 2: The limbic system is often termed the paleo*brain*, and considered to consist of primitive structures.
[ref. 4]

limb bud

Embryonic outgrowth of *mesoderm* covered in *ectoderm* that will give rise to one of the forelimbs or hindlimbs.
[ref. 5]

limit recommended

See *recommended exposure limit.*

limit test

Acute toxicity test in which, if no ill effects occur at a preselected maximum *dose*, no further testing at greater *exposures* is required.
[ref. 1]

limit value (LV)

Limit *concentration* at or below which Member States of the European Community must set their *environmental quality standard* and *emission standard* for a particular substance according to Community Directives.
[ref. 1]

limited evidence

Collection of facts and accepted scientific inferences that suggests that an agent may be causing an *effect*, when the evidence is not strong enough to be considered established fact.
Note: Limited evidence is defined by the USEPA.
[After ref. 1]

limited life-span paradigm

Model based on the assumption that the maximum life span of an individual organism is an inherent, *genetically* defined property of that organism.
[ref. 2]

limnocorral

Artificial enclosure placed in the *pelagic* region of ponds, lakes, or marine *environments*.
Note 1: Limnocorrals vary in size from as little as 2 litres to over 2.5 million litres, although most have a volume between 1,000 and 10,000 litres.
Note 2: Limnocorrals may or may not be in contact with the *profundal region*. Fish are generally excluded from these test systems.
[ref. 2]
See also *littoral enclosure*.

limnology

Study incorporating the individual studies of all aspects of inland freshwater *habitats* including lakes, ponds, rivers, streams, swamps, wetlands, groundwaters, and reservoirs that make up inland water systems.
[ref. 2]

Limulus test

Method of detecting bacterial *endotoxins* based on gelation of a *blood cell* lysate from the horseshoe crab, ***Limulus polyphemus***.
[ref. 3]
See also *pyogen test*.

linear epitope

See *epitope, linear*.

linearized multistage model

Conservative quantitative *cancer* assessment model that assumes linear extrapolation with a zero *dose* threshold from the upper confidence level of the lowest dose that produces *cancer* in an animal test or in a human *epidemiological* study.
Note: The linearized multistage model is used by the USEPA.
[*]

linkage analysis

Technique that studies patterns of heredity in high-risk families, in order to locate a *disease*-causing *gene mutation* by identifying co-inherited traits, usually by producing a *LOD score*.
[ref. 5]

linkage disequilibrium

Occurrence in members of a *population* of combinations of linked *genes* (*alleles*) in nonrandom proportions, implying that the genes are close enough together on a *chromosome* to make it unlikely that they will be separated by recombination (see *homologous recombination*) during *meiosis*.
[ref. 5]

Note: Linkage disequilbrium implies that factors other than chance - such as linkage, genetic drift, selection, or chromosomal structure - are influencing the pattern of inheritance of a *gene* within the population.
[*]

linked recognition

Requirement for a *helper T-lymphocyte* and *B-lymphocyte* to interact with separate but physically linked *epitopes* in the same *antigen*, in order to give an *immune response* to a *thymus-dependent antigen*.
[ref. 3]

lipid kinase

Any *kinase enzyme* that phosphorylates lipids in the cell, including those in the *plasma membrane* and *organelles*, often changing both the reactivity and localization of the lipid moiety.
Examples: Phosphatidylinositol kinases that phosphorylate phosphatidylinositol molecules that are important in signaling and in permitting *endocytosis* and *exocytosis*.
[*]

lipid peroxidation

Oxidative damage to lipids produced by *reactive oxygen species*, involving hydrogen abstraction and lipid peroxyl radical formation, and leading to lipid *degradation* and production of *toxic metabolites*.
Note 1: The lipid peroxidation reaction includes an initiation step in which a lipid radical is formed, a propagation step in which the lipid radical reacts with additional unsaturated lipid, and a termination step leading to degradation of lipid peroxides with formation of toxic products such as short chain aldehydes.
Note 2: Lipid peroxidation can cause harm to cells by damaging the phospholipid membrane as well as by producing toxic aldehyde species such as *4-hydroxynonenal* and malondialdehyde.
[*]
See also *oxidative stress*.

lipid raft

Cholesterol- and *glycosphingolipid*-rich membrane subdomain in which molecules involved in cellular *activation* become concentrated.
[ref. 3]
See also *caveola*.

lipidosis

Disorder of fat *metabolism* characterized by the accumulation of abnormal levels of certain lipids in the body.
[ref. 5]

lipoma

Benign *tumor* of the adipose tissue, often visible under the skin.
Note: Lipoma of the *corpus callosum* is a rare *congenital* condition that can be asymptomatic or can present with *headache, hemiplegia, dementia* and *epilepsy*.
[ref. 4]

lipophilic (adj)/**lipophilicity** (n)

See *hydrophobic.*

lipopolysaccharide (LPS)

Endotoxin, derived from Gram-negative bacterial cell walls, that has *inflammatory* and *mitogenic* actions.
[ref. 3]

liposome

1. Artificially formed lipid droplet, small enough to form a relatively stable suspension in aqueous media, useful in *membrane* transport studies and in *drug* delivery.
2. Lipid droplet in the *endoplasmic reticulum, e.g.*, of a fatty liver.

[After ref. 1]

litter

Group of *offspring* produced by a mammal from one *pregnancy*.
[ref. 5]

littoral

1. (n) Intertidal zone, sometimes referring specifically to the shallow well-lit region along the shore.
2. (adj) Belonging to the shore of a lake, river, pond, or especially the sea.

[ref. 2]

littoral enclosure

Isolated shore region of freshwater ponds used for ecotoxicological testing.
Note: Littoral enclosures are separated from the main body of the pond water by impermeable dividers. They generally have a volume of 1000 to 50,000 L with a maximum depth of 2 m.
[After ref. 2]
See also *limnocorral.*

live attenuated vaccine

See *vaccine, live attenuated.*

liver–kidney microsomal (LKM) **antibody**

See *antibody, liver–kidney microsomal.*

loading (in aquatic toxicology)

Ratio of animal biomass to the volume of test solution in an *exposure* tank.
[After ref. 2]

lobe (of cerebral cortex)

One of the four main regions of the *cerebral cortex.*
[ref. 4]
See also *lobe, frontal; lobe, occipital; lobe, parietal; lobe, temporal.*

lobe, frontal

Most anterior of the four major *lobes* of each *cerebral hemisphere*, containing the primary *motor cortex*.
[ref. 4]

lobe, occipital

One of the four major *lobe*s of each *cerebral hemisphere*, situated within the *occiput*, containing most of the *neural* apparatus of visual processing.
[ref. 4]

lobe, parietal

One of the four major *lobe*s of each *cerebral hemisphere* situated between the *frontal* and *occipital lobe*s, above the *temporal lobe*.
[ref. 4]

lobe, temporal

One of the four major *lobe*s of each *cerebral hemisphere*, situated at the base of the *brain*.
Note: The temporal lobe is involved in memory, language comprehension, emotion, and processing sensory input.
[ref. 4]

lobster-claw deformity

See *ectrodactyly*.

local effect

Change occurring at the site of contact between an organism and a *toxicant*.
[ref. 1]

local lymph node assay (LLNA)

See *murine local lymph node assay*.

locus/loci (pl) (in genetics)

Specific location of a *gene* or *DNA* sequence on a *chromosome*.
[ref. 2]

logK_{ow}

See *log*P_{ow}.

log-normal distribution

Continuous probability distribution function of a random variable whose logarithm is normally distributed, so that if the random variable x is in a normal (Gaussian) distribution and $y = f(\ln x)$, then the distribution function y is also Gaussian.
[*]

log-normal transformation

Transformation of data with a logarithmic function that results in a normal *distribution*.
[ref. 1]
See also *log-normal distribution*.

$\log P_{ow}$

$\log K_{ow}$
Logarithm (base 10) of the partition coefficient of a substance between octan-1-ol and water.
Note: This is used as an empirical measure for *lipophilicity* in calculating *bioaccumulation*, fish *toxicity*, membrane *adsorption*, and *penetration*.
[ref. 2]

logistic curve

Function, often applied to growth curves, fitting the general equation

$$y = k/(1 + e^{a+bt})$$

where y the body weight or *population* size, k the rate of growth, t is time, and a and b are positive constants.
Note: In the logistic equation the percentage rate of increase decreases linearly as size increases. The resulting logistic curve rises continually, slowly at first, more rapidly in the middle phase, and slowly again near the end of growth.
[ref. 2]

logistic growth

See *growth, logistic.*

logit

Natural logarithm of the quotient of a probability, P, and its complement, *i.e.*, $\ln[P/(1 - P)]$.
[ref. 2]

logit transformation (in toxicology)

In competitive binding assays, the *logit*-log *dose* relationship, in which the *response* R is defined by

$$R = \text{logit}(y) = \ln[y/(1 - y)]$$

where $y = b/b_0$ with b = fraction of tracer bound and b_0 = value of b with no unlabelled *ligand* in the system.
Note 1: Logit *transformation* of assay data frequently yields straight-line *dose–response* data, amenable to statistical analysis.
Note 2: More generally in *toxicology*, the logit transformation is applied to dose–response data where b_0 denotes the maximum response in the absence of a *toxic* substance.
[ref. 2]

long-term effect

See *chronic effect.*

long-term exposure

See *chronic exposure.*

long-term toxicity

See *chronic toxicity.*

longitudinal study

See *study, longitudinal cohort.*

lordosis

Forward (*ventral*) curvature of the *spine* in the *lumbar* and *cervical* regions.
Note 1: Some degree of lordosis is normal. Excessive curvature (lumbar hyperlordosis) is sometimes called swayback.
Note 2: Lordosis is also associated with a rodent being in heat.
[ref. 5]

loss of life expectancy (LLE)

Calculated estimate of loss in lifetime associated with a *risk* factor; it is estimated as the simple difference between life expectancy without the risk factor and life expectancy with the risk factor.
[ref. 2]

lotic

Related to flowing continental waters, such as rivers and streams.
[ref. 2]

lotic mesocosm/lotic microcosm

Any stream of various sizes used to evaluate the effects of substances.
Note: Unlike *lentic* systems, no standardized design for lotic *mesocosms/microcosms* has been developed for flowing, *lotic water* test systems.
[ref. 2]

lotic water

Flowing continental waters, such as rivers and streams.
[ref. 2]

lower motor neuron

Neuron that receives impulses from an *upper motor neuron* and whose *axons* innervate the skeletal muscles.
[ref. 4]

lowest-effective dose (LED)

Lowest *dose* of a chemical inducing a specified effect in a specified fraction of *exposed* individuals.
[ref. 1]

lowest lethal concentration found

See *minimum lethal concentration.*

lowest-observed-adverse-effect level (LOAEL)

Lowest *concentration* or amount of a substance (*dose*), found by experiment or observation, that causes an *adverse effect* on morphology, functional capacity, growth, development, or life span of a *target* organism, distinguishable from normal (*control*) organisms of the same *species* and strain under defined conditions of *exposure*.
[ref. 1]

lowest-observed-effect level (LOEL)

Lowest *concentration* or amount of a substance (*dose*), found by experiment or observation, that causes any alteration in morphology, functional capacity, growth, development, or life span of *target* organisms distinguishable from normal (*control*) organisms of the same *species* and strain under the same defined conditions of *exposure*.
[ref. 1]

lumbar puncture

spinal tap

Piercing into the *subarachnoid* space of the *lumbar spine* in order to obtain *cerebrospinal fluid* for diagnostic purposes or to inject a *drug*.
[ref. 5]

lumbar spine

Portion of the *vertebral column* of the lower back between the *thoracic spine* and *sacrum*, in humans consisting of five *vertebra*e designated L1 to L5.
[ref. 4]

lumen

Central cavity of a tubular or other hollow structure in an organism or *cell*.
[*]

lupus

See *systemic lupus erythematosus*.

lupus, drug-induced

Idiosyncratic drug reaction similar in character to *systemic lupus erythematosus* and having *antinuclear antibodies*, but generally milder in nature and resolving when *drug* exposure is discontinued.
[ref. 3]

lupus-like syndrome

See *drug-induced lupus*.

lupus anticoagulant

See *anticoagulant, lupus*.

lupus erythematosus

See *systemic lupus erythematosus*.

luteal phase (of menstrual cycle)

Phase of the human *menstrual cycle*, usually lasting 14 days, beginning with formation of the *corpus luteum* and ending, in the absence of *fertilization*, with the onset of *menstruation*.
[ref. 5]

luteinizing hormone (LH)

Hormone made by the *pituitary gland* that acts on the *ovary* to control *egg* maturation and to trigger *ovulation*. The same hormone acts in the *testes* to trigger production of *testosterone*.
[ref. 5]

luteinizing hormone-releasing hormone (LHRH)

See *gonadotropin-releasing hormone*.
[ref. 5]

lymph

Transparent fluid, containing chiefly lymphocytes, that bathes the tissues and drains through a system of vessels (the *lymphatic system*) into the venous bloodstream through the *thoracic duct*.
[ref. 5]
Note: Lymph plays a role in maintaining body fluid balance.
[*]

lymphadenopathy

Enlarged *lymph nodes*.
[ref. 3]

lymphangion

Morphological or functional unit of *lymphatic* vessels consisting of the region between adjacent lymphatic valves.
[ref. 3]
See also *lymphatic system.*

lymphatic

Relating to *lymph* or its secretion.
[ref. 5]

lymphatic system

Network of vessels whose special function is the collection of *lymph* and its ultimate conveyance to the *blood* circulation and *thoracic duct*.
[ref. 3]
Note 1: The lymphatic system can also transport *metastatic cancer* cells.
Note 2: Very *lipophilic xenobiotics* are bound to chylomicrons during intestinal absorption and transported from the intestine via the lymphatic system into blood, thus bypassing the *liver*.
[*]

lymphatic tissue

Tissue involved in the collection, production, and handling of *lymph*, including the lymphatic vessels and *lymph nodes*.
[ref. 3]

lymph node
lymph gland

Any of the small rounded *gland*-like structures of the *lymphatic system* that occur along the *lymphatic* vessels, that are responsible for removing bacteria, viruses, and

foreign molecules from the *lymph* stream, and for producing *lymphocytes* and *antibodies*.
[ref. 3]

lymphoblast (n)/**lymphoblastic** (adj)

Abnormal *cell* with a large nucleus and scanty *cytoplasm*, thought to be the precursor of the *lymphocyte*, found in *blood* and blood-forming *organs* in patients with lymphoblastic *leukemia*.
[ref. 3]

lymphocyte

Small *leucocyte* found in the *blood, lymph*, and *lymphoid tissues,* that has a single round nucleus and little or no granulation in the *cytoplasm*.
Note 1: Lymphocytes may be either *B-cells*, which produce *humoral immunity*, or *T-cells*, which produce *cell-mediated immunity*.
Note 2: Lymphocytes constitute about a quarter of the total leucocytes in the blood stream but occur in large numbers in the *lymph nodes* and other *lymphatic tissue*.
[ref. 3]
See also *B-lymphocyte; T-lymphocyte*.

lymphocyte, naïve

Mature *T-cell* or *B-cell* that has not yet been activated (see *lymphocyte activation*) by encounter with *antigen*.
[ref. 3]

lymphocyte, tumor-infiltrating (TIL)

Mononuclear *lymphocyte* derived from the *inflammatory* infiltrate of a solid *tumor*.
[ref. 3]

lymphocyte-activated killer cell

See *lymphokine-activated killer cell.*

lymphocyte-activating factor
interleukin-1

See *interleukin.*

lymphocyte activation

Sum of the biochemical processes necessary to stimulate a resting *lymphocyte* to become an *immune* effector *cell*, requiring *antigen* and co-stimulatory molecules.
[ref. 3]
See also *costimulation*.

lymphocyte blastogenesis assay (LBA)

See *lymphocyte transformation test*.

lymphocyte function-associated antigen-1 (LFA-1)

Adhesion molecule found on *lymphocytes, macrophages*, and *neutrophils*, involved in adhesion of lymphocytes to *antigen-presenting cells*.
[ref. 3]

lymphocyte homing

Process that directs *lymphocyte* subsets to specialized microenvironments that control their differentiation, regulate their survival, and target immune effector cells to sites of *antigenic* or microbial invasion.
[ref. 3]
See also *homing; receptor, homing.*

lymphocyte homing receptor

See *receptor, lymphocyte homing.*

lymphocyte proliferation test (LPT)

Test of *immune sensitization* in which white *blood cells* are exposed *in vitro* to an *antigen* and multiply if already sensitized (see *sensitization*) to that antigen.
[ref. 3]
See also *lymphocyte transformation test.*

lymphocyte repertoire (of *immunoglobulin* or *T-cell receptor*)

Profile of *immunoglobulins* or *T-cell receptors* (TCRs) available within a specified group of cells.
Note: Each lymphocyte repertoire is characterized by the *antigen* specificities of the *immunoglobulins* or TCRs present.
[ref. 3]

lymphocyte subpopulation

Population forming part of the whole population of *lymphocytes*, usually characterized by *sensitivity* to a given *antigen.*
[ref. 3]

lymphocyte transformation test (LTT)

lymphocyte blastogenesis assay (LBA)

Test for increased DNA synthesis followed by cell division and *differentiation* of *lymphocytes* in response to *antigens* or *mitogens*; an *in vitro* test of lymphocyte function.
[ref. 3]
See also *lymphocyte proliferation test.*

lymphocytopenia

Deficiency of *lymphocytes* in the *blood* compared with normal values.
Note: This is a characteristic feature of systemic *autoimmune diseases* (*e.g., systemic lupus erythematosus, Sjögren syndrome, mixed connective tissue disease*).
[ref. 3]

lymphocytosis

Condition characterized by an abnormal increase in the number of *lymphocytes* in *blood*, usually a result of *infection* or *inflammation.*
[ref. 3]

lymphocytotoxicity

Capability of lysing *lymphocytes.*
Note: Lymphocytotoxicity is manifest with lymphocytes having a specific cell surface *antigen* that are lysed when incubated with *antiserum* and *complement* or when attacked by *primed histoincompatible T-lymphocytes.*
[ref. 3]

lymphoid

Relating to or denoting tissue responsible for producing *lymphocytes* and *antibodies*. Note: *Lymphoid tissue* occurs throughout the body in *lymph* nodes, *thymus, tonsils*, and *spleen*.
[ref. 5]

lymphoid follicle

Region of clustered *B-cells*, allowing the selection of *antigen*-binding B-cells by *dendritic cells* during *adaptive immune responses*.
[ref. 3]

lymphoid stem cell

See *stem cell, lymphoid*.

lymphoid tissue

Vertebrate tissue that is made up predominantly of *lymphocytes, e.g., lymph, lymph nodes, spleen, thymus, Peyer's patch*es, adenoids, pharyngeal *tonsils*, and, in birds, *bursa of Fabricius* and cecal tonsils.
[ref. 3]

lymphokine

Cytokine produced by *lymphocytes*.
[ref. 3]

lymphokine-activated killer (LAK) cell
lymphocyte-activated killer cell

Killer (K) cell or *natural killer (NK) cell* activated in vitro by *interleukin*-2 to give enhanced killing of *target cells*.
[ref. 3]

lymphoma

Neoplasm, usually *malignant*, of the *lymphatic tissues*.
[ref. 3]

lymphoma, cutaneous T-cell
mycosis fungoides

Malignant growth of *T-cells* that home (see *homing*) to the skin.
[ref. 3]

lymphopenia

See *lymphocytopenia*.

lymphopoiesis

Production of *lymphocytes*.
[ref. 3]

lymphoproliferation

Proliferation of *lymphocytes* in response to stimulation with cellular activators, including *antigens* or *mitogens*.
[ref. 3]

lymphosum

Sum of *B-cells* + *T-cells* + *natural killer cells* determined separately (by *flow cytometry*), compared to the total number of *lymphocytes*.
Note: The lymphosum is used as a check on accuracy in counting the proportion of cell types, *e.g.*, a value of (100 ± 10) % being acceptable and reflecting the uncertainty of the method.
[ref. 3]

lymphotoxin (LT)

tumor necrosis factor β (TNF-β)

T-cell-derived *cytokine* that is *cytotoxic* for certain *tumor cells* and also has immunoregulatory functions.
[ref. 3]

Lyon hypothesis

Lyon law
X-inactivation
lyonization

Hypothesis (named after Mary Lyon) that random inactivation of all but one *X chromosome* occurs in each female mammalian cell in early development, thus explaining why the effect of the X chromosome on *phenotype* is the same in males with one copy as in females with two copies.
Note 1: In keeping with the Lyon law, the *Barr body*, an inactivated X chromosome, is visible in some female cells.
Note 2: X-inactivation leads to *mosaicism* for *X-linked genes* in the female, since the paternal *X chromosome* is inactivated in some cells and the maternal one in others.
Note 3: The Lyon hypothesis was designated the Lyon law by the European Molecular Biology Organization (EMBO) in 2011.
[ref. 5]

lysimeter

Laboratory column of selected representative *soil* or a protected monolith of undisturbed field soil with facilities for sampling and monitoring the movement of water and other substances through the column.
[After ref. 2]

lysosomal storage disease

One of a group of rare inherited metabolic *disorders* resulting from a defect in *lysosomal* function, commonly deficiency of *enzymes* required for the *metabolism* of lipids, *glycoproteins*, or mucopolysaccharides, resulting in their accumulation in the *cell*.
[ref. 5]

lysosome (n)/lysosomal (adj)

Membrane-bounded *cytoplasmic* *organelle* containing hydrolytic (see *hydrolysis*) *enzymes* that are involved in *phagocytosis*.
Note: Release of hydrolytic enzymes from lysosomes can cause cell *autolysis*.
[After ref. 1]

M cell

See *microfold cell.*

MacArthur–Wilson model

Model of island colonization giving the mathematical relationship

$$S(t) = S_{EQ}(1 - e^{-Gt})$$

where $S(t)$ is the number of *species* present at time t, S_{EQ} is the equilibrium number of *species* for the island, and G is the rate constant for colonization of the island.
[ref. 2]

macroautophagy

nonspecific *autophagy*

Sequestration and breakdown of *organelles* and long-lived proteins in a double-*membrane vesicle*, called an *autophagosome* or autophagic *vacuole*, inside the *cell.*
Note 1: Characteristic of macroautophagy, the outer membrane of the autophagosome fuses in the *cytoplasm* with a *lysosome* to form an autolysosome or auto*phagolysosome* where their contents are degraded by acidic lysosomal hydrolases.
Note 2: Macroautophagy is the major inducible pathway for the general turnover of cytoplasmic constituents in *eukaryotic* cells. It is also responsible for the *degradation* of active cytoplasmic *enzymes* and organelles during nutrient starvation.
[ref. 3]

macrocephaly

megacephaly
megalocephaly

Congenital disorder characterized by an abnormally large head and (or) *brain.*
[ref. 5]

macrocosm (in ecobiology)

Large multi-*species* test system.
[ref. 2]
See also *mesocosm; microcosm.*

macroglossia

Congenital disorder characterized by an abnormally enlarged tongue.
Note: This is often seen in *Down syndrome.*
[ref. 5]

macrognathia

megagnathia

Congenital disorder characterized by enlargement or elongation of the jaw.
[ref. 5]

Comprehensive Glossary of Terms Used in Toxicology
By John Duffus, Douglas M. Templeton and Michael Schwenk

Published by the Royal Society of Chemistry, www.rsc.org

macromelia
megalomelia

Congenital disorder characterized by an abnormally large limb or limbs.
[ref. 5]

macronutrient

Imprecise term referring to a *nutrient* required in relatively large amounts for normal growth and *health*.
Note: Macronutrients include carbohydrates, proteins and fats, as well as their *metabolites*, and inorganic substances such as sodium and calcium salts, and iron compounds.
[After ref. 2]
See also *trace nutrient*.

macrophage

Large (10–20 μm diameter) amoeboid and *phagocytic* cell, found in many *tissues*, especially in areas of *inflammation*, derived from *blood monocytes,* and playing an important role in *host defense* mechanisms.
[ref. 3]

macrophage, resident(ial)
macrophage, fixed

Macrophage stationed at a point where microbial invasion or accumulation of *dust* is likely to occur.
Note: Each type of resident macrophage has a specific name determined by its location, as shown in Table 1.

Table 1 Types of resident macrophages and their locations.

Name of macrophage	Location
dust cells/*alveolar* macrophages	*pulmonary* alveolus of lungs
histiocytes	*connective tissue*
Kupffer cells	liver
microglial cells	*neural* tissue
monocytes	*blood*
osteoclast	bone
sinusoidal lining cells	*spleen*

[ref. 3]

macrophage function test

Any assay suitable to characterize the effect of substances on *macrophage* function *in vivo* or *in vitro*.
Note: Common macrophage function tests are the *chromium release assay* and the *chromate uptake assay*.
[ref. 3]

macrophage mannose receptor (MMR)

Receptor involved in *pathogen* recognition, in clearance of endogenous serum *glycoproteins*, and in *antigen presentation*.
Note 1: Clusters of MMR lectin domains bind mannose residues on microbial and fungal surfaces in a Ca^{2+}-dependent manner.
Note 2: The MMR activates the C3 component of *complement*.
[ref. 3]

macrophyte

Aquatic plant large enough to be seen easily with the naked eye (as distinct from phytoplankton and small algae).
Note: The term "aquatic macrophyte" has no *taxonomic* significance.
[ref. 2]

macropinocytosis

High-volume *pinocytosis* by which cells (*e.g., dendritic cells*) engulf relatively large volumes of fluid from their surroundings, enabling them to take in many *antigens* nonspecifically.
[ref. 3]

macroscopic pathology
gross pathology

Study of *disease*-associated changes that are visible to the naked eye, without the need for a microscope.
[ref. 5]

macrosomia

Congenital disorder characterized by an abnormally large body or body part.
[ref. 5]

macrostomia

Congenital disorder characterized by an abnormally large size of the mouth.
[ref. 5]

Mad Hatter syndrome

See *mercurialism.*

magnetic resonance imaging (MRI)
nuclear magnetic resonance imaging (NMRI)
magnetic resonance tomography (MRT)

Diagnostic imaging technique that produces three-dimensional images of body structures based on the ability to detect changes in nuclear spin alignment of atomic nuclei held in a strong magnetic field and subjected to radiofrequency pulses.
Note: The basic MRI technique is based on the nuclear spin of protons in water, but MRI signals vary depending on the elements and chemical bonds in a tissue and therefore can be used to visualize other aspects of the chemical composition of organs.
[ref. 4]

magnetic resonance spectroscopy (in neurotoxicology)

Noninvasive method based on nuclear spin alignment that allows localization of levels and measurement of *kinetics* of injected labeled substances in living *tissue*.
Note: In neurology, magnetic resonance spectroscopy is used to localize the *brain* areas where increased *metabolic* activity occurs upon stimulation; it is also used to study activity and location of *neurotransmitter*s.
[ref. 4]

Magnusson and Kligman test

See *guinea-pig maximization test.*
[ref. 1]

mainstream smoke (tobacco smoking)

Smoke that is actively *inhaled* by the smoker.
[ref. 1]
See also *side stream smoke.*

major basic protein

Small basic arginine-rich peptide (pI 10.9, molecular mass of 13.8 kDa), in the granules of *eosinophils,* that kills helminths and protozoa.
[ref. 3]

major histocompatibility complex (MHC)

Cluster of genes encoding *cell* surface molecules involved in *antigen presentation* to *T-cells.*
Note 1: In humans, the MHC genes are found on chromosome 6, and in mice on chromosome 17.
Note 2: The MHC proteins are polymorphic and code for *antigens* that lead to rapid *graft rejection* between members of a single *species* that differ at these loci.
Note 3: Several classes of protein such as *MHC class I* and *class II molecules* are gene products encoded in this region. The MHC-encoded molecules are also known as *human leukocyte antigens (HLA).*
[ref. 3]
See also *H-2; H-2 complex.*

major histocompatibility complex (MHC) **class I molecule**

Surface protein encoded by the *major histocompatibility complex* expressed on all nucleated *cells* and presenting *antigen*-derived peptides.
[ref. 3]
See also *antigen presentation.*

major histocompatibility complex (MHC) **class II molecule**

Surface protein, encoded by the *major histocompatibility complex,* expressed on *antigen-presenting cells* and presenting *antigen*-derived peptides.
[ref. 3]
See also *antigen presentation.*

major histocompatibility complex (MHC) **class III molecule**

Antigen encoded by the *major histocompatibility complex*, including several *complement* factors, *tumor necrosis factor*, and *lymphotoxin.*
Note: The MHC class III genes are found on the short arm of chromosome 6 between class I and class II genes, and, although the *gene products* share no common function with the *MHC class I* and *MHC class II molecules*, they are often discussed together.
[ref. 3]

major histocompatibility complex (MHC) **molecule**

Any of the cell-surface *glycoprotein alloantigens,* encoded by the *major histocompatibility complex,* that are involved in the regulation of *immune responses,* and can cause the *rejection* of *grafted tissues, cells*, and *tumors* bearing them.
[ref. 3]

major histocompatibility complex (MHC) restriction

Necessity that *T-cells* recognize processed *antigen* only when presented by *major histocompatibility complex molecules* of the original *haplotype* associated with T-cell *priming*.
[ref. 3]

malaise

Vague feeling of bodily discomfort.
[ref. 1]

male efferent duct

See *efferent duct*.

male-mediated toxicity

Disease or *birth defects* produced by a father's *exposure* to a physical or chemical agent.
[ref. 2]

malformation

Structural defect as a result of abnormal development.
[ref. 5]

malignancy

Population of cells showing both uncontrolled growth and a tendency to invade and destroy other *tissues*.
Note: A malignancy is life-threatening.
[ref. 1]
See also *malignant*.

malignant

Opposite term: *benign*.

1. Occurring in a severe form, tending to become progressively worse, resistant to treatment, and likely to result in death.
2. (in *cancer*) *Cells* showing both uncontrolled growth and a tendency to invade and destroy other *tissues*.

[ref. 5]

Malthusian theory

Model, developed by Thomas R. Malthus (1766–1834), implying that, unchecked by *environmental* or social constraints, human *populations* would increase exponentially, eventually outstripping their food supply. Thus, if X_i denotes the population size during time period i, and r is the population *growth* rate, the Malthusian population model gives the relationship

$$X(I+1) = (1+r)X_i.$$

[After ref. 2]
See also *intrinsic (Malthusian) rate of increase*.

mammalian target of rapamycin (mTOR)

mechanistic target of rapamycin

Intracellular signaling molecule (phosphatidylinositol-3-kinase-related kinase) involved in control of *cell growth*, whose activity is negatively influenced by the *immunosuppressive drug* rapamycin.
[ref. 3]

mammary gland

Milk-producing *organ* in female mammals.
[ref. 5]

Mancini immunodiffusion

See *radial immunodiffusion*.

mandible (n)/mandibular (adj)

Jaw or jawbone, especially the lower jawbone.
[*]
See also *maxilla*.

manganism

Condition of manganese *poisoning*, usually after chronic *inhalation* exposure to manganese fumes.
Note 1: Manganism is characterized by neurological and psychiatric *disorders*, including reduced *reaction time, lethargy, tremors*, and a mask-like facies. Impotence and loss of *libido* have also been reported.
Note 2: A mild form of manganism may result from low environmental exposures to manganese that have been reported to impair *brain* development and to reduce performance in neuropsychological tests.
[After ref. 4]

mania (n)/manic (adj)

Emotional *disorder* (mental illness) characterized by an expansive and elated state (euphoria), rapid speech, flight of ideas, decreased need for sleep, distractibility, grandiosity, poor judgment, and increased motor activity.
[ref. 1]
See also *bipolar disorder*.

mannan-binding lectin-associated serine peptidase-1 and -2 (MASP1, MASP2)

mannose-binding protein-associated serine protease (MASP)

Complement-dependent bactericidal protease (EC 3.4.21.x) factors that bind to the Ra and R2 polysaccharides expressed by certain enterobacterium strains, such as Ra *chemotype* strains of ***Salmonella***.
Note 1: Alternate splicing of the MASP genes results in multiple transcript variants encoding two Ra-reactive factors (RaRF) that are involved in the *mannose-binding lectin* pathway of *complement activation*.
Note 2: MASPs are serine proteases that share about 40 % sequence identity with complement components C1r and C1s.
[ref. 3]

mannose-binding lectin (MBL)

mannan-binding lectin

See *mannose-binding protein*.

mannose-binding protein (MBP)

mannose-binding lectin (MBL)

Member of the *collectin* family of calcium-dependent *lectins*, and an *acute-phase protein.*
Note: The MBL functions as a stimulator of the *classical pathway of complement activation*, and as an *opsonin* for *phagocytosis* by binding to mannose, a sugar residue usually found in an exposed form only on the surface of microorganisms.
[ref. 3]

mantle zone

mantle
corona

Outer ring of small *lymphocytes* surrounding the center of a *lymphatic* nodule (*lymphoid follicle*).
Note: The mantle zone contains transient lymphocytes and is the location of the *lymphoma* in mantle cell lymphoma.
[ref. 3]

Mantoux test

See *tuberculin.*

Marfan syndrome

Congenital connective tissue disorder associated with *mutation* of the fibrillin-1 *gene*, FBN1.
[ref. 5]

margin of exposure (MOE)

Ratio of the *no-observed-adverse-effect level* to the theoretical or *estimated exposure dose* or *concentration.*
[ref. 1]

margin of safety (MOS)

See *margin of exposure.*

marginal zone

Outer area of the *splenic* periarteriolar *lymphoid* sheath (PALS) that is rich in *B-cells*, particularly those responding to *thymus*-independent *antigens.*
[ref. 3]

margination

Leukocyte adhesion to the *endothelium* of blood vessels in the early phase of an acute *inflammatory response.*
[ref. 3]

masculinization

Development of male characteristics, such as facial hair, either as part of normal male maturation, or pathologically by people of either sex as a result of *hormonal* imbalance.
[ref. 5]

mass balance equation

1. (in chemistry) Representation of a chemical reaction that accounts for the same number of like atoms on each side of an equilibrium.
2. (in engineering) Statement that the total mass input into a system equals the total mass output plus the accumulated mass.
3. (in ecology) Equation that expresses the total mass of a substance in terms of the sum of the mass in all the various forms and concentrations occurring in the different *environmental* compartments (including biota).

[After ref. 2]

mass mean diameter

Diameter of a spherical particle with a mass equal to the mean mass of all the particles in a population.
[ref. 1]

mass median diameter

Diameter of a spherical particle with the median mass of all the particles in a population.
[ref. 1]

mast cell

Large connective tissue cell that contains inflammatory substances such as *histamine*, proteases [including tryptases (EC 3.4.21.59), chymases (EC 3.4.21.39), and carboxypeptidase A (EC 3.4.17.1)], heparin and chondroitin sulfate proteoglycans, and eicosanoid lipid mediators (the precursors of *leukotrienes* and *prostaglandins*). These substances are released in *allergic* reactions or in response to injury or *inflammation*.
Note 1: Mast cells are bound within tissues that interface with the external world such as the skin, respiratory or intestinal tract, as well as in other areas such as heart, synovium, and *uterus*. Mast cells do not circulate.
Note 2: The mast cell has binding sites on its surface for *immunoglobulin E*.
[ref. 3]

mast cell activation disorder (syndrome) (MCAD/MCAS)

Disorder or *syndrome* in which there is evidence of *systemic*, inappropriate release of *mast cell* mediators.
Note: While people with MCAD/MCAS have a normal or near-normal tryptase (EC 3.4.21.59) level and a *bone marrow* biopsy that contains a normal number of mast cells, they experience most of the same symptoms as someone with *mastocytosis*.
[ref. 3]

mast cell degranulation

See *degranulation*.

mast cell stabilizer

Nonsteroidal medication that reduces the release of substances from *mast cells, e.g.*, sodium cromoglycate.
[ref. 3]

mastocyte

See *mast cell*.

mastocytoma

mast cell tumor

Nodule of *mast cells* that can involve the skin, subcutaneous *tissue*, and sometimes muscle.
Note: Mastocytomas are rare and are mostly seen in infants within the first three months of life.
[ref. 3]

mastocytosis

Rare *disease* characterized by the presence of too many *mast cells* in various *organs* and *tissues*.
Note 1: Mastocytosis can be a chronic, long-term illness or it can develop suddenly.
Note 2: Mastocytosis may be *systemic*, involving a variety of organs, or cutaneous, involving only the skin, also referred to as urticaria pigmentosa.
[ref. 3]

material safety data sheet (MSDS)

safety data sheet (SDS)

Compilation of information, including the identity of hazardous substances, *health* and physical *hazards*, *exposure* limits, and precautions, legally required before import, production, or marketing of any substance in most countries, and now worldwide under the *Globally Harmonized System* of regulation.
[*]

maternal serum α-fetoprotein (MSAFP)

Protein (*α-fetoprotein*), made in the *fetus,* that normally leaks in small amounts into the mother's circulation.
Note: If there is an abnormal opening in the fetus, such as a *neural tube defect*, larger amounts of MSAFP appear in the mother's serum, providing a screening test for such fetal anomalies.
[ref. 5]

matrix

Material in which something is embedded.

1. (in biology) Substance between *cells* or in which structures are embedded. See also *extracellular matrix*.
2. (in geology) Fine grained material of a sedimentary rock in which crystals, pebbles, or fossils are embedded.

[*]

maturation (in immunology)

Process by which *B-cells* produce *antibodies* with increased *affinity* for *antigen* during the course of an *immune response*.
[ref. 3]

mature B-cell

B-cell with *immunoglobulin M* and *immunoglobulin D* on its surface.
[ref. 3]

maturity index

Index of pollution based on the proportions of *species* in a *soil* nematode *community* that fall into various categories ranging from colonizers (*r-strategists*) to persisters (*K-strategists*).
[ref. 2]
See also *K-strategy; r-strategy*.

maxilla (n)/maxillary (adj)

Upper jawbone.
[ref. 5]
See also *mandible*.

maximum acceptable toxicant concentration (MATC) (in ecology)

Geometric mean of the lowest *exposure concentration* that causes a statistically significant adverse effect (*lowest-observed-effect concentration*) and the highest exposure concentration where no effect is observed (*no-observed-effect concentration*) in a *life cycle* (full *chronic*) or partial life cycle (partial chronic) test.
Note: Calculation of an MATC requires quantitative life-cycle *toxicity* data on the effects of a material on survival, growth, and *reproduction*.
[ref. 2]

maximum allowable (acceptable, admissible) concentration (MAC)

Regulatory value defining the *concentration* that, if *inhaled* daily (in the case of work people for 8 h with a working week of 40 h; in the case of the general population, 24 h), does not, in the present state of knowledge, appear capable of causing appreciable harm, however long delayed, during the working life or during subsequent life, or in subsequent generations.
[ref. 1]
See also *lowest-observed-effect concentration; no-observed-effect concentration*.

maximum average daily concentration of an atmospheric pollutant
peak daily average concentration of an air pollutant

Highest of the average daily *concentrations* recorded at a definite point of measurement during a certain period of observation.
[ref. 1]

maximum contaminant level (MCL)

Regulatory *concentration* for drinking water, under the Safe Drinking Water Act (USA).
Note 1: MCL is classified as primary and secondary.

- Primary MCL takes into account both prevention of *adverse effects* (including sensitive *populations*) and technological feasibility (including natural background levels).
- Secondary MCL is based on "welfare", such as taste and staining, rather than *health*, but also takes into account technological feasibility.

Note 2: MCL Goals (MCLG) under the Safe Drinking Water Act do not consider feasibility and are zero for all human and animal *carcinogens*.
[After ref. 1]

maximum daily intake, estimated (EMDI)

Prediction of the maximum daily intake of a potentially harmful substance based on assumptions of average food consumption per person and maximum residues in the

edible portion of a commodity, corrected for the reduction or increase in residues resulting from preparation, cooking, or commercial processing; and usually expressed in mg substance per person.
[ref. 1]

maximum daily intake, theoretical (TMDI)

Predicted maximum daily intake of a *residue*, assuming that it is present at the *maximum residue level* and that average daily consumption of foods per person is correctly represented by assessed regional diets; usually expressed in milligrams of residue per person per day.
[ref. 1]

maximum exposure limit (MEL)

Occupational *exposure* limit legally defined in the United Kingdom under COSHH as the maximum *concentration* of an airborne substance, averaged over a reference period, to which employees may be *exposed* by inhalation under any circumstances, and set on the advice of the HSC Advisory Committee on Toxic Substances.
[ref. 1]

maximum likelihood estimation (MLE)

Parametric method used to fit *dose-* or *concentration-effect* data to the *log-normal*, log-logistic, or other models.
Note: *Probit* and *logit* approaches are most often applied with MLE methods.
[ref. 2]

maximum permissible concentration (MPC)

See *maximum allowable concentration.*

maximum permissible daily dose

Maximum daily dose of a substance whose penetration into a human body during a lifetime will not cause *diseases* or *health hazards* that can be detected by current investigation methods and will not adversely affect future generations.
[ref. 1]

maximum permissible level (MPL)

Level, usually a combination of time and *concentration*, beyond which any *exposure* of humans to a chemical or physical agent in their immediate environment is unsafe.
[ref. 1]

maximum residue limit, temporary

Regulatory value established for a *pesticide* of concern over a limited time when (a) only a temporary *acceptable daily intake* for the pesticide has been established, or (b) an agreed acceptable daily intake exists but the available data are inadequate for firm maximum intake recommendations.
[ref. 1]

maximum residue limit (MRL) for pesticide residues

Maximum contents of a *pesticide* residue (expressed as mg kg^{-1} fresh weight) recommended by the *Codex Alimentarius Commission* to be legally permitted in or on food commodities and animal feeds.

Note: MRLs are based on data obtained following *good agricultural practice*. Foods derived from commodities that comply with the respective MRLs are intended to be toxicologically acceptable.
[ref. 1]

maximum residue limit (MRL) **for veterinary drugs**

Maximum contents of a *drug* residue (expressed as mg kg^{-1} or μg kg^{-1} fresh weight) recommended by the *Codex Alimentarius Commission* to be legally permitted or recognized as acceptable in or on food commodities and animal feeds.
Note: The MRL for veterinary drugs is based on the type and amount of residue considered to be without any toxicological *hazard* for human *health* as expressed by the acceptable *daily intake* (ADI) or on the basis of a temporary ADI that uses an additional uncertainty factor. It also takes into account other relevant public health *risks* as well as food technological aspects.
[ref. 1]

maximum tolerable concentration (MTC)

Highest *concentration* of a substance in an environmental medium that does not kill test organisms or species (denoted by LC_0).
[ref. 1]

maximum tolerable dose (MTD)

Highest amount of a substance that, when introduced into the body, does not kill test organisms or species (denoted by LD_0).
[ref. 1]

maximum tolerable exposure level (MTEL)

Maximum amount (*dose*) or *concentration* of a substance to which an organism can be *exposed* without leading to an *adverse effect* after prolonged *exposure* time.
[ref. 1]

maximum tolerated dose (MTD)

High *dose* used in *chronic toxicity* testing that is expected, on the basis of an adequate *subchronic* study, to produce limited *toxicity* when administered for the duration of the test period.
Note 1: The MTD should not induce

- overt toxicity, *e.g.*, appreciable death of cells or organ dysfunction
- *toxic* manifestations that are predicted materially to reduce the life span of the animals except as the result of neoplastic development
- 10 % or greater retardation of body weight gain as compared with *control* animals

Note 2: In some studies, toxicity that could interfere with a *carcinogen*ic effect is specifically excluded when determining the MTD.
[ref. 1]

maximum velocity, V_{max}

maximum rate

Term in *Michaelis–Menten kinetics* denoting the maximum rate of *conversion* of a substrate occurring when its *concentration* is not rate-limiting.
[ref. 1]

maze

Labyrinthine system, in which the ability of an animal (usually a rodent) to find a direct route from a starting point to a specific location is observed.
Note: Different mazes are available for psychological and neurotoxicity testing. Maze tests suitable for studying spatial navigation, learning, memory, cognition, anxiety and other behaviour have been developed.
[ref. 4]
See also *maze, Barnes; maze, Biel water; maze, elevated plus; maze, radial arm; maze, T/Y; water maze test.*

maze, Barnes

Circular platform equipped with some 20 equidistant holes near the outer rim, one of which is marked by visual *cues* and is an escape hole for a rodent that is placed near the middle of the platform and subjected to an adverse *stimulus, e.g.*, bright light.
Note 1: Parameters measured in a Barnes maze test include latency to escape, path length, number of errors, and velocity.
Note 2: The Barnes maze test is used to evaluate cognitive deficits.
[ref. 4]
See also *maze.*

maze, Biel water

A water labyrinth, described by Biel (1940), where rodents are forced to swim until they find a small underwater platform that allows them to escape.
Note 1: The Biel water maze test is used to study possible neurotoxic effects on spatial learning, memory and other factors.
Note 2: The Cincinnati water maze is related to the Biel water maze.
[ref. 4]
See also *maze.*

maze, elevated plus

Stage with four orthogonal side arms elevated above the floor, where two opposite arms have sidewalls and the other two arms have no walls; used as research tool for anxiety.
Note: In an elevated plus maze, rodents normally preferentially avoid the arms without walls, but during *anxiolytic* treatment they tend to spend more time on them, or enter them more often.
[ref. 4]
See also *maze.*

maze, radial arm

Apparatus with a central platform and equidistant arms (usually eight), at the end of which is a reward (*e.g.*, a food pellet).
Note: A rodent placed in the center of a radial arm maze is observed seeking the shortest way to the reward, as an indicator of spatial learning and memory.
[ref. 4]
See also *maze.*

maze, T/Y

Simple type of test apparatus with three arms shaped like the letter 'T'; after placing a rodent in the middle, how often the animal enters each arm is recorded.
Note 1: Rewards can be used for motivation in T-maze testing, or the inborn trend for alternation can be tested.

Note 2: The Y-maze is a variation of the T-maze where the apparatus is 'Y'-shaped.
[ref. 4]
See also *maze*.

mean absorption time (MAT)

Average time required for *absorption* of a substance, such as a *drug* or *contaminant*, calculated as the difference in *mean residence time* (MRT) of the substance introduced by the (noninstantaneous) route of interest and the MRT for the same substance injected intravenously.
[ref. 2]

mean generation time (*T*c)

Average time interval required for a bacterial cell to divide or for the *population* to double under a defined set of conditions.
[ref. 2]

mean life

mean time

Average lifetime of a molecule, atom, or *organelle* in a specified state.
Note: For an exponentially decaying system, mean life is the average time for the number of molecules, atoms, or organelles in a specified state to decrease by a factor of *e*, the base of natural logarithms.
[ref. 1]

mean residence time (in pharmacokinetics and toxicokinetics) (MRT)

Average time a *drug* or other potentially *toxic substance* remains in the body or in an *organ* after rapid intravenous injection.
Note 1: Like clearance, the value of MRT is independent of *dose* in most cases.
Note 2: After an intravenous bolus:
MRT = AUMC/AUC, where AUC is the *area under the curve* (plasma concentration vs time curve), and AUMC is the area under the moment curve (plasma concentration × time vs time curve)
Note 3: For a drug with one-compartment distribution characteristics (see one-compartment model), MRT equals the reciprocal of the *elimination rate constant*.
[After ref. 1]

measurement endpoint (in ecological risk assessment)

Measurable response to a stressor (*e.g.*, fledglings produced per nest each year) that is related to the valued qualities of the assessment *endpoint* (*e.g.*, reproductive success of bald eagles).
[ref. 2]

measurement uncertainty

See *uncertainty*.

mechanism of action

Detailed description of every step in the sequence of events that leads to a biological *effect*.
[*]
See also *key event*.
Compare *mode of action*.

Meckel diverticulum
ileal diverticulum

Congenital pouch in the *ileum* resulting from incomplete closure of the *yolk sac*.
[ref. 5]

meconium

First intestinal discharges of the newborn infant, greenish in color and consisting of *epithelial* cells, *mucus*, and bile.
[ref. 5]

median effective concentration (EC_{50})

Statistically derived *concentration* of a substance in an environmental medium expected to produce a certain effect in 50 % of test organisms in a given *population* under a defined set of conditions.
Note: EC_n refers to the median concentration that is effective in *n* % of the test population.
[ref. 1]

median effective dose (ED_{50})

See *dose, median effective*.

median effective time (ET_{50})

For sublethal or ambiguously lethal effects, the time until 50 % of the exposed individuals respond.
[ref. 2]

median inhibitory time (IT_{50})
inhibitory time

Time required for a *toxicant* to inhibit a specified process in 50 % of a *population* under test conditions.
See also *effect time, lethal time*.
[ref. 2]

median lethal concentration (LC_{50})

Statistically derived *concentration* of a substance in an environmental medium expected to kill 50 % of organisms in a given *population* under a defined set of conditions.
[ref. 1]

median lethal dose (LD_{50})

Statistically derived *dose* of a chemical substance or physical agent (*e.g.*, radiation) expected to kill 50 % of organisms in a given *population* under a defined set of conditions.
[ref. 1]

median lethal time (TL_{50})

Statistically derived time interval during which 50 % of a given *population* may be expected to die following *acute* administration of a chemical substance or physical agent (*e.g.*, radiation) at a given *concentration* under a defined set of conditions.
[ref. 1]

median narcotic concentration (NC_{50})

Statistically derived median *concentration* of a substance in an environmental medium expected to cause *narcotic* conditions in 50 % of a given population under a defined set of conditions.
[ref. 1]

median narcotic dose (ND_{50})

Statistically derived dose of a substance expected to cause *narcotic* conditions in 50 % of test animals under a defined set of conditions.
[ref. 1]

median teratogenic concentration (TC_{50})

Median concentration resulting in developmental malformations for 50 % of the exposed individuals within a predetermined time, *e.g.*, 96 h.
[ref. 2]

median time to death (MTTD)

Time resulting in death for 50 % of the exposed organisms.
[ref. 2]
See also *median lethal time*.

median tolerance limit (TL_m or TL_{50})

Concentration of a substance in air, water, *sediment*, or *soil* at which 50 % of the test organisms survive after a specified time of *exposure*. The TL_{50} (equivalent to the TL_m) is usually expressed as a time-dependent value (*e.g.*, 24-h or 96-h TL_{50}; the estimated concentration at which 50 % of test organisms survive after 24 or 96 h of exposure). Note: Unlike lethal concentration and *lethal dose*, the term "tolerance limit" is applicable in designating the level of any measurable lethal condition (*e.g.*, extremes in pH, temperature, dissolved oxygen). TL_m and TL_{50} have been replaced by *median lethal concentration* (LC_{50}) and *median effective concentration* (EC_{50}).
[ref. 2]

mediastinum

Region in the middle of the *thorax* between the two lungs, containing the regional vessels, *trachea*, esophagus, bronchi, *lymph* nodes, and heart.
[ref. 5]

medicine

1. Science and practice of diagnosing, treating, or preventing *disease* and other damage to the body or mind. (adj. **medical**)
2. Any *drug* or therapy used to treat disease or injury. (adj. **medicinal**)

[ref. 1]

medium/media (pl)

1. (in environmental science) Surrounding environment (air, water, *soil*, or *sediment*) in which living organisms function and thrive.
   [ref. 2]
2. (in cell biology) Aqueous solution, gel, or other laboratory environment, containing adequate concentrations of required nutrients and growth factors to sustain growth and (or) survival of living cells.
   [*]

medulla

1. medulla oblongata
   Lower part of the *brain* stem continuous with the *spinal cord*, containing neural centers regulating the autonomic functions of breathing, heart rate, and blood pressure.
2. Middle (central) part of an organ, as in *adrenal* medulla, renal medulla, or the medulla of a lymph node.

[ref. 5]

medulloblastoma

Highly malignant, invasive *brain* tumor of embryonal origin, arising in the *posterior fossa*, usually from the *cerebellum*.
Note: Medulloblastoma is the most common malignant brain tumor in children.
[ref. 4]

megacolon

Condition of extreme dilation of the colon that can be *congenital* (as in *Hirschsprung* disease) or acquired (as when children refuse to defecate).
Note: Aganglionic megacolon is a condition, where parts of the colon have abnormal motor activity, resulting in spasms and massive distension of the colon *proximal* to the spasm.
[ref. 5]

megadactyly
macrodactylia

Disorder characterized by abnormally large fingers and (or) toes.
[ref. 5]

megagametophyte

Eggproducing *gametophyte*.
[*]

megakaryocyte

Bone marrow precursor of *platelets*.
[ref. 3]

megaloblast

See *normoblast*.

meiofauna

Small *benthic* invertebrates living in interstices of *soil* or *sediment*, or in aquatic systems.
Note: The term "meiofauna" loosely defines a group of organisms by their size, larger than microfauna but smaller than macrofauna. In practice, these are usually organisms that can pass through a 1-mm mesh but will be retained by a 45-μm mesh, but the exact dimensions vary from researcher to researcher. Whether an organism will pass through a 1-mm mesh may depend upon whether it is alive or dead at the time of sorting.
[ref. 2]

meiosis

Process of "reductive" cell division, occurring in the production of *gametes*, by means of which each daughter nucleus receives half the number of *chromosome*s characteristic of the somatic cells of the species.
Note: Meiosis is not to be confused with *miosis*.
[ref. 1]

meiotic drive

Any process that causes some *allele*s to be over-represented in the gametes that are formed during *meiosis*.
Note: With normal segregation of a *Mendelian gene*, on average half of an organism's offspring inherit one of the alleles and the other half the other allele. Meiotic drive refers to rare cases in which Mendel's laws are broken, and one of the alleles is consistently found in more than half the offspring.
[ref. 2]

melanic form

Individual or subspecies with increased dark pigmentation.
[ref. 2]

melanism

Increased black or nearly black pigmentation of skin, feathers, or hair of an organism, resulting from (increased) synthesis of melanin.
[ref. 2]
See also *melanism, industrial*.

melanism, industrial

Gradual increase in *melanic forms*, often until they are predominant, in animal *populations* in industrialized regions.
[ref. 2]

membrane (n)/membranous (adj)

1. (in anatomy) Thin layer of *tissue* separating or connecting structures or organs.
2. (in cell biology) Phospholipid-based bilayer structure, surrounding and isolating cells and organelles.

[ref. 5]
See also *plasma membrane*.

membrane attack complex (MAC)

Complex of *complement* components C5b–C9 that inserts as a pore into the membrane of *target cells* leading to cell lysis.
[ref. 3]

membrane polarization

Occurrence of a potential difference across a biological *membrane*.
Note: A cell at its *resting potential* is said to be polarized.
[ref. 4]
See also *membrane potential*.

membrane potential

Difference in electric potential between the inside and the outside of a cell.
Note 1: Typical cell membrane potentials are around −70 to −80 mV.
Note 2: The ion disequilibria that give rise to the membrane potential difference are produced by the combined action of ATP-consuming ion pumps, gated *ion channels*, and ion leakage.
Note 3: During *neuronal excitation*, the membrane potential becomes transiently positive during the *action potential* before returning to the *resting potential*.
[ref. 4]
See also *depolarization; ion channel.*

memory (in immunology)

immunological memory

Characteristic of the acquired *immune response* (see *acquired immunity*) of *lymphocytes* whereby a second encounter with a given *antigen* produces a secondary immune response that is faster, greater, and longer lasting than the *primary immune response*.
[ref. 3]

memory cell

Clonally expanded *T-cell* or *B-cell* produced during a *primary immune response* and which is *primed* to mediate a *secondary immune response* to the original *antigen*.
[ref. 3]

memory lymphocyte immunostimulation assay (MELISA)

Patented modification of the *lymphocyte transformation test* based on the *enzyme-linked immunosorbent assay* principle.
[ref. 3]

menarche

First *menstrual cycle* of a woman.
[ref. 5]

Mendelian gene

See *gene, Mendelian.*

Mendelian inheritance

Inheritance in which stable and indivisible characteristics are controlled entirely or overwhelmingly by a single *genetic locus* and transmitted over many generations.
[ref. 5]

Mendelian trait

Phenotype that shows a pattern of *Mendelian inheritance*.
[ref. 5]

Mendelism

Fundamental principles of inheritance (especially the laws of segregation and independent assortment, and the existence of dominant and recessive characters), propounded originally by Gregor Mendel (1822–1884) and forming the basis for the science of classical *genetics*.
[ref. 2]

meninges

Plural of *meninx*.
[ref. 4]

meningioma

Firm, often vascular, *tumor* arising from the *meninges* of the *brain* or *spinal cord.*
Note: Meningiomas are slowly growing benign tumors and quite common.
[ref. 4]

meningitis

Inflammation or infection of the *meninges*.
Note 1: Although bacterial and viral infections are the most common causes of meningitis, there are also noninfectious causes including *cancer*s, *autoimmune disease* and head injury.
Note 2: Several common *drugs* may cause *aseptic* meningitis.
[ref. 4]

meningocele

Herniation of the *membranes* (*meninges*) of the *brain* or *spinal cord* through a defect in the *cranium* or *spinal column.*
[ref. 5]

meningoencephalitis
cerebromeningitis
encephalomeningitis

Inflammation of the *brain* and *meninges.*
[ref. 4]

meningoencephalocele

Protrusion of both the *meninges* and *brain* tissue through a defect in the skull.
Note: Meningoencephalocele is often due to a *congenital defect.*
[ref. 4]

meningomyelocele

Birth defect following failure of the *neural tube* to close, resulting in protrusion of a sac of nerve tissue and its covering *membranes* outside the spinal canal.
[ref. 5]
See also *spina bifida*.

meninx/meninges (pl)

Any *membrane*; usually referring to one of the membranes covering the *brain* and *spinal cord.*
Note: The brain and the spinal cord are enclosed by three membranes termed (from outermost to innermost) *dura mater, arachnoid* and *pia mater*; these membranes line the skull and the vertebral canal and together are called the *meninges*.
[After ref. 4,5]

menopause

Cessation of reproductive capability in a woman, marked by declining *ovarian* function and an end to *menses.*
[ref. 5]

menstrual cycle

The period, normally lasting 28 days in the human female, during which an *ovum* matures, is *ovulated*, and enters the *uterus* through the *Fallopian tubes*. If *fertilization* occurs, the *cycle* is interrupted by *pregnancy*; otherwise, the cycle ends with *menstruation*.
[ref. 5]

menstruation
menses

Cyclic *endometrial* shedding and discharge of a bloody fluid from the *uterus* during the *menstrual cycle*.
[ref. 5]

mental retardation

Formerly used term to describe intellectual disability.
[ref. 4]

mentation

Mental activity, *conscious* or *unconscious*, but especially referring to thinking and reasoning.
[ref. 4]

mercurialism
Mad Hatter syndrome

Chronic poisoning caused by *exposure* to mercury, often by breathing its vapor but also by skin absorption and, less commonly, by ingestion.
Note: *Central nervous system* damage usually predominates in mercurialism.
[ref. 1]

meromelia

Congenital absence of a part of a limb, resulting in a shrunken and deformed extremity.
[ref. 5]
See also *amelia; hemimelia; phocomelia*.

mesectoderm
ectomesenchyme

Embryonic migratory cells derived from the *neural crest* of the head that contribute to the formation of the *meninges* and give rise to pigment cells and cartilage.
[After ref. 5]

mesencephalon
midbrain

Rostral part of the *brainstem*.
Note: The mesencephalon contains nuclei of *cranial nerves* controlling shape and movement of the eye.
[ref. 4]

mesenchymal-to-epithelial transition (MET)

Process in which motile *mesenchymal* cells undergo a development to planar, polarized fixed cells, forming an *epithelium*.
Note: The MET occurs in both normal development and *tumor metastasis*.
[ref. 5]
See also *epithelial-to-mesenchymal transition*.

mesenchyme (n)/**mesenchymal** (adj)

Meshwork of *embryonic connective tissue* in the *mesoderm*, from which are formed the bone, muscular, and *connective tissues* of the body; and also the *urogenital* system, blood vessels, and *lymph* vessels.
[ref. 5]

mesenteric lymph node

Lymph node lying between layers of the *mesentery*.
[ref. 3]

mesentery

Membranous sheet attaching various *organs* to the body wall, especially the *peritoneal* fold attaching the intestine to the *dorsal* body wall.
[ref. 5]

mesocosm

Enclosed and essentially self-sufficient (but not necessarily isolated) experimental environment or *ecosystem* that is on a larger scale than a laboratory *microcosm*.
Note: A mesocosm is normally used outdoors or, in some manner, incorporated intimately with the ecosystem that it is designed to reflect.
[ref. 2]
See also *macrocosm*.

mesoderm (n)/**mesodermal** (adj)

embryonic mesoderm

Middle layer of *cells* in the *embryo*, lying between the *ectoderm* and the *endoderm*. It includes the following *tissues*:

- Lateral mesoderm: peripheral portion of intraembryonic mesoderm.
- Intermediate mesoderm: origin of the nephrogenic cord.
- *Parietal* (*somatic*) mesoderm: cell source for the formation of the lateral and *ventral* body wall.
- *Visceral* (*branchial, pharyngeal, splanchnic*) mesoderm: inner layer of lateral mesoderm that, with the *endoderm*, provides the cells from which the gut and lungs and their coverings arise.

[ref. 5]
See also *mesenchyme*.

mesogastrium

Part of the *embryonic mesentery* that is attached to the early stomach.
[ref. 5]

mesonephric duct

Wolffian duct

Embryonic duct of the *mesonephros*, which in the male becomes the *vas deferens* and in the female becomes *vestigial*.
[ref. 5]

mesonephros

Middle part of the *embryonic* kidney in *vertebrates*, becoming the *adult* kidney in fishes and amphibians and the *epididymis* in reptiles, birds, and mammals.
[ref. 5]
See also *pronephros; metanephros*.

mesothelioma

Malignant *tumor* of the *mesothelium* of the *pleura, pericardium*, or *peritoneum*, that may be caused by *exposure* to asbestos fibers and some other fibers.
[ref. 1]

mesothelium

Single layer of flattened cells forming an *epithelium* that lines *serous* cavities such as the *peritoneum, pleura*, and *pericardium*.
[ref. 5]

messenger RNA (mRNA)

See *ribonucleic acid*.

meta-analysis

Process of using statistical methods to combine the results of different studies and thus the systematic evaluation of a hypothesis using information (commonly in the form of statistical tables and other data) from a number of independent studies.
Note 1: A common application of meta-analysis in the biomedical sciences is the pooling of results from a number of small *randomized control trials*, none in itself large enough to demonstrate statistically significant differences, but capable of doing so in aggregate.
Note 2: Meta-analysis has a qualitative component, *i.e.*, application of predetermined quality criteria (*e.g.*, completeness of data, absence of bias) and a quantitative component, *i.e.*, integration of numerical information.
Note 3: Meta-analysis carries the risk of several *biases* reinforcing each other. Because of such problems inherent in the pooling of data from different studies, the results of meta-analysis must be interpreted very cautiously.
[After ref. 2]

metabolic

Associated with *metabolism*.
[*]

metabolic activation

See *activation, metabolic*.

metabolic disorder, inherited

Any *disease* caused by a defect in or absence of a *metabolically* relevant *gene*, often resulting in either the inability to synthesize a product or the accumulation of a substrate, both with adverse consequences.
Examples: Galactosemia, resulting from impaired galactose metabolism; *phenylketonuria*.
[*]

metabolic enzyme

Protein that catalyzes chemical *transformations* of body constituents and, in common usage, of *xenobiotics*.
[ref. 1]

metabolic half-life
metabolic half time

Time required for one-half of the quantity of a substance in the body to be metabolized.
Note: This definition of metabolic half-life assumes that the final quantity in the body approaches zero.
[ref. 1]
See also *half-life*.

metabolic imprinting

See *imprinting, metabolic*.

metabolic model

Analysis-based theoretical reconstruction of the way in which the body deals with a specific substance, showing the proportion that is absorbed following intake, the proportion that is stored and in what tissues, the rate of breakdown in the body, the subsequent fate of the metabolic products, and the rate at which it is eliminated (see *elimination*) by different *organs* as unchanged substance or *metabolites*.
[ref. 1]

metabolic rate

Energy expenditure per unit time, usually referring to energy derived from the digestion and *metabolism* of fats, carbohydrates and proteins by an *endothermic* animal.
Note: Basal metabolic rate (BMR) refers to energy expenditure at rest, necessary to maintain basic bodily functions. Increases in metabolic rate above the BMR occur during exercise, digestion, shivering, or other physiological demands.
[*]

metabolic syndrome
insulin resistance syndrome
syndrome X

Condition characterized by increased fasting *blood* glucose concentration, hypertriglyceridemia, low high density lipoprotein cholesterol, abdominal obesity, and increased blood pressure.
Note 1: Insulin resistance is a common factor in each of the characteristics of metabolic syndrome, often developing into *diabetes mellitus type 2*.
Note 2: Metabolic syndrome is associated with increased caloric intake, especially of carbohydrates.
[*]

metabolic transformation

Biotransformation of a substance that takes place within a living organism.
[ref. 1]

metabolism

1. Sum total of all physicochemical processes that take place within an organism.
2. In a narrower sense, biochemical changes in a substance that take place within an organism, including *biotransformation* to *metabolites*.

[After ref. 1]

metabolite

Intermediate biochemical product resulting from *metabolism*.
[After ref. 1]

metabolite, active

Metabolite (often of a *xenobiotic*), exhibiting biological, *therapeutic*, and (or) *toxicological* effects.
[After ref. 1]

metabologen

Morphogen, including *bone morphogenetic protein*, that affects *metabolism* and *homeostasis*.
[ref. 5]

metabolomics

See *metabonomics*.

metabonomics

metabolomics

Evaluation of *cells, tissues*, or biological fluids for changes in *metabolite* levels that follow *exposure* to a given substance, in order to determine the metabolic processes involved, to evaluate the disruption in intermediary metabolic processes that results from *exposure* to that substance, or to determine the part of the *genome* that is responsible for the changes.
Note: Although "metabolomics" and "metabonomics" are frequently used as synonyms, a distinction is sometimes drawn with "metabolomics" placing a greater emphasis on comprehensive metabolic profiling, while "metabonomics" is used to describe multiple (but not necessarily comprehensive) metabolic changes caused by a biological perturbation.
[ref. 1]

metallosis

Pathological effects resulting from deposition and build-up in soft tissues of metal debris following breakdown of metal-on-metal joint replacements.
[*]

metallothionein (MT)

One of a family of low-molecular mass proteins, with approximately one third of its amino acids being cysteine, that binds several metal atoms (such as zinc, copper, cadmium and mercury) per molecule.
Note 1: Metallothionein plays a role in metal *toxicology*, since it can be induced by its metal ligands and helps to lower the available concentration of some *toxic metals*.
Note 2: The cadmium-metallothionein complex is toxic to the kidney.
[After ref. 2,5]
See also *spillover hypothesis*.

metallothionein-like protein

Cysteine-rich metal-binding protein not conforming precisely to the classic properties of *metallothioneins*.
[After ref. 2]

metameter

Measurement or a *transformation* of a measurement used in the analysis of biological tests, *e.g.*, the *probit* metameter.
[ref. 2]

metamorphosis

Process of *transformation*, in insects or amphibians, from an immature form to a distinctly different mature form.
Example: Development of a tadpole into an adult frog.
[*]

metanephros

Primordium of the permanent kidney, developing later than, and *caudal* to, the *mesonephros*.
[ref. 5]

metaphase

Stage of *mitosis* or *meiosis* in which the *chromosomes* become aligned on the equatorial plate of the *cell*, separating the *centromeres*.
[ref. 5]

metaplasia

Replacement of a fully differentiated *tissue* of one kind by a differentiated tissue of another kind.
[*]

metapopulation

Set of local *populations* which interact via dispersing individuals among local populations; though not all local populations in a metapopulation need interact directly with every other local population.
Note 1: A metapopulation is generally considered to consist of several distinct populations together with areas of suitable *habitat* that are currently unoccupied. Each population *cycles* in relative independence of the other populations and eventually goes extinct as a consequence of *demographic stochasticity*.
Note 2: Individuals may immigrate to a small metapopulation and rescue that population from extinction.
[ref. 2]
See also *rescue effect*.

metastasis (n)/metastases (n,pl)/metastasize (v)

1. Movement of *cells*, especially *cancer* cells, from one part of the body to another, resulting in dissemination of a *disease*.
2. Growth of *pathogenic* microorganisms, or of abnormal cells, distant from their site of origin in the body.

[After ref. 1]

methemoglobin

Derivative of *hemoglobin* that is formed when the iron^{II} in the *heme* porphyrin is oxidized to iron^{III} and thus cannot transport dioxygen.
[ref. 1]

methemoglobinaemia

Presence of *methemoglobin* in the *blood* in greater than normal proportion.
[ref. 1]

methemoglobin-forming substance

Substance capable of oxidizing directly or indirectly the iron^{II} in *hemoglobin* to iron^{III} to form methemoglobin.
[ref. 1]

method of multiple working hypotheses

Method intended to reduce questionable explanations by testing all plausible hypotheses simultaneously, devoting equal effort and attention to each.
[After ref. 2]

N-methyl-D-aspartate (NMDA)

Excitotoxic nonessential amino acid used experimentally to identify a specific subset of *glutamate receptors.*
[ref. 4]

N-methyl-D-aspartate (NMDA)-type glutamate receptor

See *receptor,* N-*methyl-D-aspartate (NMDA)-type glutamate.*

1-methyl-4-phenyl-1,2,3,6-tetrahydropyridine (MPTP)

Synthetic substance causing *parkinsonism.*
Note: MPTP is a toxic by-product in the illicit manufacture of the synthetic *opioid* meperidine and its neurotoxicity was first detected in *drug* abusers, but now it is used as a *model* substance for studying the *pathogenesis* of *parkinsonism.*
[ref. 4]

methylation

Attachment of a methyl group to a molecule.
Note 1: Methylation of DNA on cytosine bases is an *epigenetic* event that alters *gene expression.*
[ref. 5]
Note 2: The enzyme catechol-*O*-methyl-transferase (COMT, EC 2.1.1.6) inactivates catechol *neurotransmitters* by methylation.
Note 3: Environmental and biological methylation result in formation of organometallic species of some metals, *e.g.*, mercury is methylated by microorganisms to methylmercury.
[*]

Michaelis constant, K_M

Michaelis concentration

Substance *concentration* of *substrate* at which the rate of a catalyzed or *enzymatic* reaction is equal to one-half of the limiting rate (maximum rate).
Note: The Michaelis constant may be used only when *Michaelis–Menten kinetics* are obeyed.
[ref. 1]

Michaelis–Menten kinetics

Description of the dependence of an initial rate of reaction upon the *concentration* of a *substrate* S that is present in large excess over the concentration of an *enzyme* or other catalyst (or reagent) E with the appearance of saturation behavior following the Michaelis–Menten equation:

$$\nu = V[\mathrm{S}]_0/(K_\mathrm{M} + [\mathrm{S}])$$

where v is the observed initial rate, V is its limiting value (*maximum velocity*, also termed V_{max}) at substrate saturation (*i.e.*, $[\mathrm{S}] >> K_\mathrm{M}$), and K_M the substrate concentration when $v = V/2$.
Note 1: The parameters V and K_M (the *Michaelis constant*) used in Michaelis–Menten kinetics can be evaluated from the slope and intercept of a linear plot of $1/v$ vs. $1/[\mathrm{S}]$ (a Lineweaver–Burk plot) or of a linear plot of v vs. $v/[\mathrm{S}]$ (an Eadie–Hofstee plot).
Note 2: The Michaelis–Menten kinetic equation is also applicable to the condition where E is present in large excess, in which case the total concentration $[\mathrm{E}]_0$ appears in the equation instead of $[\mathrm{S}]_0$.
Note 3: The term has sometimes been used to describe reactions that proceed according to the scheme

$$\mathrm{E} + \mathrm{S} \underset{k_{-1}}{\overset{k_1}{\rightleftharpoons}} \mathrm{ES} \xrightarrow{k_\mathrm{cat}} \mathrm{Products}$$

in which case $K_\mathrm{M} = (k_{-1} + k_\mathrm{cat})/k_1$ (Briggs–Haldane conditions). It has more usually been applied only to the special case in which $k_{-1} >> k_\mathrm{cat}$ and $K_\mathrm{M} = k_{-1}/k_1 = K_\mathrm{S}$, the dissociation constant of the complex. In this case, K_M is a true dissociation constant (Michaelis–Menten conditions).
[ref. 1]
See also *rate-controlling step*.
Note 4: Analysis of Michaelis-Menten-kinetics helps to identify the mechanism by which a *drug inhibits* an enzyme.
[*]

Michaelis–Menten mechanism

Simplest mechanism that explains *Michaelis–Menten kinetics*.
Note 1: According to the Michaelis–Menten mechanism, a substrate S first combines with a molecule of *enzyme* E, and this process is followed by a step in which the enzyme-substrate complex ES breaks down (sometimes with the participation of the *solvent*) into enzyme and reaction products.
Note 2: Other, more complicated, mechanisms lead to the Michaelis-Menten equation, adherence to which, therefore, does not require that the Michaelis-Menten mechanism applies.
[After ref. 1]

microalbuminuria

Presence of albumin in slight excess in urine.
[After ref. 1]
See also *albuminuria*.

microarray

Grid of *nucleic acid* molecules of known sequence linked to a solid substrate, which can be probed with a sample containing either m*RNA* or *complementary DNA* from a cell or tissue to reveal changes in *gene* expression relative to a *control* sample.

Note: Microarray technology, which is also a type of "gene chip" technology, allows the expression of many thousands of *genes* to be assessed in a single experiment.
[After ref. 1]

microautophagy

Process in which *lysosomes* directly engulf *cytoplasm* by invagination, protrusion, and (or) septation of the lysosomal limiting *membrane*.
[ref. 3]
See also *autophagy*.

microbiota

Entirety of microorganisms, notably bacteria, living as a collection of commensal, symbiotic (see *mutualism*), *pathogenic* and non-pathogenic organisms that share our body space.
Note 1: The pathogenic potential of the microbiota depends on competition within the community itself, and such factors as the presence of antibiotics and host *immune* status.
Note 2: The human intestinal microbiota plays an important role in mainitaining *health*.
Note 3: The intestinal microbiota can be involved in producing *toxic* products that become important when *detoxification* mechanisms are compromised, *e.g.*, during liver failure.
Note 4: Enzymes important for the formation of potentially toxic substances produced by the human colonic microbiota include azoreductase (EC 1.7.1.6) and various nitroreductases.
[*]

microcephaly

Congenital occurrence of an abnormally small head.
[ref. 5]

microcheiria

Congenital occurrence of abnormally small hands.
[ref. 5]

microcosm

Artificial multi-*species* test system that simulates major characteristics of the natural *environment* in order to identify ecotoxicological effects and carry out *risk assessment*.
Note 1: Such microcosm systems are normally terrestrial or aquatic and may contain plants, animals (vertebrates and invertebrates), and microorganisms.
Note 2: The terms *mesocosm* and *macrocosm* are used to refer to larger and more complex systems than microcosms, but the distinction is not often clearly defined.
[ref. 2]

microevolution

Evolutionary change below the *taxonomic* level of a biological *species*, and thus a small change in the *genetic* make-up of a *population* from generation to generation.
[After ref. 2]

microfold cell

M cell

Cell found in the *follicle*-associated *epithelium* of the *Peyer's patch* that has the unique ability to sample *antigen* from the *lumen* of the small intestine and deliver it via *transcytosis* to *antigen-presenting cells* and *lymphocytes* located in a unique pocket-like structure on their basolateral side.
[ref. 3]

microgametophyte

Gametophyte that produces *spermatozoa.*
[*]

microglial cell

Small *glial cell*; resident *macrophage* derived from a mononuclear *phagocyte* that populates the *brain* in early development.
Note: Microglial cells represent about 15% of all *cells* in the brain parenchyma and *spinal cord* and function in areas of neural damage or *inflammation.* They clear debris and *misfolded proteins*, assist in *synaptic stripping*, and contribute to *immune surveillance.*
[ref. 4]

microgliosis

Morphological response of *microglia* to injury, characterized by *hypertrophy* and amoeboid morphology.
Note: Microgliosis can arise from resident microglia or from infiltrating *blood*-borne *macrophages.*
[ref. 4]

microglobulin

Any small globular protein found on the surface of many *cells*, including *lymphocytes*, and in the *blood plasma,* distinct from albumin.
[ref. 3]

β_2-microglobulin

Small (12 kDa) protein forming part of the structure of *major histocompatibility complex class I*-encoded molecules.
Note: The presence of β_2-microglobulin in urine is a common indicator of *renal* tubular dysfunction.
[ref. 3]

microglossia

Congenital occurrence of an abnormally small tongue.
[ref. 5]

micrognathia

Congenital occurrence of an abnormally small jaws, especially effecting the mandible.
[ref. 5]

micromass culture

Laboratory technique in which dispersed *cells* from an *embryonic organ* or *tissue*, such as the *brain, limb bud* or *cartilage,* are allowed to reaggregate in *culture.*
[ref. 5]

micromercurialism

Early or subclinical effects of low-level *exposure* to elemental mercury.
[ref. 1]

micronucleus test

1. Test for *mutagenicity* in which animals are treated with a test agent after which time the frequency of micronucleated cells is determined.
   Note: If a micronucleus test group shows significantly increased levels of micronucleated cells compared to a *control* group, the chemical is considered capable of inducing *chromosomal* damage.
   [ref. 1]
2. Procedure to detect *clastogenic* or *aneugenic* agents by microscopic examination of chromosomes.
   Note: The micronucleus test can be performed *in vivo* in rodents, or in cell *culture* (*in vitro* mammalian cell micronucleus test).
   [ref. 5]

micronutrient

See *trace nutrient*.

microphallus

Abnormally small penis.
[ref. 5]

microphthalmia

Congenital occurrence of abnormally small eyeballs.
[ref. 5]

microphyte

Plant of microscopic size.
[ref. 2]

microproteinemia

Chronic presence of microprotein (α_1- and β_2-microglobulin) in *blood*, indicating proximal *renal* tubule damage.
[ref. 1]

microsatellite (in genetics)

short tandem repeat (STR)

Noncoding segment of DNA consisting of short nucleotide sequences (2-6 base pairs), typically occurring in 10-100 consecutive (tandem) repeats.
Note 1: The number of microsatellite repeats varies between members of any given biological *species*.
Note 2: Microsatellites are used as markers in determining *genetic* diversity, in identifying important genetic traits, in forensic science, in population studies, and in determining paternity.
[ref. 5]

microscopic polyangiitis (MPA)

ANCA-associated necrotizing, *pauci-immune vasculitis* of the small vessels (capillaries, venules, arterioles) frequently associated with rapidly progressive *glomerulonephritis* and/or hemorrhagic *alveolitis* as well as *autoantibodies* against *myeloperoxidase*.
[ref. 3]

microsome (n)/microsomal (adj)

Spherical vesicle, formed during *tissue* fractionation, that is rich in membranes of the *endoplasmatic reticulum*.
Note 1: Microsomes sediment from tissue-homogenates (usually the *S9 fraction*) when centrifuged at 100,000 g for 60 min.
Note 2: The microsomal fraction obtained in this way is often used as a source of *monooxygenase enzymes* in *drug metabolism* studies.
[After ref. 1]

microstomia

Congenital occurrence of an abnormally small opening of the mouth.
[ref. 5]

Microtox® test

Test involving luminescent marine bacteria of the ***Vibrio** sp.* [*e.g.*, ***V. (Photobacterium) phosphoreum, V. fischeri, V. harveyi***]. A decrease in bioluminescence is thought to reflect *toxic* action.
[ref. 2]

microtubule

Tubular component of the *cytoskeleton* present in the *cytoplasm* of *eukaryote cells*, composed of the monomers α- and β-tubulin.
[*]

micturition (n)/micturitic (adj)/micturate (v)

Urination.
[*]
See also *diuretic*.

midbrain

See *mesencephalon*.

midgut

mesenteron

Middle section of the digestive tract in a *vertebrate embryo*, from which the *ileum*, *jejunum*, and portions of the *duodenum* and colon develop.
[ref. 5]

midstream sampling

Taking an *aliquot* of a flowing liquid, such as urine, avoiding initial and terminal flow periods which are likely to be unrepresentative.
[ref. 1]

migraine

Recurrent *syndrome* usually characterized by unilateral head *pain* often accompanied by symptoms including nausea and vomiting, *vertigo, photophobia* and other visual phenomena.
Note: Migraine can be classified as classic migraine, common migraine, cluster *headache*, hemiplegic migraine, and ophthalm(opleg)ic migraine.
[ref. 4]
See also *aura, prodromal stage*.

migrainous infarction

Stroke that occurs in connection with a *migraine* attack.
[ref. 4]

migration

1. of *cells*: Active movement from their origin to a neighbouring or distant location.
   Note 1: Such migration of cells occurs for instance in the developing *embryo*, during *tissue* repair, or when *lymphocytes* cross an *epithelial* layer.
   Note 2: Cells often migrate in response to, and towards or away from, specific external signals, a process called *chemotaxis*.
   [After ref. 3]
   Compare *metastasis*.
2. of an individual or group: Movement into or out of a new *population* or geographical region.
   [ref. 2]
3. of a substance: Movement from one place to another.
   Note 3: Migration includes, *e.g.*, the movement of substances from food packages into food, and the downstream distribution of contaminants in river *sediments*.
   [*]

mimotope

Molecular structure, often a peptide, that mimics the structure of an *epitope*, thereby being recognized by an *antibody* to that epitope, and eliciting a similar antibody response.
[*]

Minamata disease

methylmercury poisoning

Neurological *disorder* caused by methylmercury intoxication, characterized by *tremors, dysarthria, ataxia*, and loss of peripheral sensation, hearing and vision.
Note: Minamata *disease* was first described in residents of Minamata Bay, Japan, who consumed fish that had accumulated methylmercury derived from industrial waste.
[ref. 4]

mineral

Naturally occurring substance, usually crystalline, which has a particular chemical composition and specific physical properties.
[ref. 2]

mineralization

1. Complete conversion of organic substances to inorganic derivatives, often visible as microscopic deposits that may be associated with damage to soft tissue, *e.g.*, in the kidney.
   Note: Complete mineralization involves breakdown of a complex organic compound to carbon dioxide, water, oxides, and oxidative inorganic products such as nitrate or sulfate.
   [After ref. 1]
   See also *biomineralization*.
2. Processes (*e.g.*, fossilization) occurring after death and burial of organisms within sediments, involving the total replacement of the organic material with various minerals, frequently calcite or quartz, although many other minerals, such as pyrite, may be involved.
3. (in geology) The hydrothermal deposition of economically important metals in the formation of ore bodies.
4. (in soil science) The release of inorganic compounds during complete microbial decomposition of organic materials in the *soil*.
   [ref. 2]

minimal risk level (MRL)

Estimate of the daily human *exposure* to a hazardous substance that is likely to be without appreciable risk of adverse (and generally noncancerous) *health* effects over a specified duration of exposure.
Note: This substance-specific estimate is used by ATSDR health assessors to identify *contaminants* and potential health effects that may be of concern at hazardous waste sites.
[ref. 1]

minimal time to effect or response

See *minimum time to effect or response*

minimum lethal concentration (LC_{min})

Lowest *concentration* of a *toxic* substance in an *environmental* medium that kills individual organisms or test species under a defined set of conditions.
[ref. 1]

minimum lethal dose (LD_{min})

Lowest amount of a substance that, when introduced into the body, kills individual organisms or test species under a defined set of conditions.
[ref. 1]

minimum significant difference (MSD)

Difference between groups (in tests with, *e.g.*, salmonid fish, the difference in average weights or average *mortality*) that would have to occur before it could be concluded that there was a significant difference between the groups.
Note: The MSD is provided by Dunnett's multiple range test.
[ref. 2]

minimum time to effect or response

Shortest time required after exposure to produce an effect or response.
Note: Regardless of the *toxicant* concentration, the minimum time to effect or response cannot occur any faster than the minimum time.
[ref. 2]

minimum viable population (MVP)

Smallest *population* size of a *species* allowing survival in the wild.
Note 1: More specifically, MVP is the smallest possible size at which a biological population can exist without facing extinction from natural disasters or *demographic* or *environmental* changes, or *genetic drift*.
Note 2: MVP is used in the fields of biology, *ecology*, and conservation biology/*ecology*.
[ref. 2]

minisatellite

variable number tandem repeat (VNTR)

Noncoding segment of *DNA*, found throughout the *genome*, usually near the ends of *chromosomes*, that consists of tandem repeats of sequences of about 10–100 base pairs.
Note: VNTRs are useful for *genetic* research and analysis.
[ref. 5]
See also *microsatellites*.

Minnesota multiphasic personality inventory (MMPI)

MMPI-2-RF

Psychological questionnaire for individuals aged 18 and older. The RF version has 338 true-false statements with seven validity and ten personality scales that may be used in either an individual or group format.
Note: The MMPI test has been used outside clinical psychology in legal cases, to screen applicants for certain jobs, and to evaluate treatments for substance *abuse*.
[ref. 4]

minor histocompatibility antigen

See *antigen, minor histocompatibility*.

miosis (n)/miotic (adj)

myosis

Abnormal contraction of the pupil of the eye to less than 2 mm.
Note: Miosis may indicate organophosphate poisoning or opiate intake.
[ref. 4]

miscarriage

Lay term for *spontaneous abortion.*
[ref. 5]

miscible

Liquid substances capable of mixing without separation into two phases; refers to liquid *mixtures*.
[ref. 1]

misfolded protein

Protein that has the same amino acid sequence as the normal, functional protein but exhibits a deviant tertiary structure and lacks normal function.
Note: Common *neurodegenerative diseases* (*e.g., Alzheimer disease*) are associated with the formation, aggregation and deposition of misfolded proteins in *neurons*.
[ref. 4]
See also *endoplasmic reticulum stress; inclusion body*.

miticide

Substance intended to kill mites.
[ref. 1]

mitochondrial membrane potential (Δψm)

Membrane potential across the inner membrane of the *mitochondrion* generated by the electron transport chain.
[ref. 4]

mitochondrial permeability transition

Hypothesized opening of a pore (the mitochondrial permeability transition pore (MPTP)) in response to *mitochondrial* injury, giving rise to increased permeability of the mitochondrial inner membrane; it is accompanied by dissipation of the proton gradient, a drop in *mitochondrial membrane potential*, and uncoupling of oxidative phosphorylation.
Note: The increased mitochondrial permeability results in release of pro-*apoptotic* factors such as calcium ions (Ca^{2+}), *cytochrome* c, and apoptosis-inducing factor (AIF), and thus is an important feature of the *intrinsic pathway* of cell death.
[*]

mitochondrial permeability transition pore (MPTP)

See *mitochondrial permeability transition.*
[ref. 1]

mitochondrion/mitochondria (pl)/mitochondrial (adj)

Eukaryote cytoplasmic organelle that is bounded by an outer membrane and an inner membrane; the inner membrane has folds called cristae that are the center of ATP synthesis in *oxidative phosphorylation* in the animal *cell* and supplement ATP synthesis by the chloroplasts in photosynthetic cells.
Note: The *matrix* within the inner membrane of the mitochondrion contains *ribosomes*, many oxidative *enzymes*, and a circular *DNA* molecule that carries the *genetic* information for a number of these enzymes.
[ref. 1]

mitogen (n)/mitogenic (adj)

Substance that induces *lymphocyte transformation* or, more generally, *mitosis* and cell proliferation.
Note: Mitogens most commonly employed in *immunotoxicology* assays include the *T-cell* mitogens *concanavalin A* and *phytohemagglutinin*. Mitogens routinely used for assessing *B-cell* proliferation include *pokeweed mitogen*, which can also act on T cells, and ***Escherichia coli*** *lipopolysaccharide*.
[ref. 3]

mitogen-activated protein kinase (MAPK)

Member of a *protein kinase* network in which "upstream" kinases activate "downstream" kinases that, in response to phosphorylation, translocate to the nucleus and activate transcription factors.
Note: MAPKs include the extracellular regulated kinases (Erk), stress-activated protein kinase (SAPK or p38), and the kinase of the c-jun oncoprotein (JNK).
[ref. 3]

mitophagy

Autophagy-related pathway specifically for removal of *mitochondria*; it can be subdivided into macromitophagy, triggered by starvation (mitophagy type 1) or mitochondrial damage (mitophagy type 2), and micromitophagy (mitophagy type 3), characterized by formation of mitochondria-derived *vesicles*.
[*]

mitosis (n)/mitotic (adj)

Process by which a *cell nucleus* divides into two daughter nuclei, each normally having the same *genetic* complement as the parent cell: nuclear division is usually followed by cell division.
[ref. 1]

mixed connective tissue disease (MCTD)

Sharp syndrome
Human *autoimmune disease* in which the *immune system* attacks the body, producing symptoms that combine features of polymyositis, *systemic lupus erythematosus*, and *systemic scleroderma*, and thus being considered as an overlap *syndrome*.
Note 1: MCTD commonly causes joint pain/swelling, *Raynaud phenomenon*, muscle *inflammation*, and scarring of the skin of the hand. It does not typically cause kidney disease or seizures.
Note 2: Distinguishing laboratory characteristics of MCTD are a positive, speckled *anti-nuclear antibody* and an anti-U1-RNP antibody.
[ref. 3]

mixed-function oxidase (MFO)

See *monooxygenase*.

mixed lymphocyte response/reaction (MLR)

T-cell-proliferative response induced by *cells* expressing *allogeneic major histocompatibility complex molecules*.
[ref. 3]

mixed neuropathy

Dysfunction or degeneration of both *motor* and *sensory neurons*.
[ref. 4]

mixing zone

Area where an effluent discharge undergoes initial dilution and is extended to cover the secondary mixing in the ambient water body.
Note: A mixing zone is an allocated impact zone where water quality criteria can be exceeded as long as *acutely toxic* conditions are prevented.
[ref. 2]

mixture (in toxicology)

Material, typically a liquid, composed of two or more different chemical substances.
Note: *Risk assessment* of mixtures is difficult because of possible additive effects and other types of interaction.
[*]

mode of action (MOA) (in toxicology)

Probable sequence of biochemical events (*key events*) leading to a specified *adverse effect* following exposure to a given substance or substances, under specified conditions.
Note: Exposure and all other conditions associated with the MOA must be quantitatively defined.
[*]
Compare *mechanism of action*.

model

1. (n) Simplified representation of a natural system that can be used to test a hypothesis, often expressed as a mathematical function with parameters that can be adjusted until the function closely describes a set of empirical data.
2. (v) Create such an entity as defined under definition 1. (model (n)).

Note 1: A model is often based on biological, chemical, or physical mechanisms, and its parameters are intended to represent the observable world. Alternatively, statistical models are fitted by a function whose mathematical parameters are imposed upon the data.
Note 2: Extrapolation from mechanistic models (*e.g.*, pharmacokinetic equations) and empirical models (*e.g.*, logistic extrapolations) may differ in their approximation to the real world, on the one hand, and their mathematical clarity on the other.
Note 3: A model that describes the temporal change of a system under the influence of an external force is called a dynamic model. The elements used to build dynamic models (*e.g.*, incorporating mass balance of static concentrations into a series of time-dependent differential equations) are called process models.
[After ref. 2]

model error

Elements of uncertainty associated with the discrepancy between a *model* and the real world.
[ref. 2]

modifying factor (MF)

See *uncertainty factor*.

molecular epidemiology

See *epidemiology, molecular*.

molecular intiating event (MIE)

First interaction of a substance with a biological target molecule in the chain of events leading to a specified adverse outcome.
[*]

molecular mimicry (in immunology)

Concept that identity or similarity of *epitopes* expressed by a *pathogen* and by a selfmolecule may lead to production of *antibodies* reacting to the *self-antigen*.
Note: Molecular mimicry may explain how some *autoimmune diseases* develop.
[ref. 3]

molluscicide
limacide
molluskicide

Substance intended to kill molluscs.
[ref. 1]

monitoring

Continuous or repeated observation, measurement, and evaluation of *health* and (or) environmental or technical data for defined purposes, according to prearranged schedules in space and time, using comparable methods for sensing and data collection.
Note: Evaluation of monitoring data requires comparison with appropriate reference values based on knowledge of the probable relationship between ambient *exposure* and *adverse effects*.
[ref. 1]

monitoring, biological (general)

biomonitoring

Continuous or repeated measurement of a substance, including potentially *toxic substances* or their *metabolites* or biochemical effects in *tissues*, secreta, excreta, expired air, or any combination of these in order to evaluate occupational or environmental *exposure* and *health risk* by comparison with appropriate reference values based on knowledge of the probable relationship between ambient exposure and resultant *adverse* health *effects*.
[ref. 1]

monitoring, biological (in ecotoxicology)

biomonitoring

Regular systematic use of living organisms (see *indicator species, bioindicators, sentinel species*) to evaluate changes in environmental quality, by repetitive measurements following a statistical design.
Note 1: Biomonitoring may involve the study of individuals, *species, populations*, and *communities* to understand changes due to *exposures* over extended time periods. It may involve continuous or repeated, invasive or noninvasive measurement of behavioral parameters, physiological parameters, or other *biomarkers*, in captive animals or *indigenous* species at the individual or a lower organizational level, and may contribute to the determination of *biotic indices*.
Note 2: In ecotoxicology, four types of biomonitoring are defined:

- **biomonitoring (type 1)**
  Determination of *community* changes along a gradient or among sites differing in levels of pollution.
- **biomonitoring (type 2)**
  Determination of *bioaccumulation* in organisms among sites notionally varying in the level of *contamination*.
- **biomonitoring (type 3)**
  Determination of effects on organisms using tools such as biochemical markers in sentinel *species* or some measure of diminished fitness or condition of individuals.
- **biomonitoring (type 4)**
  Determination of *genetically* based resistance in *populations* of contaminated areas.

[After ref. 2]

monitoring test

Test, designed to be applied on a routine basis, for *monitoring* the quality of an environmental *compartment*, biological endpoint, or *effluent*, in order to ensure that parameters of quality are within an acceptable range.
Note: A monitoring test implies generation of information on a regular or continuous basis.
[*]
See also *monitoring, biological*.

monoamine oxidase (MAO)

Any member of a family of several flavoprotein enzymes (E.C. 1.4.3.4) that use dioxygen and flavin adenine dinucleotide to bring about oxidative deamination of a substrate.
Note 1: The MAOs are involved in the metabolism of a number of *neurotransmitters* and neuroactive metabolites, often causing their inactivation.
Note 2: Deficiencies in MAO activity can lead to various neurological and mental *disorders*.
[*]

monoclonal

Pertaining to a specific protein from a single *clone* of cells, all molecules of this protein being identical.
[ref. 1]

monoclonal antibody

See *antibody, monoclonal*.

monocyte

Mononuclear *phagocyte* found in *blood* that is the precursor of the tissue *macrophage*.
Note 1: Monocytes are formed from promonocytes in the *bone marrow*, and then transported to *tissues* such as the lung and liver, where they develop into macrophages.
Note 2: Monocytes were formerly called large mononuclear *leukocytes* and hyalin or transitional leukocytes.
[ref. 3]

monokine

Alternative name for a *cytokine* produced by *monocytes*.
[ref. 3]

mononuclear phagocyte system (MPS)

reticuloendothelial system (RES)

Network of *phagocytic* cells throughout the body, comprised of *blood monocytes* and tissue *macrophages*.
[ref. 3]

monooxygenase

mixed-function oxidase (MFO)

One of a group of *enzymes* that catalyze reactions between an organic compound and dioxygen in which one atom of the dioxygen molecule is incorporated into the organic compound and one atom is reduced to water using NADPH.
Note 1: Monooxygenases are involved in the *metabolism* of many endogenous and foreign compounds. The products are generally more water soluble and less reactive than the mother compounds, but nevertheless, products of different or increased *toxicity* from that of the parent compound occur.
Note 2: Monooxygenases are the main catalysts of *phase I reactions of biotransformation* in the metabolism of *xenobiotics*. They are located on the *endoplasmic reticulum* and are enriched in preparations of *microsomes*.
[After ref. 1]

monophthalmos

Congenital absence of one eye.
[ref. 5]

monosomy

Disorder in which body cells have only one pair instead of the normal two pairs of a particular *chromosome*.
[ref. 5]

monozygotic twin

See *identical twin*.

Monro-Kellie hypothesis

Monro-Kellie doctrine
Monro doctrine

Hypothesis that the intra*cranial* volume is unchangeable and therefore a constant *intracranial pressure* requires that the sum of the volumes of the three compartments *blood, brain* tissue and *cerebrospinal fluid* remains constant.
[ref. 4]

Monte Carlo simulation

Analysis of a sequence of events using random numbers to generate possible outcomes in an iterative process.
[ref. 1]

Montreal Protocol

Officially the "Protocol on Substances That Deplete the Ozone Layer", a treaty signed in Montreal on 16 September 1987 by 25 nations.
Note 1: The Montreal protocol is, as of 2016, ratified by nearly 200 nations, including all United Nations members.
Note 2: The Montreal protocol sets limits on the production of *chlorofluorocarbons* (CFCs), halons, and related substances that release chlorine or bromine to the ozone layer of the atmosphere.
[After ref. 2]

morbidity (n)/morbid (adj)

Any departure, subjective or objective, from a state of physiological or psychological well-being.
Note: The terms "sickness", "illness", "*disease*", and "morbid condition" also denote morbidity.
[After ref. 1]

morbidity rate

Term used to refer to *incidence* or *prevalence* rates of *disease*.
Note: The term is used loosely and should be avoided.
[After ref. 1]

morbidity survey

Method for the estimation of the *prevalence* and (or) *incidence* of a *disease* or diseases in a *population*.
[ref. 1]

mordant

Substance that fixes a dyestuff in or on a material by combining with the dye to form an insoluble compound, used to fix or intensify stains in a *tissue* or *cell* preparation.
[ref. 1]

Moro reflex

See *startle reflex.*

morphine

The major phenanthrene alkaloid of *opium*, used as an *analgesic, sedative*, and *anxiolytic.*
Note 1: Morphine and its analogues exert their action by binding to morphine *receptors* in the *brain* and nervous tissues. The natural *ligands* of these receptors are peptide *neurotransmitter*s such as *endorphin.*
Note 2: While *chronic* consumption of morphine leads to the development of tolerance and physical dependence (see *addiction*), the artificial morphine derivative heroin can cause severe *addiction* after only few *doses.*
[ref. 4]
Note 3: Acute overdosing with morphine causes potentially lethal respiratory depression.
[*]

morphodynamics (in physical geography)

Study of the interaction and adjustment of the seafloor topography and fluid hydrodynamic processes, seafloor *morphologies*, and sequences of changes involving the motion of *sediment.*
[ref. 2]

morphogen (n)/morphogenetic (adj)

Any of various signalling factors in *embryonic* tissue that influences the movement and organization of cells during *morphogenesis* by forming a concentration gradient.
[ref. 5]

morphogenesis

Shaping of an organism during *embryological* development by *differentiation* of *cells, tissues, organs* and organ systems, according to the *genetic* program of the organism, and influenced by *morphogens* and *environmental* conditions.
[ref. 5]

morphology (n)/morphological (adj)

Pertaining to structure or form.
[ref. 5]

Morris water maze

See *water maze test.*

mortality

Death rate, thus the number of individuals dying per unit time.
Note: Data from *natality* and mortality graphs together can be used to construct a *life table.*
[ref. 2]
See also *carrying capacity.*

mortality rate

See *death rate.*

mortality study

See *study, mortality.*

morula

Early multi-celled stage of the *embryo* from which the *blastocyst* is formed.
[ref. 5]

mosaicism

Condition in which an individual or an organism that develops from a single *zygote* has two or more cell populations that differ in *genetic* constitution.
Note: Mosaicism is seen in humans in *Down syndrome*, *Turner syndrome* and *Kleinfelter syndrome.*
[ref. 5]

most-sensitive-species approach

Ecotoxicological approach in which results for the most sensitive of all tested *species* are used as an indicator of the *toxicant concentration* below which the entire *community* is protected from *adverse effects.*
[ref. 2]

motility, sperm

Energy-dependent forward movement of the *sperm*, allowing it to reach and *penetrate* the *egg.*
Note: Decreased sperm motility is an indicator of reduced *fertility.*
[ref. 5]

motor activity

Physical activity and performance of an animal.
Note: In performance tests, motor activity includes locomotor or ambulatory activity, both referring to the linear movement of an animal. Ambulatory and *rearing* movements together are referred to as total activity.
[ref. 4]

motor coordination

Cooperation of the *motor neurons* and the involved muscles to perform a body movement precisely according to spatiotemporal requirements.
Note 1: Motor coordination involves signals from the *organ of equilibrium*, the visual system and the *cerebellum* as well as other neural inputs.
Note 2: Impaired motor coordination results in *ataxia.*
[ref. 4]

motor cortex

See *cortex, motor.*

motor endplate

Complex structure by which the *axon* of a *motor neuron* establishes *synaptic* contact with a skeletal muscle fiber.
[ref. 4]

motor neuron

Nerve cell in the *spinal cord* having an *axon* that leaves the *central nervous system* to establish a functional connection with an effector (muscle or *glandular*) *tissue*.
[ref. 4]

motor neuron disease (MND)

Generic term for a heterogenous group of *disorders*, all affecting *motor neurons* in the *brain, spinal cord*, or both.
Examples: Spinal muscle atrophy, *amyotrophic lateral sclerosis*, progressive bulbar paralysis, and primary lateral sclerosis.
[ref. 4]

motor system

Part of the *central nervous system* responsible for control of movement, consisting of the *pyramidal system* controlling voluntary movement and the *extrapyramidal system* coordinating involuntary movement.
[ref. 4]

mouse IgE test (MIGET)

Procedure in which serum *immunoglobulin E (IgE)* levels are measured in mice following topical exposure to a test substance. Substances that cause a significant increase in IgE are considered to be potential *allergens*.
[ref. 3]

mouse ear-swelling test (MEST)

Test for *sensitization* in which the test substance is applied *topically* to the ear of a mouse for three consecutive days. The change in ear thickness is then measured on day 8 following *challenge*.
[ref. 3]

mouthing behaviour

hand-to-mouth activity

Tendency, most notable in toddlers, to take objects, including dirt and *dust*, into the mouth, potentially leading to *hazardous* exposures.
[*]

moving average method

Method of estimating LC_{50}, EC_{50}, or LD_{50} in experimental animals. It can be implemented with straightforward equations if the *toxicant concentrations* are set in a geometric series and there are equal numbers of individuals exposed in each treatment.
[ref. 2]
See also *median effective concentration; median lethal concentration; median lethal dose.*

mucociliary escalator

mucociliary ladder

Defense mechanism against microbial *infection* in the mammalian airways, in which mucus and particulate matter are cleared from the lungs through the bronchi and *trachea* by the sweeping motion of motile *cilia* on the columnar *epithelium* that lines them.

Note: *Metaplastic transition* of ciliated columnar epithelium to squamous epithelium upon *chronic exposure* to tobacco smoke causes loss of the mucociliary escalator, and predisposes the individual smoker to bronchitis and lung infections.
[*]
See also *mucociliary transport.*

mucociliary transport

Process of removal of inhaled particles from the bronchi of the lungs in a *mucus* stream moved upward by cilia.
Note: Mucociliary transport contributes to *uptake* from the *gastrointestinal tract* because after reaching the throat, mucus tends to be swallowed.
[After ref. 1]
See also *mucociliary escalator.*

mucocutaneous

Pertaining to or affecting the *mucous membranes* and/or the skin.
[ref. 3]

mucosa (n)/mucosal (adj)

Moist *tissue* that lines some *organs* and body cavities, including the nose, mouth, lungs, and digestive tract.
[ref. 3]
See also *mucous membrane; mucus.*

mucosa-associated lymphoid tissue (MALT)

Secondary lymphoid tissue present in the surface *mucosa* of the respiratory tract and bronchus (*BALT*), *gastrointestinal tract* (*GALT*), nasal passages (*NALT*), larynx (LALT), conjunctiva (CALT), and genitourinary tract, and in the skin sub-epidermis (SALT).
Note: MALT plays an important part in limiting entry of *pathogens* through the mucosal surfaces.
[ref. 3]

mucosal addressin cell adhesion molecule-1 (MAdCAM-1)

Protein involved in trafficking of *lymphocytes* to *mucosal* endothelium.
Note: Expression of MAdCAM-1 is induced in the murine endothelial cell line bEnd.3 by *tumor necrosis factor* α, *interleukin*-1, and bacterial *lipopolysaccharide.*
[ref. 3]

mucosal tolerance

State of *lymphocyte* hyporesponsiveness to protein *antigens* applied across *mucosal* surfaces by oral or nasal instillation.
[ref. 3]

mucous membrane

Layer of *epithelial* tissue with a thin underlying layer of *connective tissue* (the *lamina propria*) that lines many body cavities, including the gut, respiratory passages, and tubular *organs*; it secretes, and is covered in, *mucus.*
[ref. 5]

mucus (n)/**mucosal** (adj)/**mucous** (adj)

Slippery viscous fluid, consisting largely of water and *glycoproteins*, secreted by *mucous membranes*.
[ref. 5]

Müllerian duct

See *paramesonephric duct*.

Müllerian inhibiting factor (MIF)

See *anti-Müllerian hormone*.

Müllerian-inhibiting hormone (MIH)

See *anti-Müllerian hormone*.

Müllerian inhibiting substance (MIS)

See *anti-Müllerian hormone*.

Mulliken population analysis

Partitioning scheme based on the use of density and overlap matrices, at one time used for allocating the electrons of a molecule in some fractional manner among its various parts (atoms, bonds, orbitals).
[ref. 1]

multicompartment model

Formal or graphical representation of the *pharmacokinetic* or *toxicokinetic* behaviour of a substance, based on a *compartmental analysis* requiring more than two *compartments*.
[After ref. 1]

multicotyledonary placentation

Formation of a *placenta* with many lobes.
[ref. 5]

multidrug resistance

1. (in chemotherapy) Phenomenon characterized by the efficiency of chemo-*therapeutics* tending to decrease with time.
   Note: One reason for chemotherapeutic multidrug resistance is the *induction* of membrane *transporters, e.g.*, the *ABC-transporter* multidrug resistance protein-1 (MDR1) in the target cells that export the *drug* out of the cell.
2. (in antibacterial therapy) Occurrence of a strain of a *pathogenic* bacterium that has developed resistance to previously effective antibiotics.

[*]

multifactorial disease

Illness with *pathogenesis* dependent on complex interplay of *genetic* and (or) *environmental* factors.
[ref. 1]

multifactorial inheritance

Transmission from parents to *offspring* of a trait that is determined by multiple *genetic* factors in combination with *environmental* factors, each factor having a small effect on its own.
[After ref. 5]

multigenerational study

1. Animal test of reproductive *toxicity* in which two to three generations of the test organism are exposed to the substance being assessed.
2. Animal test of reproductive toxicity in which only one generation is exposed and effects on subsequent generations are assessed.

[ref. 5]

multiple chemical sensitivity (MCS)

environmental illness
idiopathic environmental intolerance

Intolerance condition attributed to extreme *sensitivity* of an individual to various *environmental* chemicals, found in air, food, water, building materials, or fabrics.
Note 1: This *syndrome* is characterized by the patient's belief that his or her *symptoms* are caused by very low-level exposure to environmental chemicals. The term "chemical" is used to refer broadly to many natural and man-made substances, some of which have several chemical constituents.
Note 2: Several theories have been advanced to explain the cause of multiple chemical sensitivity, including *allergy, toxic* effects, neurobiological sensitization and psychosomatic illness. There is insufficient scientific evidence to confirm a relationship between any of these possible causes and symptoms.
[After ref. 1]

multiple heterosis

Higher fitness of an individual as a composite or summed effect of *heterozygote advantage* (*heterosis*) at each of a series of *loci*.
[ref. 2]

multiple myeloma

Plasma cell malignancy resulting in high levels of monoclonal *immunoglobulin* in *serum* and of free *light chains* (*Bence-Jones protein*) in urine.
[ref. 3]
See also *myeloma*.

multiple sclerosis (MS)

Common *demyelinating disorder* of the *central nervous system*, causing patches of *sclerosis* (plaques) in the *brain* and *spinal cord*.
Note: *Autoantibodies* targeting *myelin basic protein* are believed to play an important role.
[ref. 4]

multiple screening

multiphasic screening

Administration of a number of tests, in combination, to large groups of people.
[After ref. 1]

multiplex immunoassay

Type of particle *immunoassay* employing sets of microspheres with various physicochemical features, each labeled with a different *antibody*. The method allows detection in a single measurement of an array of 100 or more proteins.
[ref. 3]
See also *particle immunoassay*.

multiplicative growth factor per generation

See *finite rate of increase*.

multipotent

Of a *cell*, capable of giving rise to several different kinds of structures or types of cell.
[ref. 1]

multipotent progenitor cell

Undifferentiated *stem cell*, obtained from adult *bone marrow* or other non*embryonic tissue* sources, that possesses the ability to differentiate into a variety of *cell* types, especially into cells of a closely related family of cells that are expanded *in vitro* and deposited in master cell banks for "off-the-shelf" use, with potential *hematopoiesis*-inducing and *immunomodulating* activities.
Note 1: *Allogeneic* multipotent adult progenitor cells (MAPCs) are non*immunogenic* due to the lack of *major histocompatibility complex molecule* expression, and so elicit no *immune response* upon administration.
Note 2: *In vivo, bone marrow*-derived *adult stem cells* are capable of maturing into a broad range of cell types and may help to restore the *immune system* by producing multiple *therapeutic* molecules in response to *inflammation* and *tissue* damage.
[ref. 3]

multistage model

Dose–response model for *cancer* death estimation of the form

$$P = 1 - \exp[-(q_o + q_1 d_1 + \ q_2 d_2 \ \ldots + q_k d_k)]$$

where P is the probability of *cancer* death from a continuous *dose* rate, d_i, of group (or stage) $i = 0, 1, 2\ldots$, the q's are constants, and k is the number of dose groups (or, if less than the number of dose groups, k is the number of biological stages believed to be required in the *carcinogen*esis process).
Note: With the *multistage model*, it is assumed that cancer is initiated by cell *mutations* in a finite series of steps. Additional stages are tumor *promotion* (selective growth of initiated cells), tumor *progression* (time-dependent expansion of the initiated *clone*) and a potentially counteracting *immunological* defense.
[ref. 1]

multistage sampling

Type of sampling in which the *sample* is selected by stages, the sampling units at each stage being subsampled from the larger units chosen at the previous stage.
[ref. 1]

multivariate statistics

Set of statistical tools to analyze data matrices using regression and (or) pattern recognition techniques.
[ref. 1]

murine

Of or belonging to the family ***Muridae*** that includes rats, mice, and gerbils.
[ref. 1]

murine local lymph node assay (LLNA)

Predictive test of sensitization in which a test substance is applied topically to the skin of mice (usually three times at daily intervals) and the weight of the local *draining lymph nodes* is measured at six days.
Note: Usually in the LLNA, *lymphoproliferation* in the nodes is measured following injection of [^{3}H]thymidine or bromodeoxyuridine.
[ref. 3]

muscarinic

Referring to agents that stimulate the post*ganglionic parasympathetic receptor*, named after the prototypical mushroom alkaloid, muscarine [2,5-anhydro-1,4,6-trideoxy-6-(trimethylammonio)-D-*ribo*-hexitol].
Note 1: The *muscarinic receptor* has a recognition site for *acetylcholine*.
Note 2: Muscarinic receptors are distinguished from *nicotinic receptor*s, thus allowing classification of *cholinergic* receptors as muscarinic and nicotinic.
Note 3: *Drugs* that bind with muscarinic cholinergic receptors but do not activate them, thus preventing access to acetylcholine, include atropine [(*RS*)-(8-methyl-8-azabicyclo[3.2.1]oct-3-yl) 3-hydroxy-2-phenylpropanoate] and scopolamine [(−)-(*S*)-3-hydroxy-2-phenylpropionic acid (1*R*,2*R*,4*S*,7*S*,9*S*)-9-methyl-3-oxa-9-azatricyclo[3.3.1.0^{2,4}]-non-7-yl ester].
[ref. 4]

muscarinic receptor

One of the two main classes of *acetylcholine receptors* (the other being *nicotinic receptors*) that responds to *muscarinic* agents.
[ref. 4]

muscle spindle
neuromuscular spindle

Sensory organ in the body of a striated muscle containing *afferent* and *efferent nerve fibers* that detect passive muscle stretch and convey information to the *central nervous system* to cause *reflex* resistance to this stretch.
[ref. 4]

mutagen (n)/mutagenic (adj)

Agent that can induce (or generate) heritable changes (*mutations*) in the *genotype* of a *cell*, as a consequence of alterations in, or loss of, *genetic* material.
[ref. 5]

mutagenesis

Induction (or generation) of heritable changes (*mutation*s) of the *genotype* in a cell as a consequence of alterations or loss of *genes* or *chromosome*s (or parts thereof).
[ref. 1]

mutagenicity

Ability of a physical, chemical, or biological agent to induce (or generate) heritable changes (*mutation*s) in the *genotype* in a cell as a consequence of alterations or loss of *genes* or *chromosome*s (or parts thereof).
[ref. 1]

mutation

Any relatively stable heritable change in *genetic* material that may be a chemical *transformation* of an individual *gene* (gene or *point mutation*), altering its function; or a rearrangement, gain, or loss of part of a *chromosome*, which may be microscopically visible (chromosomal mutation).
Note: A mutation can be either germinal and inherited by subsequent generations, or *somatic* and passed through cell lineage by cell division.
[ref. 5]

mutation (in immunology)

See *somatic hypermutation*.

mutation, back

Process that reverses the effect of a *mutation* that has modified a *gene*, restoring the wild phenotype.
[ref. 1]

mutation, dominant lethal

Genetic change occurring in a *germ cell* that does not cause dysfunction of the *gamete* but which is lethal to the fertilized *egg* or developing *embryo* that develops from it.
Note: Induction of a dominant lethal event after *exposure* to a chemical substance (called a dominant lethal test) indicates that the substance has affected germinal tissue of the test species.
[ref. 1]

mutation, point

Change in a single base pair in *DNA*.
[ref. 1]

mutation, reverse

Second or subsequent *mutation* in a mutant *allele* that makes it capable of producing the nonmutant *phenotype*.
Note: Reverse mutation may result from restoration of the original *DNA* sequence of the *gene* or from production of a new DNA sequence that has the same effect.
[ref. 1]

mutualism

Interaction between two or more *species*, giving fitness benefit to all the involved species, *e.g.*, increased *carrying capacity*.
Note 1: Beneficial interactions within one species are not, strictly speaking, mutualism and are called cooperation.
Note 2: Symbiosis is the form of mutualism leading to the closest spatial or physical association. The process may be obligate, meaning the involved species cannot survive alone.
Examples: Cleaner fish, pollination and seed dispersal, gut flora, and nitrogen fixation by fungi.
[ref. 2]

myalgia

Pain or tenderness in a muscle or group of muscles.
[ref. 1]

myasthenia

Muscular weakness.
[ref. 1]

myasthenia gravis, acquired

Autoimmune disease characterized by muscle weakness usually affecting *ocular* and oropharyngeal muscles due to an *autoimmune* attack against components of the *neuromuscular junction* (*e.g.*, the *nicotinic acetylcholine receptor*).
Note: Acquired myasthenia gravis may be *idiopathic*, paraneoplastic [*thymic tumor* or lung (*Lambert–Eaton myasthenic syndrome*) tumor, *etc.*], or *drug*-induced (*e.g.*, D-penicillamine).
[ref. 3]

mycoplasma

Very small infectious microorganism, related to bacteria, but without a *cell* wall.
Note: *Genital* mycoplasma infections may lead to spontaneous preterm *labor* or *perinatal morbidity* and *mortality.*
[ref. 5]

mycotoxin

Toxin produced by a fungus.
Examples: Aflatoxins, tricothecenes, ochratoxin, patulin.
[ref. 1]

mydriasis

Dilation of the pupil.
Note: Mydriasis can be a physiological response to low light, a sign of *brain* trauma, or caused by *drugs* such as *atropine.*
[ref. 4]
See also *miosis.*

myelencephalon

Part of the *brain* in the *embryo* that gives rise to the *medulla oblongata.*
[ref. 5]

myelin (n)/myelinated (adj)

Electrically insulating lipoprotein layers that are produced by *glial cell*s and surround the *axon*s of the *neuron*s.
Note: Myelin is produced by *oligodendrocytes* in the *central nervous system* and by *Schwann cells* in the *peripheral nervous system.*
[ref. 4]
See also *myelin sheath.*

myelin-associated glycoprotein

Transmembrane *glycoprotein* that plays an important role in the interaction between *axon*s and *myelin* and affects *myelination* during *nerve* regeneration.
[ref. 4]

myelin basic protein

Major component of *myelin*, that helps organizing the correct assembly of the lipids and proteins in myelin sheets.
Note 1: Absence of myelin basic protein in animals causes *seizure*s.

Note 2: Myelin basic protein levels in the *cerebrospinal fluid* are elevated in various *demyelinizing disorders*, including *multiple sclerosis* where *autoantibodies* against myelin basic protein are believed to play a role.
[ref. 4]

myelin sheath

Concentric layers of *myelin* surrounding the *axons* of some *neurons*.
Note: The myelin sheath increases the conduction velocity of electrical impulses.
[ref. 4]

myelination (n)/myelinated (adj)

Acquisition, development, or formation of a *myelin sheath* around a *nerve fiber*.
[ref. 5]
See also *demyelination*.

myelinopathy

Neuropathy affecting only or primarily the *myelin sheath*.
[*]

myeloblast (n)/myeloblastic (adj)

Immature *bone marrow cell* that is a precursor of the *granulocyte* series.
[ref. 5]

myelodysplastic syndrome
preleukemia (obsolete)

Diverse collection of hematological conditions united by ineffective production (or dysplasia) of *myeloid blood cells* and risk of *transformation* to *acute myelogenous leukemia*.
Note: *Anemia* requiring chronic blood *transfusion* is frequently present in myelodysplastic syndrome.
[ref. 3]

myelogram

X-ray of the *spinal* canal following injection of a contrast material into the surrounding *cerebrospinal fluid* spaces.
[ref. 4]

myeloid
myelogenous

Referring to the non*lymphocytic* groups of white *blood cells*, including *granulocytes, monocytes*, and *platelets*.
Note: *Acute myelogenous leukemia* is also known as acute myeloid leukemia.
[ref. 3]

myeloid stem cell

See *stem cell, myeloid*.

myeloid tissue

Tissue within red *bone marrow* that produces the *blood cells*.
Note: Myeloid tissue is found around the blood vessels and contains various cell types that are precursors of the blood cells.
[ref. 3]

myeloma

Tumor composed of cells derived from hematopoietic cells (see *hematopoiesis*) of the *bone marrow*, or from *mast cells.*
[ref. 3]
See also *Bence-Jones protein; multiple myeloma.*

myeloma protein

Monoclonal antibody secreted by *myeloma cells.*
[ref. 3]

myelomeningocele

Protrusion of the *spinal cord* and its coverings through a defect in the *vertebral column.*
[ref. 4]

myelopathy

1. Any functional or pathologic disturbance in the *spinal cord.*
2. *Disorder* of the *myelopoietic* tissues of the bone marrow.

[ref. 4]

myeloperoxidase (MPO)

Enzyme found in azurophilic granules of *neutrophils*, the major target of *anti-neutrophil cytoplasmic autoantibody.*
Note 1: MPO *autoantibodies* are diagnostic markers for microscopic polyangiitis, rapidly progressive *glomerulonephritis*, and *Goodpasture disease* or *syndrome.*
Note 2: MPO autoantibodies are also found in patients exposed to silica or *drugs* (*e.g.*, hydralazine, propylthiouracil, D-penicillamine) as well as in some patients with *Wegener granulomatosis* and other *autoimmune diseases.*
[ref. 3]

myelopoiesis (n)/myelopoietic (adj)

Process of formation and development of *myeloid blood cells* in the *bone marrow.*
[ref. 3]

myelosuppression

Reduction of *bone marrow* activity leading to a lower *concentration* of *platelets, erythrocytes*, and *leukocytes* in the *blood.*
[ref. 1]

myelotoxic

Harming *bone marrow* or any of its components.
[ref. 5]

myoblast

Mononucleate cell that is committed to *differentiate* into muscle.
[ref. 5]

myocarditis

Inflammation of the heart muscle.
[ref. 5]

myocardium

Muscle of the heart
[ref. 5]

myoglobin

Dioxygen-binding *heme* protein of muscle, related to *hemoglobin*.
Note: With *necrosis* of muscle *tissue*, release of myoglobin into the bloodstream can result in a high load of the protein reaching the kidney, where its breakdown results in *toxicity* to the *tubular epithelium*.
[*]

myometrium

Muscular wall of the *uterus*.
[ref. 5]

myopathy

Any *disease* of muscle.
[ref. 4]

myositis

Inflammation of muscle.
[ref. 5]

myositis, autoimmune

Rare *systemic inflammatory myopathy*, including primary polymyositis, primary dermatomyositis, myositis associated with malignancy, childhood dermatomyositis, and myositis with multisystem *autoimmune disease* [*e.g., mixed connective tissue disease, systemic sclerosis*].
Note: *Autoantibodies* in autoimmune myositis, directed against aminoacyl-tRNA synthetases (*e.g.*, anti-Jo-1), signal recognition particles (*e.g.*, anti-SRP54), nuclear helicase (anti-Mi-2), tRNA and tRNA–protein complexes (*e.g.*, anti-Mas), and translation factor (anti-KJ), have been described as myositis-specific.
[ref. 3]

myotome

In the *embryo*, that part of a *somite* that develops into skeletal muscle.
[ref. 5]

myotonia

Prolonged *contraction* or delayed *relaxation* of a muscle after mechanical or brief electrical *stimulus*.
Note: Myotonia is indicative of an abnormality of *ion channel*s of the muscle membrane, and is often an example of an *ion channelopathy*.
[ref. 4]

NACHT domain-, leucine-rich repeat (LRR)-, and pyrin (N-terminal homology) domain (PYD)-containing protein 3 (NALP3, NLRP3)
cryopyrin

NOD-like receptor, found in certain *inflammasomes*, that binds to aggregated proteins and the peptides that compose them.
Note 1: Its activation leads to the generation of *inflammatory cytokines*, such as *interleukin*-1, and neurotoxic factors.
Note 2: Mutations in NALP3 are responsible for the autoinflammatory *diseases* familial cold autoinflammatory *syndrome*, Muckle–Wells syndrome, and neonatal onset multisystem inflammatory disease.
[ref. 3]

NADPH oxidase

See *respiratory burst.*

NG2 cell
polydendrocyte

Glial cell of the *central nervous system*, distinct from an *oligodendrocyte* or *astrocyte*, that may serve as a precursor of oligodendrocytes, and that takes its name from expression of proteoglycan NG2.
[ref. 4]

NIMBY principle

Acceptance by members of the public of change (*e.g.*, waste incinerators) only if it does not adversely affect their living space.
Note: "NIMBY" is an acronym derived from "not in my backyard".
[ref. 2]

NK cell

See *natural killer cell.*

NKT cell

See *natural killer T-cell.*

N-nucleotide

Nontemplated nucleotide added to the junctions between *antibody* and *T-cell receptor variable (V) gene, diversity (D) gene Tr1*, and *joining (J) gene* segments during *gene rearrangement.*
[ref. 3]

NOD-like receptor (NLR)

See *receptor, nucleotide-binding oligomerization domain-containing protein (NOD)-like.*

N-region

Highly *variable region* on the *heavy chain* of *immunoglobulins.*
[ref. 3]

Comprehensive Glossary of Terms Used in Toxicology
By John Duffus, Douglas M. Templeton and Michael Schwenk

Published by the Royal Society of Chemistry, www.rsc.org

naïve lymphocyte

See *lymphocyte, naïve.*

nanomaterial

Substance in particulate form that has at least one spatial dimension in the size range from 1 to 100 nanometers.
[*]

nanoparticle

Particle with all three spatial dimensions in the size range from 1 to 100 nanometers.
Note: Naturally occurring nanoparticles (*e.g., dusts*) or particulate byproducts of combustion (*e.g.*, from diesel engines) are usually physically and chemically heterogeneous and are often termed *ultrafine particles.*
Note: The term "nanosized particle" is sometimes used to describe any particle with an *aerodynamic diameter* <100 nm.
[*]

nanotoxicology

Scientific discipline involving the study of the actual or potential harmful effects of *nanoparticles* on living organisms and *ecosystems*, of the relationship of such harmful effects to *exposure*, and of the mechanisms of action, diagnosis, prevention, and treatment of *intoxications.*
[After ref. 1]

narcosis

Nonspecific, reversible depression of *central nervous system* function, marked by *stupor* or *unconscious*ness.
[ref. 4]

narcotic

1. (nonspecific usage) Agent that produces insensibility or *stupor.*
2. (specific usage) Any natural or synthetic substance that has *morphine*-like actions.

[ref. 4]
See also *opioid.*

nasal

Relating to the nose.
[ref. 5]

nasal-associated lymphoid tissue (NALT)

See *mucosa-associated lymphoid tissue.*

natality

Rate of birth (see *birth rate*), thus the number of newborn individuals per unit time.
Note: Natality and *mortality* graphs together constitute the basis for a *life table.*
[ref. 2]

National Academy of Sciences (NAS) paradigm of risk assessment

Model for *risk assessment* with four components—*hazard identification, exposure assessment, dose*–response assessment, and *risk characterization.*
Note: The NAS paradigm model is used for both human and *ecological* risk assessments.
[ref. 2]

natriuretic

Substance increasing the rate of *excretion* of sodium ion in the urine.
[ref. 1]

natural autoantibody (NAA)

See *autoantibody, natural.*

natural immunity

See *immunity, natural.*

natural killer (NK) cell

Large granular *lymphocyte* that does not rearrange nor express either *immunoglobulin* or *T-cell receptor genes* but is able to recognize and destroy certain *tumor* and virally infected *cells* in a *major histocompatibility complex molecule-* and *antibody*-independent manner.
[ref. 3]

natural killer cell activity assay

Immunotoxicity test in which *lymphoid tissue* or *blood* that has been treated with a test compound is co-incubated with target cells. The *cytotoxic* effect on target cells is measured, *e.g.*, with the *chromium release assay.*
Note: The natural killer cell activity assay is used under circumstances where differences from untreated cells are attributed to *natural killer cell* activity.
[ref. 3]

natural killer T (NKT) cell

Lymphoid cells with a morphology and granule content intermediate between *T-cells* and *natural killer (NK) cells.*
Note: NKT cells express low levels of $\alpha{:}\beta$ *T-cell receptor* with an invariant α chain and very restricted β chain specificity, recognize lipid and glycolipid *antigens* presented by the nonclassical *major histocompatibility molecule*-like molecule CD1d, and are potent producers of *interleukin (IL)*-4 and *IFN*-γ.
[ref. 3]

natural occurrence

Presence of a substance in nature, as distinct from presence resulting from inputs from human activities.
Note: The contamination of the natural environment by some man-made substances may be so widespread that it is practically impossible to get access to biota with a truly natural level.
[ref. 1]

natural regulatory T-cell (Treg)

See *regulatory T-cell.*

natural resistance-associated macrophage protein 1 (NRAMP-1)

Iron *transporter* that plays a critical role in *macrophage activation* and differentiation.
Note: *Allele* 3 of the NRAMP-1 promoter is associated with *autoimmune disorders* (*e.g., rheumatoid arthritis*, juvenile rheumatoid arthritis, *diabetes mellitus type 1, multiple sclerosis*).
[ref. 3]

natural selection

Process whereby organisms that are better adapted to their *environment* show higher survival rates and produce more *offspring*.
Note: Natural selection is a result of various events such as *mutation, species* migration, and genetic drift, and is a key component of Darwinian *evolution.*
[*]
See also *selection components.*

natural radiation background

natural background radiation

Sum of cosmic radiation emitted from stars, long-lived terrestrial radionuclides that are ubiquitously present at varying amounts in the Earth's *crust,* and radiation arising from radioactive isotopes in the organism itself (notably ^{40}K).
[*]

navel

See *umbilicus.*

necrapoptosis

necroptosis

Hybrid term derived from *necrosis* and *apoptosis*, describing a mechanism of *cell* death showing features of both, including altered cell calcium ion (Ca^{2+}) *homeostasis* and opening of the *mitochondrial permeability transition pore.*
Note 1: In necrapoptosis, it is not clear whether features of both necrosis and apoptosis evolve together during the cell death process, or whether apoptosis is initiated first and then aborted, leading to necrotic cell death by default, for instance if the cell becomes depleted of sufficient ATP to sustain energy-dependent steps in apoptosis.
Note 2: The term aponecrosis may describe an identical or very similar phenomenon to necrapoptosis.
[*]

necropsy

Postmortem examination of the *organs* and body tissue of a nonhuman animal to determine cause of death or pathological condition.
[ref. 5]
Compare *autopsy.*

necrosis (n)/necrotic (adj)

Sum of *morphological* changes resulting from *cell* death by lysis and (or) *enzymatic degradation*, usually accompanied by *inflammation* and affecting groups of cells in a *tissue.*
Note: Necrosis is distinct from *apoptosis, autophagy*, and other modes of cell death.
[ref. 5]

negative control

See *control, negative.*

negative selection (immunology)

Deletion by *apoptosis* in the *thymus* of *T-cells* that recognize self-peptides presented by self-*major histocompatibility complex molecules*, thus preventing the development of *autoimmune* T-cells.
Note: Negative selection of developing *B-cells* is also thought to occur if they encounter high levels of *selfantigen* in the *bone marrow*.
[ref. 3]

negligible risk

1. Probability of *adverse effects* occurring that can reasonably be described as trivial.
2. Probability of adverse effects occurring that is so low that it cannot be reduced appreciably by increased regulation or investment of resources.

[ref. 1]

nekton (n)/nektonic (adj)

Aggregate of actively swimming animals in a body of water, ranging from microscopic organisms to whales.
[ref. 2]

nematicide
nematocide

Substance intended to kill nematodes.
[ref. 1]

neoantigen

Antigen newly expressed on a *tumor* or virally infected *cell*, or arising after macromolecule-*hapten* binding.
[ref. 3]

neocortex

Outer layer of the *cerebral cortex* that supports higher *brain* functions, especially *cognitive function* and language in humans.
Note: The neocortex includes most of the *cerebral cortex* except for the *hippocampus*.
[ref. 4]

neo-Darwinism

Theory of biological *evolution* (widely accepted since the 1920s) based on Darwin's theory of *natural selection* but incorporating the theories of later biologists regarding *genes*, inheritance, and *mutation*, particularly those of Weismann and Mendel.
[ref. 4]
See also *Mendelism; Weismannism.*

neonatal tolerance

See *tolerance, neonatal.*

neonate (n)/**neonatal** (adj)

Newborn animal or human infant during the first four weeks of *postnatal* life.
Note: For statistical purposes, some scientists have defined the period as the first seven days of human postnatal life. The precise definition varies from species to species.
[ref. 5]

neophyte

Plant found newly in an area where it had not been recorded previously.
[ref. 2]

neoplasia

Occurrence of a *neoplasm*.
[*]

neoplasm (n)/**neoplastic** (adj)

New and abnormal formation of *tissue* as a consequence of growth by *cell* proliferation, which may continue after the initial *stimulus* that initiated the proliferation has ceased, and may develop into a *tumor*.
[ref. 5]

nephritis/nepritides (pl)

Inflammation of the kidney, usually accompanied by *proteinuria, hematuria, edema*, and *hypertension*, potentially leading to kidney failure.
[After ref. 1]

nephritis, autoimmune

Inflammation of the kidney due to *immunological* reaction to renal *antigens*.
Note: Common examples are anti-*glomerular basement membrane disease* (*Goodpasture disease* or *syndrome*), *autoimmune* tubulointerstitial *nephritis* with *antibody* to tubular basement membrane, or occurring as part of *systemic autoimmune diseases* independent of renal *autoantigens* (*lupus* nephritis in *systemic lupus erythematosus*, interstitial nephritis in *Sjögren syndrome*, nephritis in *ANCA-associated vasculitis, cryoglobulinemic vasculitis*, or hypo*complement*emic urticarial vasculitis syndrome).
[ref. 3]

nephron

Functional subunit of the kidney, each having a filtering apparatus (*glomerulus*) and an extended tubular system (renal tubule) rich in membrane *transporters*, where water, electrolytes, *xenobiotics* and other low molecular mass substances are partly *excreted* or partly *reabsorbed*, to form urine.
Note 1: Each human kidney has about 1 million nephrons.
Note 2: Decreased nephron function (*e.g.*, in connection with *nephropathy* or aging) results in decreased ability to eliminate *metabolites* and *xenobiotics*.
[*]

nephropathy
renopathy

Any *disease* or abnormality of the kidney.
[ref. 1]

nephrosis

Disease of the kidneys marked by degeneration of renal tubular epithelium.
[ref. 1]

nephrotoxin (n)/nephrotoxic (adj)

Substance harmful to the *cells* of the kidney.
[ref. 1]

nerve

Ensheathed bundle of *nerve fibers* that conveys information between the *central nervous system* and other regions of the body.
[ref. 4]
See also *peripheral nervous system.*

nerve, cranial

Each of the twelve pairs of *nerve*s that arise directly from the *brain*, not from the *spinal cord*, and pass through separate apertures in the skull.
[ref. 4]

nerve, trigeminal

Fifth *cranial nerve*, supplying sensation to the face and controlling *motor activity* of mastication.
[ref. 4]

nerve, vagus

Tenth *cranial nerve*, arising from the *medulla oblongata.*
Note: The vagus nerve carries *parasympathetic* and motor impulses (see *motor activity*) to the *larynx* and *pharynx, thoracic* organs and *abdominal* viscera, as well as containing *afferent* fibres that supply information about the state of the organs to the *central nervous system.*
Note: The vagus nerve is primarily *cholinergic.*
[ref. 4]

nerve conduction study

Measure of the functional integrity of a *nerve* with a stimulating electrode, placed on the skin over the nerve, and a more distal recording electrode, to determine the velocity of the impulse that passes along the nerve between the electrodes.
[ref. 4]
See also *nerve conduction velocity.*

nerve conduction velocity

Rate of progression of a *nerve* impulse in a peripheral nerve or in its largest component *nerve fibers*
Note: Nerve conduction velocity is measured in a *nerve conduction study* to provide information on the intactness of the nerve.
[ref. 4]

nerve fiber

Axon with its surrounding *myelin sheath.*
[ref. 4]

nerve gas

nerve agent

Volatile substance with *neurotoxic* features intended for use in warfare to disable or kill the organism rapidly after inhalation or skin contact, and classified as a prohibited weapon of mass destruction by The Chemical Weapons Convention (CWC).
Note: Some *organophosphates* are characteristic representatives of nerve gases, including the G series (*e.g.*, sarin, tabun), the V series (*e.g.*, VX, VG), and some *insecticides*.
[ref. 4]

nerve cell

See *neuron*.

nerve growth factor (NGF)

One of a family of proteins known as *neurotropins* that function as signaling molecules to induce *axon* growth, branching, elongation and survival of *neurons*.
[ref. 4]

nerve root

Proximal end of a *spinal nerve* nearest its attachment to the *spinal cord*.
[ref. 4]

nervous system

The entire *neuronal* apparatus, composed of both the *central nervous system* and the *peripheral nervous system*.
[ref. 4]

net reproductive rate, R_0

Expected number of females to be produced during the lifetime of a newborn female as estimated with a *life table*.
[ref. 2]

nettle rash

See *hives*.

neural

1. Pertaining to a nerve or to the nervous system.
2. Pertaining to the *dorsal* side of the *vertebral* bodies or to their precursors.

[ref. 5]
Compare *hemal*.

neural activity

Metabolic and electrical activity of *neurons*.
Note: *Brain* regions showing neural activity during task performance can be studied with implanted electrodes or with noninvasive methods such as *electroencephalography* and functional *magnetic resonance imaging*.
[ref. 4]

neural arch

1. *Dorsal* bony covering of the *spinal cord*, also called the *vertebral* arch.
2. *Cartilaginous* structures surrounding the *embryonic* spinal cord.

[ref. 5]

neural crest

Band of cells on either side of the *neural tube*.
Note: Cells from the region of the neural crest migrate to form parts of the *nervous system*, face, skin, and heart.
[ref. 5]

neural network
neuronal network

A functionally interconnected set of *neurons*, generally in the *central nervous system*.
Note: In computer science, the term "neural network" refers to an interconnected set of electronic components designed to mimic or exploit functional aspects of the human *brain*.
[ref. 4]

neural plate

Area in the middle of the early *embryo* that rolls up to form the *neural tube*.
[ref. 5]

neural stem cell

See *stem cell, neural*.

neural tube

Embryonic tubular structure that becomes the *brain* and *spinal cord*.
[ref. 5]

neural tube defect

Failure of the *neural tube* to close properly during *gastrulation*.
[ref. 5]
See also *anencephaly; spina bifida*.

neuralgia

Paroxysmal *pain* extending along the course of one or more *nerves*.
[ref. 4]

neuralgia, trigeminal
tic douloureux

Severe, paroxysmal bursts of *pain* in one or more branches of the *trigeminal nerve*, often induced by touching trigger points in or about the mouth.
[ref. 4]
See also *neuralgia*.

neurectomy

Excision of a *nerve* or part of a nerve.
[ref. 4]

neurite

Outgrowth or projection of either an *axon* or a *dendrite* from the *neuron* cell body that is the structural basis of the *neural network.*
[ref. 4]

neurite outgrowth

Phenomenon in which *neurons* tend to send out *neurites* to make contact with other *nerve* cells.
Note: These outgrowths can be induced by electrical stimulation, *neurotropic* factors, and other stimuli.
[ref. 4]

neuritic plaque

See *amyloid plaque.*

neuritis

Inflammation of a *nerve.*
Note: Neuritis may also be used to denote noninflammatory nerve lesions of the *peripheral nervous system.*
[ref. 4]

neurobehavior core test battery (NCTB)

A set of seven tests, recommended by the World Health Organization (WHO) in 1983, to detect *neurotoxicity* in human populations.
Note: The NCBT consists of *digit symbol*, *digit span*, *pursuit aiming*, *Benton visual memory*, *simple reaction time*, *Santa Ana dexterity*, and *profile of mood states tests.*
[ref. 4]

neurobehavioral

Pertaining to the function of the *nervous system* as it relates to behavior.
[ref. 5]

neuroblast

Cell derived from *neural stem cell* that will *differentiate* into a *neuron.*
[ref. 5]
See also *neuroblastoma.*

neuroblastoma

Malignant neoplasm consisting of poorly *differentiated embryonic nerve cells* (*neuroblasts*).
Note: Neuroblastoma occurs mostly in infants and children.
[After ref. 4,5]

neurodegenerative disease

Disease of the *brain* and (or) *peripheral nervous system* with progressive loss of *neuronal* function, accompanied by changes in *morphology* and subcellular organization of the *nervous system.*
[ref. 4]

neurodevelopmental toxicity

1. Adverse effect of a substance that disrupts developmental processes of the *nervous system*.
2. *Toxicity* in which the developing nervous system shows heightened *sensitivity* compared with the *adult* nervous system.

[ref. 4]

neuroectoderm

Central region of the early *embryonic ectoderm* that will give rise to the *brain* and *spinal cord*, together with the *neural crest* cells that will form the peripheral nervous system.
[ref. 5]

neuroendocrine

Pertaining to the *endocrine* and *nervous systems* in anatomical or functional relationship.
[ref. 5]

neuroendocrine system

Combined and cooperating network of the *nervous system* and *hormonal* system.
Note: An example of a component of the neuroendocrine system is the action of the *pituitary gland*, which responds to *neuronal* signals from the *hypothalamus* by secreting hormones into the circulation.
[ref. 4]

neurofibril

Part of a filamentous structure found in the cell body, *axons, dendrites*, and sometimes *synaptic* endings of *neurons*, consisting of bundles of *neurofilaments* and *neurotubules*.
[ref. 4]

neurofibrillary tangle

Intracellular accumulation of aggregates of hyperphosphorylated *tau protein* or *paired helical filaments* consisting of the tau protein, a *microtubule*-associated protein that normally stabilizes the *cytoskeleton*.
Note: Neurofibrillary tangles are characteristically found in *neuron*s of the *cerebral cortex* of patients with *Alzheimer disease*.
[ref. 4]

neurofibroma

Tumor of the *peripheral nervous system* representing an abnormal collection of *Schwann cell*s and connective tissue.
[ref. 4]

neurofilament

Class of *intermediate filament* of the *neuronal cytoskeleton*, providing support for the *axon* and *dendrites*.
See also *neurofibril*.
[ref. 4]

neurogenesis

Formation of *nerve* cells or of the *nervous system.*
[ref. 4]

neurogenic

1. Originating in, starting from, or caused by, the *nervous system* or *nerve* impulses.
2. Relating to *neurogenesis.*

[ref. 4]

neurogenic shock

Condition of decreased blood pressure, slow heart rate and insufficient perfusion of the body with *blood*, caused by loss of autonomic control (see *autonomic nervous system*) following *acute* trauma to the *brain* or *spinal cord.*
[ref. 4]

neurohypophysis

Posterior lobe of the *pituitary gland*, involved in the storage and secretion of *oxytocin* and *vasopressin.*
[ref. 5]

neuroimaging

Process of producing images of the structure or activity of the *brain* or other parts of the *nervous system.*
Note: Current neuroimaging techniques include *magnetic resonance imaging* and *computerized tomography.*
[ref. 4]

neuroinflammation

Complex series of local *immune responses* within the *nervous system* to deal with a threat to the *neural* environment from infection, injury, or trauma.
Note: In the *brain*, the process is initiated by *microglial* release of *cytokines*, often leading to increased *blood-brain barrier* permeability and a secondary *lymphocyte*-mediated *inflammation.*
[ref. 4]

neuroleptic

Any of a class of *psychotropic drugs* used to treat *psychosis*, particularly *schizophrenia.*
Note: Neuroleptics include the phenothiazines, thioxanthene, and butyrophenone derivatives and the dihydroindolones.
[ref. 4]

neurologic shellfish poisoning (NSP)

See *neurotoxic shellfish poisoning*

neurolysis

1. Breakdown of *neural tissue* from *disease* or injury.
2. *Therapeutic* destruction of a *nerve* or nerves to treat intractable *pain.*
3. Surgical freeing of a nerve from adhesions of the neural sheath.

[ref. 4]

neuroma

Tumor made up largely of *nerve cells*.
[ref. 4]

neuromuscular junction (NMJ)

See *motor endplate.*

neuron (n)/neuronal (adj)
nerve cell

Electrically *excitable cell* type consisting of a cell body, *axon*, and *dendrites* that is the basis of *brain* function and of peripheral sensory and *motor activity.*
Note: Neurons cooperate in *neural networks* via chemical *neurotransmitters* at the *synapses.*
[ref. 4]

neuron, upper motor

Neuron whose cell body lies in the *cerebral cortex* or *brainstem* and whose *axon* carries impulses to a *lower motor neuron.*
[ref. 4]

neuron-specific enolase (NSE)
enolase 2 (ENO2)
phosphopyruvate hydratase

Enzyme (EC 4.2.1.11) of glucose *metabolism*, normally found in *neural tissue*, that catalyzes the dehydration of 2-phosphoglycerate.
Note: Increased *concentrations* of NSE in the *blood* are associated with various *diseases*, including *neuroblastoma* and non*neuronal tumors*.
[ref. 4]

neuronopathy

Disorder involving destruction of the *cell* bodies of *neurons.*
[ref. 4]

neuropathological examination

Application of gross and *histopathologic* methods to study *toxic* changes in the *morphology* and *histology* of the *neural tissues* and the *brain.*
Note: This can be a very detailed part of *neurotoxicity* evaluation that may reveal mechanisms of action.
[ref. 4]

neuropathy (n)/neuropathic (adj)

Pathological change in the *peripheral nervous system.*
Note: It may occur as a localized lesion, or secondary to systemic *toxicity* (*e.g.*, from alcohol consumption) or a generalized medical condition (*e.g., diabetes*).
[ref. 4]

neuropathy, autoimmune

Autoimmune disease of the *nervous system.*
Note 1: More neuropathies are being described as autoimmune or possibly autoimmune in nature. Little is known about *xenobiotics* in their *pathogenesis*, but infections may play an important role in the initiation of some *diseases.*

Note 2: Autoimmune neuropathies may be manifested at the *neuromuscular junction*, as *central nervous system* diseases (*e.g., multiple sclerosis, paraneoplastic autoimmune syndromes*, stiff-person *syndrome*, as well as manifestations of *systemic* autoimmune diseases), and diseases of the *peripheral nervous system* (*e.g.*, various forms of *acute* and *chronic demyelinating* neuropathies).
[ref. 3]

neuropathy target esterase (NTE)

neurotoxic esterase

Enzyme (EC 3.1.1.5) that is phosphorylated by *organophosphate* compounds and is believed to be involved in the delayed *neuropathy* of organophosphates.
[ref. 4]

neuropeptide

One of a group of small proteins (peptides) that serve as *neurotransmitter*s in the *brain, autonomic nervous system* and *neuroendocrine system.*
[ref. 4]
See also *endorphin, enkephalin.*

neuropore

Opening at either the *cranial* (*caudal*) or anterior (*rostral*) end of the *neural tube* before it completes closure in the early *embryonic stage.*
[ref. 5]

neuroprogenitor cell

Precursor *cell* that is capable of differentiating into specific cell types of the *nervous system.*
Note 1: The term "neuroprogenitor cell" typically refers to a cell that has further committed beyond an early *neural stem cell*, either by being located in a particular region of the nervous system or destined for a particular type of *neuron.*
Note 2: The renewal potential of neuroprogenitor cells is typically reduced relative to *neural stem cells.*
[ref. 4]

neuroprotective

Agent or property of an agent that protects *neuron*s from damage and (or) from the process of aging or degeneration of the *brain.*
[ref. 4]

neuropsychological testing

Assessment, under standardized conditions, of an individual's *brain* function as it impacts upon *cognitive function*, thought processes, behavior and personality.
Note 1: Neuropsychological tests are designed to measure a psychological function known to be linked to a particular brain structure or *pathway* and often measure *reaction time*s, motor performance or cognitive association (see *motor activity, cognitive function*).
Note 2: An initial training period may be required before neuropsychological testing so that each individual starts the testing at an optimized performance level, although most neuropsychological assessments compare an individual's raw score to a normative sample score of the population.
[ref. 4]

neurotoxic esterase (NTE) **assay**

Test in which delayed *neuropathy* resulting from hydrolytic cleavage of *organophosphate* esters is studied with measurement of the responsible *enzyme* activity.
[ref. 4]
See also *hen test; neuropathy target esterase*

neurotoxicant

Substance that can produce functional or structural damage to the *nervous system.*
[ref. 4]

neurotoxicity (n)/**neurotoxic** (adj)

Production of an *adverse effect* on structures or functions of the *nervous system*: such effects may be subdivided into two types.
Note: Neurotoxicity includes

- *Central nervous system* effects (including transient effects on mood or performance and *pre-senile dementia* such as *Alzheimer disease*).
- *Peripheral nervous system* effects (such as the inhibitory effects of organophosphorus compounds at the neuromuscular junction).

[After ref. 1]

neurotoxicology

Discipline applying principles of both neuroscience and *toxicology* to study the ability of certain substances to alter *nervous system* structure or function.
[ref. 4]

neurotoxic shellfish poisoning (NSP)

Toxic shellfish poisoning characterized by nausea, vomiting, and mild neurological symptoms such as *dysarthria, paresthesia, ataxia*, and *vertigo* caused by ingestion of shellfish (specifically, bivalve molluscs) contaminated with the polyether brevetoxin and its derivatives produced by the dinoflagellate ***Karenia brevis***.
[ref. 4]

neurotoxin

Any substance that has the potential to damage the *nervous system.*
Note: In the narrower sense, neurotoxins are of biological origin, as used for *toxins* in general. However, the term neurotoxin is also in general use for nonbiological substances that are toxic to any part of the nervous system.
[ref. 4]

neurotransmission

Process by which a *presynaptic neuron*, upon *excitation*, releases a specific agent (a *neurotransmitter*) that crosses the *synaptic cleft* to stimulate or inhibit the *postsynaptic neuron.*
[ref. 4]
See also *neurotransmission, retrograde.*

neurotransmission, retrograde

Neurotransmission wherein a *neurotransmitter* is sent from the *postsynaptic* to the *presynaptic membrane* in order to modify a signal.
[ref. 4]

neurotransmitter

Biochemical that is released upon *excitation* from a *presynaptic membrane*, crosses the *synaptic* space and binds to a receptor on the *postsynaptic* membrane, where it induces a signal that may be either stimulatory or inhibitory.
[ref. 4]

neurotropic

neurotrophic

Having an *affinity* for *nerve cell*s or *tissues* of the *nervous system*.
[ref. 3]

neurotropin

neurotrophin

Family of secreted proteins that promote the survival, *differentiation*, and function of *neurons*.
[ref. 4]
See also *nerve growth factor*.

neurotubule

Microtubule found in *neurons*.
[ref. 4]
See also *neurofibril*.

neurovascular

1. Relating to both the *nervous system* and the *vascular* system.
2. Relating to the vasomotor nerves that supply the walls of the blood vessels.

[ref. 4]

neurulation

Formation of the *embryonic neural plate* and its rolling up into the *neural tube*.
[ref. 5]

neutralization (in immunology)

Blocking by an *antibody* of the effects of a *pathogen* such as a virus.
[ref. 3]

neutropenia

Abnormally low concentration of *neutrophils* in the *blood*.
Note: Neutropenia is associated with an increased risk of infection.
[ref. 3]

neutrophil

polymorphonuclear leucocyte

Granular *leukocyte*, the major circulating *phagocytic* polymorphonuclear *granulocyte*, having a *nucleus* with three to five lobes and fine *cytoplasmic* granules stainable by neutral dyes.
Note 1: Neutrophils have properties of *chemotaxis*, adherence to *immune complexes*, and *phagocytosis*.

Note 2: Neutrophils are involved in a variety of *inflammatory* processes including late-phase *allergic* reactions and are also able to mediate *antibody-dependent cellular cytotoxicity*.
[ref. 3]
See also *phagocyte*.

neutrophil activation

See *activation, neutrophil*.

niche (in ecology)

Group of conditions and resources, facilitating but limiting survival, growth, and *reproduction* of a defined group of organisms or *species*.
Note 1: The niche influences how a *population* responds to the *abundance* of its resources and enemies.
Note 2: The niche is influenced by its inhabiting populations.
Note 3: The abiotic or physical environment is part of the niche because it influences how populations affect, and are affected by, resources and enemies.
[ref. 2]
See also *niche, complementary; niche, fundamental; niche, Hutchinsonian; niche, realized; niche preemption*.

niche, complementary

Niche where coexisting *species* occupy a similar position along one niche dimension, *e.g.*, altitude, but differ along another, *e.g.*, diet.
[ref. 2]

niche, fundamental

Environmental conditions under which a *species* can thrive.
[ref. 2]
See also *niche; niche, Hutchinsonian; niche, realized*.

niche, Hutchinsonian

Intersection of ranges of *tolerances* for sets of resources utilized by organisms, represented mathematically by multidimensional spatial coordinates whose dimensions correspond to *environmental* variables. Any *species* is considered unimodally distributed, *i.e.*, confined to a *habitat* in the *niche*.
Note 1: The Hutchinsonian niche is perhaps the most accepted, quantifiable concept of the niche in use today. In practice, it is impossible to identify and quantify all the resources utilized by an organism. Thus, typically the limiting factors receive most attention.
Note 2: Two aspects of the Hutchinsonian niche can be visualized: A *realized niche* for a species is the sum of niche dimensions unique to that particular species. A *fundamental niche* is the total sum of the species niche dimensions including parts shared with other species and parts unshared.
[ref. 2]

niche, realized

Portion of a *species' fundamental niche* that it actually occupies.
Note: The realized niche is narrower than the fundamental niche owing to pressure from, and interactions with, other organisms (*e.g.*, superior competitors).
[ref. 2]
See also *niche; niche, Hutchinsonian*.

niche preemption

Rapid use and preemption of resources by a biological *species* that exploits them to the exclusion or severe disadvantage of another species.
[ref. 2]
See also *niche.*

niche width

Term referring to the area that a *species* could physically inhabit.
Note: Niche width is defined by suitable climate and available food sources appropriate to the species of interest as well as other factors such as temperature and air or water pressure levels. The niche width often differs from the *realized niche.*
[ref. 2]

nicotinic

Referring to a substance or effect that mimics *acetylcholine* at the *neuromuscular junction*, at *autonomic ganglia* and at other locations in the *brain.*
Note 1: Nicotinic substances bind to a specific class of *cholinergic receptor*s denoted nicotinic *acetylcholine receptors.*
Note 2: The prototype nicotinic substance is the *parasympathomimetic* alkaloid, nicotine [(*S*)-3-(1-methylpyrrolidin-2-yl)pyridine].
[ref. 4]
See also *muscarinic.*

nicotinic receptor

See *receptor, nicotinic.*

nine aspects of disease association

Nine aspects of evidence, defined by Bradford-Hill (1965), reflecting the accuracy of linkage between a risk factor and *disease*: strength of association, consistency of association, specificity of association, temporal association, biological gradient (*dose*-response) in the association, biological plausibility, coherence of the association, experimental support of association, and analogy.
[ref. 2]

nine-hole box test

5-9 hole attention box test

Behavioral test based on the five-choice serial *reaction time* task, which allows the study of attention based on a test animal learning from which hole (typically one of five open holes in an arc of nine) a visual (light) cue was given, with a food pellet reward for nose-poking the correct hole.
[ref. 4]
See also *nose-poke test.*

nipple

Projection on the apex of the breast through which the *ducts* of the milk-producing *glands* open.
[ref. 5]

Nissl body

Nissl granule
Nissl substance

Granular structure consisting of rough *endoplasmic reticulum*, found in *neurons*.
[ref. 4]
See also *chromatolysis*.

nitric oxide

Generic term for nitrogen monoxide species, including nitrosonium (NO^+), nitric oxide radical ($NO^\bullet$), and nitroxyl (NO^-), that can function in a cell-signaling capacity.
[After ref. 3]
See also *reactive nitrogen species*.

nitrification

Sequential oxidation of ammonium salts to nitrite and nitrate by microorganisms.
[ref. 1]

nitrosation (in toxicology):

Non*enzymatic* reaction of secondary amines with nitrate under acidic conditions to yield nitrosamines as products.
Note 1: Nitrosation may occur in the stomach, where secondary amines from food and nitrate from saliva meet.
Note 2: Nitrosation is an endogenous toxification reaction, since most nitrosamines are mutagenic and carcinogenic.
[*]

nitrosative stress

Adverse effects occurring when the generation of *reactive nitrogen species* in a system exceeds the system's ability to neutralize and eliminate them.
Note: Nitrosative stress may lead to nitrosylation reactions that can alter protein structure, thus inhibiting normal function.
[ref. 1]

no-acceptable-daily-intake-allocated

Expression applied to a substance for which the available information is not sufficient to establish its *safety*, or when the specifications for identity and purity are not adequate, or when the available data show that the substance is *hazardous* and should not be used.
Note: The basis for the designation "no-acceptable-daily-intake-allocated" should be determined before action is taken; in the first two cases above, not being able to allocate an acceptable daily intake does not mean that the substance is unsafe.
[After ref. 1]

"no action" alternative (to remediation of a site)

Scenario in which one assesses if the contaminants at a waste site pose, or will pose in the future, a *risk* if left alone.
[ref. 2]

nociception

Physiological response to harmful stimuli by specialized *nerve* endings that transmit a signal perceived as *pain* by the *brain*.
[ref. 4]
See also *antinociception*.

nodal (protein)

Growth factor of the transforming growth factor β (TGF-β) superfamily, coded by a *gene* designated NODAL, that plays crucial roles in *embryogenesis*, particularly in signalling from the *primitive streak* to the *mesoderm* to establish left-right asymmetry as well as aspects of *stem cell* differentiation.
Note: Nodal derives from *expression* of the gene in the *primitive node*.
[ref. 5]

node of Ranvier

Short interval in the *myelin sheath* of a *nerve* fiber where the *axon* is invested only by scant cytoplasmic processes of the neighboring *Schwann cell*s or, in the *central nervous system*, of *oligodendroglia* cells.
Note: At a node of Ranvier the *axon*al membrane is not insulated and contains a high density of voltage-gated Na^+ channels (see *voltage-gated ion channel*) that generate *action potentials*.
[ref. 4]

nodule

Small node or boss that is solid and can be detected by touch.
[ref. 1]

no-effect dose (NED)
subthreshold dose

Amount of a substance that has no effect on the organism.
Note: The NED is lower than the *threshold* of harmful effect and is estimated while establishing the threshold of harmful effect.
[ref. 1]

no-effect level (NEL)

Maximum dose of a substance that produces no detectable changes under defined conditions of *exposure*.
Note: NEL tends to be substituted by *no-observed-adverse-effect level* or *no-observed-effect level*.
[ref. 1]

noggin (NOG)

Signaling protein released by the *notochord*, important in *somite* patterning and nervous system development.
[ref. 5]
See also *Spemann organizer*.

nonalcoholic fatty liver (disease) (NAFL(D))

See *fatty liver*.

nonbioenvironmental transformation

Change in the chemical or physical nature of a substance in the natural *environment* occurring as a result of physicochemical conditions and independent of any biological system.
[ref. 1]

noncoding RNA (ncRNA)

See *ribonucleic acid, noncoding.*

nondepleting antibody

See *antibody, nondepleting.*

nondisjunction

Failure of *chromosomes* to separate during *meiosis*, resulting in an uneven distribution of chromosomes in the two *gametes* (24 and 22 in humans).
[ref. 5]

nonenzymatic glycosylation

nonenzymatic glycation

Covalent addition of a sugar to an endogenous biomolecule without the need for *enzyme* catalysis.
Note: In conditions of increased glucose levels, nonenzymatic glycation of proteins or *hemoglobin* may occur.
[*]
See also *advanced glycation end product; covalent binding; hemoglobin adduct.*

non-Hodgkin lymphoma

Any of various malignant *lymphomas* characterized by the absence of *Reed–Sternberg cells* and producing *symptoms* similar to those of *Hodgkin disease.*
[ref. 3]

nonionizing radiation

Electromagnetic radiation of sufficiently low energy that is not capable of causing ionization.
[ref. 1]

nonobese diabetic (NOD) mouse

Genetically modified mouse with a susceptibility to spontaneous development of *automimmune diabetes mellitus type I.*
[ref. 3]

nonoccupational exposure

Environmental *exposure* to substances that may be associated with particular work environments and (or) associated activities and processes, but that may also occur in the environment outside the workplace.
[After ref. 1]

nonself

Of, relating to, or designating a *cell* or *tissue* that has not been produced by the individual organism.
Note: Nonself molecules are identified by the *immune system* as foreign or abnormal, thus provoking an *immune response.*
[ref. 3]

nonstochastic

See *deterministic.*

nonstochastic health effects

Effects that are dependent on the magnitude of the *dose* in excess of a threshold.
[ref. 2]

nontarget organism

Organism that is not the intended target of a particular use of a *pesticide,* but is potentially affected by its use.
[After ref. 2]

no-observed-adverse-effect level (NOAEL)

Greatest *concentration* or amount of a substance, found by experiment or observation, which causes no detectable *adverse change* in morphology, functional capacity, growth, development, or life span of the *target* organism under defined conditions of *exposure.*
[ref. 1]

no-observed-effect concentration (NOEC) (in aquatic toxicology)

Special case of the *no-observed-effect level*, commonly used in aquatic toxicology.
Note: When derived from a *life-cycle* or partial life-cycle test, the NOEC is numerically the same as the lower limit of the *maximum acceptable toxicant concentration.*
[ref. 2]

no-observed-effect level (NOEL)

Greatest *concentration* or amount of a substance, found by experiment or observation, that causes no alterations of morphology, functional capacity, growth, development, or life span of *target* organisms distinguishable from those observed in normal (*control*) organisms of the same *species* and strain under the same defined conditions of *exposure.*
[ref. 1]

noradrenaline

noradrenalin
norepinephrine (INN)
4-[(1*R*)-2-amino-1-hydroxyethyl]benzene-1,2-diol

Catecholamine hormone and *neurotransmitter* acting as a post*ganglionic adrenergic* mediator at α- and β-*adrenergic receptors.*
Note 1: Noradrenaline is stored in, and released from, *chromaffin* granules in the adrenal medulla (see *adrenal gland*).
Note 2: Noradrenaline has strong *vasoconstrictive* effects.
[ref. 5]

norepinephrine

See *noradrenaline.*

no-response level (NRL)

Maximum *dose* of a substance at which no specified response is observed in a defined *population* and under defined conditions of *exposure.*
[ref. 1]

normal equivalent deviation (NED)

Proportion dying in a *toxicity* test expressed in terms of standard deviations from the mean of a normal
curve.
[ref. 2]

normit

Metameter equal to the *normal equivalent deviation.*
Note: The resulting analysis of *dose-effect* or *concentration*-effect data with the normit metameter is often called normit analysis and is essentially equivalent to *probit* analysis.
[ref. 2]

normoblast

erythroblast

Nucleated precursor of the *erythrocyte* (red blood cell), which in humans has no *nucleus.*
Note: In some usages, the normoblast refers only to an erythroblast that is developing normally into an erythrocyte, and then the term megaloblast is used for an erythroblast that is enlarged and developing abnormally.
[*]

nose-poke test

Test allowing study of attention deficit based on noting the success of a test animal in gaining a food pellet reward for nosing the correct hole in a box, *e.g.*, the *nine-hole box test.*
[ref. 4]

nosocomial

Associated with a hospital or infirmary, especially used of a *disease* that results from care in such an institution.
[ref. 1]

notochord

Rod-shaped structure of cells derived from *mesoderm*, lying *ventral* to the *neural tube* and defining the *primitive axis* of the *embryo.*
[ref. 5]

noxious substance

See *harmful substance.*

nuclear envelope

Outer and inner *membranes* of the *cell nucleus*, intermembrane space, and associated structures.
[*]

nuclear factor kappa-light-chain-enhancer of activated B-cells (NFκB)

Protein complex that controls the *transcription* of *genes* involved in *cytokine* production, *cellular adhesion, inflammation*, and *apoptosis.*

Note: NFκB is found in almost all animal *cell* types and is involved in cellular responses to stimuli such as stress, cytokines, free radicals, ultraviolet irradiation, oxidized low-density lipoprotein (LDL), and bacterial or viral *antigens*.
[ref. 3]

nuclear factor of activated T-cells (NFAT)

Transcription factor involved in rapid *cell* response to *stress*, such as injury or invading *pathogens*, and in cell proliferation and survival.
[ref. 3]

nuclear spindle

mitotic spindle

Microtubular structure that draws newly duplicated *chromosomes* apart during *mitosis* and *meiosis*.
[ref. 5]

nuclear type I receptor

See *receptor, nuclear type I.*

nuclear type II receptor

See *receptor, nuclear type II.*

nucleic acid

See *deoxyribonucleic acid; ribonucleic acid.*

nucleolus

Dense spherical structure, found in the *nucleus* of a *cell* during *interphase*, and responsible for *ribosome* synthesis and assembly.
[*]

nucleotide-binding oligomerization domain-containing protein 1, 2 (NOD1, NOD2)

Members of a family of human intracellular proteins involved in the detection of invasive bacteria and activation of the *NFκB transcription factor* pathway.
Note: In *epithelial cells*, NOD1 is essential for sensing intracellular Gram-negative bacteria through a tripeptide motif in the bacterial peptidoglycan.
[ref. 3]

nucleotide-binding oligomerization domain-containing protein (NOD)-like receptor (NLR)

See *receptor, nucleotide-binding oligomerization domain-containing protein (NOD)-like.*

nucleus (n)/nuclei (n, pl)/nuclear (adj) (in cell biology)

Compartment in the *interphase eukaryotic cell* bounded by a double *membrane* and containing most of the *genomic DNA*, with the associated functions of transcription and processing.
[ref. 1]

nude mouse

Mouse that is *T-cell*-deficient owing to a *homozygous gene* defect (*nu/nu*) resulting in the absence of a *thymus* (and also lack of body hair).
[ref. 3]

nuisance threshold

Lowest *concentration* of an air *pollutant*, or lowest level of a physical agent such as light or noise, that can be considered objectionable.
[*]

null cell

Lymphocyte with neither *T*- nor *B-cell differentiation antigens* on its surface.
[ref. 3]

nulligravida

Never having been *pregnant*.
[ref. 5]
Compare *nulliparous*.

nulliparous

Never having given *birth* to a live baby.
[ref. 5]
Compare *nulligravida*.

numbness

Imprecise term for absent or reduced touch perception.
[ref. 4]
See also *paresthesia*.

numerical response

Change in *predator* or grazer number through increased reproductive output, decreased *mortality*, or increased immigration in response to changes in prey or food densities.
[ref. 2]

nutrient

See *nutrient, essential*.

nutrient, essential

Substance that is absolutely required for the normal growth and development of a defined organism throughout a complete *life cycle*.
Note 1: Terms related to "essential nutrient" are "essential element" and "essential metal", which may be given the same definition by substituting "element" or "metal" for "nutrient".
Note 2: The term "essential nutrient" is meaningless unless accompanied by a statement of which organisms show a requirement for the nutrient.
[ref. 2]

nutrient, trace

micronutrient

Substance required in very small quantities by a defined organism, in order to maintain health.
Note: The organism and the quantity required for health should be stated for the term 'trace nutrient' to be meaningful.
[After ref. 2]

nutritional table method

Procedure for evaluating the dietary intake of a defined group of people.
Note 1: The accuracy of the nutritional table method depends on the accuracy with which records of the food consumption can be established, in addition to the accuracy of the nutritional tables specifying the *concentration* of various nutrients, vitamins, and other essential and nonessential substances, including *pesticide residues*.
Note 2: For each record of quantity of food consumed during a certain time period, the daily intake of the substance in question is calculated by multiplying the substance concentration in the food item (as obtained from the nutritional table) by the quantity of food consumed and dividing by the time of observation.
[ref. 1]

nychthemeral

See *circadian*.

nychthemeron

Time period of 24 consecutive hours.
[*]

nystagmus

Involuntary, rapid, rhythmic movement (horizontal, vertical, rotary, or mixed) of the eyeball, usually caused by a *disorder* of the labyrinth of the inner ear or a malfunction of the *central nervous system*.
[ref. 1]

OKT3

Brand name for muromonab-CD3, an *immunosuppressant drug* given intravenously to reverse *acute rejection* of transplanted organs, including the heart, kidneys, and liver. Note: OKT3 was the first *monoclonal antibody* used to treat patients.
[ref. 3]
See also *antibody therapy*.

objective environment

Actual physical, chemical, and social *environment* as described by objective measurements, such as noise levels in decibels and *concentration*s of air *pollutants*.
[ref. 1]

occipital lobe

See *lobe, occipital*.

occiput (n)/occipital (adj)

Back part of the head or skull.
[ref. 5]

occupational environment

Surrounding conditions at a workplace.
[ref. 1]

occupational exposure

Experience of substances, radiation, or other conditions such as noise or odor, while at work.
[After ref. 1]

occupational exposure limit (OEL)

Regulatory level of *exposure* to substances, intensities of radiation, or other conditions, specified in relevant government legislation or related codes of practice.
[ref. 1]

occupational exposure standard (OES)

1. Level of *exposure* to substances, intensities of radiation, or other conditions considered to represent specified good practice and a realistic criterion for the control of exposure by appropriate plant design, engineering controls, and, if necessary, the addition and use of personal protective devices.
2. In the U.K., *health*-based exposure limit defined under COSHH Regulations as the *concentration* of any airborne substance, averaged over a reference period, at which, according to current knowledge, there is no evidence that it is likely to be injurious to employees, if they are *exposed* by inhalation, day after day, to that concentration, and set on the advice of the HSE Advisory Committee on Toxic Substances.

[ref. 1]

Comprehensive Glossary of Terms Used in Toxicology
By John Duffus, Douglas M. Templeton and Michael Schwenk

Published by the Royal Society of Chemistry, www.rsc.org

occupational hygiene

Identification, assessment, and control of physicochemical and biological factors in the workplace that may affect the *health* or well-being of those at work and in the surrounding community.
[ref. 1]

occupational medicine

Specialty devoted to the prevention and management of occupational injury, illness, and disability, and the promotion of the *health* of workers, their families, and their communities.
[ref. 1]

occupational safety and health

See *occupational hygiene.*

octanol-air partition coefficient, P_{OA}, K_{OA}

Partition coefficient for a compound between octan-1-ol and air at equilibrium.
Note: Like K_{ow}, it is a measure of *lipophilicity*.
[ref. 2]

octanol–water partition coefficient, P_{OW}, K_{OW}

Ratio of the solubility of a chemical in octan-1-ol divided by its solubility in water at *equilibrium*.
Note: Measure of *lipophilicity*, used in the assessment of both the uptake and physiological distribution of organic chemicals and prediction of their environmental fate.
[ref. 1]

octaves (in environmental science)

Log2 classes (*e.g.*, 1–2, 2–4, 4–8, 8–16, 16–32, . . . individuals) used in *species-abundance* curves and representing doublings of the numbers of individuals in a species.
[ref. 2]

ocular

Pertaining to the eye.
[ref. 1]

odds

Probability of the occurrence of an event divided by that of its nonoccurrence; or more generally the probability that something is so, divided by the probability that it is not so.
[After ref. 1]

odds ratio (OR)

cross-product ratio
relative odds

Quotient obtained by dividing one set of *odds* by another.
Note 1: The concept of "odds ratio" is important in *environmental health* research because it allows identification of *disease*-associated factors in human *populations*.
Note 2: Several different types of odds ratio can be defined. Consider the following notation for the distribution of a binary *exposure* and a disease in a population or a *sample*. From Table 2 the odds ratio (cross-product ratio) is *ad*/*bc*.

Table 2 Variables assigned for the distribution of a binary exposure and a disease in a population or sample.

Subjects	Exposed	Nonexposed
Disease	*a*	*b*
No disease	*c*	*d*

A) The *exposure*-odds ratio for a set of *case control* data is the odds in favor of exposure among the cases (*a/b*) divided by the odds in favor of exposure among noncases (*c/d*), which is equal to *ad/bc*. With incident cases, unbiased subject selection, and a "rare" disease (say, under 2 % cumulative *incidence* rate over the study period), *ad/bc* is an approximate estimate of the *risk* ratio. With incident cases, unbiased subject selection, and density sampling of *controls*, *ad/bc* is an estimate of the ratio of the person-time incidence rates in the *exposed* and unexposed. No rarity assumption is required for this.
B) The disease-odds (rate-odds) ratio for a cohort or cross-section is the the odds in favor of disease among the exposed population (*a/c*) divided by the odds in favor of disease among the unexposed (*b/d*), which is equal to *ad/bc* and hence is equal to the exposure odds ratio for the cohort or cross-section.
C) The *prevalence*-odds ratio refers to an odds ratio derived cross-sectionally, as, for example, an odds ratio derived from studies of prevalent (rather than incident) cases.
D) The *risk*-odds ratio is the odds in favor of getting disease, if exposed, divided by the odds in favor of getting disease if not *exposed*. The odds ratio derived from a *cohort study* is an estimate of this.

[After ref. 1]

odontoblast

Dentin-forming cell of the pulp *cavity* of a tooth, arising from the *mesenchyme* of the *neural crest*.
[ref. 5]

odor threshold
odor detection threshold

In principle, the lowest *concentration* of an odorant in the air that can be detected by a human being.
Note: In practice, a panel of "sniffers" is often used, and the odor *threshold* is taken as the concentration at which 50 % of the panel can detect the odorant (although some workers have also used 100 % thresholds). The odor concentration at the detection threshold may be defined as one odor unit.
[ref. 1]
See also *olf*.

oedema

See *edema*.

offspring
progeny

Child or children of a person, or the young of an animal, in relation to the parent(s).
[ref. 5]

Oklo natural reactors

Naturally occurring nuclear reactors arising through geochemical processes approximately 1.8 billion years ago in Oklo (Gabon, Africa).
Note: Because the current abundance of fissible ^{235}U in natural uranium deposits is too low to sustain nuclear fission, conditions for active natural reactors do not exist on Earth today.
[After ref. 2]

olf

Unit used to measure scent emission of people and objects; one olf is defined as the scent emission of an "average person", a sitting adult who takes an average of 0.7 baths per day and whose skin has a total area of 1.8 m^2; the scent emission of an object or person is measured by specially trained personnel comparing it to normed scents.
Note: The olf should not be confused with the unit of scent immission (as opposed to emission), the *decipol*, which also takes into account the ventilation system's air volume flow.
[ref. 1]
See also *odor threshold*.

olfaction

Detection of odors.
[ref. 4]

olfactometer

Apparatus for testing the power of the sense of smell.
[ref. 1]

olfactory bulb

Region of the *frontal lobe* of the *brain*, receiving input from *neurons* of the nasal mucosa and involved in the sense of smell.
[ref. 4]

oligoclonal

Having a few different *clones*, or the product of a few different clones.
[ref. 3]

oligodactyly

Congenital occurrence of fewer than the usual number of digits, resulting in humans having fewer than five fingers or toes on a hand or foot.
[ref. 5]

oligodendrocyte
oligodendroglial cell

Type of *glial cell* that produces the *myelin sheath* in the *central nervous system*.
Note: *Schwann cells* perform a comparable function in the *peripheral nervous system*.
[ref. 4]

oligodendroglial cell

See *oligodendrocyte*.

oligodendroglioma

Glioma arising from the *oligodendrocytes*.
Note: An oligodendroglioma is usually a slow-growing, well-circumscribed *tumor*.
[ref. 4]

oligodontia

Congenital absence of some of the teeth.
[ref. 5]

oligomenorrhea

Infrequent or scanty *menstruation*.
[ref. 5]

oligospermia
oligospermatism
oligozoospermia

Subnormal concentration of *sperm* in the male ejaculate (see *ejaculation*).
[ref. 5]

oligotrophic

Describing an environment having a low concentration of nutrients.
Note: The term is usually used to describe bodies of water or *soils* with very low nutrient levels and low rates of biological production.
[ref. 2]
See also *eutrophic*.

oligotrophy

1. State of being oligotrophic.
2. Obligate or facultative capacity to live in low-nutrient *habitats*.

[ref. 2]
See also *eutrophy*.

oligozoospermia

Sperm *concentration* less than a *reference value*.
[ref. 1]

oliguria

Excretion of a diminished amount of urine in relation to fluid intake.
[ref. 1]

-ome (n)/-omics (n)/-omic (adj)

Referring to a field of study in biology ending in the suffix -omics, such as *genomics* or *proteomics*; the related -omes neologisms refer to the objects of study of the field such as the *genome* or *proteome*, respectively.
[After ref. 1]

omentum

Fold of *peritoneal membrane* passing between the stomach and another abdominal organ.
[ref. 5]
See also *omentum, greater; omentum, lesser.*

omentum, greater

Omentum passing from the greater curvature of the stomach in front of the small intestine, folding back on itself to fuse into four layers of *peritoneal membrane*, and ascending to the transverse colon.
Note: The greater omentum functions in fat deposition, contains islands of *macrophages* that contribute to immune function, and can delimit areas of traumatic tissue damage or *infection*.
[ref. 5]

omentum, lesser

Double-layer of *peritoneal membrane* (*omentum*) passing between the lesser curvature of the stomach and the duodenum.
[ref. 5]

omphalocele
exomphalos

*Congenital hernia*tion of *abdominal viscera* (bowel or *omentum*) through the abdominal wall under the skin at the base of the *umbilical cord*.
[ref. 5]
Compare *gastroschisis*.

omphalosite

Lesser developed of two *monozygotic twins* that failed to separate completely during *embryogenesis*.
Note: The omphalosite is joined to the other twin (the *autosite*) by the *umbilical* vessels, receives its blood supply from the *placenta*, and is incapable of survival after separation from the placenta.
[ref. 5]

oncofetal antigen

See *antigen, oncofetal*.

oncogene

Gene that can cause *neoplastic transformation* of a cell.
Note: Oncogenes are slightly changed equivalents of normal genes known as proto-oncogenes.
[ref. 1]

oncogene, ABL

Gene resulting from a *chromosomal translocation* (9;22) that fuses sequences from the BCR (breakpoint cluster region) gene with the ABL gene.
Note 1: The DCR/ABL translocation creates the *Philadelphia chromosome*, found in most human patients with *chronic myelogenous leukemia*.
Note 2: The fusion protein encoded by BCR-ABL possesses unregulated *tyrosine kinase* activity.
Note 3: The term ABL derives from the Abelson murine leukemia virus, from which the gene was first isolated.
[ref. 3]

oncogenesis

Production or causation of *tumors*.
[ref. 1]

oncogenic

Capable of producing *tumors* in animals, either *benign* (noncancerous) or *malignant* (*cancerous*).
[ref. 1]

one-compartment model

Kinetic *model* of substance distribution, in which the whole body is thought of as a single *compartment* where the substance distributes rapidly, achieving an *equilibrium* between *blood* and *tissue* immediately.
[After ref. 1]

one-generation reproductive toxicity study

Procedure in which male rodents are dosed with a test substance for at least one *spermatogenic cycle* and females for two *estrous cycles*, and then further exposed during mating, *pregnancy* and nursing; adverse effects on reproduction, *parturition, lactation* and *postnatal* growth are studied.
[ref. 5]
Compare *extended one-generation reproductive toxicity study.*
See also *two-generation reproductive toxicity study*.

one-hit model

Dose–response model of the form

$$P = 1 - e^{-bd}$$

where P is the probability of *cancer* death from a continuous *dose* rate, d, and b is a constant.
[ref. 1]

onycholysis

Loosening or detachment of the nail from the nail bed following some destructive process.
[ref. 1]

oocyte

ovocyte

Immature precursor of the *ovum* resident in the *ovary*.
[ref. 5]

oocyte, primary

Oocyte during growth phase before completion of the first *meiotic* division.
Note: The primary oocyte is *diploid* and becomes a *secondary oocyte* before *birth*.
[ref. 5]

oocyte, secondary

Oocyte in which the first meiotic division to a *haploid* cell has been completed.
[ref. 5]
Compare *oocyte, primary*.

oogenesis

Process of formation and development of an *ovum*.
[ref. 5]
See also *oocyte; oocyte, primary; oocyte, secondary; oogonium*.

oogonium

Primitive *germ cell* that proliferates by *mitosis* and develops into a *primary oocyte* prior to *birth*.
[ref. 5]

open field test

Procedure to observe changes in *motor activity* and *rearing*, in which a rodent is placed on a surface and distance and patterns of movement are recorded.
Note 1: In a typical open field test, the animal is placed within a circular enclosure with grid lines marking the floor and the number of line crossing and rearing events are counted within a defined period of time.
Note 2: Automated procedures for the open field test include video capture methods using photocell devices to measure activity as photocell beam breaks.
[ref. 4]

open reading frame (ORF)

DNA sequence, that begins with an initiation codon and ends with a termination codon, that codes for and is potentially translatable into polypeptide.
[ref. 5]

operant behavior, schedule-controlled

See *schedule-controlled operant behavior*.

operon

Complete unit of *gene* expression and regulation, including structural genes, regulatory gene(s), and control elements in *DNA*, that are recognized by regulatory *gene product*(s).
[ref. 1]

ophthalmic

Pertaining to the eye.
[ref. 1]

opiate receptor

One of a group of *G-protein-coupled receptor*s that bind *morphine* and endogenous substances that have morphine-like effects.
Note: Opiate receptor-binding endogenous substances include *endorphins* and *enkephalins*.
[ref. 4]

opioid

Synthetic *narcotic* having properties consistent with binding to *opiate receptor*s, but not derived from *opium*.
[ref. 4]

opium

Extract of the opium poppy, ***Papaver somniferum***, containing *morphine* as a major *psychoactive* component.
[ref. 4]

opportunistic

1. (in medicine) Of a microorganism or related *infection*, causing illness mainly when the *immune system* is not functioning properly.
2. (in ecology) Of an organism, able to occupy rapidly any suitable new habitat.

[*]

opsonin

Molecule, *e.g., antibody* or C3b, that enhances *phagocytosis* by binding to the *antigen* promoting its adhesion to the *phagocyte*.
[ref. 3]

opsonization

Coating of *antigen* with an *opsonin* to enhance *phagocytosis*.
Note: Opsonization leads to interaction of opsonized complexes with *Fc receptors* or *complement receptors* that facilitates their uptake by the receptor-bearing *phagocytic cells*.
[ref. 3]

optic

Relating to the eye or vision.
[ref. 5]

optimal-foraging theory

Idea that the ideal food gatherer will obtain a maximum net rate of energy gain by optimally allocating its time and energy to the various components of the food acquisition process.
[After ref. 2]

optimal stress response

Process that maximizes *Darwinian fitness* under *stressful* conditions by shifting the balance of energy allocation between *somatic growth rate* and longevity (survival).
[After ref. 2]

oral tolerance

Orally induced and *immune*-mediated nonresponsiveness.
[ref. 3]
See also *tolerance*.

oral vaccination

Immunization against a *pathogen* with a *vaccine* administered by mouth.
[ref. 3]

orbit (in anatomy)

eye socket

Cavity in the skull of a *vertebrate* that contains the eye.
[ref. 5]

organ (in biology)

Structural unit consisting of *tissues* and *extracellular matrix* organized to perform as a functional entity (*e.g.*, liver or kidney).
[*]

organ culture

See *culture*.

organ dose

Amount of a substance or physical agent (radiation) absorbed by an *organ*.
[ref. 1]

organ of Corti

spiral organ

Specialized collection of *epithelial* hair cells in the inner ear, involved in hearing.
[ref. 5]

organelle

Microstructure or separated compartment within a *cell* that has a specialized function, *e.g., ribosome, peroxisome, lysosome, Golgi apparatus, mitochondrion, nucleolus*, or *nucleus*.
[ref. 1]

organic carbon partition coefficient, K_{oc}

Measure of the tendency for organic substances to be adsorbed by *soil* or *sediment*, expressed as:

$$K_{oc} = \frac{(\text{mass adsorbed substance})/(\text{mass organic carbon})}{(\text{mass concentration of adsorbed substance})}$$

Note: The K_{oc} is substance-specific and is largely independent of soil properties.
[ref. 1]

organogenesis

Formation and development of organs.
[ref. 5]

organoleptic

1. Relating to perception by a sensory *organ*.
2. Involving the use of sensory organs, *e.g.*, organoleptic tests.

[ref. 1]

organ-on-a-chip

In vitro diagnostic system with modular, microchip-based technology, using *cell cultures*, co-cultures, and tissue-like constructs approximating to an *organ*, allowing study of simulated organ *toxicity* without using an animal.
[*]
See also *body-on-a-chip; lab-on-a-chip*.

organometallic compound

Compound having *covalent bonds* between one or more metal atoms and one or more carbon atoms of an organyl group.
Note: Conversion of metals such as manganese, lead, tin and mercury to lipid-soluble organometallic species ("organification") often enhances their *neurotoxicity*.
[ref. 4]

organophosphate

Organic ester of phosphoric acid.
Note: Organophosphates are often *acetylcholinesterase inhibitor*s used as *pesticide*s or prohibited agents in chemical warfare.
[ref. 4]

organophosphate-induced delayed neuropathy (OPIDN)

Disorder, typically with *symptoms* of *pain* and weakness in the extremities, resulting from *neuron*al death associated with *organophosphate* poisoning (either *chronic* or a late effect of *acute poison*ing).
[ref. 4]

organotropy (n)/organotropic (adj) (in toxicology)

Feature of a substance exerting a *toxic* effect on a specific *organ*.
Note: Organs typically affected by organotropy include the *nervous system*, liver, lungs, *blood*, and kidneys.
[*]

orofacial cleft

Failure of the lip or *palate* to fuse properly.
[ref. 5]
See also *facial cleft*.

oropharyngeal membrane

See *buccopharyngeal membrane*.

osmophobia

olfactophobia
Morbid fear of odors.
[ref. 4]

osmosis (n)/osmotic (adj)

Net movement of *solvent* molecules through a semipermeable membrane into a compartment of higher solute *concentration* to equalise the solute chemical activity on both sides of the membrane.
Note 1: The osmotic force driving solvent movement is called osmotic pressure and is dependent only on the molar concentration of solutes present, *i.e.*, it is a *colligative* property of the solutes.
Note 2: Osmosis plays a role in absorption, renal elimination and permeation of substances through biological membranes.
[*]

ossification

See *osteogenesis*.

osteo-

Prefix meaning pertaining to bone.
[ref. 1]

osteoblast

Fibroblast-derived bone-forming cell that produces a collagen type-I-rich *matrix*; this matrix calcifies to become bone.
[ref. 5]

osteoclast

Large multinucleate cell that resorbs bone, allowing for the deposition of new bone.
Note: Osteoclasts secrete *enzymes* and acids that dissolve the calcium phosphate *matrix* of old bone tissue.
[ref. 5]

osteodystrophy

Abnormal development of bone.
[ref. 1]

osteogenesis

Formation or development of bone or bony tissue.
[ref. 5]

osteomalacia

Condition marked by softening of the bones due to impaired *mineralization*, with excess accumulation of osteoid.
Note: Osteomalacia results from deficiency of vitamin D and calcium, and is characterized by bone pain and tenderness, muscle weakness, *anorexia*, and weight loss.
[After ref. 1]

osteoporosis

Significant decrease in bone mass with increased bone porosity and an increased tendency to fracture.
[ref. 1]

ostium/ostia (pl)

Opening into a vessel or *cavity* of the body.
[ref. 5]

otic

auricular

Pertaining to, or located near, the ear.
[ref. 5]

otocephaly

Congenital anomaly characterized by the absence or extreme underdevelopment of the lower jaw, producing closeness of the ears below the face.
[ref. 5]
See also *agnathia; synotia.*

Ouchterlony technique

Ouchterlony double diffusion assay

Double-radial immunodiffusion procedure for the detection of *precipitating antibodies.*

Note: The Ouchterlony technique is a method of high diagnostic *specificity* but low *sensitivity*.
[ref. 3]

ovarian cycle

Sequence of recurring events in the *ovary* involved in *ovulation*.
Note 1: The ovarian *cycle* consists of the *follicular phase* with maturation of the *ovarian follicle* under control of *follicle stimulating hormone* (FSH), *ovulation* with release of the *secondary oocyte*, and the *luteal phase* in which FSH and *luteinizing hormone* drive formation of the *progesterone*-producing *corpus luteum*.
Note 2: Together with the *uterine cycle*, the ovarian cycle comprises the *menstrual cycle*.
[ref. 5]

ovarian follicle

Cavity in the *ovary* containing a maturing *ovum*, at any stage of development, surrounded by its encasing *cells*.
[ref. 5]

ovary (n)/ovarian (adj)

One of the paired female reproductive *glands* containing the ova (see *ovum*).
[ref. 5]

ovicide

Substance intended to kill *eggs*.
[ref. 1]

ovotestis

Abnormal *gonad* in which both *ovarian* and *testicular* tissues are present, and thus a form of *hermaphroditism*.
[ref. 5]

ovulation

Release of a mature *ovum* from an *ovary* into a *Fallopian tube*.
[ref. 5]

ovum

Mature female sex *cell*, capable of undergoing *fertilization*.
[ref. 5]
See also *egg; gamete; oocyte*.

oxidative burst

See *respiratory burst*.

oxidative phosphorylation

Process in which energy derived from the *enzymatic* oxidation of nutrients is coupled to the production of *ATP*, generally occurring in the *mitochondria* of *eukaryotic cells*.
[*]

oxidative stress

Adverse effects occurring when the generation of *reactive oxygen species* (ROS) in a system exceeds the system's ability to neutralize and eliminate them; excess ROS can then damage a *cell*'s lipids, protein, and (or) *DNA*.
[ref. 1]
Note 1: Oxidative products such as those resulting from carbonylation, *DNA adducts*, and glutathionylation reactions (see *glutathione*), and sulfenic acid derivatives, are biomarkers for oxidative stress.
Note 2: Oxidative stress and resultant tissue modifications are believed to play a role in the *pathogenesis* of aging and various chronic *diseases*.
[*]

oxytocin

Peptide *hormone* secreted by the *neurohypophysis* that stimulates contraction of the *myometrium* during *labor* and secretion of milk during *lactation*.
Note: Oxytocin is used clinically in the induction of labor and in the management of *postpartum hemorrhage*.
[ref. 5]

ozone hole

Extreme thinning of the *ozone layer* above the Antarctic, thought to be largely a consequence of ozone (O_3) destruction by *chlorofluorocarbon* accumulation in the stratosphere.
[After ref. 2]

ozone layer

ozonosphere

Part of the Earth's atmosphere, mainly located in the lower portion of the stratosphere, approximately 15–35 km above the Earth's surface, containing higher concentrations (μM) of ozone (O_3) than the lower atmosphere.
Note 1: The thickness of the ozone layer varies seasonally and geographically.
Note 2: The intact ozone layer absorbs a considerable fraction of the sun's ultraviolet radiation, thus protecting the biosphere from hazardous radiation intensities.
[After ref. 2]
See also *Dobson unit; ozone hole*.

ozonosphere

See *ozone layer*.

PC-12 cell

Cell of an established line originally derived from a *pheochromocytoma* of the rat adrenal medulla (see *adrenal gland*).
Note: PC-12 cells dividing in *culture* will terminally differentiate into *neuron*-like cells under an appropriate *stimulus* (*e.g.*, *nerve growth factor*), making them a common *model* for studying neuronal *differentiation* and properties in culture.
[ref. 4]

pH-partition hypothesis

Idea that *bioavailability* is governed by the *diffusion* through the *gastrointestinal lumen* of the unionized form of an ionizable substance, as determined by p*K*a and pH.
[ref. 2]

P-nucleotides

Palindromic nucleotide sequences generated at the junctions between *antibody* and *T-cell receptor variable (V), diversity (D)*, and *joining (J) gene* segments during *gene rearrangement*.
[ref. 3]

P-selectin

Cell adhesion molecule expressed on the surface of activated *endothelial* cells and *platelets*.
[ref. 3]

pacemaker cell

See *sinoatrial node*.

pain

1. *Conscious* awareness of an unpleasant sensation mediated by *nerve* conduction of a *stimulus* from a site of *tissue disorder*, such as injury, *inflammation* or muscle tension, to the *brain*.
   Note 1: Local chemical mediators of pain include *histamine, bradykinins*, and *prostaglandins*.
   Note 2: The sensation of pain may occur or persist when an injured tissue is no longer present, as in *phantom pain*.
2. Sensation of being hurt in body or mind.

[After ref. 4]

pain, neuropathic

Pain initiated by *nerve* injury, not mediated by *nociception*.
[ref. 4]

pain, nociceptive

See *nociception*.

Comprehensive Glossary of Terms Used in Toxicology
By John Duffus, Douglas M. Templeton and Michael Schwenk

Published by the Royal Society of Chemistry, www.rsc.org

pain, phantom
phantom limb pain

Sensation that an amputated limb is still present, often associated with *pain*.
[ref. 4]

pain receptor

See *nociception*.

paired helical filament (PHF)

Describing the aggregation of hyperphosphorylated *tau protein* into *neurofibrillary tangles*.
[ref. 4]
See also *neurofilament*.

palaeontology

Branch of science that deals with fossilized remains of animals and plants, or more generally with evidence of extinct organic life during the geological past.
[After ref. 2]

palate (n)/palatine (adj)

Roof of the mouth, separating the oral and *nasal* cavities.
Note 1: In *embryonic* development an anterior, primary palate is distinguished from a posterior, secondary palate.
Note 2: The embryonic primary palate gives rise to an anterior bony part called the hard palate, and a posterior muscular part called the soft palate.
[ref. 5]
See also *orofacial cleft*.

palatine raphe

Medial central ridge of the *palate*.
[ref. 5]

palatoschisis

See *cleft palate*.

palpitation

1. Unduly rapid or throbbing heartbeat that may be regular or irregular and is noted by a person.
2. Undue awareness by a person of a heartbeat that is otherwise normal.

[After ref. 1]

pancytopenia

Abnormally low numerical concentration of all the cellular components of *blood* (*erythrocytes, leukocytes*, and *platelets*).
Note: Pancytopenia can be caused by *drugs* that suppress *bone marrow* function.
[*]

Papanicolaou smear
Papanicolaou stain
Pap smear
Pap test
cervical smear

Examination by light microscopy of a sample of *cells* scraped from the *uterine cervix*, used to screen for cervical *cancer*.
[ref. 5]

papilledema

Edema of the region of the head of the *optic* nerve in the *retina* (the optic disc).
Note: Papilledema is often caused by increased *intracranial pressure*.
[ref. 4]

paracellular

Situated alongside or between *cells*.
[*]
Compare *transcellular*.
See also *transport, paracellular*.

paracortex

See *paracortical area*.

paracortical area

paracortex

Region of a *lymph node* enriched in *T-lymphocytes*.
[ref. 3]

paracrine

1. Type of signaling in which a *cell* secretes into the intercellular space a molecular messenger that diffuses and binds to *receptors* on nearby target cells, producing a signal in those cells.
2. Describing or relating to a regulatory cell that secretes an *agonist* into intercellular spaces in which it diffuses to a target cell other than that which produces it.

[ref. 3,5]
See also *autocrine*.

paradigm

1. *Model* or template.
2. Body of concepts that, in a particular branch of science, has withstood rigorous testing, and is generally accepted by scientists working in that field as offering true explanations of fact and observation.

Note: The usage of paradigm as a body of concepts in a branch of science is derived from the work of the philosopher T. S. Kuhn.
[After ref. 2]

parafollicular cell

C cell

Neuroendocrine cell that migrates into the *thyroid gland* during *embryo*nic development and secretes the *hormone* calcitonin.
[ref. 5]

paralysis

Total or partial loss of *motor activity*.
Note: Paralysis may occur as a consequence of *disease* or injury to the muscle, or impairment of its *nerve* supply.
[ref. 4]

paralytic shellfish poisoning (PSP)

Illness that is a consequence of consumption of bivalve molluscs such as mussels, oysters, and clams that have ingested large quantities of microalgae containing the *neurotoxin saxitoxin* or its derivatives.
Note: PSP is characterized by initial tingling, numbness, and burning of the tongue and lips, which spreads to the face, neck, arms, fingertips, legs, and toes; this is followed by weakness of the upper and lower limbs, loss of *motor coordination*, and, in severe cases, *paralysis*.
[ref. 4]

paramesonephric duct

Müllerian duct

One of two paired *embryonic ducts* of *mesodermal* origin that will become the *Fallopian tubes, uterus, cervix* and upper part of the *vagina* in the female, and will regress in the male.
[ref. 5]

parametrium

Connective tissue of the floor of the female pelvis that lies in front of the *uterine cervix* and separates it from the bladder.
[ref. 5]

paramone

Paracrine agonist.
[ref. 3]

paraneoplastic autoimmune syndrome

See *autoimmune syndrome, paraneoplastic.*

para-occupational exposure

1. *Exposure* of a worker's family to substances carried from the workplace to the home.
2. Exposure of visitors to substances in the workplace.

[ref. 1]

paraoxonase

Any of several related enzymes that hydrolyze aryl esters and lactones, notably *organophosphate* pesticides including the *acetylcholinesterase* inhibitor, paraoxon.
Note: The most studied, PON1 (EC 3.1.8.1), is associated with high density lipoprotein and is considered to have beneficial antioxidant properties, including anti-atherosclerotic effects.
[ref. 4]

paraplegia

Paralysis of both lower limbs.
[ref. 4]

parasitic twin

Smaller of unequal *conjoined twins*.
[ref. 5]
See also *autosite*.

parasympathetic

Of, relating to, or affecting the *parasympathetic nervous system.*
[ref. 1]
See also *sympathetic nervous system.*

parasympathetic nervous system

Division of the *autonomic nervous system* involved in regulation of most inner *organs*, such as stimulating digestive *secretions*, slowing heart rate, constricting the pupils of the eyes, and dilating blood vessels.
Note: The principle nerve conducting impulses of the parasympathetic nervous system is the tenth *cranial nerve* (*vagus nerve*).
[After ref. 4]
See also *sympathetic nervous system.*

parasympatholytic

Producing effects resembling those caused by interruption of the *parasympathetic nerve*; also called *anticholinergic.*
[ref. 1]

parasympathomimetic
cholinomimetic

1. (n) Substance that produces effects resembling those of impulses transmitted by the post*ganglion*ic fibers of the *parasympathetic nervous system.*
2. (adj) Producing effects resembling those of impulses transmitted by the postganglionic fibers of the parasympathetic nervous system.

[ref. 4]

paratope

Site in the *variable region* of an *antibody* or *T-cell receptor* that binds to an *epitope* of an *antigen.*
[ref. 3]

paraxial mesoderm
somitic mesoderm

Area of *mesoderm* in the *embryo* that forms during *neurulation*, lies along both sides of the *neural tube*, and gives rise to the *somites.*
[ref. 5]

parenchymal cell

1. (in animals) Distinguishing or specific type of *cell* of an *organ* or *gland* (*e.g.*, hepatocyte, pancreatic islet cell), contained in, or supported by, the *connective tissue* framework provided by the *stromal cell*s.
2. (in plants) Thin-walled cell forming the bulk of *tissue* of the roots, stems, leaves and fruit of a plant

[ref. 5]

parenteral dosage

Introduction of substances into an organism avoiding the *gastrointestinal tract*, *e.g.*, subcutaneous, intravenous, or intramuscular administration.
[ref. 1]

paresis

Slight or incomplete *paralysis*.
[ref. 1]

paresthesia

Abnormal or unexplained tingling, pricking, or burning sensation on the skin.
[ref. 1]

parietal

Relating to or denoting the wall of the body or of a body *cavity* or hollow structure.
[ref. 5]

parietal cell, gastric

Acid-producing cell in the stomach.
[ref. 5]

parietal lobe

See *lobe, parietal*.

Parkinson disease

idiopathic parkinsonism
primary parkinsonism

Degenerative *disorder* of the *central nervous system* resulting from decreased production of the *neurotransmitter dopamine* in the *basal ganglia* (notably the *substantia nigra*).
Note 1: Parkinson *disease* is characterized by rhythmic muscle *tremor*, rigidity of movement, and a mask-like *facies*.
Note 2: Parkinson disease is usually idiopathic, although inherited cases occur.
[ref. 4]

parkinsonism, secondary

Neurological *syndrome* resembling *Parkinson disease* and often resulting from decreased *dopamine* production as a consequence of neurodegenerative changes in the *substantia nigra*.
Note: There are a number of known causes for secondary parkinsonism, including exposure to various *neurotoxic* substances.
[ref. 4]

parthanatos

Mechanism of *programmed cell death*, distinct from *apoptosis*, resulting from *genomic stress*, accumulation of poly(ADP-ribose), and release of apoptosis-inducing factor from *mitochondria*.
[*]

parthenogenesis

apogamia
Type of a*sexual reproduction* in which an un*fertilized ovum* develops into an *embryo*.
Note 1: Parthenogenesis occurs in lower plants, invertebrate species (water fleas, aphids, some bees, and parasitic wasps), and *vertebrates* (some reptiles, fish, and, very rarely, birds and sharks).

Note 2: Parthenogenesis is used to describe reproduction in self-fertilizing *hermaphroditic* species.
[*]

partial kill

Treatment in a *toxicity* test in which some, but not all, exposed individuals are killed.
[ref. 2]

particle immunoassay

Immunoassay in which *antibody* is bound to the surface of microspheres. After incubation with the *antigen*-containing biological fluid, and subsequent manipulation, detection is usually performed by *flow cytometry*.
[ref. 3]

particulate matter (in atmospheric chemistry)

1. General term used to describe airborne solid or liquid particles of all sizes. Note: The term *aerosol* is used to describe airborne particulate matter.
2. Particles in air, usually of a defined size range and specified as PM*n*, where *n* is the maximum *aerodynamic diameter* (usually expressed in µm) of at least 50 % of the particles.

[ref. 1]

partition coefficient

Concentration of a substance in one phase divided by the concentration of the substance in the other phase when the heterogeneous system of two phases is in *equilibrium*.
Note 1: The ratio of concentrations (or, strictly speaking, activities), represented by the partition coefficient of the same molecular species in the two phases, is constant at constant temperature.
Note 2: The *octanol–water partition coefficient* is often used as a measure of the *bioconcentration* factor for *modeling* purposes.
Note 3: The term "partition coefficient" is in common usage in *toxicology* but is not recommended by IUPAC for use in chemistry and should not be used as a synonym for partition constant, partition ratio, or distribution ratio.
[ref. 1]

partition ratio, K_D

Concentration of a substance in a single definite form, A, in an extract divided by its concentration in the same form in another phase at *equilibrium*. For example, for an aqueous/organic system $K_D(A) = [A]_{org}/[A]_{aq}$.
[ref. 1]

parturition

Process of giving *birth*.
[ref. 5]

passive avoidance test

Fear-motivated test in which rodents learn to avoid an otherwise preferred environment in which they are exposed to an *adverse event*.

Note: The latency to avoid the adverse *stimulus* in the passive avoidance test indicates changes of learning and (or) memory.
[ref. 4]

passive cutaneous anaphylaxis (PCA) test

Assay for *allergen*icity in which an *antibody* is injected intradermally into a test animal followed at a later time (anywhere from 3 to 48 h) with an intravenous injection of a mixture of a test *antigen* and a dye (typically Evans blue); increased vascular permeability at the site of antigen–antibody reaction is visualized by *extravasation* of the dye.
[ref. 3]

passive hemagglutination

See *hemagglutination, passive.*

passive immunization

See *immunization, passive.*

passive sampler

Device for taking samples of *environmental* media without the use of a pump, by diffusional or sedimentational adherence of the analyte to a suitable collecting device.
[*]
See also *personal sampler.*

passive smoking

Inhalation of *sidestream smoke* by people who themselves do not smoke.
[ref. 1]
See also *sidestream smoke.*

passive transport

Opposite term: *active transport.*

Transfer of a substance across a *cell membrane* without input of energy.
Note 1: Passive transport is driven by the difference in chemical activity across the cell membrane and may reflect a concentration gradient and (or) an electrical gradient.
Note 2: The main forms of passive transport are simple *diffusion, facilitated diffusion*, filtration and *osmosis.*
[*]

patch test

Test for *allergy* that is performed by placing the suspected *allergen* in direct contact with the skin or *mucosa.*
[ref. 3]

patent ductus arteriosus

Congenital disorder wherein the *ductus arteriosus* fails to close after *birth.*
Note: Patent ductus arteriosus may lead to failure to thrive and increased breathing rate in early life.
[ref. 5]

pathobiology

Study of *disease* mechanisms and processes.
Note: Whereas *pathology* is concerned with understanding causal relationships and diagnosing disease, pathobiology more broadly encompasses the mechanistic basis of disease, stressing the stepwise biological events, as well as the medical aspects, of *pathogenesis*.
[*]

pathogen (n)/pathogenic (adj)

Any organism that can cause *disease*, commonly restricted to fungi and micro-organisms such as yeasts, bacteria, and viruses.
[*]

pathogen-associated molecular pattern (PAMP)

Describing repetitive motifs of molecules, such as *lipopolysaccharide*, peptidoglycan, lipoteichoic acids, and mannans, that are widely expressed by microbial pathogens but are not present on *host* tissues.
Note: PAMPs are utilized by the *pattern recognition receptors* of the *immune system* to distinguish pathogens from *self-antigens*.
[ref. 3]

pathogenesis

Sequence of molecular and cellular mechanisms involved in the departure of an organism from its normal or *healthy* state, leading to the development of a *disease*.
[*]

pathognomonic

Denoting one or more *symptoms* or findings characteristic of, and unique to, a specific *disease*.
[*]

pathology (n)/pathological (adj)

1. Study of cause and effect of *disease* states.
2. Characteristic features of a disease state.
3. Medical discipline concerned with diagnosis of disease by the examination of body fluids, *tissues* and *organs*, as well as *postmortem* examination to determine cause of death.

[*]
Compare *pathobiology*.
See also *pathogenesis*.

pathway

1. (in biology) Sequence of *enzymatic* or other reactions by which one biological material is converted to another.
   [ref. 2]
2. (in toxicology) Sequence of enzymatic or other reactions by which an *adverse effect* is produced.
   [*]

See also *adverse outcome pathway*.

pathway perturbation

Alteration of a *toxicity pathway* that is large enough to change a normal biological process and produce an *adverse effect.*
[*]

pattern recognition receptor (PRR)

See *receptor, pattern recognition.*

pauci-immune

Referring to *vasculitis* characterized by relatively little deposition of *immunoglobulin* and *complement* factors, usually describing a form of *glomerulonephritis.*
[ref. 3]

paw-reaching test

staircase test
Test used to reveal motor deficits, usually of central origin, exhibited on the contralateral side by reduced ability of a test animal to extend the forelimb.
Note 1: Typically the paw-reaching test is performed with rodents in an apparatus resembling a staircase on which reward food pellets are placed on steps of increasing distance, or with larger animals reaching under a barrier for a reward.
Note 2: The paw-reaching test is often used to assess traumatic *brain* injury deficits or recovery.
[ref. 4]

peak daily average concentration of an air pollutant

See *maximum average daily concentration of an atmospheric pollutant.*

pedosphere

Part of the Earth made up of *soils* and where important soil processes are occurring.
[ref. 2]

pelagic (in ecology)

Designating, relating to, or inhabiting that region of the sea which consists of open water of any depth, away from or independent of both the shore and the sea floor (and so contrasted with the *littoral* and *benthic* regions).
[ref. 2]

pelvic kidney

ectopic kidney

Congenital abnormality in which a kidney develops and remains in the pelvic area.
Note: Pelvic kidney is generally asymptomatic but may produce complications.
[ref. 5]

pemphigus

pemphigus vulgaris

Rare, serious *autoimmune disease* marked by successive outbreaks of blisters, which appear suddenly and disappear, leaving pigmented spots.
Note: In pemphigus, other mucous membranes, as well as the skin, are usually affected and the disease may be fatal.
[ref. 3]

penetration (n)/penetrate (v) (in cell biology)

Action of entering or passing through a biological membrane.
[ref. 1]

peptide-binding groove

Structural feature found in *major histocompatibility complex class I* and *class II* heterodimeric proteins that can bind endogenous peptides.
[ref. 3]
See also *antigen-presenting groove*.

peptide tetramer

Structure consisting of four identical *major histocompatability complex (MHC)*-encoded peptides, presenting four binding sites for biotin attached to the tail of the MHC molecule, and held together by fluorescent streptavidin.
[ref. 3]

peptide vaccine

Preparation of an immunologically active peptide found in a *disease*-causing organism or substance, or any of their products, which is specially treated for use in *vaccination*.
[ref. 3]

per capita

In relation to the number of individuals; literally, by heads.
[*]

per capita birth rate (*b*)

See *birth rate, per capita*.

per capita death rate (*m*)

See *death rate, per capita*.

per capita rate of increase (*r*)

Relative increase, r, in the *population* per unit of time expressed *per capita*, thus $r = b - m$ where b is *per capita birth rate* and m is *per capita death rate*.
[ref. 2]

perceived environment

See *subjective environment*.

percutaneous

Through the skin.
[ref. 1]

perforin

Molecule produced by *cytotoxic T-cells* and *natural killer cells* that, like *complement* component C9, polymerizes to form a pore in the *membrane* of the *target cell* leading to cell death.
[ref. 3]

perfusion (in physiology)

Act of pouring over or through, especially the passage of a fluid through the vessels of a specific *organ.*
[ref. 1]
Note: Experiments with isolated organs require a continuous perfusion of the organ via blood vessels with *blood* or with oxygenated physiological fluid containing nutrients in order to maintain tissue viability.
[*]

periarteriolar lymphoid sheath (PALS)

Lymphoid tissue that forms the *white pulp* of the *spleen.*
[ref. 3]

pericardium

Serous membranous sac that surrounds the heart, consisting of an inner *visceral* layer (the *epicardium*), and an outer *parietal* pericardium that is attached to the sternum and *diaphragm.*
[ref. 5]

pericyte
perivascular cell
Rouget cell

Contractile cell that wraps around the abluminal surface of capillaries and venules.
Note: Pericytes and vascular smooth muscle cells together are called mural cells.
[*]

perinatal

Relating to the period shortly before and after *birth*, usually from the 20th to the 29th week of *gestation* to 1 to 4 weeks after birth.
[ref. 1]

perineum

Muscular structure of the lower pelvis, between the legs and extending from the anus to the *pubic symphysis*, or alternatively including the *anus* and *vagina* in the female and the region from the anus to the base of the *scrotum* in the male.
[ref. 5]

periodontitis

Inflammatory reaction of the tissues surrounding a tooth (periodontium), usually resulting from the extension of gingival *inflammation* (gingivitis) into the periodontium, and involving inflammation and *infection* of the ligaments and bones that support the teeth.
[ref. 3]

peripheral blood leukocyte (PBL)

See *leukocyte, peripheral blood.*

peripheral blood mononuclear cell (PBMC)

Monocyte produced by the *bone marrow* from *hematopoietic stem cell* precursors, circulating in the bloodstream for about one to three days before moving into tissues throughout the body.

Note: PBMCs constitute between 3 to 8 % of the *leukocytes* in the *blood*. In the tissues monocytes mature into different types of *macrophages* at different anatomical locations
[ref. 3]
See also *macrophage, resident(ial)*.

peripheral lymphoid organ

Any of the *lymphoid* organs other than the *thymus*.
[ref. 3]

peripheral nervous system (PNS)

One of the two major divisions of the *nervous system*, made up of the *nerves* and *ganglia* lying outside the *brain* and *spinal cord* that transmit sensory and motor signals to and from the *central nervous system*.
[ref. 4]

peripheral neuropathy

Neuropathy affecting *nerves* of the *peripheral nervous system*.
[ref. 4]

peripheral neuropathy, autoimmune

Acute or *chronic inflammatory neuropathy* leading to *demyelination* and *axonal* damage of *nerves* and *nerve roots* associated with high-*titere*d *autoantibodies* against *gangliosides* (*e.g., Guillain–Barré syndrome*, Miller–Fisher syndrome, acute sensory ataxic neuropathy).
[ref. 3]

peripheral tolerance

Specific immunological *tolerance* occurring outside of the *primary lymphoid organs*.
[ref. 3]

periphyton

Matrix of *algae*, microbes, and *detritus* attached to submerged surfaces in aquatic *ecosystems*.
[ref. 2]
See also *aufwuchs*.

peristalsis

Progression of a wave of smooth muscle contraction followed by relaxation along the length of a muscular tube.
Note: Typically occurring in the *gastrointestinal tract* and ureter.
[ref. 5]

peritoneal cavity

Potential space between the two layers (*visceral* and *parietal*) of the *peritoneum*.
[ref. 5]

peritoneal dialysis

Method of artificial *detoxication* in which a *toxic* substance from the body is transferred into liquid that is instilled into the *peritoneum*.

Note: Effectively, peritoneal dialysis represents the employment of the peritoneum as a dialyzing membrane for the purpose of removing *waste* products or *toxic* substances accumulated as a result of *renal* failure.
[ref. 1]

peritoneal membrane

See *peritoneum*.

peritoneum (n)/peritoneal (adj)

Thin double layer of *mesothelium* and irregular *connective tissue* that lines the *abdominal cavity* and covers most of the abdominal *organs*.
Note: The two layers of the peritoneum consist of the *parietal* peritoneum that lines the abdominal wall and the *visceral* peritoneum that covers the abdominal organs.
[ref. 5]
See also *peritoneal cavity*.

permeability

Ability to enter or pass through a porous material, such as a *cell membrane* or *epithelial* layer.
[*]

permeability coefficient, *P*

Quantity defining the permeability of molecules across a cell membrane and expressed as $P = k\mathrm{D}/\Delta x$ where K is the partition coefficient, D is the diffusion coefficient, and Δx is the thickness of the *cell membrane*.
[ref. 1]

permeable

Of a membrane, allowing a given substance to pass through.
Note: When applied to nonbiological membranes with no qualification, the term "permeable" normally refers to water.
[ref. 1]

permeation

Action of entering or passing through a *cell membrane*.
[ref. 1]

permissible exposure limit (PEL)

Recommendation by U.S. OSHA for a *time-weighted average concentration* that must not be exceeded during any 8-h work shift of a 40-h working week.
[ref. 1]

pernicious anemia

Disease in which the *erythrocytes* are abnormally formed, due to an inability of the GI-tract to absorb vitamin B12. True pernicious anemia refers specifically to a *disorder* of atrophied parietal cells leading to absent *intrinsic factor*, resulting in an inability to absorb vitamin B12.
Note 1: Pernicious anemia is the end stage of 10 to 15 % of cases of *autoimmune* gastritis.

Note 2: Pernicious anemia is associated with a variety of autoimmune endocrine diseases (*e.g., Hashimoto thyroiditis, Addison disease*, and autoimmune myasthenic *syndromes*).
[ref. 3]

peroxidase

Any enzyme (EC 1.11.1.x) catalyzing the reduction of peroxides, notably hydrogen peroxide and lipid peroxides.
Note: Peroxidase reactions serve to remove reactive peroxides from the cell, and may regenerate reduced *glutathione* from oxidized glutathione.
[*]
See also *reactive oxygen species*.

peroxisome

Organelle involved in the oxidation of long chain fatty acids, characterized by its content of *catalase* (EC 1.11.1.6), *peroxidase* (EC 1.11.1.7), and other oxidative *enzymes*.
[*]

persistence (n)/persistent (adj)

Attribute of a substance that describes the length of time that the substance remains in a particular environment before it is physically removed or chemically or biologically transformed.
[ref. 1]

persistent inorganic pollutant (PIP)

Inorganic substance that is stable in the *environment*, is liable to long-range transport, may *bioaccumulate* in human and animal *tissue*, and may have significant impacts on human *health* and the environment.
Examples: Arsenides, fluorides, cadmium salts, mercury/methylmercury and lead salts.
Note: Some inorganic chemicals, like crocidolite asbestos, are persistent in almost all circumstances, but others, like metal sulfides, are persistent only in unreactive environments; sulfides can be converted to hydrogen sulfide in a reducing environment or sulfates and sulfuric acid in oxidizing environments. Thus, as with organic substances, persistence of PIPs is a function of *chemical speciation*.
[ref. 1]
See also *persistent organic pollutant*.

persistent organic pollutant (POP)

Organic chemical that is stable in the *environment*, is liable to long-range transport, may *bioaccumulate* in human and animal tissue, and may have significant impacts on human health and the environment.
Examples: Dioxins, polychlorinated biphenyls, dichlorodiphenyltrichloroethane, tributyltin oxide.
Note: The Stockholm Convention on Persistent Organic Pollutants was adopted at a Conference of Plenipotentiaries held in 2001 in Stockholm, Sweden; by signing this convention, governments have agreed to take measures to eliminate or reduce the release of POPs into the environment.
[ref. 1]
See also *persistent inorganic pollutant*.

person-time

Measurement based on summing number of individuals multiplied by the time each is exposed or at *risk*, used as the denominator in *incidence* and *mortality rate* calculations.
[*]

personal monitoring

Type of *environmental monitoring* in which an individual's *exposure* to a substance is measured and evaluated.
Note: Personal monitoring is normally carried out using a *personal sampler*.
[ref. 1]

personal protective device (PPD)
individual protective device (IPD)
personal protective equipment (PPE)

Equipment (clothing, gloves, hard hat, respirator, *etc.*) worn by an individual to prevent *exposure* to a potentially *toxic* substance.
[ref. 1]

personal sampler
individual sampler

Compact, portable instrument for individual air sampling, measuring, or both, the content of a harmful substance in the respiration zone of a working person.
[ref. 1]
See also *passive sampler*.

perspire (v)

See *sweat*.

perspiration (n)

See *sweat*.

pest

Organism that may harm public *health*, attacks food and other materials essential to mankind, or otherwise affects human beings adversely.
[ref. 1]

pesticide

Substance intended to kill pests.
Note: In common usage, any substance used for controlling, preventing, or destroying animal, microbiological, or plant pests.
[ref. 1]

pesticide, botanical

Substance with lethal activity against *pests*, that is produced naturally within a plant and may act as a defense against *predators*.
[After ref. 1]
See also *pesticide*.

pesticide residue

Any substance or *mixture* of substances found in humans or animals or in food and water following use of a *pesticide*, including any specified derivatives, such as *degradation* and conversion products, *metabolites*, reaction products, and impurities considered to be of *toxicological* significance.
[ref. 1]

pexophagy

Autophagy selective for *degradation* of *peroxisomes*: pexophagy may be subdivided into macropexophagy and micropexophagy.
[ref. 3]

Peyer's patch

Part of the *gut-associated lymphoid tissue* and found as distinct lymphoid nodules, mainly in the small intestine.
[ref. 3]

phage antibody library

Collection of *cloned antibody variable (V) region* gene sequences that can be expressed as *Fab* or scFv fusion proteins with bacteriophage coat proteins. These can be displayed on the surface of the phages. The gene encoding a recombinant *monoclonal antibody* is enclosed in the phage particle and can be selected from the library by binding of the phage to specific *antigen*.
[ref. 3]

phage display

Method that enables the presentation of large peptide libraries on the surface of bacterial virus (phage) particles, from which proteins with desired functional properties can be selected rapidly.
[ref. 5]

phage display library

See *phage antibody library*.

phagocyte (n)/phagocytic (adj)

Cell, especially of *monocyte/macrophage* or *neutrophil* lineage, that is specialized for the engulfment of cellular and particulate matter.
Note: Phagocytes play an important role in removing particles from tissues, *e.g.*, in the lower airways.
[After ref. 3]

phagocytic activity assay
phagocytosis assay

Method of quantifying *phagocytosis* in which yeast cells, stained with May-Grünwald Giemsa stain, are incubated with *macrophages*, and subsequently, after a fixed time, yeast cells engulfed in the *macrophages* are counted.
[ref. 3]

phagocytosis (n)/phagocytose (v)

Process by which particulate material is endocytosed by a cell.
[ref. 1]
See also *endocytosis; pinocytosis.*

phagocytosis assay

See *phagocytic activity assay*.

phagolysosome

Intracellular vacuole where killing and digestion of *phagocytosed* material occurs following the fusion of a *phagosome* with a *lysosome*.
[ref. 3]

phagosome

Intracellular vacuole produced following invagination of the cell membrane around phagocytosed material.
[ref. 3]
See also *phagocytosis*.

phantom risk

See *risk, phantom.*

pharmaceutical

Drug with *medicinal* properties.
[ref. 1]

pharmacodynamics

Process of interaction of *pharmacologically* active substances with *target* sites in living systems, and the biochemical and physiological consequences leading to *therapeutic* or *adverse effects*.
[ref. 1]
See also *therapeutic index*.

pharmacogenetics

Study of the influence of *genetic* factors on the effects of *drugs* on individual organisms.
[ref. 1]
Note: *Genetic polymorphisms* of *biotransformation enzymes* and of *receptor* targets may affect the *therapeutic* efficiency and *toxicity* of a *drug*/compound in an individual.
[*]

pharmacogenomics

Methods and science permitting identification of the *genes* that influence individual variation in the efficacy or *toxicity* of *therapeutic* agents, and the application of this information in clinical practice.
[ref. 1]

pharmacokinetics

1. Process of the *uptake* of *drugs* by the body, the *biotransformation* they undergo, the *distribution* of the drugs and their *metabolites* in the *tissues*, and the *elimination* of the drugs and their metabolites from the body.
2. Study of such processes.

[ref. 1]

pharmacology (n)/**pharmacological** (adj)

Science of the use and *effects* of *drugs*: it may be subdivided into *pharmacokinetics* and *pharmacodynamics*.
[ref. 1]

pharyngeal groove

One of several paired grooves in the *embryonic endoderm,* lateral to the corresponding *pharyngeal pouch* in the *ectoderm.*
[ref. 5]

pharyngeal pouch
branchial pouch

One of several paired evaginations in the *embryonic endoderm* that develop into *epithelial* tissues and organs such as the *thymus* and *thyroid gland.*
[ref. 5]

pharynx (n)/**pharyngeal** (adj)

Part of the digestive tube lying between the esophagus below, and the mouth and *nasal cavity* above and anterior.
Note: The pharynx is subdivided into the nasopharynx lying at the base of the nasal cavity, the oropharynx behind the mouth, and the laryngopharynx posterior to the larynx.
[ref. 5]

phase (in toxicology)

In clinical trials: See *clinical trial.*
In xenobiotic metabolism: *See phase I reaction of biotransformation; phase II reaction of biotransformation; phase III reaction of biotransformation.*

phase I reaction of biotransformation

Enzymatic modification of a substance by oxidation, reduction, hydrolysis, hydration, dehydrochlorination, or other reactions catalyzed by *enzymes* of the cytosol, of the *endoplasmic reticulum* (microsomal enzymes), or of other cell *organelles.*
[ref. 1]
See also *cytochrome P450.*

phase II reaction of biotransformation

Enzyme-catalyzed binding of a substance, or its *metabolites* from a *phase I reaction,* to an *endogenous* molecule (*conjugation*), making more water-soluble derivatives that may be excreted in the urine or *bile.*
Note: Phase II reactions include glucuronidation, sulfation, acetylation, amino acid (*e.g.*, glycine) binding, and *glutathione* conjugation.
[After ref. 1]
See also *"covalent binding".*

phase III reaction of biotransformation

Further *metabolism of conjugated metabolites* produced by *phase II reactions of biotransformation.*
[ref. 1]

phenology

Life history.
[ref. 2]

phenome

Complete *phenotypic* description of an organism (by analogy with *genome*).
[ref. 1]

phenotype (n)/phenotypic (adj)

Observable characteristics or traits of an organism, including those at a biochemical level, resulting from interaction of its *genotype* with *epigenetic* and *environmental* factors.
[ref. 5]

phenylketonuria (PKU)

Autosomal recessive disorder resulting from *mutations* that impair the function of the enzyme phenylalanine 4-monooxygenase (EC 1.14.16.1).
Note 1: The resulting failure of phenylalanine metabolism in the liver leads to its accumulation, causing intellectual disability, *seizures*, and other neurological disorders in untreated individuals with PKU.
Note 2: Excess phenylalanine accumulating in PKU is metabolized to phenyl pyruvate (2-oxo-3-phenylpropanoic acid, or "phenylketone") that is detected in the urine and is used for screening newborns.
[ref. 5]

pheochromocytoma

Tumor of the *chromaffin cells* of the *adrenal medulla* that results in excessive secretion of *norepinephrine* and other *catecholamines*, causing a severe rise in blood pressure.
[After ref. 4]

pheromone

Substance used in olfactory communication between organisms of the same species, eliciting a change in sexual or social behavior.
[ref. 1]
See also *ectohormone*.

Philadelphia chromosome

Chromosome resulting from a *reciprocal translocation* between human chromosomes 9 and 22, most commonly associated with *chronic myelogenous leukemia*.
[ref. 3]
See also *ABL oncogene*.

philtrum

Groove in the midline of the upper lip below the nose.
[ref. 5]

phocomelia

Congenital abnormality in which one or more of the hands or feet is attached to an underdeveloped limb, and therefore too close to the body.
Note: Phocomelia is a very rare *disorder* and is associated with prenatal exposure to *thalidomide*.
[ref. 5]

phonophobia

Abnormal fear of, or *sensitivity* to, loud sound, or occasionally of voices.
[After ref. 4]

phorbol 13-acetate 12-myristate

tetradecanoyl phorbol acetate (TPA)

Mitogenic phorbol ester that directly stimulates *protein kinase C* and acts as a *tumor promoter*.
Note: Commonly referred to less correctly as phorbol 12-myristate 13-acetate and abbreveviated PMA.
[ref. 3]

phospholipase Cγ (PLC-γ)

Enzyme (EC 3.4.1.11) that cleaves phosphatidylinositol bisphosphate into diacylglycerol and inositol trisphosphate, leading to the activation of two major cell signaling pathways.
Note: One consequence of PLC-γ signaling is *B*- and *T-lymphocyte activation*.
[ref. 3]

photoallergy

Type IV hypersensitivity reaction in which photoactivation of a substance produces a *hapten* that then acts as a *sensitizer*.
[ref. 3]

photochemical smog

summer smog

Mixture of highly reactive and *toxic* substances, including ozone, produced by the action of sunlight on hydrocarbons, nitrogen oxides, and other *pollutant*s.
[ref. 2]

photocontact dermatitis

See *dermatitis, photocontact.*

photodegradation

Any breakdown reaction of a chemical that is initiated by sunlight (UV light), or more accurately, by the influence of a high-energy photon.
Note: Photodegradation can be either i) direct, in which the photon photolyzes or ionizes the target molecule itself, which then may react with other molecules in its vicinity, or ii) indirect, in which the relevant molecule reacts with ions or radicals created by *photolysis* of other molecules.
[ref. 2]
See also *degradation; indirect photolysis; photolysis.*

photo-induced toxicity

Toxicity of a chemical in the presence of light due to the production of toxic *photolysis* products.
[ref. 2]

photoirritation

phototoxicity

Reaction of the skin, often inflammatory, induced by light in the presence of a substance.
Note 1: Photoirritation may be a consequence of photoreactivity of the substance converting it to a *species* that reacts with biomolecules in the skin, or alternatively may result from changes in *metabolic* pathways in the skin following exposure to light.
Note 2: Photoirritation is induced by contact with some plants (*e.g.*, giant hogweed), various cosmetics, and some *drugs* (*e.g.*, tetracyclines).
[*]

photolysis

Cleavage of one or more *covalent bonds* in a molecule resulting from *absorption* of light, or a photochemical process in which such cleavage is an essential part.
[ref. 1]

photooxidation

Oxidation reaction induced by light.
Note 1: Common photooxidation processes are:

1. Loss of one or more electrons from a chemical *species* as a result of photoexcitation of that species.
2. Reaction of a substance with oxygen under the influence of ultraviolet, visible, or infrared light.

Note 2: When oxygen remains in the product, this latter process is also called photooxygenation. Reactions in which neither the substrate nor the oxygen are electronically excited (*i.e.*, photosensitized oxidations) are sometimes called photoinitiated oxidations.
[ref. 1]
Note 3: Photooxidation of outdoor air contaminants is a major mechanism in the formation of *photochemical smog*.
[*]

photophobia

Abnormal visual intolerance of light.
[ref. 1]
Note: Photophobia often occurs in connection with a *migraine* attack or a febrile *infection*, but there are many other causes.
[*]

photoperiod

Cycle of illumination and darkness over a 24-h day.
[After ref. 2]

photoreceptor cell

Specialized *neuron* found in the *retina*, involved in detecting light and transducing the signals (see *signal transduction*) of vision.
Note: The two main types of photoreceptor cells are rod cells, responsible for vision at low light intensities, and cone cells, responsible for colour and high acuity vision at higher light intensities.
[ref. 4]

photosensitivity

Abnormal erythematous reaction of the skin to sunlight.
Note: Possible causes of photosensitivity are an inherited skin sensitivity, photoxicity, photoallergy, or one of a number of *diseases* such as *systemic autoimmune diseases* (*e.g., systemic lupus erythematosus, mixed connective tissue disease*).
[ref. 3]

phototoxicity test

Procedure used to identify the phototoxic potential of a test substance. The substance is administered either *systemically* or *topically* on the skin, and light is subsequently shone on the skin to photoexcite the substance.
Note: There is an *in vitro* phototoxicity test using photoexposure of treated Balb c/3T3 cells followed by measurement of *cell viability*.
[ref. 3]

phylogenetic tree

See *cladogram*.

phylogenetics

Branch of biology that deals with *phylogeny*, especially with the deduction of the historical relationships between groups of organisms.
[ref. 2]
See also *cladistics; systematics*.

phylogeny
phylogenesis

Pattern of historical relationships between *species* or other groups resulting from divergence during evolution.
Note 1: Phylogenetic relationships are shown in diagrams such as *cladograms, phylogenetic trees,* and *evolutionary trees*.
Note 2: *Paleontology* is important for understanding phylogeny. Without the *fossils* of the many groups of organisms now extinct, it could not be understood how present life forms are interrelated.
Note 3: Phylogenetics, the science of phylogeny, is part of the larger field of *systematics,* also including *taxonomy*.
[ref. 2]
See also *cladogram; phylogenetics*.

phylum

Taxonomic rank at the level below Kingdom and above Class.
Note: Formally, the term phylum can be used for any biological *species*, but traditionally it was used for animals, whereas "division" was often used for other species such as plants and fungi.
[After ref. 2]

physical map (in genetics)

Map showing how much *DNA*, measured in base pairs, separates two *genes*.
Note: The physical map is not to be confused with a genetic map which shows the position of genes in relation to each other, based on the frequency of cross-over events.
[ref. 1]

physiological adaptation

See *adaptation.*

physiological availability

See *bioavailability.*

physiological pharmacokinetic model

See *physiologically based pharmacokinetic modeling.*

physiologically based pharmacokinetic (PBPK) modeling

toxicologically based pharmacokinetic modeling

Mathematical *modeling* of *kinetic* behavior of a substance in an organism, based on measured physiological parameters and *concentration* measurements of the substance and its *metabolites.*
Note 1: Physiological parameters used in PBPK modeling include rates of *absorption,* dynamics of *blood* flow in respective organs, and *biotransformation* patterns.
Note 2: PBPK models subdivide the organism into *compartments.*
[*]

phytochelatin

Class of cysteine-rich peptides in plants that are induced by and bind to some metals, and can function in the regulation and *detoxification* of metals by plants.
[ref. 2]
See also *metallothionein-like protein.*

phytoestrogen

Non*steroidal* natural product from a plant that, because of a structural similarity to 17β-*estradiol* can exert mild *estrogenic* effects, or antagonize them.
Examples: Isoflavones, coumestans.
Note: Phytoestrogens are sometimes called "dietary estrogens" and foods containing them are often promoted as beneficial, although there is insufficient evidence of their *medical* benefits.
[After ref. 5]

phytohemagglutinin (PHA)

Plant *lectin* that acts as a *T-cell mitogen.*
[ref. 3]

phytoplankton

Photosynthesizing organisms found in the *plankton.*
[ref. 2]

phytotoxic

Toxic to plants.
[ref. 2]

pia

pia mater

Innermost of three membranous layers, together composing the meninges (see *meninx*), that surrounds and adheres to the *brain* and *spinal cord.*
[ref. 4]

piebaldism (n)/**piebald** (adj)

Patchy absence of pigmentation of the hair or skin or, depending on the *species*, of feathers, scales, or other body surfaces.
[ref. 5]

Pielou's *J*

Pielou's J evenness

Measure of *species evenness* for a sample from a *community*, calculated as $J = H'/\ln S$ where H' is the *Shannon–Wiener* diversity measure of the community and S is its average *species richness*.
[After ref. 2]

pineal gland

epiphysis

Pea-sized conical mass of tissue behind the third *ventricle* of the *brain*, secreting the *hormone*-like substance melatonin (*N*-[2-(5-methoxy-1*H*-indol-3-yl)ethyl]acetamide) in some mammals.
[ref. 4]

pinna

1. Externally visible portion of the ear.
   See also *auricle*.
2. Feather or fin.

[ref. 5]

pinnipeds

Seals, sea lions, and walruses.
[ref. 2]

pinocytosis

Type of *endocytosis* in which soluble material is taken up by the *cell* in a liquid phase and incorporated into *vesicles*.
[ref. 3]

piscicide

Substance intended to kill fish.
[ref. 1]

piscivorous

Feeding on fish.
[ref. 2]

pituitary

hypophysis
pituitary gland

Small *endocrine gland* sitting in a bony *cavity* (the *sella turcica*) at the base of the *brain* and connected to the *hypothalamus*.
Note 1: The pituitary is structurally and functionally divided into anterior and posterior lobes. The anterior lobe secretes *growth hormone* (*somatotropin*), *thyroid-stimulating hormone, adrenocortocotropic hormone, prolactin, luteinizing hormone*, and

follicle-stimulating hormone. The posterior lobe develops from the hypothalamus and secretes *oxytocin* and *antidiuretic hormone* (also called arginine *vasopressin*). An intermediate lobe (indistinct in humans) secretes melanocyte-stimulating hormone (MSH).
[ref. 4]
Note 2: The pituitary is a major structure through which the brain influences various *somatic* functions.
[*]

pivotal study

Key study used in the decision making process for *drug* approval, usually in phase III *clinical trials* and of a *randomized control trial* design.
[*]
See also *critical study*.

placebo

Substance or procedure that has no *therapeutic* effect, but is used as a control in testing new *drugs*.
[*]

placenta (n)/placental (adj)

Organ of exchange of nutrients and waste products between mother and *fetus*, having parts derived from both.
[ref. 5]
See also *placental barrier*.

placental barrier

See *barrier, placental*.

placental circulation

Circulation of *blood* through the *placenta* during *intrauterine* life, serving the needs of the *fetus* for oxygenation, nutrition, and elimination of waste.
[ref. 5]

placental insufficiency

Inadequate *blood* flow through the *placenta* to maintain the needs of the *fetus* for oxygenation and metabolic balance.
[ref. 5]
See also *placental circulation*.

placental membrane

See *barrier, placental*.

placental transfer

Delivery of substances from the maternal circulation to the *fetus*, across the *placental barrier*.
[ref. 5]

placentation

1. Formation of a *placenta* in the *uterus*.
2. Arrangement of ovules within the pistil of a plant.

[After ref. 1]

planktivorous

Feeding on *plankton.*
[ref. 2]

plankton

Organisms living suspended in the water column and incapable of moving against water currents.
[ref. 2]

planktotrophic larva

Developmental stage of an organism between the ovum and the juvenile that must, during that stage, feed on *plankton.*
[*]

plantibody

Animal *antibody* (or fragment thereof), expressed in a genetically modified plant.
[ref. 3]
See also *geneticaly modified organism.*

plaque assay

See *anti-sheep red blood cell IgM response assay.*

plaque-forming cell (PFC)

Antibody-secreting *plasma cell* detected *in vitro* by its ability to produce a "plaque" of lysed *antigen*-sensitized *erythrocytes* in the presence of *complement.*
[ref. 3]
See also *plaque assay.*

plasma (in biology)

1. Fluid component of *blood*, containing salts, *antibodies*, clotting factors, other proteins and *metabolites*, in which the blood cells and *platelets* are suspended. Compare *serum.*
2. Fluid component of *semen* produced by the *accessory sex glands*, such as the *seminal vesicles*, the *prostate*, and the *bulbourethral glands.*
3. *Cell* substance outside the *nucleus* (*i.e.*, the *cytoplasm*).

[ref. 1]

plasmablast

Highly proliferative *cell* that is a developmental intermediate between small *B-lymphocytes* and *immunoglobulin*-secreting mature *plasma cells.*
[ref. 3]

plasma cell

Terminally differentiated *B-lymphocyte*, with little or no capacity for *mitotic* division, that actively *secretes* large amounts of *antibody.*
Note: Plasma cells have eccentric nuclei, abundant *cytoplasm*, and distinct perinuclear haloes. Their cytoplasm contains dense rough *endoplasmic reticulum* and a large Golgi complex.
[ref. 3]

plasmacytoid dendritic cell

See *dendritic cell, plasmacytoid.*

plasmacytoma

Mass of *neoplastic monoclonal plasma cells* growing in bone or soft tissue.
[ref. 3]

plasma exchange

See *plasmapheresis.*

plasma half-life

See *elimination half-life.*

plasma membrane

cell membrane
External *membrane* of a *cell*, delimiting its *cytoplasm.*
[*]

plasmapheresis

plasma exchange
Technique of extracorporeal separation of *blood cells* from *plasma*, with return of the cells to the patient.
Note: Plasmapheresis is used to remove *antibodies* in *autoimmune disease* and to remove *toxic* substances or *metabolites* in some cases of severe *intoxication.*
[After ref. 3]

plasmid

Autonomous self-replicating extra-*chromosomal* circular *DNA* molecule present in bacteria and yeast.
Note 1: Plasmids replicate autonomously each time a bacterium divides, and are transmitted to the daughter cells.
Note 2: DNA segments are commonly cloned using plasmid *vectors.*
[ref. 1]

platelet

thrombocyte
Small irregular or disc-shaped cell found in large numbers in mammalian *blood*, essential for blood clotting.
[ref. 3]

platelet-activating factor (PAF)

Alkyl phospholipid, released by a variety of cell types (including *mast cells, endothelium* and *basophils*), that has immunoregulatory effects on *lymphocytes* and *monocytes/macrophages*, can cause *platelet* aggregation and *degranulation,* activates the *respiratory burst*, and functions as a mediator in *sepsis*, shock, and *bronchoconstriction.*
[After ref. 3]

platelet-derived growth factor (PDGF)

Protein synthesized by *platelets* that is released into the *serum* during *blood* clotting.
Note: PDGF is a major *growth factor* in human *serum* and is a potent *mitogen* for *connective tissue* and *glial cells.*
[ref. 3]

pleiotropism (n)/**pleiotropic** (adj)

1. Having more than one effect.
2. Relating to a *gene, expression* of which gives rise to multiple *phenotypic* traits.

[ref. 5]

pleura (n)/**pleural** (adj)

Each of a pair of *serous membranes* lining the *thorax* and enveloping the lungs in humans and other mammals.
Note: The pleural membrane covering the lungs and extending into the fissures of the lobes is called the *visceral* pleura and lacks a *nerve* supply. That lining the chest *cavity, mediastinum* and *diaphragm* is called the *parietal* pleura; it is innervated and sensitive to *pain*.
[ref. 5]

pleural cavity

Potential space between the *pleural* membranes lining the chest *cavity* (*parietal* pleura) and covering the lungs (*visceral* pleura).
Note: In pathological conditions, fluid may accumulate in the pleural cavity, between the visceral and parietal pleura.
[ref. 5]

plexus

Network of interconnecting *nerves*, blood vessels or *lymphatic* vessels.
[ref. 4]
See also *ganglion*.

ploidy

Number of *haploid* sets of *chromosome*s in a *cell*.
[ref. 5]

plumbism

saturnism
Chronic poisoning caused by *absorption* of lead or lead salts.
[ref. 1]

pluripotent

Able to *differentiate* into a variety of *cell* types.
Examples: The *ovum, embryonic stem cells*.
[ref. 5]

pluripotent stem cell

See *stem cell, pluripotent*.

pneumoconiosis

Usually fibrosis of the lungs that develops owing to (prolonged) inhalation of inorganic or organic dusts.
Note: Cause-specific types of pneumoconiosis include *anthracosis* (from coal dust), *asbestosis* (from asbestos dust), *byssinosis* (from cotton dust), *siderosis* (from iron dust, although the term siderosis can also refer more generally to deposition of iron in any tissue), *silicosis* (from silica dust), and stannosis (from tin dust).
[After ref. 1]

pneumonitis

Inflammation of the lung.
[ref. 1]

pneumonitis, hypersensitivity (HPS)

extrinsic allergic alveolitis
Immune-mediated *inflammatory disease* of the lung *parenchymal cells* caused by exposure to an inhaled chemical *allergen* or organic *dust*.
[ref. 3]
See also *pneumonitis*.

pneumotaxic center

pontine respiratory group
Neural network in the *brainstem* involved in regulating respiration.
[ref. 4]

poikilotherm (n)/poikilothermal (adj)/poikilothermic

Organism whose internal temperature is not constant but varies with the ambient *environmental* temperature.
[*]
See also *ectotherm; endotherm; heterotherm; homeotherm*.

poikilothermy

Absence of regulation of the internal body temperature of an organism allowing temperature variation that reflects the ambient *environmental* temperature.
[*]
See also *ectothermy; endothermy; heterothermy; homeothermy*.

point mutation

See *mutation, point*.

point source

Single *emission* source in a defined location.
[ref. 1]

poison (n)/poisonous (adj)

Substance that, taken into or formed within the organism, impairs the *health* of the organism and may kill it.
[ref. 1]

poison-bearing

Containing a *poison*.
[ref. 1]

poisoning

intoxication
Morbid condition produced by a *poison*.
[ref. 1]

pokeweed mitogen (PWM)

Plant *lectin* that is a *T-cell*-dependent *B-cell mitogen*.
[ref. 3]

polarization

See *membrane polarization*.

polarized cell

See *cell polarity*.

pollen

Male *microgametophytes* of seed plants that produce *sperm*.
Note: Many airborne pollens are strong *allergens*.
[*]

pollenosis

See *hay fever*.

pollutant

Any undesirable substance occurring, often as a result of human activities, in the *environment* and capable of causing adverse effects.
Note 1: Undesirability of a pollutant, like *toxicity*, is *concentration*-dependent, low concentrations of some substances being tolerable or even essential in some cases.
Note 2: A primary pollutant is one emitted directly into the atmosphere, water, *sediments*, or *soil* from an identifiable source.
Note 3: A secondary pollutant is a pollutant formed by chemical reaction in the atmosphere, water, sediments, or soil.
Note 4: "Pollutant" should be distinguished from *contaminant*, the latter implying presence above background, usually in a technical or agricultural product.
[After ref. 2]

pollution

Introduction and (or) presence of *pollutants* in an *environment*, or any undesirable modification of the composition of an environmental *medium*.
[*]

pollution-induced community tolerance (PICT)

Increase in tolerance to *pollution* resulting from a shift *species* composition of a *community, acclimatization* of individuals, or genetic changes in *populations* in the community.
[ref. 2]

pollution tolerance index (PTI)

See *tolerance index, pollution*.

poly I:C

Double stranded polymer consisting of hydrogen-bonded chains of poly(inosinic acid) and poly(cytidylic acid), that acts as a synthetic *immunostimulant* by mimicking viral double-stranded *RNA*.
[ref. 3]
See also *polyICLC*.

poly ICLC

Complex of poly(**i**nosinic acid):poly(**c**ytidylic acid) [*poly I:C*], poly(L-**l**ysine), and (**c**arboxymethyl)cellulose (letter roots of the acronym underlined), that acts as a synthetic *immunostimulant* by mimicking viral double-stranded *RNA*.
[ref. 3]

poly-Ig receptor

See *receptor, poly-Ig*.

polyarteritis nodosa

disseminated necrotizing periarteritis
panarteritis
periarteritis
periarteritis nodosa
Systemic *disease* characterized by widespread *inflammation* of small and medium-sized arteries in which many of the foci are nodular.
[ref. 3]

polyclonal

Many different *clones*, or the product of many different clones, *e.g.*, polyclonal *antiserum*.
[ref. 3]

polyclonal activator

Substance that induces *activation* of multiple clones of *B-lymphocytes* or *T-lymphocytes*.
[ref. 3]
See also *mitogen*.

polyclonal antibody

See *antibody, polyclonal*.

polycystic

Composed of, or having, many *cysts*.
[After ref. 5]

polycythemia

Abnormal increase in the number concentration of *erythrocytes* in *blood*.
Note 1: Polycythemia may result from a reduction of plasma volume or an increase in red cell number.
Note 2: Polycythemia may cause respiratory or circulatory *diseases*, may be associated with *cancer*, or may reflect *toxicity* or another disease process.
[*]

polydactyly

Congenital occurrence of *supernumerary* fingers or toes.
[ref. 5]

polydendrocyte

See *NG2 cell*.

polydipsia

Chronic excessive thirst that may be *symptomatic* of *disease* (*e.g.*, *diabetes*) or may be a behavioral *disorder*.
[*]

polyendocrinopathy, autoimmune

Autoimmune disease affecting multiple endocrine organs.
Note: Autoimmune polyendocrinopathy includes two types of polyglandular *syndromes*:

(i) Autoimmune polyglandular syndrome type 1 is characterized by mucocutaneous candidiasis in association with endocrine manifestation (also called APECED syndrome, autoimmune polyendocrinopathy-candidiasis-ectodermal dystrophy).
(ii) Autoimmune polyglandular syndrome type 2 exhibits any combination of adrenal insufficiency (see *Addison disease*), *diabetes mellitus type 1*, lymphocytic thyroiditis (see *thyroiditis, autoimmune*), *hypoparathyroidism*, and gonadal failure.

In both types, organ-specific *autoantibodies* against a variety of *endocrine glands* are detectable.
[ref. 3]

polygenic control

Control of a *phenotypic* trait by several *genes*.
[ref. 2]

polymerase chain reaction (PCR)

Technique by which specific *DNA* segments are amplified selectively using *cycles* of annealing, chain extension, and thermal dissociation.
[ref. 1]

polymorphism (n)/polymorphic (adj)

1. Occurrence of a *gene* in more than one distinct nucleotide sequence in a *population*, resulting from *mutation*(s) and potentially producing *gene products* with different levels of function.
   Note 1: It is sometimes considered that the least frequent of polymorphic gene sequences should be present in at least 1% of the population; otherwise the variant is a *mutation* rather than a polymorphism.
   Note 2: Polymorphisms of *drug* metabolizing *enzymes* are common, causing interindividual differences in drug metabolism, sometimes leading to enhanced side effects, idiosyncratic drug toxicity (see *idiosyncratic drug reaction*), or differences in clinical effects (as in variation in *metabolism* of *steroid hormones*).
2. Occurrence of different *phenotypes* of a single trait.

After [3,5]

polymorphism, genetic

Existence of inter-individual differences in *DNA* sequences coding for one specific *gene*, giving rise to different functional and (or) *morphological* traits.
[ref. 1]
Note 1: Genetic polymorphism may be a cause of rare and serious *diseases*, as well as of common *metabolic* variations (*e.g.*, in lipid metabolism).

Note 2: Genetic polymorphism of *cytochrome P448* and *cytochrome P450* enzymes is a cause for interindividual differences of *biotransformation* rates and *toxicokinetics*.
[*]

polymorphonuclear granulocyte

See *leukocyte, polymorphonuclear*.

polymorphonuclear leukocyte

See *leukocyte, polymorphonuclear*.

polymyositis

Disorder characterized by *inflammation* and degeneration of skeletal muscle, causing *pain*, weakness, and wasting in affected (usually proximal) muscles.
[ref. 3]

polyneuritis

Inflammation of several *peripheral nerves* simultaneously.
[ref. 4]

polyneuropathy

Neuropathy (distal *axonopathy*) of the *peripheral nervous system*, often affecting the extremities in a bilateral distribution, and characterized by numbness, tingling, and *paresthesia*.
Note: Polyneuropathy may be caused by *infections* or *toxic substances* (notably alcohol *abuse*), may be associated with *chronic diseases* such as *diabetes*, or may be *idiopathic*.
[ref. 4]

polyploidy

Occurrence of more than two complete sets of *chromosomes*.
[ref. 5]
See also *ploidy*.

polyuria

Excessive production and discharge of urine.
[ref. 1]

pontine respiratory group

See *pneumotaxic center*.

poor metabolizer

Individual, in whom *biotransformation* of a certain *drug* or *xenobiotic* is considerably slower than in the average population, usually as a consequence of *polymorphism* of a *drug metabolizing enzyme* such as an isoform of *cytochrome P448* or *P450*.
Note: Individuals classifiable as poor metabolizers must be identified before prescription of the *pharmaceuticals* that they metabolize poorly, in order to prevent *adverse effects* of overdose.
[*]
See also *polymorphism*.

popliteal lymph node assay (PLNA)

Test for immunosensitization (see *immunosensitizer*) measuring popliteal *lymph node hyperplasia* after subcutaneous injection of a test substance into the footpad of the hindpaw of a rodent.
[ref. 3]

population

1. (in epidemiology) Assemblage of individuals with defined characteristics. Note: A clearly defined part of a population is called a subpopulation. The term "population segment" is sometimes used as a synonym for subpopulation.
2. (in ecology) Any group of interacting and interbreeding organisms of the same *species* occupying a given area at the same time.

[1,2]

population at risk

Group of individuals who are liable to develop an adverse *health* effect when *exposed* to a substance causing such an effect.
Note: People already having chronic *disease* are often excluded when designing studies to determine populations at risk.
[*]

population biomass

Total mass of organisms in a *population, i.e.*, the sum of the masses of all the individual members of the population.
[After ref. 2]

population critical concentration (PCC)

Concentration of a substance in the *critical organ* at which a specified percentage of an *exposed population* has reached the individual *critical organ concentration.*
Note: The PCC percentage is indicated by, *e.g.*, PCC-10 for 10 %, similar to the convention used with the term LD_{50}.
[ref. 1]

population cycle

Oscillation in the number of individuals in a *population* between periods of high and low *population density*.
[After ref. 2]

population density (PD)

Number of individuals in a *population* divided by the area (m^2) or volume (m^3) it inhabits.
[After ref. 2]

population dynamics

Variations in time and space in the sizes, composition, and densities of *populations*.
[ref. 2]

population ecology

Study of the nature of and factors determining *population dynamics*.
[*]

population effect

Absolute number or *incidence* rate of cases occurring in a group of people.
[ref. 1]

population fluctuation

Variations over time in the number of individuals of a *population.*
[ref. 2]

population growth rate

Change in number of individuals in a *population,* ΔN, during a specified time period, Δt, given by the equation

$$\Delta N/\Delta t = (b - d)N$$

where N is the number of individuals, b is *per capita birth rate*, and d is *per capita death rate.*
[ref. 2]
See also *per capita rate of increase.*

population pyramid

Diagrammatic illustration of the age structure of a *population* by depicting the youngest age class at the base and stacking successive age classes above it.
[ref. 2]
Note 1: The depiction of a "population pyramid" is in reality often a triangle with its apex at the top (△) if the number of individuals decreases progressively with age.
Note 2: If the birth rate declines in a given population, and older individuals accumulate, the population pyramid may more resemble a triangle with its base at the top (▽) and is referred to as an "inverted triangle (pyramid)".
[*]

population risk

See *risk, societal.*

population size

Total number of organisms in a *population.*
[ref. 1]

pore water

See *interstitial water.*

porencephaly

Occurrence of a *cyst* in the substance of the *brain* that usually communicates with one of the lateral *ventricles.*
Note: The abnormal porencephalic cavities may result either from brain tissue destruction or from abnormal brain development.
[ref. 5]

porous pot test

Procedure to evaluate *biodegradation* by simulating a continuous *activated sludge* (sewage treatment) system.
[After ref. 2]

porphin(e)

Molecular skeleton of four pyrrole nuclei united through the α-positions by four methine groups to form a macrocyclic structure; parent compound of *porphyrins*.
[*]

porphyria

One of a group of hereditary *diseases* resulting from a disturbance of *porphyrin metabolism*, characterized by increased formation, accumulation, and excretion of porphyrins and their precursors.
Note: Acute porphyria can be triggered by intake of any of several *therapeutic drugs*.
[*]

porphyrin

Substituted *porphin* occurring naturally in pigments and cofactors such as *hemoglobin* and *cytochromes*.
[*]

Porsolt test

See *swimming test*.

positive control

See *control,* positive.

positive selection

1. (in biology) Process by which a new advantageous *genetic* variant tends to expand in a *population*.
2. (in immunology) Selection of those developing *T-cells* in the *thymus* that are able to recognize self-*major histocompatibility complex molecules*.

Note: Immunological positive selection occurs by preventing *apoptosis* in these cells.
[*]

posology

Pharmacological study of the choice of appropriate *dose* of a *drug* in relation to the physiological factors, such as age, that may influence its effect.
[ref. 1]

posterior fossa

Pocket in the back of the skull that accommodates the *cerebellum* and the *midbrain*.
[ref. 4]

post-implantation

Occurring after the early *embryo* embeds in the lining of the *uterus*.
[ref. 5]

postmortem

Opposite term: *antemortem*.
Occurring after death.
[ref. 5]

postnatal

Referring to events in the life of the mother or infant following *birth*.
[After ref. 5]

postpartum

Period following the *birth* of an infant, often considered to be about six weeks in the human.
[ref. 5]

postsynaptic

Describing an event or structure at the *distal* side of a *synaptic cleft*.
[ref. 4]

post-translational modification

Processes by which proteins are biochemically modified within a cell subsequent to their synthesis on the *ribosomes*.
[ref. 1]

potency (in toxicology)

Quantitative expression of *toxicity* of an agent as compared to a given or implied standard or *reference dose*.
[ref. 1]

potency factor

See *slope factor*.

potentiation (in toxicology)

Dependent action in which a substance or physical agent at a *concentration* or *dose* that does not itself have an *adverse effect* enhances the harm done by another substance or physical agent.
[ref. 1]
See also *synergism*.

potentiation (in neurology)

post-tetanic potentiation
Increase in strength of *synaptic transmission* between two *neurons* after repetitive stimulation of the *presynaptic* partner.
Note 1: The typical duration of potentiation is minutes.
Note 2: Potentiation is attributed to various mechanisms including *presynaptic* biochemical changes, *e.g.*, kinase activation or increased Ca^{2+} availability.
[ref. 4]

potentiation, long-term

Potentiation lasting up to several months.
Note: Long-term potentiation is considered to be a major mechanism involved in learning and memory.
[ref. 4]

practical certainty (of safety)

Numerically specified low *risk* of *exposure* to a potentially *toxic* substance or socially acceptable low *risk* of *adverse effects* from such an exposure applied to decision making in regard to chemical safety.
[ref. 1]

pre-B-cell

Cell in the *B-lymphocyte* lineage that has rearranged *heavy chain* but not *light chain* genes; it expresses surrogate light chains and μ heavy chain at its surface in conjunction with *immunoglobulins* Ig α and Ig β.
Note: All these molecules comprise the pre-*B-cell receptor*.
[ref. 3]

precautionary principle

Approach to risk management that can be applied in circumstances of scientific uncertainty, reflecting a perceived need to take action in the face of a potentially serious risk without waiting for definitive results of scientific research.
Note: The 1992 Rio Declaration on Environment and Development says: "In order to protect the environment, the precautionary approach shall be widely applied by states according to their capabilities. Where there are threats of serious or irreversible damage, lack of full scientific certainty shall not be used as a reason for postponing cost-effective measures to prevent environmental *degradation*."
[ref. 1]

precipitating antibody

See *antibody, precipitating*.

precipitin

Precipitate of *antibody* and multivalent *antigen* due to the formation of high-molecular-weight complexes.
[ref. 3]

precision (in metrology)

Closeness of agreement between *indications* obtained by replicate measurements on the same or similar objects under specified conditions.
Note: Precision of a measurement is usually expressed numerically by measures of imprecision, such as standard deviation, variance, or coefficient of variation under the specified conditions of measurement.
[ref. 1]

precordial

Pertaining to the region over the heart and lower *thorax*.
[ref. 1]

precursor

Substance participating in a chemical reaction in which another chemical structure is formed; in toxicology the second structure is usually more biologically active.
[*]

predator

Animal that hunts and kills other animals for food.
[*]

predatory mite test

Procedure in which *adult* females of the predatory mite (***Hypoaspis (Geolaelaps) aculeifer***, considered representative of *soil* fauna) are exposed to a test substance in artificial soil and the number of surviving females and of juveniles is determined.
[ref. 5]

predicted environmental concentration (PEC)

See *estimated environmental concentration.*

predicted exposure concentration (PEC)

See *estimated environmental concentration.*

predicted no-effect concentration (PNEC)

Concentration that is expected to cause no adverse effect to any naturally occurring *population* in an *environment* at *risk* from *exposure* to a given substance.
[ref. 1]

predictive risk assessment

See *risk assessment, predictive.*

predictive validity

Reliability of a measurement expressed in terms of its ability to predict the criterion. Example: An academic aptitude test that is validated against subsequent academic performance.
[ref. 1]

predictive value

Percentage of positive results that are true positives or of negative results that are true negatives.
[ref. 1]
See also *false negative; false poasitive.*

pre-eclampsia

toxemia of pregnancy
Pathological condition in late *pregnancy* with symptoms of high blood pressure, kidney dysfunction, *proteinuria*, and *edema.*
[ref. 5]
See also *eclampsia.*

pre-embryo

Fertilized *ovum* up to 14 days of age and before *implantation.*
[ref. 5]

pregnancy (n)/pregnant (adj)

State of a female between *conception* and the termination of *gestation.*
[ref. 5]
See also *pseudopregnancy.*

pre-implantation

Occurring before the early *embryo* embeds in the lining of the *uterus.*
[ref. 5]

preliminary test

See *screening test.*

premature birth

Delivery before the expected length of *gestation* for the species; in humans taken as *birth* before a gestational age of 37 weeks.
[ref. 5]

premature ovarian failure

Follicular depletion by the age of 35 years.
[ref. 1]

prenatal

antenatal
Referring to events in the life of the mother or *fetus* preceding *birth.*
[ref. 5]

prenatal development study

Procedure in which a substance is administered to *pregnant* animals (usually rodents or rabbits) from the time of *implantation* until closure of the hard *palate*. The animals are killed one-to-two days before a scheduled delivery, whereupon *uterine* contents and the *fetuses* are evaluated for abnormalities.
[ref. 5]

preneoplastic

Before the formation of a *tumor.*
[ref. 1]

preneoplastic island

preneoplastic focus
Group of slightly altered *cells* in a *tissue*, developing after treatment of an organism with a *carcinogenic* substance, that is characterized by altered *enzyme* activities and usually different tissue architecture compared to the healthy surrounding cells.
Note: Preneoplastic island cells can further degenerate to *tumor* cells and are used in *toxicological pathology* as an early (preneoplastic) marker for *tumorigenesis.*
[*]

preoptic area

preoptic region
Region of the anterior *hypothalamus* primarily involved in regulating body temperature.
[ref. 5]

prepubertal

Stage of human development before the onset of *puberty.*
[ref. 5]
Compare *prepubescence.*

prepubescence

Period before *pubescence.*
Note: Whereas *prepubertal* refers to any time before *puberty*, prepubescence refers more specifically to a time closely preceding early puberty.
[ref. 5]

prepuce

Skin protecting the *glans penis* in the male (foreskin) or the *clitoris* in the female (clitoral hood).
[ref. 5]

preputial separation

Separation of the *prepuce* from the *glans penis.*
[ref. 5]

presynaptic

Event or structure at the proximal (transmitting) side of a *synaptic cleft.*
[ref. 4]

pre-T-cell

thymocyte
Cell differentiating into a *T-lymphocyte* in the *thymus* gland.
Note 1: During maturation, thymocytes express on their surface a precursor *T-cell receptor* called a pre-T-cell receptor, along with both *CD8* and *CD4* proteins (*double-positive cells*). At the same time they migrate from the outer cortex of the *thymus* to the inner medullary region.
Note 2: Only the 2 % of thymocytes capable of distinguishing *self-antigen* survive to maturity in the *medulla*, where they become *single-positive cells*, expressing CD4 or CD8 surface proteins, and are exported from the thymus into the bloodstream to become *helper T-cells* and *cytotoxic T-cells*, respectively.
[ref. 3]

prethalamus

See *subthalamus.*

prevalence

Number of existing cases of a given *disease* or other condition in a given *population* at a given time; sometimes used to mean *prevalence rate.*
Note: When used without qualification, prevalence usually refers to the situation at a specified time (point prevalence).
[ref. 1]

prevalence rate (ratio)

Total number of individuals who have an attribute or *disease* at a particular time (or during a particular period) divided by the number of individuals in the *population* at *risk* of having the attribute or disease at this point in time, or midway through the period.
[ref. 1]

prick test

Test carried out by placing a drop of a suspected *allergenic* extract on the skin of the forearm and gently pricking it into the upper layer of skin, *sensitivity* to a substance being indicated if the spot swells slightly and becomes red within about 15 min.
Note: A positive prick test result is far from conclusive and, at best, gives a vague indication of allergenicity. The prick test is inappropriate as a test for food allergens.
[ref. 3]

primary biliary cirrhosis (PBC)

Autoimmune liver *disease* that results in the destruction of *bile* ducts, leading to *fibrosis* and *cirrhosis.*
Note: Primary biliary cirrhosis-specific *antibodies* are *antimitochondrial antibodies* directed against proteins of the pyruvate dehydrogenase complex (mainly the E2 subunit).
[ref. 3]

primary challenge

See *primary immune response.*

primary immune response

Immune response to the first encounter with an *antigen*, characterized by slow production of *antibody* molecules and the *priming* of *lymphoid tissue* in readiness for the production of a *secondary immune response* on subsequent *challenge* with the same antigen.
Note: The primary response is generally weak, has a long induction phase or lag period, consists primarily of the release of *immunoglobulin M* antibodies, and generates immunologic *memory.*
[ref. 3]

primary immunization

See *immunization, primary.*

primary lamella

Gill structure in fish that extends outward at right angles from the *branchial arch* and is involved in gas exchange with the *blood.*
Note: Secondary lamellae branch from the primary lamellae to increase the surface area for gas exchange.
[*]

primary lymphoid follicle

Region of a *secondary lymphoid organ* containing predominantly unstimulated *B-lymphocytes* that develops into a *germinal center* following *antigen* stimulation.
[ref. 3]
See also *lymphoid follicle.*

primary lymphoid organ

Site at which *immunocompetent lymphocytes* develop, *i.e., bone marrow* and *thymus* in mammals.
[ref. 3]

primary myxedema

Atrophic form of diffuse *autoimmune thyroiditis.*
[ref. 3]

primary pollutant

See *pollutant.*

primary producer

Organism capable of deriving energy from light or a chemical substance in order to manufacture energy-rich organic compounds.
[ref. 2]

primary protection standard

Accepted maximum level of a *pollutant* (or its indicator) in the *target* organism, or some part thereof, or an accepted maximum intake of a pollutant or nuisance into the target under specified circumstances.
[ref. 1]

primary response

See *primary immune response.*

primary sclerosing cholangitis (PSC)

Chronic, nonbacterial, inflammatory narrowing of the *bile* ducts.
Note: PSC is often associated with ulcerative colitis (see *inflammatory bowel disease).*
[ref. 3]

primary sex organ

Gonad, which forms *gametes; ovary* in the female and *testis* in the male.
[ref. 5]
See also *accessory sex organ.*

primary succession

See *succession, primary.*

prime (v)

Process of giving an initial *sensitization* to *antigen.*
[ref. 3]

priming (v)

See *prime.*

primitive groove

Shallow depression in the *primitive streak* that extends anteriorly to communicate with the *yolk sac.*
[ref. 5]

primitive node

primitive knot
Group of cells at the anterior end of the *primitive streak*, involved in secreting chemical signals that regulate differentiation of the *germ layers* during *gastrulation.*
[ref. 5]

primitive pit

Depression in the *primitive node* contiguous with the *notochord*.
[ref. 5]

primitive streak

Structure forming in the *blastula* during early *embryogenesis* that establishes bilateral symmetry and determines the site of *gastrulation* and *germ layer* formation.
[ref. 5]

primordial follicle

Early stage of the *oocyte* in which it is surrounded by a single layer of *follicular* cells.
[ref. 5]
See also *follicle*.

primordial germ cell

Germ cell in the earliest stages of development.
[ref. 5]

primordium

Organ or *tissue* at its earliest recognizable stage of development.
[ref. 5]

principle of allocation

Concept that there exists a cost or trade-off to every allocation of energy resources, such that energy spent by an individual organism on one function, process, or structure cannot be spent on another.
Note: The principle of allocation is associated with the idea that optimal allocation of resources enhances *Darwinian fitness*.
[After ref. 2]

prior informed consent (PIC)

Concept in law and medicine that states that before one is subjected to a *risk*, especially a risk of bodily harm, one is entitled to be fully apprised, in advance, of the nature of that risk in order to make an informed decision about whether to accept it or not.
[ref. 1]
Note: In most jurisdictions, PIC must be considered before starting an invasive clinical procedure or before including a volunteer in a *clinical trial*.
[*]

privileged site

See *immunologically privileged site*.

probability sample

See *random sample*.

probit

Portmanteau of the words "probability unit", describing a unit derived from a regression *model* in which only two outcomes are allowed, *e.g.*, *diseased* or not diseased.

Note: A plot of probit against the logarithm of the *concentration* or *dose* of a substance when a *quantal* or *graded response* has been measured is a probit (log) transform. Linearity of such a plot is evidence that the response follows a log normal distribution, and permits straightforward estimates of the $L(E)C_{50}$ and $L(E)D_{50}$, as well as the standard deviation for the distribution, to be made.
[*]

problem formulation (in ecological risk assessment)

Planning and scoping phase of a *risk assessment* that establishes the framework in which the assessment is to be done.
[After ref. 2]

procarcinogen

Substance that becomes a *carcinogen* only after it is *metabolized*.
[ref. 1]

proctodeum

anal pit
Ectodermal depression of the *caudal* end of the *embryo*, where later the *anus* is formed.
[ref. 5]

prodromal stage

Phase before the onset of full-blown *disease*.
Note: Often used in referring to visual disturbances and (or) mood changes before the further development of a *migraine headache* or *epileptic seizure*.
[ref. 4]
See also *prodrome*.

prodrome

Symptom(s) heralding impending onset of a *disease*.
[ref. 4]
See also *prodromal stage*.

prodrug

Precursor converted to an active form of a *drug* within the body.
[ref. 2]

product-limit method

Kaplan–Meier method
Nonparametric method for analyzing time-to-death or *survival time* data that does not require a specific *model* for the *survival curve*.
[ref. 2]

productivity

Rate at which *biomass* is produced per unit area, usually specified by class of organism.
[ref. 2]

professional antigen-presenting cell

Highly efficient *antigen-presenting cell*, generally referring to *dendritic cells, B-cells*, or *macrophages*.
Note: In contrast to professional antigen-presenting cells, other cells, that do not constitutively express *major histocompatibility complex class II molecules* (*e.g., fibroblasts* and endothelial cells), may be induced to do so by certain *cytokines* and are sometimes referred to as nonprofessional antigen-presenting cells.
[ref. 3]

profile of mood state (POMS) test

Procedure in which a test subject is asked to indicate his/her mood during the past week, by quickly marking specified emotional words on a scale between "not at all" and "extremely".
Note: Tested moods in the POMS test typically include tension, anxiety, depression, hostility, vigor, fatigue and confusion.
[ref. 4]

profundal region

profundal zone
Deep zone of an inland body of freestanding water, such as a lake or pond, that is below the range of effective light penetration.
Note: The profundal region is usually below the *thermocline*.
[*]

progeny

See *offspring*.

progesterone

pregn-4-ene-3,20-dione
Steroidal hormone produced in the *ovary* by the *corpus luteum*.
Note: Progesterone is involved in sexual development and the *ovarian cycle*, and essential for maintenance of *pregnancy*.
[ref. 5]

progestin

Synthetic variant of *progesterone*, often used in oral *contraceptive* pills or to suppress *hyperplasia* of the *endometrium*.
[ref. 5]

progestogen

gestagen
Member of a family of *hormones*, based on the 21-carbon pregnane skeleton, involved in maintaining *gestation* and regulating the *ovarian cycle*.
[ref. 5]
See also *progesterone; progestin*.

programmed cell death

Referring to the organized death of a cell by one of several defined pathways, including *apoptosis* and *autophagy*, and, in some circumstances, possibly by a "programmed *necrosis*".
[*]

progression (in oncology)

Increase in the size of a *tumor* often associated with increased *malignancy* and spread of *cancer* in the body.
Note: Progression is the third phase of tumor development, after *initiation* and *promotion*.
[*]

progressive systemic sclerosis

Systemic autoimmune disease marked by formation of *hyalinized* and thickened *collagenous* fibrous *tissue*, with thickening and adhesion of skin to underlying tissues, especially of the hands and face and *vascular* alterations.
[ref. 3]
See also *scleroderma*.

proinflammatory cytokine

Cytokine that initiates or enhances *inflammation*.
[ref. 3]

prokaryote (n)/prokaryotic (adj)

Unicellular organism, characterized by the absence of a *membrane*-enclosed *nucleus*.
Note: Prokaryotes include bacteria, blue-green algae, and *mycoplasmas*.
[ref. 1]
See also *eukaryote*.

prolactin

Hormone released from the anterior *pituitary gland* that stimulates milk production after childbirth; it also regulates *proliferation* and *differentiation* of a variety of *cells* in the *immune system* and can modulate mood.
[3,5]

prolapse

Falling or slipping out of place of an *organ* or other body part.
Note: *Uterine* prolapse occurs when the ligaments holding the uterus weaken and the uterus slips down into, or even protrudes from, the *vagina*.
[ref. 5]

proliferation (in biology)

Multiplication or increase by frequent and repeated reproduction or *growth* by *cell* division.
[ref. 2]

proliferation assay

Any test that determines the effect on increase in *cell* number of a test agent such as a *cytokine* or *mitogen*.
[ref. 3]
See also *proliferation*.

promoter

1. (in molecular genetics) Sequence of nucleotides in a *DNA* molecule to which *RNA* polymerase binds so as to start *transcription*.
2. (in oncology) Agent that stimulates growth of a *cancer* when administered to an animal or human being who has been *exposed* to a cancer *initiator*.

[After ref. 1]

promotor

Erroneous spelling of *promoter* (in molecular genetics), found in some literature.
[ref. 1]

pronephros

Collection of cells in the *vertebrate embryo* that represents the earliest stage of development of the kidney.
[ref. 5]

pronucleus

Haploid nucleus formed by either the head of the *sperm* or the nucleus of the *oocyte* after *fertilization* but before their *nuclei* fuse to form the *diploid zygotic* nucleus.
[ref. 5]

propagule

1. Portion of a plant or fungus (*e.g.*, a cutting, leaf bud, bulbil, seed, or spore) that can be excised and cultivated to give rise to a new individual by asexual reproduction.
2. Less commonly, any of the products of asexual reproduction in certain invertebrates.

[After ref. 2]

propagule rain

In *metapopulation* dynamics, the presence of a seed bank or dormant stage for a *species* that continually introduces individuals to the patch regardless of the density of occupancy in the surrounding patches.
Note: Propagule rain increases the likelihood of *population* reappearance and decreases the likelihood of patch extinction.
[ref. 2]

properdin

Relatively heat-labile, normal *serum* protein (a *euglobulin*) that, in the presence of *complement* component C3 and magnesium ions, is involved in the *alternative pathway of complement activation*.
Note 1: Properdin acts nonspecifically against Gram-negative bacteria and viruses and may contribute to the lysis of *erythrocytes*.
Note 2: Properdin migrates on electrophoresis as a β_3-*globulin* and, although not an *antibody*, may act in conjunction with complement-fixing antibody.
[ref. 3]

pro-pesticide

Substance applied in a form that is not active as a *pesticide* and that becomes active once it enters an organism and undergoes chemical modification.
[ref. 1]

prophage

Latent state of a phage *genome* in a lysogenic bacterium.
[ref. 1]

propharynx

See *pharynx.*

prophase

First stage of *meiosis* or *mitosis* in which thickening and orientation of the *chromosomes* occurs.
[ref. 5]

proportional mortality rate (ratio)

Proportion of observed deaths from a specified condition in a defined *population* divided by the proportion of deaths expected from this condition in a standard population, expressed either on an age-specific basis or after age adjustment.
[ref. 1]

proprioception

Sense of the movement or position of the body independent of vision.
Note: Proprioception is often gained from input from *nerve* terminals in the muscles, tendons, and joint capsules.
[ref. 4]
See also *proprioceptor.*

proprioceptor

Sensory organ in a muscle, tendon or joint capsule that senses position or state of *contraction.*
[ref. 4]

prosencephalon

forebrain
Most forward part of the *brain* that includes most of the *cerebral cortex*, the *thalamus* and *hypothalamus*, and the *basal ganglia.*
[ref. 5]

prospective cohort study

See *study, prospective cohort.*

prospective risk assessment

See *risk assessment, predictive.*

prostaglandin

Any of a group of acidic lipids derived by cylooxygenase (EC 1.14.99.1) activity from arachidonic acid.
Note 1: Prostaglandins act as *autocrine* and *paracrine* mediators of various biological functions, such as *vascular* permeability, fever, *inflammation*, and *pain.*
Note 2: Nonsteroidal antiinflammatory *drugs* inhibit prostaglandin synthesis.
[*]

prostate (n)/prostatic (adj)

Male *exocrine gland* whose secretion contributes alkaline fluid to the ejaculate (see *ejaculation*).
Note: The alkaline nature of the prostatic secretion facilitates *sperm* transport and prolongs the survival of sperm in the acidic environment of the *vagina*.
[ref. 5]

prosthetic group

Nonprotein entity essential for an *enzyme's* activity and tightly bound to the enzyme molecule in its active form.
[ref. 1]

protamine

Small, basic (arginine-rich) protein involved in *sperm* maturation and *DNA* packaging during *spermatogenesis*.
[ref. 5]

protease

Enzyme catalyzing proteolytic cleavage.
[*]
See also *proteolysis*.

protectin

CD59
Member of the *Ly-6* family of cell surface molecules that prevents insertion of the *membrane attack complex* into the *membrane*, thereby protecting cells from *complement*-induced lysis.
[ref. 3]

protective immunity

Protection against *infectious* agents conferred by *vaccination*.
[ref. 3]

protein A

Staphylococcus aureus cell wall protein that binds to the *Fc region* of *immunoglobulin G*.
[ref. 3]

protein G

Streptococcal cell wall protein that binds to the *Fc region* of *immunoglobulin G*, with wider species specificity than *protein A*.
[ref. 3]

protein kinase

Enzyme that catalyzes the transfer of a phosphate group from a donor (almost always *ATP*) to a protein acceptor.
Note 1: Phosphorylation of the target protein by the kinase is a regulatory mechanism that may either activate or inactivate the protein substrate, which itself may be another enzyme.

Note 2: The kinase reaction is a key feature of *signal transduction* pathways, wherein the newly phosphorylated protein is activated to act in turn upon its own downstream substrate.
[*]

protein kinase C (PKC)

Member (EC 2.7.11.13) of a kinase family with broad substrate specificity, activated by calcium, diacylglycerol, and (or) *phorbol 12-myristate 13-acetate.*
Note: Protein kinase C is activated during *B-lymphocyte* and *T-lymphocyte* activation.
[ref. 3]

proteinase 3 (PR3)

Multifunctional *enzyme* (EC 3.4.21.x) of azurophilic granules of *neutrophils* and *monocytes* and the major target of *antineutrophil cytoplasmic autoantibodies.*
Note: PR3 *autoantibodies* are diagnostic markers for *Wegener granulomatosis* and are involved in the *pathogenesis* of this *disease*. They are also found in patients with other *autoimmune systemic* vasculitic diseases.
[ref. 3]

proteinuria

Excretion of excessive amounts of protein (derived from *blood plasma* or kidney tubules) in the urine.
[ref. 1]

proteolysis (n)/**proteolytic** (adj)

proteolytic cleavage
proteolytic degradation
Breakdown of a protein to shorter polypeptides or to individual amino acids by cleavage of *covalent* peptide bonds.
Note: The peptide bond is stable under physiological conditions, and uncatalyzed hydrolysis of peptides is very slow. Thus, proteolysis usually refers to protein cleavage catalyzed by an *enzyme* that is then classified as a protease.
[*]

proteome

Description of the complete set of proteins encoded by the *genome.*
[ref. 1]
See also *-ome.*

proteomics

Global analysis of *gene expression* using a variety of techniques to identify and characterize proteins.
Note: In *toxicology*, proteomics can be used to study changes caused by exposure to substances and to determine if changes in m*RNA* expression correlate with changes in protein expression (see *gene expression*). The analysis may also show changes in *post-translational modification*, which cannot be distinguished by mRNA analysis alone.
[ref. 5]
See also *-ome.*

proto-oncogene

See *oncogene.*

provisional tolerable weekly intake (PTWI)

See *tolerable weekly intake.*

proximal (in anatomy)

Opposite term: *distal.*
Nearer to an anatomical point of origin or attachment, or to the midline of the body.
[ref. 5]

proximal tubule

proximal convoluted tubule (PCT).
Portion of the tubular system of the *nephron* closest to the *glomerulus.*
Note: The PCT is exposed to the newly formed *plasma* filtrate leaving the glomerulus, and so is a common *target* for filtered substances such as potentially *toxic metal* ions.
[*]

prozone effect

Loss of *immunoprecipitation* or *agglutination* that occurs when *antibody* concentration is increased to an extent that the antibody is in such excess that it is no longer able to effectively cross-link the *antigen.*
Note: A similar phenomenon to the prozone effect may occur in states of antigen excess.
[ref. 3]

pruritis (n)/**pruritic** (adj)

Itching of the skin.
[*]
See also *pruritogen.*

pruritogen (n)/**pruritogenic** (adj)

Substance that causes *pruritis.*
[*]

pseudo-acceptable daily intake (PADI)

Approximate *acceptable daily intake* for a substance derived by applying a thousand-fold *uncertainty factor* to the lowest low-effect level for non*carcinogenic* endpoints.
[ref. 1]

pseudoadaptation

Apparent *adaptation* of an organism to changing conditions of the *environment* associated with *stresses* (often from chemical substances) in biochemical systems that exceed the limits of normal (*homeostatic*) mechanisms.
Note: In pseudoadaptation, there is often a temporary concealed *pathology* that later can be manifested in the form of explicit pathological changes, sometimes referred to as "decompensation".
[ref. 1]

pseudoallergy

pseudoallergic reaction
Inflammatory or *anaphylactic* reaction with *symptoms* similar to an *allergy* but not involving an *antigen-* specific *immune response, e.g.*, salicylate intolerance, reaction to contrast reagents.

Note: Causes of pseudoallergy include direct *histamine* release and (or) *complement* activation.
[ref. 3]

pseudobulbar affect (PBA)

Involuntary emotional outburst (typically crying or laughing).
Note: PBA is a result of neurological injury or *disease*, but the precise mechanism is unknown.
[ref. 4]

pseudocholinesterase

See *butyrylcholinesterase*.

pseudocyesis

See *pseudopregnancy*.

pseudohermaphrodite

Organism possessing either male (*testes*) or female (*ovaries*) *gonads*, but with ambiguous *external genitalia*.
[ref. 5]
Compare *hermaphrodite*.

pseudomeningocele

Part of the *cerebrospinal fluid* that, in contrast to a *meningiocele*, is not surrounded by *dura*.
[ref. 4]

pseudopregnancy

pseudocyesis
false pregnancy
Development of signs of *pregnancy* in the absence of an *embryo*.
Note: Commonly, the term pseudocyesis is used for false pregnancy occurring in humans and pseudopregnancy then refers to its occurrence in other mammals.
[ref. 5]

pseudotumor cerebri

idiopathic intracranial hypertension
Disorder with increased *intracranial pressure, cerebral* edema, and frequently *papilledema*, symptoms that resemble the effects of a *tumor* but without a tumor present.
[ref. 4]

psoriasis (n)/**psoriatic** (adj)

Skin *disorder* that has a hereditary component and is characterized by erythematous patches covered with silvery scales, especially on the elbows, knees, and scalp.
Note: Psoriasis is associated with excessively rapid proliferation of *keratinocytes* that mature in less than a week.
[ref. 3]

psychoactive

Having the ability to alter mood, behavior, *cognitive function* or mental state.
Note: Usually referring to a *pharmacologic* agent or a recreational *drug*.
[ref. 4]
Compare *psychotropic*.

psychomotor retardation

Delayed development of both *cognitive function* and *motor function*.
[ref. 5]

psychoneuroimmunology (PNI)

Study of links between the *brain* and the immune system, recognizing an interaction between psychological states and the outcome of *immune responses* to *disease*.
[ref. 4]

psychosis

Any major mental *disorder* characterized by derangement of the personality, *cognitive function*, perception, belief, behaviour or mood; loss of contact with or awareness of reality.
[1,4]
Note: Psychosis may occur in an individual *acutely, chronically* or recurrently.
[*]

psychosis, organic

organic brain syndrome
Psychosis with a known physical (anatomic, *disease*-related or *toxic*) cause.
[ref. 4]

psychotropic

Capable of affecting the mental activity, emotions and behavior.
Note: Psychotropic is often used to describe a *drug* effective in treating a relevant mental illness.
[ref. 4]
Compare *psychoactive*.

puberty

Process in which an youngster undergoes sexual development, including the onset of *gametogenesis*, changes in *hormonal* secretions, *secondary sexual characteristic*s, and reproductive competence.
[ref. 5]

pubescence (n)/pubescent (adj)

Being in the early stage of *puberty*.
[ref. 5]

pubic

Relating to the region of the most *ventral* bone of the pelvis (the pubic bone), and thus the region around the *genital* area, normally showing hair growth (pubic hair) in the *adult*.
[ref. 5]

pubic symphysis

Cartilaginous joint between the *pubic* bones forming the front of the pelvis.
[ref. 5]

public health impact assessment

Applying *risk assessment* to a specific *target population* of known size, giving as the end product a quantitative statement about the number of people likely to be affected in a particular population.
[ref. 1]

public T-cell response

Phenomenon in which multiple individuals share identical *T-cell receptor* sequences in responding to the same *antigenic epitope*.
[*]
See also *public T-cell receptor sequence*.

public T-cell receptor sequence

Identical *T-cell receptor* amino acid sequence shared by many *major histocompatibility complex*-matched individuals in a *population*.
[*]

puffer fish

Marine fish of the order ***Tetraodontiformes*** and family ***Tetraodontidae***.
[ref. 4]
See also *tetrodotoxin*.

pulmonary

Pertaining to the lung(s).
[ref. 1]

pulmonary artery

Large vessel that transports *blood* from the heart to the lungs.
[ref. 5]

pulmonary valve stenosis

Condition in which the flow of *blood* from the heart to the lungs is slowed by a deformity on or near the *pulmonary* valve that controls the blood flow from the right heart to the lungs.
[ref. 5]
See also *stenosis*.

pup

1. (n) Young or newborn dog, rat or seal.
2. (v) Give birth to a pup.

[ref. 5]

purgative

See *laxative*.

purified protein derivative (PPD)

Partially purified derivative of *tuberculin* used in the *Mantoux test* for tuberculosis.
[ref. 3]

Purkinje cell

Large *neuron* forming part of a layer of *cells* in the *cerebellum*.
Note: By releasing *γ-aminobutyric acid*, the inhibitory *GABAergic* Purkinje cells regulate and coordinate *motor activity*.
[ref. 4]

purpura

Purple discoloration occurring in patches on the skin, *mucous membranes*, or organs.
See also *idiopathic thrombocytopenic purpura.*
[ref. 3]

pursuit aiming test

Procedure in which a subject is instructed to place a dot in defined sites (such as a number of circles), as quickly as possible.
Note: The pursuit aiming test provides information about eye-to-hand coordination.
[ref. 4]
See also *neurobehavior core test battery*.

putamen

Part of the *basal ganglia* that plays a role in coordinating movement and learning.
Note: The putamen is involved in *neurodegenerative diseases* such as *Parkinson disease*.
[ref. 4]

pyknosis

Clumping of *nuclear chromatin* and shrinkage of the cell nucleus during cell degeneration.
[ref. 4]

pyloric stenosis

Narrowing of the *sphincter* (the pylorus) between the stomach and *duodenum*.
[ref. 5]
See also *stenosis*.

pyramidal cell

Large *neuron* of the *cerebral cortex* having a triangular cell body in *histological* section with several *dendrites* at the base and one large apical *axon*.
Note 1: Pyramidal cells are also found in other *brain* areas such as the *hippocampus*.
Note 2: Pyramidal cells are thought to play a role in *cognitive function*.
[ref. 4]

pyramidal system

See *motor system*.

pyrethrin

See *pyrethroid*.

pyrethroid

Synthetic molecule with structural similarity to the natural pyrethrins found in plants of the genus ***Chrysanthemum***.
Note: Pyrethroids are a major class of *insecticide* and cause *paralysis* by blocking closure of *axonal* sodium *ion channels*, thus leading to the *depolarization* of *neurons*.
[ref. 4]

pyrexia

Condition in which the temperature of a human being or mammal is above normal.
[ref. 1]

pyrogen

Any substance that produces fever.
[ref. 1]

pyrogen test

Any of various tests used to determine whether an agent, usually an infusion or injection fluid, is free of *pyrogens*.
Examples: (i) the rabbit test, observing whether the body temperature of the animal increases after administration of the agent, (ii) the ***Limulus*** *test*, measuring the effects of *endotoxins* on a biological system, and (iii) in vitro tests, observing the release of *interleukin*-1β from human *blood cells* during incubation with the test fluid.
[ref. 3]

Qa antigen

See *antigen, Qa.*

QT-interval

Time between the features designated Q and T in an *electrocardiogram*, the Q spike representing the peak of electrical activity associated with *depolarization*, and the T feature representing a wave of ventricular repolarization.
Note 1: The QT-interval, usually reported in msec, represents a phase in which the heart is *depolarized* during systole and thus more susceptible to further electrical stimulation.
Note 2: A prolongation of the QT interval beyond normal, known as "long QT (LQT) *syndrome*", presents an increased risk for potentially life-threatening *arrhythmias*. It may arise from a variety of *genetic mutations* affecting cardiac Na^+ and K^+ channels, or from various *drug toxicities*.
[*]

quadriplegia

Paralysis of both upper and both lower limbs.
[ref. 4]

quality assurance

All those planned and systematic actions necessary to provide adequate confidence that a product or service will satisfy given requirements for quality.
[ref. 1]
See also *quality control.*

quality control

1. Operational techniques and activities that are used to fulfill requirements for quality.
2. In *toxicology*, procedures incorporated in experimental protocols and documentation to reduce the possibility of error, especially human error.

Note: Quality control is a requirement of *good laboratory practice.*
[ref. 1]
See also *quality assurance.*

quality criterion

One of a set of consensual rules, processes, tests and controls, based on scientific data and sufficient to achieve a desired level of quality.
Note: Quality criteria are the basis for both internal and external *quality control.*
[*]
See also *quality guideline; quality objective; quality standard.*

quality guideline

One of a set of consensual rules and (or) numerical limits, usually with official character and adopted by a national or international agency.

Comprehensive Glossary of Terms Used in Toxicology
By John Duffus, Douglas M. Templeton and Michael Schwenk

Published by the Royal Society of Chemistry, www.rsc.org

Note: In *toxicology*, quality guidelines are intended to protect the environment and human health, and include those for drinking water, outdoor air quality, and conditions in the workplace.
[*]
See also *quality criterion; quality objective; quality standard.*

quality objective

One of a set of consensual aims and purposes of a *quality control* procedure.
Note: In toxicology, quality objectives include accuracy, *precision*, repeatability and documentation.
[*]
See also *quality criterion; quality guideline; quality standard.*

quality standard (in environmental toxicology)

One of a set of consensual fixed upper limits for *exposure* to certain substances recognized under law by one or more levels of government.
Examples: Air, water, and *soil* quality standard; *threshold limit value* for an air *pollutant* in the workplace.
Note: A quality standard may be subject to change with time.
[After ref. 2]
See also *quality criterion; quality guideline; quality objective.*

quantal

Describing a condition that can be expressed only as "occurring" or "not occurring", such as death.
[ref. 1]

quantal effect

all-or-none effect
Opposite term: *graded effect.*

Effect that can be expressed only as "occurring" or "not occurring", such as death or occurrence of a *tumor* after an exposure.
[ref. 1]

quantitative structure–activity relationship (QSAR)

1. Quantitative *model* relating chemical structure of organic compounds to biological activity (including *toxicity*), derived using *regression analysis* and containing as parameters physicochemical constants, indicator variables, or theoretically calculated values.
   Note: QSAR is used as a method of predicting toxicity by *read-across*. It is also used to design molecules with a specified biological activity prior to their synthesis for use as *drugs, pesticides*, and other bioactive compounds, and for assessing the *environmental* fate of chemicals.
2. Quantitative *model* relating chemical structure of compounds to chemical activity in the environment.

[After ref. 2]

quantitative structure–metabolism relationship (QSMR)

Quantitative association between the physicochemical and (or) the structural properties of a substance and its *metabolic* behavior.
[ref. 2]

quickening

Initial awareness of *fetal* movement by the *pregnant* mother, usually occurring early in the second *trimester*.
[ref. 5]

quotient method

Calculation of the value of the measured or *predicted environmental concentration* of a *contaminant* divided by the *predicted no-effect level*, used as an expression of *hazard* or *risk*.
Note: Higher quotients constitute greater evidence of a hazard or a greater risk.
[After ref. 2]
See also *hazard quotient*.

r/K selection theory

See *K-strategy; r-strategy.*

RNA

See *ribonucleic acid.*

RNA interference (RNAi)

See *ribonucleic acid interference.*

r-strategist

Organism that reproduces rapidly in large numbers; usually a colonizing species with high *fecundity* and low competitive ability.
Note: Species of r-strategists are usually found in unstable biological *communities.*
[*]
Compare *K-strategist.*
See also *r-strategy.*

r-strategy

Opportunistic strategy favoring biological *species* that establish themselves quickly, grow quickly to exploit as many resources as possible, and produce many *offspring.*
[ref. 2]
Compare *K-strategy.*
See also *Verhulst equation.*

rachischisis

Failure of the *neural tube* to close *in utero*, resulting in a *birth defect* that leaves a fissure in the *vertebral* column with part of the *spinal cord* exposed.
[ref. 5]

radial arm maze

See *maze, radial arm.*

radial immunodiffusion

Mancini immunodiffusion

Method for quantifying an *antigen* by measuring the diameters of circular precipitates around an antigen-spiked *cavity* in an *antibody*-containing agar gel.
[ref. 3]

radiant power, P_λ

Energy emitted, transferred, or received as electromagnetic radiation per unit time.
[ref. 1]

radiation toxicology

Scientific study involving research, education, prevention, and treatment of *diseases* caused by ionizing or nonionizing electromagnetic radiation.
[*]

Comprehensive Glossary of Terms Used in Toxicology
By John Duffus, Douglas M. Templeton and Michael Schwenk

Published by the Royal Society of Chemistry, www.rsc.org

radiculitis

Inflammation of the *spinal nerve* roots leading to *pain* and *hyperesthesia* radiating along the *nerve*.
[ref. 4]

radioallergosorbent test (RAST)

Solid-phase *radioimmunoassay (RIA)* for detecting *immunoglobulin E (IgE) antibody* specific for a particular *antigen*.
[ref. 3]

radioimmunoassay (RIA)

Technique for measuring the level of a substance in a sample, by measuring the binding of *antigen* to radioactively labeled *antibody* (or vice versa).
[ref. 3]

radioimmunoconjugate

Biochemical *conjugate* consisting of a targeting molecule such as an *antibody* or antibody fragment together with a *cytotoxic* or diagnostic radionuclide.
[After ref. 3]

radiotoxicity

Property of an incorporated radioactive substance to produce *adverse effects* on the organism and its *tissues* due to its *ionizing radiation*.
[*]

rain-out

Removal of *pollutants* from air by incorporation into developing rain droplets in clouds.
[ref. 2]

rales

See *crepitation*.

random sample

probability sample
Opposite term: *biased sample*

Subset of elements of a *population* that is arrived at by selecting elements in such a way that each element has an equal probability of selection.
[*]

randomized control trial

randomized controlled trial

Study in which subjects are divided at random into two or more groups, one of which serves as a *control group* and receives either no treatment, a standard treatment, or a *placebo*, while the remainder receive a treatment or drug, the effectiveness of which is being tested.
[*]

range-finding test

See *screening test*.

rarefaction estimate of richness

Estimate of *species richness* expressed relative to that of a *sample* having a standard number of individuals.
[ref. 2]

rate (in epidemiology)

Frequency of occurrence, a measure of the frequency with which an event occurs in a defined *population* in a specified period of time.
Note 1: Most rates in epidemiology are ratios, calculated by dividing a numerator (*e.g.*, the number of deaths or newly occurring cases of a *disease* in a given period), by a denominator, (*e.g.*, the average population during that period).
See also *birth rate, per capita; death rate, per capita.*
Note 2: Some rates in epidemiology are proportions, *i.e.*, the numerator is contained within the denominator (as when a number of patients with a given disease is divided by the total population from which they come).
Note 3: The term "rate" has different meanings depending on the scientific context. In chemistry it usually means "velocity" and in mathematics a "quotient".
[*]
See also *birth rate; death rate.*

rate constant, k

rate coefficient

Numerical constant in a rate-of-reaction (v) equation; for example,

$$v = k\,[\mathrm{A}]\alpha[\mathrm{B}]\beta\ \ldots$$

where [A], [B] *etc.* are reactant concentrations, k is the rate constant, and α, β, *etc.* are corresponding empirical constants.
[ref. 1]

rate constant-based model

Compartment model that employs rate constants to quantify the rate of change in *concentration* or amount of a *toxicant.*
[ref. 2]

rate-controlling step

rate-determining step
rate-limiting step

Reaction in a sequence of chemical reactions that most restricts the overall velocity of product formation.
Note: In biochemistry, a rate-determining step can be due to low availability (*concentration*) of a substrate, cofactor, or catalyst (*enzyme*), or depend upon the turnover rate of the responsible enzyme.
[*]

rate-determining step

See *rate-controlling step.*

rate difference (RD) (in epidemiology)

Absolute difference between two *rates.*
Example: Difference in *incidence* rate between a population group *exposed* to a causal factor and a population group not exposed to the factor.

Note: In comparisons of exposed and unexposed groups, the term *excess rate* may be used as a synonym for rate difference.
[After ref. 1]

rate-limiting step

See *rate-controlling step.*

rate-of-living theory of aging

See *aging, rate-of-living theory of.*

rate ratio (in epidemiology) (RR)

Value obtained by dividing the *rate* in an *exposed population* by the rate in an unexposed population.
[ref. 1]

rate, vital

See *vital rate.*

raticide

Substance intended to kill rats.
[ref. 1]
Compare *rodenticide.*

Raynaud phenomenon

Intermittent bilateral attacks of *vasospasm* and *ischemia* of the fingers or toes, and sometimes of the ears and nose, marked by a severe pallor and often accompanied by *paresthesia* and *pain.*
Note 1: The Raynaud phenomenon is brought on characteristically by cold or emotional stimuli and relieved by heat, and may be due to an underlying *disease* or anatomic abnormality.
Note 2: The Raynaud phenomenon is more common in women than men and occurs in most patients with *progressive systemic sclerosis, mixed connective tissue disease*, and polymyositis/scleroderma overlap *syndrome.*
Note 3: When the condition is *idiopathic* or primary, it is termed Raynaud *disease.*
[ref. 3]

reabsorption (in biology)

Absorption by a living organism of a substance that it has previously absorbed and then released (*e.g.*, the uptake of a substance from the proximal renal tubule following *glomerular* filtration).
[ref. 1]

reaction time

Time between an inducing sensory *stimulus* and a measured physiological response.
[ref. 4]
See also *simple reaction time test.*

reactive airways dysfunction syndrome (RADS)

Syndrome characterized by reversible airflow limitation and complicating bronchial hyperresponsiveness induced by acute exposure to high *concentrations* of non-*sensitizer* irritant gases.
[ref. 3]

reactive intermediate

Unstable, short lived, reaction product, such as a radical or a carbocation.
Note: Reactive intermediates formed during *phase I reactions of biotransformation* of some *xenobiotics* tend to react nonspecifically with surrounding biomolecules, including *DNA*, thus leading to *cell* damage, organ *necrosis,* and potentially *tumor* initiation.
[*]
See also *reactive intermediate.*

reactive metabolite

Chemically *reactive intermediate* (*e.g.*, a radical species) formed during the *phase I reaction of biotransformation* of a *xenobiotic* or endogenous compound.
Note 1: Reactive metabolites may bind to *biomolecules* such as proteins and DNA, potentially leading to *cell* damage and *somatic mutations.*
Note 2: Some chemicals, such as nitrosamines and chlorinated aliphatic compounds, release large amounts of reactive *metabolites* during biotransformation in the liver and other *drug*-metabolizing *organs*; they are often potent *carcinogens.*
[*]

reactive nitrogen species (RNS)

Any small oxygen/nitrogen-based molecule with biological activity or that can facilitate biological nitrosylation reactions.
Note: Reactive nitrogen species include dioxidonitrogen (NO_2), nitryl ($NO_2^{\bullet}$), oxidonitrogen (nitrogen monoxide, nitrosyl radical; $NO^{\bullet}$), oxidonitrogen (nitrosyl cation; NO^+), hydroxyoxidonitrogen (nitrous acid; HNO_2), and oxidonitrate (NO^-).
[*]
See also *reactive oxygen species.*

reactive oxygen intermediate (ROI)

See *reactive oxygen species.*

reactive oxygen species (ROS)

Chemically reactive inorganic *species* of oxygen, often used in a biological context where such species play roles in *oxidative stress* and normal *cell* physiology.
Note 1: ROS are often considered to be the intermediates in the biological reduction of dioxygen to water; superoxide ($O_2^{-\bullet}$), hydrogen peroxide (H_2O_2), and hydroxyl ($HO^{\bullet}$).
Note 2: Sometimes ROS is also used as a term to include other oxygen-containing molecules, including *reactive nitrogen species.*
[*]

read-across (in toxicology)

Prediction of *toxicity* of untested substances with specific molecular structure(s), based on known toxicity of other substances that contain these same structures and that have been tested.
[*]
See also *quantitative structure–activity relationship.*

readily biodegradable

Arbitrary classification of substances that have passed certain specified screening tests for ultimate biodegradability; these tests are so stringent that such compounds will be rapidly and completely biodegraded in a wide variety of *aerobic* environments.
[ref. 1]
See also *biodegradation.*

reagin

Historic term for *antibodies* of the *immunoglobulin E* class.
[ref. 1]

realized niche

See *niche, realized.*

rear

1. Of a rodent or other animal, to lift both its front legs simultaneously off a surface upon which it is standing.
2. Of an animal, to care for its young until they are mature.
3. To breed and raise animals to maturity.

[*]

reasonable maximum exposure (RME)

Highest *exposure* that is reasonably expected to occur.
Note: Typically, the 95 % upper confidence limit of the *toxicant* distribution is used, but if only a few data points (say less than 10) are available, the maximum detected *concentration* is used.
[ref. 2]

reasonable worst case

Semiquantitative term referring to the lower portion of the high end of the *exposure*, dose, or *risk* distribution.
[ref. 2]

rebound (in medicine)

Reappearance of original symptom(s), often exacerbated, following cessation of treatment.
[ref. 4]
See also *headache, rebound.*

recalcitrant residue

Substance that does not degrade under normal *environmental* conditions.
Note: The recalcitrant residue may be very stable and insoluble in water or *hydrophobic solvents* and, as a result, it may not be *bioaccessible, bioavailable*, or *biodegradable.*
[*]

recall antigen

See *antigen, recall.*

receiving water

See *water, receiving.*

receptor

Molecular component, in or on a cell, that is specifically recognized by and binds a molecular structure (*ligand*), leading to physiological *signal transduction* or mediation of an effect.
[ref. 5]

β-receptor

See *receptor, β-adrenergic.*

receptor, acetylcholine

Integral *membrane* protein that enables responsiveness of a *cell* to the binding of *acetylcholine*.
[After ref. 4]

receptor, α-adrenergic

Class of *adrenergic receptor* mainly functioning in *vasoconstriction* and modulation of *glandular secretions*.
[ref. 4]
See also *sympathomimetic*.

receptor, β-adrenergic

adrenergic receptor
adrenoceptor
β-receptor

Member of a class of *G protein-coupled receptors* that are targets of the *catecholamines*, especially *adrenaline, noradrenaline*, and related substances.
[ref. 4]
See also *β-blocker*.

receptor, γ-aminobutyric acid (GABA)

Transmembrane *receptor* protein that binds and responds to the inhibitory *neurotransmitter γ-aminobutyric acid*.
Note 1: GABA receptors are found in different parts of the *central nervous system*.
Note 2: There are two different receptor types with different *signal transduction* pathways:

- GABA-A receptors are *ion channels*.
- GABA-B receptors are *G-protein-coupled* signal transducers.

[ref. 4]

receptor, 2-amino-3-(3-hydroxy-5-methyl-1,2-oxazol-4-yl)propanoic acid (AMPA receptor)

Glutamate receptor in the *central nervous system* activated by the synthetic glutamate analog, AMPA.
[ref. 4]
See also *excitotoxicity*.

receptor, antigen

Specific *antigen*-binding *receptor* on *T* or *B-lymphocytes* that is transcribed and translated following rearrangements and translocation of *V, D*, and *J genes*.
[ref. 3]

receptor, aryl hydrocarbon (AHR)

Ligand-activated *transcription factor* involved in the regulation of biological responses to planar aromatic hydrocarbons.
Note 1: The AHR has been shown to regulate *xenobiotic*-metabolizing *enzymes* such as various forms of *cytochrome P450* family 1 members.

Note 2: The AHR also appears to play a role in cell *proliferation* and *differentiation* during *vertebrate* development, including *hematopoiesis* and development of the *lymphoid* and *immune systems.*
[ref. 5]
See also *receptor.*

receptor, B-cell (BCR)

Receptor on the surface of a *B-cell* consisting of transmembrane *immunoglobulin* that recognizes a specific *antigen.*
[ref. 3]

receptor, complement (CR)

Cell-surface protein that recognizes and binds *complement* proteins that have bound an *antigen.*
Note 1: CRs on *phagocytes* allow them to identify *pathogens* coated with complement proteins for uptake and destruction.
Note 2: CRs include CR1, CR2, CR3, CR4, and the receptor for Clq.
[ref. 3]

receptor, G-protein coupled

Seven-transmembrane-domain receptor that, after receiving a signal through ligand-binding, interacts with guanosine triphosphate/diphosphate (GTP/GDP) binding proteins (G proteins) to initiate *signal transduction.*
[ref. 4]

receptor, homing

Cell-surface molecule that directs *leukocytes* to specific locations in the body.
[ref. 3]

receptor, lymphocyte homing

Cell-surface *glycoprotein* on *lymphocyte*s and other *leukocyte*s that mediates adhesion to specialized blood vessels, the *high endothelial venules.*
Note: Several different classes of lymphocyte *homing receptors* have been identified, and they appear to bind to different surface molecules (*addressins*) on high *endothelial* venules in different *tissues.*
[ref. 3]

receptor, *N*-methyl-D-aspartate (NMDA)-type glutamate

One of the various types of *receptor*s of the *neurotransmitter glutamate.*
Note 1: The NMDA-type glutamate receptor is both a *ligand-gated* and *voltage-gated* cation channel.
Note 2: The NMDA-type glutamate receptor is believed to be involved in memory and learning.
[ref. 4]
See also *receptor, α-amino-3-hydroxy-5-methyl-4-isoxazole propionic acid; ion channel;* N-*methyl-D-aspartate.*

receptor, nicotinic

One of the two main classes of *acetylcholine receptor*s (see also *muscarinic receptor*), *ligand-gated ion channel*s that open upon binding nicotine as well as *acetylcholine.*
[ref. 4]

receptor, nuclear

Receptor that encounters its ligand in the cytosol and translocates to the nucleus, where it binds DNA and acts as a factor regulating *gene transcription*.
[ref. 5]

receptor, nuclear type I

Steroid hormone receptor, found in the cytosol, that upon ligand binding translocates into the *nucleus* and interacts with *DNA* as a homodimer to drive specific *gene transcription*.
[ref. 5]
Compare *receptor, nuclear type II*.

receptor, nuclear type II

Steroid hormone receptor, found in the nucleus, that upon ligand binding interacts with *DNA* as a heterodimer (usually with the *retinoid* X receptor, RXR) to drive *transcription* of specific *genes*.
[ref. 5]
Compare *receptor, nuclear type I*.

receptor, nucleotide-binding oligomerization domain-containing protein (NOD)-like (NLR)

NOD-like receptor protein (NLRP)
Cytosolic protein that contains a central nucleotide-binding oligomerization domain, an N-terminal effector-binding domain and C-terminal leucine-rich repeats (LRRs).
Note 1: NOD-like receptors are involved in regulation of *inflammation* and *apoptosis*; many family members are thought to function as *pattern recognition receptors*.
Note 2: NOD-like *receptors* have been implicated as medications for protective *immune responses* against intracellular *pathogens*.
Note 3: *Genetic* associations of *polymorphisms* in NOD-like receptor genes with complex *chronic* inflammatory barrier *diseases*, such as *Crohn disease* and *asthma*, and with rare auto-inflammatory *syndromes* including familial cold *urticaria*, Muckle–Wells syndrome and *Blau syndrome* have been described.
[ref. 3]
See also *NACHT domain-, leucine-rich repeat-, and PYD-containing protein 3 (NALP3, NLRP3)*.

receptor, pattern recognition (PRR)

Receptor found on many different cell types in the *immune system* that enables them to recognize *pathogen-associated molecular patterns*.
Note 1: Among the large number of different PRRs are the mannose receptor (CD206), *macrophage* scavenger receptor (CD204), and the *toll-like receptors*.
Note 2: Many of the *NOD-like receptors* are thought to serve as PRRs.
[ref. 3]

receptor, poly-Ig

Receptor molecule that specifically binds *J chain*-containing polymeric *immunoglobulin, i.e.*, dimeric secretory *immunoglobulin A* and pentameric *immunoglobulin M*, and transports it across *mucosal* epithelium.
[ref. 3]
Note: The poly-Ig receptor contributes to an important mechanism for *immunological* defense against microorganisms at the intestinal barrier.
[*]

receptor, T-cell (TCR)

Antigen-specific *receptor* on *T-cells* composed of one set of heterodimeric chains; two types of TCR heterodimers are known (α/β and γ/δ).
Note: Functional binding for TCR requires a complex of *major histocompatibility complex molecule, antigenic* peptide, and TCR.
[ref. 3]

receptor, α:β T-cell

T-cell receptor consisting of a heterodimer of two different *glycoprotein* chains, designated α and β, assembled into an α:β heterodimer.
[ref. 3]

receptor, γ:δ T-cell

T-cell receptor composed of two different *glycoprotein* chains, designated γ and δ, assembled into a heterodimer.
Note: Cells bearing γ:δ T-cell receptors are called *γ:δ T-cells*. The group of γ:δ T-cells is much less common than *α:β T-cells*, and is usually found in the gut *mucosa*, in a population of *lymphocytes* known as *intra-epithelial lymphocytes*.

receptor, thyroid-stimulating hormone (TSHR)

Receptor in the *thyroid gland* for *thyroid-stimulating hormone*, found to be the main *autoantigenic* target in patients with *Graves disease*.
Note: Most TSHR *autoantibodies* are stimulatory, acting as *agonists* of thyroid-stimulating hormone, but *receptor*-blocking *antibodies* are also found.
[ref. 3]

receptor, toll-like (TLR)

Member of a family of *pattern recognition receptors* involved in the detection of structures associated with *pathogens* or damaged *host* tissues.
[ref. 3]

receptor-mediated endocytosis

Endocytosis of a substance together with its *receptor* following receptor binding.
[ref. 1]

recessive (in genetics)

Referring to or denoting heritable characteristics controlled by *genes* that are expressed in *offspring* only when inherited from both parents.
[ref. 5]
Compare *dominant*.
See also *autosomal recessive mutation*.

recessive gene

See *gene, recessive*.

reciprocal mesenchymal-epithelial interaction

Process in *tissue* or *organ* development in which *epithelium* induces changes in the *mesenchyme* and the mesenchyme also induces changes in the epithelium, through *paracrine signaling*.
Note: An example of the reciprocal interaction occurs during development of the *prostate*, in which mesenchyme of the *urogenital sinus* influences differentiation and

patterning of the prostatic epithelium, and the developing epithelium induces prostatic mesenchymal cells to differentiate into smooth muscle and other prostatic *stromal cells*.
[ref. 5]
See also *epithelial-to-mesenchymal transition; mesenchymal-to-epithelial transition*.

reciprocal translocation

Chromosomal translocation in which crossing over between two non*homologous* chromosomes leads to each carrying genetic material from the other.
Note: If the translocation is equal (*i.e.*, no *genetic* material is missing following reciprocal translocation) it is called a balanced translocation, and may be without severe consequences for the developing *embryo*. If extra or missing genetic material results from the process, it is called an unbalanced translocation, and the consequences are often harmful.
[ref. 5]

recombinant antibody

See *antibody, recombinant*.

recombinant DNA

New *DNA* made by transplanting or *splicing* a DNA sequence into the DNA of host cells in such a way that the modified DNA can be replicated in the host cells in a normal fashion.
[ref. 1]

recombinant DNA technology

Methods involving the use of *restriction enzymes* to cleave *DNA* at specific sites, allowing sections of DNA molecules to be inserted into *plasmid* or other vectors and cloned in an appropriate host organism (*e.g.*, a bacterial or yeast cell).
[ref. 1]

recombination, genetic

1. Referring to new *gene* sequences, and thus to new heritable information, caused by gene crossovers, occurring naturally in either *meiosis* or *mitosis*, or constructed artificially, for the purpose of introducing a new trait into an organism or *cell line*.
   See also *recombination, homologous*.
2. In immunology, random scrambling of specific gene sequences to produce the vast array of possible *immunoglobulin* and *T-cell receptor* sequences required to recognize, potentially, all possible *antigens*.

[ref. 5]

recombination, homologous

Crossing over between two similar or identical strands of *DNA*, resulting in exchange of corresponding stretches of DNA between two sister *chromosomes*.
[ref. 5]

recombination-activating gene (RAG)

See *gene, recombination-activating*.

recombination signal sequence (RSS)

Any conserved heptamer (7-nucleotide)-nonamer (9-nucleotide) sequence, separated by a 12 or 23 base spacer, which occurs 3′ of variable gene segments, 5′ and 3′ of *diversity gene* segments, and 5′ of *joining gene* segments, in both *immunoglobulin* and *T-cell receptor genes.*
Note: The RSS functions as a recognition sequence for the recombinase *enzymes* that mediate the *gene rearrangement* process involved in the generation of *lymphocyte antigen receptor* diversity.
[ref. 3]

recommended exposure level (REL) (in toxicology)

Highest allowable airborne *concentration* of a regulated substance.
Note: *Exposure* at the REL is expected to be noninjurious to workers. It may be expressed as a ceiling limit or as a *time-weighted average.*
[ref. 1]

recommended limit

Maximum concentration of a potentially *toxic* substance that is expected to be *safe.*
Note: Recommended limits are rarely defined as legal limits to be enforced. They are analogous to guidelines, which have only advisory status.
[ref. 2]

reconstituted water

Deionized or glass-distilled water to which reagent-grade chemicals have been added.
Note: Reconstituted water is expected to be free from *contaminants* and to have desired pH and *hardness* characteristics.
[ref. 2]

reconstitution

Restoration to original form of a substance previously altered for preservation and storage.
[ref. 1]

recovery

1. Process leading to partial or complete restoration of a *cell, tissue, organ*, or organism following its damage from *exposure* to a harmful substance or agent.
2. Term used in analytical and preparative chemistry to denote the fraction of the total quantity of a substance that can be separated by a specified chemical procedure.

[ref. 1]

recovery factor

Fraction or percentage of the total quantity of a substance extracted or separated from a sample under specified conditions.
[ref. 1]

rectum (n)/**rectal** (adj)

Terminal part of the large intestine, ending at the *anus.*
[ref. 5]

recycling (of waste)

Process or method achieving recovery of some value from a *waste*, either as reusable material or as energy.
[ref. 1]

red pulp

splenic pulp

Parenchymal tissue of the *spleen* consisting of cords of *cells* and *sinuses* infiltrated with *erythrocytes* and responsible for removal of aged or damaged erythrocytes.
[ref. 3]
See also *white pulp*.

5α-reductase

alpha-reductase

Enzyme (EC 1.3.99.5) that converts *testosterone* to 5α-dihydrotestosterone in peripheral tissues.
[ref. 5]

5α-reductase deficiency

Condition caused by a *mutation* of the *5α-reductase* type II gene, with *autosomal recessive* inheritance.
Note: The resulting deficiency of 5α-dihydrotestosterone leads to varying degrees of feminization in genetic males.
[After ref. 3]

redundancy hypothesis

Hypothesis that many biological *species* are redundant, and their loss will not influence *community* function as long as crucial (*e.g.*, *keystone* and *dominant*) species *populations* are maintained.
[ref. 2]

Reed–Sternberg cell

Large transformed *lymphocyte*, often binucleate, considered pathognomonic of *Hodgkin lymphoma*.
[ref. 3]

reference concentration (RfC) (for inhalational exposure)

Estimate of *exposure* of the human population (including sensitive subgroups that include children, *asthmatics*, and the elderly) by continuous *inhalation* that is likely to be without an appreciable risk of deleterious effects to *health* during a lifetime.
Note 1: The RfC can be derived from various types of human or animal data such as the *no-observed-adverse-effect level, lowest-observed-adverse-effect level*, or the *benchmark concentration*, with *uncertainty factors* generally applied to reflect the limitations of the data. Uncertainty in the estimate may span perhaps an order of magnitude.
Note 2: The RfC is used in USEPA's non*cancer* health assessments.
[ref. 1]

reference distribution

Statistical distribution of *reference values*.
[ref. 1]

reference dose (RfD)

Estimate of a daily *exposure* of the human *population* (including sensitive subgroups) to a defined substance, that is likely to be without an appreciable risk of deleterious effects to *health* during a lifetime.
Note 1: The RfD can be derived from a *no-observed-adverse-effect level, lowest-observed-adverse-effect level*, or the *benchmark dose*, with *uncertainty factors* generally applied to reflect limitations of the data used.
Note 2: The RfD is usually reported in units of mg of substance/kg body weight/day for oral *exposures* and may carry an uncertainty of perhaps an order of magnitude.
Note 3: The RfD is used in the EPA's non*cancer* health assessments.
[After ref. 1]

reference environment

Generalized description of the *environment* into which *contaminants* will be released, and in which organisms will be exposed.
Note: Reference environments are used when there is no specific site at risk.
[ref. 2]

reference group

See *reference sample group.*

reference individual

Person selected with the use of defined criteria for comparative purposes in a clinical *study*.
[ref. 1]

reference interval

Region between, and including, two reference limits, for example, between the percentiles 2.5 and 97.5.
[ref. 1]

reference limit

Boundary value defined so that a stated fraction of the *reference values* is either less than or exceeds that boundary value with a stated probability.
[ref. 1]

reference material (RM)

calibration material
reference standard
standard material
standard

Material sufficiently homogeneous and stable regarding one or more properties, for use in *calibration*, in assignment of a *traceable* value to another material, or in *quality assurance*.
[ref. 1]

reference population

Group of all *reference individuals* used to establish criteria against which a *population* that is being studied can be compared.
[ref. 1]

reference sample group

Selected *reference individuals*, statistically adequate numerically, to represent the *reference population.*
[ref. 1]

reference sediment

Whole *sediment* collected near a site of interest, used to assess sediment conditions in the absence of the substance(s) of concern that is (are) present at the site itself.
Note: Reference sediment should represent the background conditions in sediment free of the substance(s) of concern.
[ref. 2]

reference site

Relatively unpolluted site used for comparison with *polluted* sites in *environmental monitoring* studies, often incorrectly referred to as a *control* site.
[ref. 2]

reference toxicant

Substance used as a *positive control* in a *toxicity* test, in contrast to the *negative control* provided by a sample free of the substance being tested.
Note: The term "positive control" is used here to describe a situation (sample and procedure) that is very similar to that of the actual experimental test and that is known from previous experience to give a positive result (*e.g.*, a defined *toxic* effect).
[After ref. 2]

reference toxicity test

Assay conducted with a *reference toxicant* to determine:

- possible changes of the *sensitivity* of a test organism (*e.g.*, an aquatic organism that lived in contaminated water)
- in-lab problems with a test procedure.
- deviations between different laboratories.

[ref. 1]

reference value

Value of a quantity generally accepted as having a sufficiently small measurement uncertainty that it can be used reliably as a basis for comparison with values of quantities of the same kind.
[After ref. 1]

reflex

Involuntary reaction in response to a *stimulus* applied to the *peripheral nervous system* followed by its transmission to the nervous centers in the *brain* or *spinal cord.*
Note: The reflex response is often the *contraction* of a muscle due to a stimulus applied to its *proprioceptors.*
[ref. 4]

reflex sympathetic dystrophy (RSD)

Diffuse persistent *pain*, usually in an extremity.
Note: RSD is often associated with vasomotor disturbances, interruption of the *nerve* supply, and limitation of joint movement, frequently following local injury.
[ref. 4]

region (in geography)

Area of the Earth's surface differentiated by its specific natural or artificial features.
[After ref. 2]

regioselectivity (n)/**regioselective** (adj)

Referring to a chemical reaction in which bond making or breaking occurs preferentially at one atom over all other atoms.
Note: A reaction is termed completely (100 %) regioselective if the discrimination is complete; otherwise it is partially (<100 %) regioselective.
[*]
See also *stereoselectivity*.

regression analysis

Statistical approach including modeling techniques to describe a set of dependent variables, *Y*, in terms of combinations of predictors, *X*.
[After ref. 1]

regulated upon activation normal T-cell expressed and secreted (RANTES)

Chemokine, which is secreted by *T-cells* and *macrophages* upon stimulation by *mitogens*, and that acts as a chemoattractant and stimulates *eosinophils* and *basophils*.
[ref. 3]

regulatory dose

Expected *dose* resulting from human *exposure* to a substance at the level at which it is regulated in the *environment*.
[ref. 1]

regulatory idiotope

Antibody or *T-cell receptor idiotope* capable of regulating *immune responses* via interaction with *lymphocytes* bearing complementary *idiotopes* (anti-idiotopes).
[ref. 3]

regulatory sequence

DNA sequence to which specific proteins bind to activate or repress the expression of a *gene*.
[ref. 1]

regulatory T-cell (Treg)

See *T-cell, regulatory*.

regulatory toxicology

Branch of *toxicology* that deals with the evidence-based generation of laws and *guidelines*, methods of adherence to rules and regulations, and related *risk assessment* and *risk management*.
[*]

reinforcement (in psychology)

Use of a *stimulus* in *operant conditioning* to increase the likelihood that a particular behavior will occur.

Note 1: Reinforcement may be positive (using a desirable stimulus) or negative (removing or withholding an adverse stimulus).
Note 2: In contrast to reinforcement, use of stimuli to decrease a behavior is called punishment.
[ref. 4]

rejection (in immunology)

Immune response leading to destruction of a *transplanted organ* or *tissue*.
[ref. 3]
See also *rejection, acute; chronic rejection; graft rejection*.

rejection, acute

Rejection of a tissue or *organ graft* from a genetically unrelated donor, typically occurring within 10 to 13 days of *transplantation*.
[ref. 3]

rejection, chronic

Immunologically triggered reaction occurring in a *transplanted organ* or *tissue*, leading to progressive destruction and finally failure of the transplanted organ occurring two months to many years after *transplantation*.
Note: In contrast to chronic rejection, hyperacute rejection caused by preformed *antibodies* starts within minutes after organ transplantation, and acute rejection occurs within 2 to 60 days.
[ref. 3]

rejection, graft

Destruction of *grafted* tissue by *host lymphocytes* following an *adaptive immune response*.
[ref. 3]
See also *rejection*.

relative bioavailability

See *bioavailability, relative*.

relative excess risk (RER)

See *risk, relative excess*.

relative fitness

See *fitness*.

relative odds

See *odds ratio*.

relative risk (RR)

See *risk ratio*.

relative systemic availability

Area under the curve following nonintravenous administration of one substance divided by that of another, or of the same substance given in a different formulation, corrected for *dose*.

Note: *First-pass metabolism* in the intestine, liver, or lung may affect relative *systemic* availability.
[*]
See also *bioavailability, relative*.

relaxant

Agent that reduces muscle tension.
[ref. 4]
See also *relaxation*.

relaxation (in neurobiology)

Reduction in or release of tension, as in, *e.g.*, reversal of muscle *contraction* or relief of anxiety.
[ref. 4]

remedial investigation (RI)

Study, preceding remediation activities, that has three parts: (1) characterization of the type and degree of pollution or *contamination*, (2) human *risk assessment*, and (3) ecological *risk assessment*.
[ref. 2]

remedial investigation and feasibility study (RI/FS)

Study of an EPA *Superfund* site that has as its goal the implementation of "remedies that reduce, control, or eliminate risks to human *health* and the *environment*" or, more specifically, the accumulation of "information sufficient to support an informed *risk management* decision regarding which remedy appears to be most appropriate for a given site".
[ref. 2]
See also *remediation*.

remediation

Removal of *pollution* or *contaminants* from *environmental* media such as *soil*, groundwater, *sediment*, or surface water for the general protection of human *health* and the *environment*.
[After ref. 1]
See also *remedy*.

remote sensing

Technology that allows the acquisition and analysis of data without requiring physical contact with the land or water surface being studied.
Note: Most remote sensing determines qualities or characteristics of areas of interest based on measurements of visible light, infrared radiation, or radio energy coming from them.
[ref. 2]

renal

Pertaining to the kidneys.
[ref. 1]

renal tubule

See *nephron*.

renewed static test

See *static-renewal test.*

renal plasma flow

Volume of *plasma* passing through the kidneys in unit time.
[ref. 1]

renopathy

See *nephropathy.*

remedy

Anything, such as a medicine or therapy, that relieves *pain*, cures *disease*, or corrects a *disorder*.
[ref. 1]

repeatability

measurement repeatability

Measurement precision under *repeatability conditions* of measurement.
[ref. 1]

repeatability condition

repeatability condition of measurement

Measurement under a set of conditions that includes the same measurement procedure, operator, measuring system, operating conditions, and location, with the measurement replicated one or more times over a short period of time.
[ref. 1]

repellent

Substance used mainly to repel *blood*-sucking insects (*e.g.*, mosquitoes) in order to protect humans and animals.
Note: The term "repellent" may also be applied to substances used to repel other biological organisms, *e.g.*, mammals, birds, rodents, mites, and plant pests.
[ref. 1]

reperfusion

Restoration of the *blood* supply to an *organ* or *tissue* following a period of *ischemia*.
Note: Reperfusion itself may cause further injury to the tissue (*ischemia-reperfusion injury*), for instance, by production of *reactive oxygen species* or excessive Ca^{2+} influx.
[ref. 4]
See also *ischemia-reperfusion injury*.

reperfusion injury

See *ischemia-reperfusion injury*.

replicate sampling

Act of taking multiple *sample*s concurrently under comparable conditions.
Note: Replicate sampling may be accomplished by taking samples adjacent in time or space.
[ref. 1]

replication

1. Duplication or repetition of an experiment under similar (controlled) conditions to reduce to a minimum the error and to estimate the variation, thus obtaining a more precise result
   Note: Each determination, including the first, is called a replicate (see *replicate sampling*).
2. Process whereby the *genetic* material of an organism is duplicated.

[ref. 1]

repolarization

Returning of a cell's *membrane potential* to its *resting potential* following *depolarization*.
[ref. 4]

reproducibility

measurement reproducibility

Measurement precision under *reproducibility conditions of measurement*.
[ref. 1]
See also *repeatability*.

reproducibility condition

reproducibility condition of measurement
Specified condition of measurement selected from a range of conditions that include different locations, operators, and measuring systems.
Note 1: The different measuring systems may use different measurement procedures.
Note 2: As far as possible, specification of reproducibility conditions should include all the relevant conditions, whether changed or unchanged.
[ref. 1]

reproduction (n)/reproduce (v) (in biology)

Generation of offspring by living organisms.
[*]

reproductive assessment by continuous breeding (RACB)

fertility assessment by continuous breeding (FACB)

Reproductive toxicity test in rodents in which female animals are repeatedly mated, and frequency and size of *litters* and other parameters are measured; second or later generation *fertility* is also studied.
[ref. 5]

reproductive cycle

Cycle of physiological changes in the female reproductive organs, from the time of *fertilization* of the *oocyte* through *gestation* and *parturition*.
[ref. 5]

reproductive senescence

Progressive decline in reproductive capacity with age, marked by *menopause* in females.
[ref. 5]

reproductive toxicant

Agent that interferes with reproductive function, including sexual performance, *fertility*, and development of the *fetus* and *embryo*.
Note 1: Effects of reproductive toxicants on fertility may include effects on *sperm* count and sperm *viability, oogenesis* and *ovulation, placental* function, *lactation*, male erectile function (see *erectile dysfunction*), and *genetic* intactness.
Note 2: Effects of reproductive toxicants on development may include, but are not limited to, effects on embryo *viability*, fetal growth, *morphogenesis*, and functional integrity.
Note 3: Reproductive toxicants may show long-term effects not detectable before the second or later generations.
[ref. 5]
See also *developmental toxicology*.

reproductive toxicity test

Procedure based on specific guidelines in which *adverse effects* of a substance on reproduction and development are studied either in animals or by use of *in vitro assays*.
[ref. 5]

reproductive toxicology

Study of the *adverse effects* of substances on male and female reproductive function or capacity and on resultant *offspring*.
[ref. 1]

reproductive value, V_A

Expected contribution of an individual to the *growth* of the *population* based on both current and future reproduction expected for an individual of that age taken from a *life table*, and sometimes restricted to the female population (mothers and their rates of giving birth to girls).
[*]

rescue effect

Increased probability of a vacated-patch reoccupation in a *metapopulation* as the number of nearby occupied patches increases.
[ref. 2]

reserve capacity

Physiological or biochemical cushion that may be available to maintain *homeostasis* when the body or an organism adapts to an *environmental* change.
[After ref. 1]

reservoir (in biology)

Storage *compartment* from which a substance may be released with subsequent biological effects.
[ref. 1]

residence time

See *mean residence time*.

residual risk

See *risk, residual.*

residual time

See *mean residence time.*

residue

Contaminant remaining in an organism or in other material such as *soil*, plants, food or packaging, following *exposure*.
[ref. 1]

residue level of an antibiotic, acceptable

Acceptable *concentration* of a residue that has been established for an *antibiotic* found in human or animal foods.
[ref. 1]

resilience (of a community)

Ability of a *community* to maintain its structure and function in the face of disturbance, and to reorganize following disturbance-driven change.
[ref. 1]

resistance (in immunology)

Ability of an organism to withstand an *infection.*
Note: Bacterial resistance is the ability of a bacterium to grow and divide despite the presence of an *antibiotic.*
[ref. 3]

resistance (in physiology and toxicology)

Ability to withstand the effect of various factors including potentially *toxic* substances.
Examples: Resistance of bacteria to *antibiotics*, resistance of insects towards *pesticides.*
Note: The term "resistance" is often reserved for the enhanced ability to cope with a factor due to *genetic adaptation*. The term "*tolerance*" is often reserved for enhanced abilities associated with physiological *acclimation*. Tolerance may be used for both acclimation and genetic adaptation.
[ref. 2]

resolution phase

Return to a sexually unexcited state following orgasm.
[ref. 4]

resorption

1. Removal of *mineralized* or *necrotic tissue* by natural processes, as in breakdown of bone by *osteoclasts*, or disappearance of a tooth.
2. Disintegration and assimilation of an *embryo* or *fetus*, through a natural process involving lysis and removal of all the products of *conception* by cells of the maternal *immune system.*
3. In multi*gestational* pregnancies, death of one fetus followed by absorption of its *tissue* by another, sometimes referred to as "vanishing twin".

[ref. 5]

resorptive effect

Action of a substance after its *reabsorption* from the *gastrointestinal tract* into the *blood*.
[ref. 1]

respirable dust

respirable particles
Mass fraction of *dust* (particles) that penetrates to the unciliated (see *cilium*) airways of the lung (the *alveolar* region).
Note: The respirable dust fraction may be represented by the lower part of a cumulative log-normal curve having a median *aerodynamic diameter* of 4 μm with a standard deviation of 2 μm (values for human lungs).
[ref. 1]

respiratory burst

Generation of *cytotoxic* superoxide from dioxygen due to increased NADPH oxidase (EC 1.6.3.1) activity, typically occurring in activated *neutrophils*.
[ref. 3]
See also *neutrophil activation*.

respiratory cycle

Repetitive pattern of breathing, based on a *cycle* of *inhalation* and *exhalation*, usually with a pause before inhalation.
Note: The respiratory cycle is controlled by sensors in the respiratory system that initiate the repetition of the process.
[*]

respiratory hypersensitivity assay

Test of the ability of a substance to induce *hyperreactivity* in the airways, typically measured as an increase in the rate of respiration of guinea pigs during *inhalation* of the substance.
[ref. 3]

respiratory lamellae

See *secondary lamellae*.

response (in populations)

Proportion of an *exposed population* with a defined effect or the proportion of a group of individuals that demonstrates a defined effect in a given time at a given *dose rate*.
[ref. 1]

response, adaptive

Reaction of a biological system to *stress* by alteration of *tissue* structure, *cell phenotype*, or *metabolic homeostasis* to establish a more resistant state.
Note 1: *Adaptive response* to *exposure* to potential toxicants may occur at subtoxic doses and may involve both beneficial and (or) *adverse effects*.
Note 2: In *pathology*, *hypertrophy*, *hyperplasia*, *atrophy* and *metaplasia* are considered to be *adaptive responses*.
[*]

response, benchmark (BMR)

Response, expressed as an excess of background, at which a *benchmark dose* or *benchmark concentration* is set.
[ref. 1]

resting potential

Baseline *membrane potential.*
[ref. 4]

resting tremor

See *tremor*.

restriction (in immunology)

See *major histocompatibility complex (MHC) restriction.*

restriction endonuclease
restriction enzyme

Endonuclease from bacteria or archaea that recognizes specific short sequences of *DNA*, and cleaves the DNA molecule at that site, creating a double-strand break of DNA.
Note 1: Restriction enzymes are widely used as laboratory reagents to manipulate DNA sequences, *e.g.*, in molecular cloning, and can be used together with ligase enzymes that can join the newly exposed ends of the cut polymer chain to other polynucleotides.
Note 2: Type I restriction *enzymes* bind to these recognition sites but subsequently cut the DNA at different sites. Type II restriction enzymes both bind and cut within their recognition or *target* sites.
[*]
See also *restriction site*.

restriction enzyme

See *restriction endonuclease.*

restriction fragment length polymorphism (RFLP)

Variations in *DNA* nucleotide sequence that are indicated by the presence or absence of particular *restriction sites* in the DNA.
Note: RFLP analysis is a common method used for DNA profiling.
[ref. 5]

restriction site

Short *DNA* nucleotide sequence that is recognized by a sequence-specific *enzyme* (*restriction enzyme*) that cleaves the double stranded DNA.
[ref. 5]

rete

Fibrous mesh or network.
[ref. 5]

rete testis

Rete in the *testis* that carries *sperm* from the *seminiferous tubules*.
[ref. 5]

retention

1. Amount of a substance that is left from the total amount absorbed at a certain time after *exposure*.
2. Voluntary or involuntary holding back within the body or within an *organ, tissue*, or *cell* of matter that is normally eliminated (*e.g.*, urinary retention).

[After ref. 1]

retention effect, environmental

Consequence of the high *lipophilicity* of some *persistent organic pollutants* (POPs) that causes them to be bound more firmly than less lipophilic POPs in solid phases (such as *soil* and vegetation), and thus to spend less time in the atmosphere while also being less available for transport in the solid phase.
[After ref. 2]

reticuloendothelial system (RES)

See *mononuclear phagocyte system*.

reticulosis

Abnormal increase in *cells* related to the *reticuloendothelial system*.
[*]

retina

Multicell-layer *membrane* in the back of the eye containing *photoreceptor cells* and other *neural* components that make it sensitive to light and capable of transducing (see *signal transduction*) incoming optical information into neuronal signals that are necessary for vision.
[ref. 4,5]

retinoic acid

(2*E*,4*E*,6*E*,8*E*)-3,7-dimethyl-9-(2,6,6-trimethylcyclohex-1-en-1-yl)nona-2,4,6,8-tetraenoic acid

Acidic metabolite of vitamin A.
Note 1: Retinoic acid binds to the retinoic acid *receptor*, which then acts as a *transcription factor*.
Note 2: The role of the retinoic acid receptor in development (*e.g.*, in regulating *homeobox genes*) accounts for the *teratogenicity* of related *pharmaceuticals*.
[ref. 5]

retinoid

Member of a class of substances structurally related to vitamin A.
Note: Retinoids play roles in *cell growth* and *differentiation, tumor* suppression (see *tumor suppressor gene*), *immune* function, and vision. At higher concentrations they cause multiple *toxicities*, including effects on the long bones, spleen and *lymph* nodes, and *retina*.
[ref. 5]

retinopathy

Non*inflammatory degenerative disease* of the *retina*.
Note: Retinopathy of prematurity (see *premature birth*) is a risk for preterm infants, possibly induced by oxygen therapy and related to disorganized *retinal* blood vessels.
[ref. 5]

retinoschisis, congenital
juvenile retinoschisis
X-linked retinoschisis

Congenital splitting of the *retina* into two layers.
[ref. 5]

retroactive risk assessment
See *risk assessment, retrospective.*

retrograde axonal transport
See *axonal transport, retrograde.*

retroperitoneal
Outside of and posterior to the *peritoneum.*
[ref. 5]

retrospective cohort study
See *study, retrospective cohort.*

retrospective risk assessment
See *risk assessment, retrospective.*

retrospective study
See *study, retrospective cohort.*

returned effect of poisons
Enhancement of the *dose–effect relationship* for a poison following repeated *exposure* to decreasing doses.
[ref. 1]

reuptake
Transporter-dependent resequestration of a *neurotransmitter* by a *presynaptic neuron*, terminating *synaptic transmission.*
[ref. 4]

reverse genetics
See *genetics, reverse.*

reverse immunology
See *immunology, reverse.*

reverse mutation
See *mutation, reverse.*

reverse transcription
See *transcription, reverse.*

reversible alteration

Change from normal structure or function, induced by a substance or other agent(s), that returns to normal status or within normal limits after cessation of *exposure*.
[ref. 1]

Rey-Osterrieth complex figure (ROCF) test

Procedure in which the test subject first copies a complicated drawing and then is asked to draw it from memory.
Note: This tests several aspects of *cognitive* ability, including visuospatial perception and memory.
[ref. 4]

rhabdomyolysis

Acute, fulminating, potentially lethal *disease* of skeletal muscle that causes disintegration of striated muscle fibers, as evidenced by *myoglobin* in the *blood* and urine.
[ref. 1]
Note: Rhabdomyolysis is known to occur as a side-effect of treatment with statins.
[*]

rhesus (Rh) factor

Antigen that occurs on the *erythrocytes*, especially the D *antigen* of the Rh *blood group*, of about 85 per cent of humans.
Note 1: The Rh antigen is a common cause of *hemolytic disease of the newborn* (*erythroblastosis fetalis*), and of hemolytic *transfusion* reactions.
Note 2: The Rh factor was first identified in the *blood* of a rhesus monkey (***Mucaca mulatta***).
[ref. 3,5]

rheumatic fever

Inflammatory *disease* that may develop following a ***Streptococcal*** infection such as strep throat, and may affect the heart, joints, skin, and *brain*.
[ref. 3]

rheumatoid arthritis (RA)

Episodic *inflammatory systemic disease* with *autoimmune pathogenic* mechanisms.
Note: RA primarily affects the joints, causing symmetrical lesions and severe damage to the affected joints. It is the most common form of inflammatory joint disease (prevalence about 0.5 to 1 %).
[ref. 3]

rheumatoid factor

Immunoglobulins IgM, IgG, and *IgA autoantibodies* to the *Fc region* of IgG.
Note: Although detectable in various *diseases*, rheumatoid factor is used as a classification criterion of *rheumatoid arthritis (RA)*.
[ref. 3]

rhinitis

Inflammation of the *mucous membrane* of the nose.
[ref. 3]

rhinitis, allergic

Nasal discharge resulting from an *allergic* response.
[ref. 3]

rhombencephalon

hindbrain
Posterior portion of the *brain* that includes the *cerebellum, pons*, and *medulla.*
[ref. 5]

rhonchus/rhonchi (pl)

Harsh *crepitation* in the throat, sometimes resembling snoring and usually caused by bronchial *secretions.*
[After ref. 1]

ribonucleic acid (RNA)

Linear, usually single-stranded, polymer of ribonucleotides, each containing the sugar ribose in association with a phosphate group and one of four nitrogenous bases: adenine, guanine, cytosine, or uracil.
Note: Messenger RNA (mRNA) encodes the information for the sequence of amino acids in proteins synthesized using it as a template.
[ref. 1]
See also *ribonucleic acid, noncoding; ribonucleic acid interference.*

ribonucleic acid, micro (miRNA)

See *ribonucleic acid interference.*

ribonucleic acid, noncoding (ncRNA)

RNA that is *transcribed* from a *DNA* sequence (sometimes called an RNA gene) but is not *translated* into protein.
Note: ncRNAs include transfer RNAs (tRNAs) carrying amino acids for translation, *ribosomal RNAs* (rRNAs) that are structural components of the *ribosome*, and a large number of RNA sequences that serve as either cis- or *trans-acting factors* regulating the expression of other genes.
[*]

ribonucleic acid interference (RNAi)

Effect of small, often double-stranded *RNA* that targets a specific *messenger RNA*, blocking its *translation*, and thereby silencing *expression* of the corresponding *gene.*
Note 1: Cells produce two types of small RNA, microRNA (miRNA) and small interfering RNA (siRNA) that are both involved in regulation of *gene expression.*
Note 2: As an experimental technique, RNAi uses designed sequences to silence a gene of interest.
Note 3: Short hairpin RNAs (shRNA) are sequences, designed for improved effect in RNAi experiments, that have a base-paired stem representing the double-stranded portion and an intervening unpaired loop.
[ref. 5]

ribosomal RNA (rRNA)

See *ribonucleic acid, noncoding.*

ribosome

Small *organelle*, made up largely of *RNA* and proteins, that is the site of synthesis of polypeptides and proteins in the *cell*.
[*]

righting test, elevated

See *rotarod test*.

righting test, surface

Procedure in which a test animal is placed on its back and the time to achieve and retain an upright position with four paws in contact with the surface is measured.
Note: The surface righting test may be used to study development.
[ref. 4]

ring test

See *round-robin test*.

riparian

Interface between land and a flowing body of surface water.
Note: Plant *communities* along river margins are called riparian vegetation.
[ref. 2]

risk (in toxicology)

Probability that *adverse effects* may occur following exposure of a biological organism, *population*, or *ecological* system to a potentially harmful agent under specified conditions.
Note: In *risk assessment* and *risk characterization*, the likely severity of the adverse effects must be taken into consideration.
[*]
See also *hazard*.

risk, absolute

Risk to an *individual* of experiencing an incident (*e.g.*, an illness or an *adverse event*) over a period of time (often over a lifetime).
[*]
See also *risk, relative*.

risk, acceptable

Probability of suffering *disease* or injury that is considered to be sufficiently small as to be negligible.
Note: Calculated risk of an increase of one case in a million people per year for cancer is usually considered to be negligible and therefore acceptable.
[ref. 1]

risk, accepted

Probability of suffering *disease* or injury that is accepted by an individual or group.
[ref. 1]

risk, added

Difference between an increased *incidence* of an *adverse effect* in an exposure group compared to the background incidence in *control groups* of organisms.
[After ref. 1]

risk, cumulative

1. Probability of a common harmful effect associated with concurrent *exposure* by all relevant pathways and routes of exposure to a group of substances that share a common chemical mechanism of *toxicity*.
2. Total probability of a harmful effect over time.

[ref. 1]

risk, extra

Probability that an agent produces an observed *response*, as distinguished from the probability that the response is caused by a spontaneous event unrelated to the agent.
[ref. 1]

risk, genetic

Risk to the *progeny* of an exposed individual of an *adverse effect* associated with heritable *genetic* damage.
Examples: Damage to germ cells leading to a nonviable fetus, an offspring with a birth defect.
[ref. 2]

risk, individual

Probability that an individual will experience a defined *adverse effect*.
[ref. 1]

risk, phantom

Concern for having a harmful exposure, when the supposed exposure is in reality either absent or present at a nontoxic level.
Note: Phantom risk must be considered in *risk management* of possible *environmental* exposures.
[*]

risk, population

See *risk, societal*.

risk, relative

risk ratio
rate ratio

1. Ratio of the *risk* of *disease* or death among the *exposed* to the risk among the less exposed or unexposed.
2. Ratio of the *cumulative incidence rate* in the exposed to the cumulative *incidence rate* in the unexposed.

[ref. 1]

risk, relative excess

Measure that can be used in comparison of *adverse drug reactions*, or other *exposures*, based solely on the component of *risk* due to the exposure or drug under investigation, removing the *risk* due to background exposure experienced by every individual in the *population*. The *relative excess risk, R*, is given by

$$R = (R_1 - R_0)/(R_2 - R_0)$$

where R_1 is the *rate* in the study population, R_2 is the rate in the comparison population, and R_0 is the rate in the general population.
[ref. 1]

risk, residual

Health risk remaining after risk reduction actions are implemented.
[ref. 1]

risk, societal

population risk

Total probability of *harm* to a human *population* including the probability of *adverse effects* to *health* of descendants and the probability of disruption resulting from loss of services such as industrial plant or loss of material goods and electricity.
[ref. 1]

risk, tolerable

Probability of suffering *disease* or injury that can be tolerated for the time being, taking into account the associated benefits of the exposure or activity, and assuming that the *risk* is minimized by appropriate control procedures.
[After ref. 1]

risk, unit

Upper-bound excess lifetime *cancer risk* estimated to result from continuous exposure to an agent at a *concentration* of 1 $\mu g\,L^{-1}$ in water, or 1 $\mu g\,m^{-3}$ in air.
Example: If the unit risk of a substance $= 1.5 \times 10^{-6}$ $\mu g\,L^{-1}$, then an excess of 1.5 *tumors* are expected to develop per 1 000 000 (10^6) people if they are exposed daily for a lifetime to 1 μg of the substance in 1 litre of drinking water.
[ref. 1]

risk analysis

Process consisting of three components: *risk assessment, risk management*, and *risk communication*.
Note 1: Risk analysis is used for controlling situations where an organism, system, or sub*population* could be exposed to a *hazard*.
Note 2: The term risk analysis may be misleading because "analysis" has a fundamental meaning of resolving a complex situation or entity into its simpler elements, whereas risk analysis is a process of synthesis of three aspects of risk.
[After ref. 2]

risk analysis, environmental

Determination of the probability of *adverse effects* on humans and other *biota* resulting from an *environmental hazard* (a chemical, physical, or biological agent occurring in or mediated by the environment).
[ref. 2]

risk assessment

Identification and quantification of the *risk* resulting from a specific use or occurrence of a substance or physical agent, taking into account possible *harmful* effects on individuals or *populations* exposed to the agent in the amount and manner proposed and all the possible routes of *exposure*.
Note 1: Risk assessment is generally considered to involve four steps: *hazard identification*, *hazard characterization*, *exposure assessment*, and *risk characterization*.
Note 2: Quantification ideally requires the establishment of *dose–effect* and *dose–response relationships* in likely target individuals and populations.
[ref. 2]

risk assessment, environmental

Estimate of the probability that *harm* will result from a defined *exposure* to a substance in an *environmental* medium.
Note: The estimate of probability of harm is valid only for given biological *species* and the set of conditions that were used in the environmental risk assessment.
[ref. 1]

risk assessment, predictive
prospective risk assessment

Risk assessment for a proposed future situation, such as the use of a new chemical or the release of a new *effluent*.
[ref. 2]

risk assessment, retrospective
retroactive risk assessment

Risk assessment addressing a pre-existing condition.
[After ref. 2]

risk assessment management process

Global term for the whole process from *hazard identification* to *risk reduction* and *risk management*.
[ref. 1]

risk associated with a lifetime exposure

Probability of the occurrence of a specified undesirable event following *exposure* of an individual person from a given *population* to a specified substance at a defined level for the expected lifetime of the average member of that population.
[ref. 1]

risk aversion

Tendency of an individual person to avoid *risk*.
[ref. 1]

risk characterization

Outcome of *hazard identification* and *risk estimation* applied to a specific use of a substance or occurrence of an environmental *health* hazard.
Note: Risk characterization requires quantitative data on the *exposure* of the organisms or people at risk in the specific situation. The end product is a quantitative statement about the proportion of organisms or people affected in a *target population*.
[ref. 1]

risk communication

Interpretation and communication of *risk assessments* in terms that are comprehensible to the general public, including the dialogue and discourse with shareholders and the public
[ref. 1]

risk cycle

Iterative series of steps that leads from risk awareness, to *risk assessment*, to *risk reduction management,* to subsequent risk review, and finally to starting a new *cycle* to generate continuing improvement of *risk management* and *risk reduction.*
[*]

risk *de minimis*

negligible risk
"virtually safe"

Risk that is negligible or too small to be of societal concern (usually assumed to be a probability below 10^{-5} or 10^{-6} of an *adverse effect* occurring).
Note: In the United States, this is a legal term used to mean "negligible risk to the individual".
[ref. 1]

risk estimation

Assessment, with or without mathematical modeling, of the probability and nature of effects of *exposure* to a substance based on quantification of *dose–effect* and *dose–response* relationships for that substance and the population(s) and environmental components likely to be *exposed,* as well as on assessment of the levels of potential exposure of people, biological organisms, and environments at *risk.*
[ref. 1]

risk evaluation

Establishment of a qualitative or quantitative relationship between *risks* and *benefits*, involving the complex process of determining the significance of the identified *hazards* and estimated risks to those organisms or people concerned with or affected by them.
[ref. 1]

risk factor

Exposure or circumstance associated with an increased *risk* of an *adverse effect.*
[*]

risk hypothesis

Clear statement of postulated or predicted *adverse effect* of a *toxicant* on an *assessment endpoint.*
[ref. 1]

risk identification

Recognition of potential *exposure* of biological organisms to a *hazard*, and of harm that may result from such exposure.
[After ref. 1]
Note: To be effective in risk prevention, risk identification should include definition of the factors determining the probability of harm occurring from exposure to the hazard.
[*]

risk indicator

See *risk marker.*

risk management

Decision-making process involving considerations of political, social, economic, and engineering factors with relevant *risk assessments* relating to a potential *hazard,* so as to develop, analyze, and compare regulatory options, and to select the optimal regulatory response for *safety* from that hazard.
Note: Risk management is essentially the combination of three steps: *risk evaluation, emission* and *exposure* control, and *risk monitoring.*
[ref. 1]

risk marker

risk indicator

Attribute that is associated with an increased probability of occurrence of a *disease* or other specified outcome, and that can be used as an indicator of increased *risk.*
Note: A risk marker is not necessarily a causal factor.
[ref. 1]

risk monitoring

Process of following up on the decisions and actions taken in a *risk management* process in order to check whether the aims of reduced *exposure* and *risk* are being achieved.
[ref. 1]

risk perception

Person's subjective view of the gravity or importance of a specific *risk,* based on that person's self-perceived knowledge of different risks, and on his or her moral, economic, and political judgment of the implications of the risk.
[After ref. 1]

risk phrase

Word group identifying potential *health* or environmental *hazards* that may be incorporated into *safety data sheets.*
[After ref. 1]

risk quotient

Quantity calculated as the *predicted environmental concentration* divided by the *predicted no-effect concentration.*
Note: The greater the risk quotient than 1, the greater the risk. If the value is below 1, there should be no risk as a result of the predicted *exposure.*
[ref. 1]

risk ratio

relative risk

Value calculated as the probability of occurrence of a specific effect in one group divided by the probability of occurrence of the same effect in another group; alternatively as the probability of occurrence of one potentially hazardous event divided by the probability of occurrence of another.
Note: Calculation of a risk ratio is used in choosing between options in *risk management.*
[ref. 1]

risk reduction

Measures taken to protect people or the *environment* against an identified *risk*.
[ref. 2]

risk source

Agent, substance, medium, process, procedure, or site with the potential to cause an *adverse effect* or effects.
[ref. 2]
See also *hazard*.

risk-specific dose

Quantitated *exposure* corresponding to a specified level of *risk*.
[ref. 1]

rivet popper hypothesis

Proposition that each *species* in a *community* contributes to its proper functioning.
Note: The rivet popper hypothesis is derived from the metaphor that the species can be compared to rivets that hold an airplane together, with the loss of each rivet weakening the structure until a critical point is reached at which a catastrophic failure of the structure occurs.
[ref. 2]

Robertsonian translocation

Chromosomal translocation in which *chromosomes* with *acrocentric centromeres* break the centromere to fuse the long arms into a new large chromosome and the short arms into another small one that may be lost, leaving a *karyotype* in the human of 45 chromosomes.
[ref. 5]

rocket electrophoresis

Technique in which a test *antigen* is electrophoretically driven through an *antibody*-containing gel.
Note: The rocket-shaped tails of precipitation give information on the antigen *concentration*.
[ref. 3]

rod cell

See *photoreceptor cell*.

rodenticide

Substance intended to kill rodents.
[ref. 1]

rosette

Structure formed when particles or cells (usually erythrocytes) bind to cover the surface of a *lymphocyte* (*e.g.*, sheep *erythrocytes* organizing around a human *T-cell*).
[After ref. 3]

rostral

Opposite term: *caudal*.

1. Closer to the head.
2. Pertaining to, resembling, or having a rostrum or beak.
3. Situated toward the beak (thus, oral and nasal region); this location may be superior (in relationship to areas of the *spinal cord*) or anterior or *ventral* (in relationships to *brain* areas).

[ref. 5]

rotarod test

Experimental observation of an animal's (usually a rodent's) ability to stay on a rotating rod without falling off.
Note 1: The length of time the animal stays on the rod is a relative measure of *motor coordination*, balance and resistance to fatigue.
Note 2: Maintaining an upright position on the rod involves the *righting reflex*.
[ref. 4]

round-robin test
ring test

Part of an external *quality assurance* program for assessment of an analytical method or test, in which a reference institute sends identical samples that have to be analyzed or tested for specified parameters, to a number of different laboratories.
Note 1: The reference institute sets a deadline before which test results must be provided for statistical evaluation and interpretation of the results, permitting assessment of the reliability of the methods used and a comparison of the testing laboratories' proficiency.
Note 2: For accreditation of laboratories, regular participation in ring tests is obligatory.
[ref. 2]

route of exposure
Means by which a *toxic* agent gains access to an organism, *e.g.*, by administration through the *gastrointestinal tract* (ingestion), nose and lungs (*inhalation*), or skin (*topical*); or by other routes such as intravenous, subcutaneous, intramuscular, or intraperitoneal routes, or through the eyes.
[ref. 1]

rules of practical causal inference (in ecotoxicology)

Considerations applied in *ecotoxicology* and *environmental epidemiology* to infer causality for *scenarios* of *toxicant exposures* and their *effects*.
Note: The rules of practical causal interference apply the following criteria for objectively evaluating the relationship between a suspected cause and a *chronic effect*: (1) probability, (2) time order, (3) strength of association, (4) specificity, (5) consistency on replication, (6) predictive performance, and (7) coherence.
[ref. 2]

run-off (in ecology)

Portion of the wet precipitation on land that reaches streams, rivers, lakes, and, ultimately, the sea.
[ref. 2]

runt

Smallest and weakest animal of a *litter*.
Note: A runt may be disadvantaged in competing with its siblings for resources and for its mother's attention.
[ref. 5]

S9 fraction

Supernatant fraction obtained from a *cell* or *tissue* (usually liver) homogenate by centrifuging at 9000 *g* for 20 min in a suitable medium; this fraction contains *cytosol* and *microsomes*.
[ref. 1]

scFv

Single-chain molecule composed of the *variable (V) regions* of an *antibody's heavy* and *light chains* joined together by a flexible linker.
[ref. 3]

siRNA

See *ribonucleic acid interference*.

SLUDDE syndrome
SLUDGE syndrome

Acronym for the constellation of signs **s**alivation, ***l**achrymation*, **u**rination, **d**efecation, ***d**yspnea/**g**astrointestinal* upset, and ***e**mesis*.
Note 1: These are consequences of stimulation of the *parasympathetic nervous system* by some *poisons* such as mushroom *toxins*, *nerve gases*, or *organophosphate insecticides*.
Note 2: Sometimes used as an acronym to remember functions of the parasympathetic nervous system.
[ref. 4]

saccadic eye movement

Rapid or jerky movement of the eyes from one line of sight to another, as in reading or correction of a jerky *nystagmus*.
[ref. 4]

sacral agenesis
caudal regression syndrome

Absence or significant underdevelopment of the lower part of the *spine* and the lower limbs.
Note: Sacral agenesis is associated with maternal *diabetes*.
[ref. 5]

saddle back

See *lordosis*.

safe concentration

Concentration of a specified substance to which prolonged *exposure* will cause no *adverse effect*.
[ref. 2]

Comprehensive Glossary of Terms Used in Toxicology
By John Duffus, Douglas M. Templeton and Michael Schwenk

Published by the Royal Society of Chemistry, www.rsc.org

safety (n)/**safe** (adj)

Practical certainty that injury will not result from a *hazard* under defined conditions; a reciprocal of *risk*.
Note 1: Safety of a *drug* or other substance in the context of human *health* governs the extent to which a substance may be used in the amount necessary for the intended *therapeutic* purpose with a minimal risk of *adverse* health *effects*.
Note 2: Safety in *toxicology* denotes a high probability that injury will not result from *exposure* to a substance under defined conditions of quantity and manner of use, ideally when use is controlled to minimize exposure.
[ref. 1]

safety data sheet

See *material safety data sheet.*

safety factor (SF)

See *uncertainty factor.*

safety pharmacology

Science directed to the discovery, development, and *safe therapeutic* use of biologically active substances as a result of the identification, monitoring, and characterization of potentially undesirable *pharmacodynamic* activities of these substances in nonclinical studies.
[ref. 1]

sagittal

Vertical (longitudinal) plane dividing the body into right and left sections.
[ref. 4]

Saint Anthony fire

1. See *ergotism.*
2. Referring to *inflammatory* conditions of the skin such as erysipelas.

[ref. 4]

salinity, *S*

Mass of dissolved salts in water divided by the mass of the solution.
Note 1: In *ecotoxicology, S* is an important parameter for describing seawater, brackish water, brine, or other saline solutions.
Note 2: In practice, *S* is not measured directly in seawater or other natural waters because of the impracticality of recovering the salts from these waters by drying, and is usually calculated from another property (*e.g., chlorinity* or electrical conductivity) whose relationship to salinity is well known.
Note 3: In oceanography, where precise and reproducible determination of seawater density is needed, practical salinity is defined as the electrical conductivity of the seawater sample at 15 °C and 1 atm divided by that of a potassium chloride solution in which the mass fraction of KCl is 32.453×10^{-3} at the same temperature and pressure.
[ref. 2]

Salmonella **test**

See *Ames test.*

salpingectomy

Surgical removal of the *Fallopian tubes.*
[ref. 5]

salt tolerance index (STI)

See *tolerance index, salt.*

saluretic

See *natriuretic.*

sample (in statistics)

1. Group of individuals taken from a *population*, often at random, for research purposes.
2. Subset of items taken from a population and intended to provide information on the population as a whole.
3. Material selected from a larger quantity so as to be representative of the whole.

[After ref. 1]

sampling error

That part of the total error (the difference between the value estimated from a *sample* and the value for whole *population*) associated with using only a fraction of the population and extrapolating to the whole, as distinct from analytical or test error.
Note: Sampling error arises from a lack of homogeneity in the parent population.
[ref. 1]

Santa Ana dexterity test

Santa Ana pegboard test

Procedure in which a test subject stands in front of a plate with 48 square holes and an equal number of fitted pegs, each having a cylindrical upper part and square base. Initially the cylindrical end is in the hole, and the subject is asked to turn the pegs 180° to fit the square ends into the holes, as quickly as possible, first with one hand and in a subsequent trial with the other hand.
Note: Performance of the Santa Ana test relies on finger and hand dexterity, as well as visual guidance.
[ref. 4]

sandwich immunoassay

Analytical test using an immobilized primary antibody to bind a target *antigen* from the test sample, followed by addition of a second, mobile *antibody* that detects the trapped antigen.
[*]

saprobe (n)/saprobic (adj)

1. Organism living on dead or decaying organic matter.
2. Describing an *environment* rich in dead or decaying organic matter and relatively poor in dioxygen, or containing a high number of *species* living under such conditions.

[*]
See also *index, saprobic; saprobic water classification.*

saprobian spectrum

Characteristic change in *community* composition at different distances below the discharge into a river or stream of organic waste susceptible to, or capable of, putrifying or decaying.
[ref. 2]

saprobic index

See *index, saprobic.*

saprophyte
saprotroph

Organism that carries out external digestion of nonliving organic matter and absorbs the products across the *plasma membrane* of its *cells* (*e.g.*, fungi).
[ref. 2]

sarcoid

See *sarcoidosis.*

sarcoidosis
sarcoid

Chronic, progressive, generalized *granulomatous reticulosis* of unknown etiology, involving almost any *organ* or *tissue*, including the skin, lungs, *lymph nodes*, liver, *spleen*, eyes, and small bones of the hands and feet; it is characterized histologically by the presence in all affected organs or tissues of noncaseating *epithelioid cell* tubercles.
Note: In sarcoidosis, there is usually diminished or absent reactivity to *tuberculin*, and in most active cases, a positive *Kveim reaction.*
[ref. 3]

sarcoma

Malignant tumor arising in a *connective tissue* and composed primarily of *anaplastic cells* resembling supportive tissue.
[ref. 1]

satellite group (in toxicology)

Organism or group of organisms treated in a similar fashion to those in the main *toxicity* test group, but intended for the purpose of additional studies, often of a *chronic* nature.
[ref. 2]

saturable elimination

Elimination that becomes *concentration*-independent at a concentration at which the elimination process is functioning maximally.
[ref. 1]

saturation mutagenesis

Mutagenesis screening in which a large number of *mutations* are introduced in a target area of the *genome* with the aim of identifying all the *genes* or their functions that are associated with that area.
[ref. 5]

saturnia

Pain in a joint resulting from lead poisoning.
[ref. 1]

saturnism

plumbism

Intoxication caused by lead.
[ref. 1]

scaling

allometric scaling

1. Mathematical *transformation* of *allometric* data to produce a quantitative relationship between organism (or *species*) size and some characteristic such as *metabolic rate*, gill surface area, lung ventilation rate, or biochemical activity.
2. Adjustment of data to allow for change in proportion between an organ or organs and other body parts during the growth of an organism.
3. Adjustment of data to allow for differences and make comparisons between species having dissimilar characteristics (*e.g.*, in size, shape, and metabolism).

[1,2]
See also *allometric*.

scaphocephaly (n)/scaphocephalic (adj)

Elongated and narrow head with decrease of the *parietal* regions and conspicuous frontal and *occipital* protrusions; a type of *craniosynostosis*.
Note: Scaphocephaly is a result of premature closure of the *sagittal* suture and usually accompanied by intellectual disability.
[ref. 5]

Scatchard plot

Method for analyzing data for freely reversible *ligand/receptor* binding interactions.
Note: The graphical plot is of [bound ligand]/[free ligand] against [bound ligand], which has a slope equal to the negative reciprocal of the dissociation constant ($-1/K_d$) and an intercept on the x-axis equal to the number of bound ligands.
[ref. 1]

scavenger receptor

Cell surface *receptor*, for example on *phagocytes*, that recognizes cells or molecules that require *clearance* from the body.
[ref. 3]

scenario, behavior

Model incorporating all activities of an individual during a day (*e.g.*, sleeping, driving, working), and their locations (*e.g.*, indoor, countryside), attempting to serve as a basis to quantify residence time in *exposure* areas.
[*]
See also *scenario, exposure*.

scenario, exposure

1. (in human exposure) Model of the likely qualitative and quantitative *exposure* of selected *populations* following handling and possible release of a substance in the workplace or other human environment.

2. (in regulatory toxicology) Document on chemical safety required in the European Union for substances that are manufactured or imported by member countries in higher quantities (presently greater than 10^4 kg y^{-1}).
   Note: The exposure scenario is intended to give an assessment of human and environmental exposure to the substance throughout its *life cycle*, from manufacture and use to disposal, with the aim of reducing *risk*.
3. (in ecotoxicology) Set of assumptions concerning how an exposure may take place, including assumptions about the exposure setting, stressor characteristics, and activities that may lead to exposure.

[*]

schedule-controlled operant behavior (SCOB)

Experimental procedure in which operant behavior (see *conditioning, operant*) is assessed following a conditioning *stimulus* delivered at a pre-determined duration and frequency ('*schedule of reinforcement*'), thus allowing comparison of the effects of magnitude, frequency and duration of the stimulus.
[ref. 4]

schedule of reinforcement

Frequency, duration, dose, and (or) intensity of a conditioning *stimulus* (see *stimulus, conditioned*).
See also *schedule-controlled operant behavior.*
[ref. 4]

Schwann cell

Glial cell in the *peripheral nervous system* that produces *myelin* for the *axons* of the peripheral nerves.
[ref. 4]

scleroderma

Chronic progressive *autoimmune disease* characterized by *systemic fibrosis* and *vascular* changes.
Note: There are two types: *progressive systemic sclerosis*, and a more limited and less rapidly progressive form known as CREST *syndrome*, referring to Calcinosis, *Raynaud phenomenon*, Esophageal dysfunction, Sclerodactyly, and Telangiectasias.
[ref. 3]

sclerosis (n)/**sclerotic** (adj)

Hardening of an *organ* or *tissue*, especially that due to excessive deposition of fibrous tissue.
[ref. 1]

scoliosis (n)/**scoliotic** (adj)

Abnormal lateral and rotational curvature of the *vertebral spinal column*.
[ref. 5]
See also *lordosis*.

Scombroid poisoning

Constellation of symptoms resembling an *allergic* reaction, caused by eating the meat of decaying fish that have high levels of *histamine* (in this context sometimes referred to as scombrotoxin).

Note: Scombroid poisoning is typically, but not exclusively, caused by fish of the ***Scombridae*** family, such as tuna, albacore, and mackerel.
[ref. 4]

scope for growth

Index of production (P) calculated as the amount of energy taken into the organism in its food (A) minus the energy used for respiration (R) and excretion (U): $P = A - (R + U)$.
Note: Scope for growth is an indicator of the amount of energy available for *growth* or production of *offspring*.
[ref. 2]

scope of activity

Difference between the rates of oxygen consumption of an organism under maximal and minimal activity levels.
Note: Scope of activity reflects the respiratory capacity available for the diverse demands on and activities of an organism.
[ref. 2]

scotoma

Area of diminished or lost vision within the visual field, surrounded by an area of less affected or normal vision.
Note: A scintillating scotoma is characterized by moving zigzag patterns, often occuring transiently before onset of a *migraine* attack.
[ref. 1]

screening

1. (v) Carrying out a test(s), examination(s), or procedure(s) in order to expose undetected abnormalities, unrecognized (incipient) *diseases*, or defects.
   Examples: Population-based X-rays, cervical smears, or detection of the internal load of *environmental* substances (*biomonitoring*) in different populations.
2. (adj) Describing a testing procedure designed to separate people or objects according to a fixed characteristic or property.
3. (v) *Pharmacological* or *toxicological* screening consists of carrying out a specified set of procedures to which the respective compounds are subjected to characterize pharmacological and toxicological properties and to establish *dose–effect* and *dose–response* relationships.

[ref. 1,2]

screening level

Decision limit or cut-off point at which a *screening* test is regarded as positive.
[ref. 1]

scrotum

Pouch of skin containing the *testicles* and their accessory tissues.
[ref. 5]

second messenger

secondary messenger

Substance inside a *cell* responsible for communicating a chemical signal from another substance that cannot itself enter the cell, but acts through binding to cell surface *receptors*.

Note: Common second messengers are cyclic AMP, Ca^{2+}, and inositol-1,4,5-trisphosphate.
[ref. 3]

second set rejection

Accelerated *rejection* of an *allograft* in a *primed* recipient.
[ref. 3]

secondary challenge

Second exposure of *primed lymphocytes* to a given *antigen*.
[ref. 3]
See also *immune response, secondary.*

secondary immune response

See *immune response, secondary*.

secondary lamella/lamellae (pl)

respiratory lamella

One in a row of parallel projections on the *dorsal* and *ventral* sides of each *primary lamella* of the fish gill.
Note: The secondary lamellae are the primary sites of gas exchange in the gills.
[ref. 2]

secondary lymphoid tissue (organ)

Tissue or *organ* in which *antigen*-driven proliferation and differentiation of *mature B-lymphocytes* and *T-lymphocytes* take place following *antigen recognition*.
Examples: Lymph nodes, Peyer's patches, the *spleen*.
[ref. 3]
See also *mucosa-associated lymphoid tissue; primary lymphoid organ*.

secondary metabolite

Product of biochemical processes other than the normal *metabolic* pathways, mostly found in microorganisms or plants.
[ref. 1]
Note: Plant pigments, flavors and *pharmacological* substances such as digoxin are generally secondary metabolites.
[*]

secondary poisoning

Poisoning of a *predator* as a result of eating prey that has accumulated a *toxicant* by *biomagnification* through its *food chain*.
[ref. 2]

secondary sexual characteristic

secondary sex characteristic
Feature of the *adult* animal, appearing during *puberty* in humans and distinct between the sexes, although it is not part of the reproductive system.
Examples: Enlargement of the female breasts, sex-specific patterns of body hair such as facial hair in the male, the male or female *pubic* escutcheon.
[ref. 5]

secondary spermatocyte

See *spermatocyte.*

secondary substrate metabolism

Microbial growth on a nutrient substrate that is accompanied by *transformation* of another substrate that yields no energetic benefit.
Note: Secondary substrate metabolism has proved difficult to demonstrate in nature, although it can be demonstrated in pure *cultures.*
[ref. 2]
See also *cometabolism.*

secondary succession

See *succession, secondary.*

secondhand smoke

See *sidestream smoke.*

secretion (n,v)/**secrete** (v)

1. (v) Passage of a substance such as a *hormone, enzyme* or *metabolic* waste product produced in a *cell,* through a *plasma membrane* to the outside of the cell, for example, into the intestinal *lumen* or the *blood* (internal secretion).
2. (n) Solid, liquid, or gaseous material passed from the inside of a cell through a plasma membrane to the outside as a result of cell activity.

[After ref. 1]

secretory component

Proteolytic cleavage product of the poly-Ig *receptor* that remains associated with dimeric *immunoglobulin A* in *seromucus* secretions.
[ref. 3]

secretory immunoglobulin A (IgA)

Dimeric *immunoglobulin A* found in *seromucus* secretions.
Note: This is an important mechanism of defence against microorganisms at their site of entry.
[ref. 3]

sedative

1. (n) Substance that exerts a soothing or tranquillizing effect.
2. (adj) Describing an effect that is soothing or tranquillizing.

[ref. 4]
Compare *tranquilizer.*

sediment (n)

1. (n) Matter that settles to the bottom of a liquid.
2. (n) (in geology) Matter deposited anywhere by water or wind.
3. (v) Deposit.

[After ref. 2]

sediment, whole

Sample of *sediment* and associated *interstitial water* that has undergone minimal manipulation after collection.
[ref. 2]

seizure

Sudden change in *neural activity*, leading to *convulsions* and (or) changes in *consciousness* of varying degrees of severity.
[ref. 4]
See also *epilepsy*.

selectin

Any member of a family of cell-surface *adhesion molecules* that are found on *leukocytes* and *endothelial cells*, and that bind to sugars on *glycoproteins*.
[ref. 3]

selection components

Facets of the *life cycle* of an individual upon which *natural selection* can act.
Note: Selection components can be subdivided into *viability selection*, *sexual selection*, *meiotic drive*, *gametic selection*, and *fecundity* selection.
[ref. 2]

selection theory (in immunology)

See *clonal selection*.

selective IgA deficiency (SIgAD)

Most common form of primary *immunodeficiency*.
Note: *Autoimmunity* is the most prevalent manifestation of SIgAD. Individuals with SIgAD have an increased risk of developing *systemic* (*e.g., systemic lupus erythematosus, rheumatoid arthritis*) and *organ*-specific (*e.g., celiac disease*) *autoimmune disorders*.
[ref. 3]

selective serotonin reuptake inhibitor (SSRI)

Drug in a subclass of substances that interfere with the resequestration of *serotonin* by the *presynaptic* membrane.
Note: The SSRI subclass is used in the treatment of clinical *depression*.
[ref. 4]

selector gene

Member of a group of *genes* that code for factors driving *embryonic differentiation* and regional patterning during development.
[ref. 5]

self-antigen

See *autoantigen*.

self-cleaning of water (in a reservoir)

Water purification by natural biological and physicochemical processes.
[ref. 1]

self-purification of the atmosphere

Cleansing of the atmosphere of *contaminants*, occurring by natural physicochemical processes (*e.g.*, rain).
[ref. 1]

self-tolerance

Specific *immunological* unresponsiveness to a defined *autoantigen*.
Note 1: Primary (*clonal deletion, anergy, clonal indifference*) and secondary or regulatory (interclonal competition, suppression, *immune deviation, vetoing*, feedback regulation by the *idiotypic network*) mechanisms are involved in the induction and maintenance of self-tolerance.
Note 2: Breaking self-tolerance may lead to pathological *autoimmunity* and development of *autoimmune disease*.
[ref. 3]

sella turcica

Depression on the upper surface of the *sphenoid bone*, accommodating the *pituitary gland*.
[ref. 5]

Selyean stress

See *stress, Selyean*.

semelparous species

Species capable of reproducing only once.
[ref. 2]

semen (n)/seminal (adj)

ejaculate (n)
seminal fluid
Fluid, containing *spermatozoa*, that is expelled from the penis during *ejaculation*.
[ref. 5]

semichronic

See *subchronic*.

semi-continuous activated sludge (SCAS) test

Test for inherent biodegradability (see *biodegradation*) of organic substances in *activated sludge* by measurement of the decrease in *dissolved oxygen content* in the test system.
[ref. 2]

seminal fluid

See *semen*.

seminal vesicle

One of a pair of *glands* of the male reproductive system that together produce many components of the *semen*.
Note: Seminal vesicle *secretion* does not contain *spermatozoa*, but provides nutrients and an alkaline environment that prolongs their survival.
[ref. 5]

seminiferous tubule

One of numerous coiled tubes, found in the *testis*, in the walls of which *spermatogenesis* occurs.
[ref. 5]

semiochemical

Substance produced by plants or animals, or a synthetic analogue thereof, that evokes a behavioral response in individuals of the producing species or in other species (*e.g., allomones, kairomones, pheromones*, and *synomones*).
[ref. 1]

semipermeable membrane

differentially permeable membrane
selectively permeable membrane
Membrane that will preferentially allow certain molecules or ions to pass through it while preventing the passage of others.
[ref. 1]

semi-static test

See *static-renewal test.*

senile plaque

See *amyloid plaque.*

senility (n)/senile (adj)

Characteristics of physiological deterioration typically associated with old age, especially relating to memory loss and other mental impairment.
[ref. 4]
See also *dementia.*

sensibilization

See *sensitization.*

sensitivity

1. (in metrology and analytical chemistry)
    1.1. Change in the *indication* divided by the corresponding change in the value of the quantity being measured.
    1.2. Slope of the calibration curve.
    Note 1: If the curve is nonlinear, then sensitivity will be a function of analyte *concentration* or amount.
    Note 2: If sensitivity is to be a unique performance characteristic, it must depend only on the measurement process, not upon scale factors.
    [ref. 1]
2. (of a screening test)
    Extent (usually expressed as a percentage) to which a method gives results that are free from *false negatives*.
    Note 1: The fewer the false negatives, the greater the sensitivity.
    Note 2: Quantitatively, sensitivity is the proportion of truly affected (*e.g.*, diseased) persons in the screened population who are identified as affected by the *screening* test.
    [ref. 1]

Compare *specificity*.
3. (to a toxicant or other agent)
Susceptibility to *adverse effects*.
[*]

sensitization (in immunology)

Alteration of a body's responsiveness to a foreign *antigen*, usually an *allergen*, such that upon subsequent exposures to the allergen there is a heightened *immune response*.
[ref. 3]

sensitized strain

Model organism containing a *mutation* in a pathway (*e.g.*, a *metabolic* or a *signal transducing* pathway) that does not itself cause a change in *phenotype*, but makes the organism more sensitive to another change elsewhere in the pathway.
[ref. 5]

sensitizer (in immunology)

Substance that brings about *sensitization*.
[ref. 3]

sensory effect level

1. Intensity of a *stimulus*, where the detection *threshold* level is defined as the lower limit of the perceived intensity range (by convention, the lowest *concentration* that can be detected in 50 % of the cases in which it is present).
2. Quality of a stimulus, where the recognition threshold level is defined as the lowest concentration at which the sensory effect can be recognized correctly in 50 % of the cases.
3. Acceptability and annoyance levels of a stimulus, where the nuisance threshold level is defined as the concentration at which not more than a small proportion of the *population* (*e.g.*, less than 5 %) experiences annoyance for a small part of the time (*e.g.*, less than 2 %).

Note: Since annoyance will be influenced by a number of factors, a nuisance threshold level cannot be set on the basis of concentration alone.
[After ref. 1]

sensory neuron

Neuron specialized for detecting and (or) transducing signals from external or *somatic* stimuli.
[ref. 4]

sensory system

Part of the *nervous system* that receives, by way of *receptors*, physical information from outside and inside the body, evaluates that information and thus allows perception of the surrounding *environment*.
Note: The sensory system includes vision, hearing, taste, smell, balance, touch and pain.
[*]

sentinel species

Species (feral, caged, or endemic) used to measure or indicate the level of *contamination* or effect during a *biomonitoring* exercise.
[ref. 2]

sepsis (n)/septic (adj)

Opposite term: asepsis.

Spread of bacteria or bacterial products throughout the *blood*, eliciting a life-threatening, *systemic inflammatory response*.
[ref. 3]

septum (n)/septal (adj) (in anatomy)

Thin wall dividing two *cavities* or masses of softer *tissue*.
[ref. 5]

septum, ventricular

Dividing wall between the two lower chambers (*ventricle*s) of the heart.
[ref. 5]

sero-

Prefix denoting *serum* or *serous*.
[*]

seroconversion

The appearance in the *blood serum* of detectable *antibodies* against a specific infectious agent.
[ref. 3]

serology

Study of *serum*, especially *blood* serum, frequently used to detect *antibodies* to microorganisms.
[ref. 3]

seromucous

1. Describing a gland or other tissue having both *serous* and *mucus*-secreting *cells*.
2. Secreted substance (see *secretion*) intermediate between a watery serous fluid and a more viscous mucus.

[*]

serotonin

3-(2-aminoethyl)-1H-indol-5-ol

Neurotransmitter found in the digestive tract, platelets and *central nervous system*.
Note: In the central nervous system, serotonin influences mood, appetite and sleep.
[ref. 4]

serotonin syndrome

Potentially life threatening condition caused by excess of *serotonin* resulting in neuromuscular, autonomic, and behavioral changes including confusion, *ataxia*, excitement, hyperthermia, and *tremor*.
[*]

serotoninergic

Relating to a nerve that releases or responds to *serotonin* as a *neurotransmitter*.
[ref. 4]

serous

Containing, resembling, or *secreting serum*.
[ref. 5]

Sertoli cell

Somatic cell in the *seminiferous tubule* that supports *spermatogenesis*.
Note: Tight junctions between Sertoli cells contribute to the *blood-testis barrier*.
[ref. 5]

Sertoli-Leydig cell tumor

Ovarian tumor composed of both *Sertoli* and *Leydig cells*.
Note: The tumor may secrete *androgens*, thus causing *masculinization*.
[ref. 5]

serum

1. Clear watery fluid (serous fluid), especially that which moistens the surface of *serous membranes* or that exudes through *inflammation* of any of these membranes.
2. Blood serum; watery proteinaceous portion of the *blood* that remains after clotting.

[ref. 3]

serum sickness

Hypersensitivity reaction to the administration of a foreign *serum*, characterized by fever, swelling, skin rash, and enlargement of the *lymph nodes*.
[ref. 3]

seston

Minute living organisms and particles of nonliving matter that float in water and contribute to *turbidity*.
[ref. 2]

severe combined immunodeficiency (SCID)

Immunodeficiency affecting both *T-lymphocytes* and *B-lymphocytes*.
[ref. 3]

sex chromatin

Barr body

Condensed mass of one inactivated *X chromosome* seen inside the nuclear *membrane* of an *interphase cell*.
Note 1: Sex *chromatin* is not seen in normal male cells (XY), but one body may be seen in normal female cells (XX).
Note 2: In *chromosomal* abnormalities, the number seen is one less than the number of X chromosomes.
[ref. 5]
See also *Lyon hypothesis*.

sex chromosome

One of the pair of *chromosomes* determining sex; in humans designated an *X chromosome* and a *Y chromosome*, with females having an XX *genotype* and males an XY genotype.
[ref. 5]

sex-determining region Y (SRY) protein

testis-determining factor (TDF)

Transcription factor coded by a gene on the *Y chromosome* that initiates development of the male sex organs (*i.e., testicular differentiation*) in the *embryo*.
[ref. 5]

sex-linked

Trait determined by a *gene* carried on one of the sex chromosomes, and thus inherited in a gender-dependent manner.
[*]
See also *X-linked*.

sexual dimorphism

Phenotypic difference between the sexes of a *species*.
[ref. 5]

sexual dysfunction

Difficulty of a person to engage in normal sexual activity, including desire, arousal, or orgasm with a partner.
[*]
See also *impotence*.

sexual maturation

Process of reaching *sexual maturity*, the age or stage when an organism can reproduce sexually.
[ref. 5]

sexual maturity

Age or stage when an organism can reproduce sexually.
[ref. 5]

sexual reproduction

Creation of a new organism requiring combination of the *genetic* material from two different sexes.
Note: There exists asexual reproduction in lower organisms that does not require participation of two sexes.
[ref. 5]

sexual selection

Natural selection involving differential mating success of individuals.
[ref. 2]

sexually dimorphic nucleus (SDN)

Compact area of large cells in the anterior *hypothalamus*, larger in men than women, and believed to influence sexual behaviour.
[ref. 5]
See also *sexual dimorphism*.

Shannon–Wiener diversity index, *H*

See *index, Shannon–Wiener diversity*.

sheep red blood cell (SRBC) **antigen**

See antigen, sheep red blood cell.

Shelford's law of tolerance

Species' tolerance(s) along an environmental gradient (or series of environmental gradients) will determine its *population* distribution and size in the *environment*.
[ref. 2]

shellfish poisoning

Illness associated with consumption of molluscan or crustacean seafood *contaminated* with *toxins*.
Note 1: Shellfish poisoning is primarily associated with consumption of bivalve molluscs such as mussels, clams, oysters and scallops that have accumulated, by filter feeding, toxins produced by microscopic *algae* such as dinoflagellates and diatoms, and by cyanobacteria.
Note 2: Four *syndromes* of shellfish poisoning with overlapping features are recognized. These are *amnesic shellfish poisoning*, *diarrheal shellfish poisoning*, *neurotoxic shellfish poisoning*, and *paralytic shellfish poisoning*.
[ref. 4]

short-term effect

See *acute effect*.

short-term exposure limit (STEL)

Fifteen-minute *time-weighted average* (TWA) *exposure* recommended by ACGIH that should not be exceeded at any time during a workday, even if the 8-h TWA is within the *threshold limit value–timeweighted average*, TLV®-TWA.
Note: Workers can be exposed to a maximum of four periods per 8 h shift at the STEL, with at least 60 min between exposure periods.
[ref. 1]

short-term toxicity

See *acute toxicity*.

shunt

1. (n) *Fistula* or prosthetic device that diverts fluid from one system to another.
2. (v) To bypass or divert.

[ref. 4]

shunt, arteriovenous

Connection between the arterial and venous sides of the circulation that bypasses the capillary beds.
[ref. 5]

shunt, ventriculo-atrial

Surgical *shunt* draining *cerebrospinal fluid* into a cardiac *atrium*, to relieve pressure in *hydrocephalus*.
[ref. 4]
See also *ventriculo-peritoneal shunt*.

shunt, ventriculo-peritoneal

Surgical *shunt* draining *cerebrospinal fluid* into the peritoneum of the *abdominal cavity*, to relieve pressure in *hydrocephalus*.
[ref. 4]
See also *shunt, ventriculo-atrial*.

Siamese twin

See *conjoined twin*.

sibling
sib

One of two or more individuals with a common pair of parents.
[ref. 5]

siccative

Drying agent.
[*]

sick building syndrome

Adverse effects on *health* or loss of a sense of wellbeing associated, by those who experience it, with time spent in a certain building or room.
Note 1: *Neurological* symptoms include *headache*, irritability, and *fatigue*.
Note 2: Potential causes include poor ventilation and indoor air quality, outgassing of volatile substances from building materials, molds, and ozone build-up from office machines. Psychological factors may play a role.
[ref. 4]

side-effect

Action of a *drug* other than that desired for a beneficial *pharmacological* effect.
[ref. 1]

side product

Unwanted product that is formed during synthesis or processing of a given substance.
Example: Polychlorinated dibenzodioxins (common side products of the synthesis of aromatic chlorinated compounds) found as contaminants in the defoliant Agent Orange.
[*]

siderosis

1. Excess of iron in the urine, *blood*, or *tissues*, characterized by *hemosiderin* granules in urine and iron deposits in tissues.
2. *Pneumoconiosis* resulting from the *inhalation* of iron *dust*.

[ref. 1]

sidestream smoke

environmental tobacco smoke (ETS)
secondhand smoke

Cloud of small particles and gases, given off from the end of a burning tobacco product (cigarette, pipe, cigar) between puffs and, in contrast to *mainstream smoke,* not directly inhaled by the smoker.
Note: Sidestream smoke gives rise to passive *inhalation* on the part of bystanders (see *bystander exposure).*
[ref. 1]

sign

Objective evidence of a *disease*, deformity, or an effect induced by an agent, perceptible to an examining physician.
[ref. 1]
Compare *symptom.*

signal peptide

signal sequence

Any sequence of amino acid residues that, when linked to a newly synthesized protein, identifies it to transport mechanisms that guide the protein to a specific location among the *organelles* of a *eukaryotic cell*, or from the *cytoplasm* to the periplasmic space of *prokaryotic* cells.
[ref. 3]

signal sequence

See *signal peptide.*

signal transducer and activator of transcription (STAT)

Any member of a specific family of *cytoplasmic* proteins that act as *second messengers* to activate *gene transcription* in response to *cytokines* and *growth factors.*
[ref. 3]
See also *JAK/STAT signaling pathway.*

signal transduction

Process whereby a signal arising outside the *cell* is converted through a series of intermediate biochemical reactions inside the cell to produce a functional change in the cell.
[ref. 3]
See also *cytokine; growth factor; receptor; second messenger.*

signaling lectin (SIGLEC)

Any member of a large family of *lectins* that binds sialylated glycans.
Note: Most SIGLECs associated with cells of the *immune system.*
[ref. 3]

silicosis

Pneumoconiosis resulting from *inhalation* of silica *dust.*
[ref. 1]

silt

Sediment particles with a grain size between 0.004 and 0.062 mm, *i.e.*, coarser than clay particles but finer than sand.
[ref. 2]

silver staining

Method for visualization of macromolecules such as nucleic acids and proteins, typically in electrophoretic gels or formalin-fixed histological sections, based on the reduction of silver salts to metallic silver or the formation of crystalline silver compounds.
[ref. 4]
See also *Golgi staining.*

simple reaction time test

Procedure to assess psychomotor speed in which a test subject is presented at irregular intervals with a visual *stimulus*, such as a coloured dot on a screen, and is asked to press a button immediately after noticing the stimulus.
Note 1: Premature or untimely late reactions should be minimized during an initial practise phase.
Note 2: Many variations of the simple reaction time test exist.
[ref. 4]
See also *neurobehavior core test battery.*

Simpson's diversity index, *D*

See *index, Simpson's diversity.*

simulated field study

Ecological impact study conducted on an experimental *ecosystem* that fulfills the following criteria: physically confined, self-maintaining, multitrophic, having a duration exceeding the generation time of the penultimate *trophic level* present, and of sufficient size to enable pertinent sampling and measurements to be made without seriously influencing the structure and dynamics of the system.
[ref. 2]

simulation study

Study in which real circumstances are simulated, either mathematically or by construction, to examine the probabilities of various outcomes.
[*]

simulation test (environmental)

Procedure designed to predict the outcome of *environmental* influences on living systems (and vice versa), *e.g.*, the rate of *biodegradation* of a substance in *soil* under relevant environmental conditions.
Note: Such tests are either practically performed in technical institutes, or, when there are sufficient data for model-building, with computer software.
[ref. 1]

single-chain antibody (SCA)

See *antibody, single chain.*

single-nucleotide polymorphism (SNP)

Single base variation at a *chromosomal locus*, which exists stably within populations (typically defined as each variant form being present in at least 1 to 2 % of individuals).
[ref. 5]
See also *polymorphism; polymorphism, genetic.*

single-positive cell

See *pre-T-cell.*

sink (in ecotoxicology)

Area or part of the *environment* in which, or a process by which, one or more *pollutants* is removed from the medium in which it is dispersed.
Example: Moist ground acts as a sink for atmospheric sulfur dioxide.
[ref. 1]
See also *sink function.*

sink function

Ability of an *environment* to absorb and render harmless waste and *pollution*: when waste output exceeds the *sink* capacity, environmental damage occurs.
Note: Many current methods of disposing of waste materials are based on the incorrect idea that the global environment has an infinite sink function.
[*]

sinoatrial node
sinuatrial node

Mass of specialized *cardiac* muscle cells ("pacemaker cells") that spontaneously *depolarize* to initiate rhythmic *contraction* of the heart.
[ref. 5]

sinus

1. Hollow or *cavity*.
2. Channel for the passage of fluid, lacking the usual lining of a *blood* or *lymphatic* vessel; especially a dilatation for the passage of venous blood.

[ref. 5]

sinus, urogenital

Embryonic structure that forms in the *ventral* part of the *cloaca* when it separates from the *anal canal* to give rise to the *genitourinary* organs.
Note: A rare urogenital sinus anomaly occurs as a birth defect in the female when the *urethra* and *vagina* open into a common channel.
[ref. 5]

sinus venosus
venous sinus

Cavity at the *caudal* end of the developing *embryonic* heart where intra- and extra-*embryonic* veins meet.

Note: The sinus venosus develops into the portion of the right *atrium* in the *adult* heart that receives *blood* from the *vena cava*.
[ref. 5]

sister chromatid

See *chromatid*.

sister chromatid exchange (SCE)

Reciprocal exchange of *chromatin* between two replicated *chromosomes* that remain attached to each other until *anaphase* of *mitosis*.
Note: SCE is used as a measure of *mutagenicity* of substances that produce this effect.
[ref. 1]

situs inversus

Developmental anomaly in which major *visceral organs* are found in a mirrored position to their normal location.
[ref. 5]
See also *dextrocardia*.

Sjögren syndrome

Chronic *inflammation* of the lachrymal and salivary glands, often accompanied by *rheumatoid arthritis* and the presence of *autoantibodies* in the *blood*, occurring chiefly among women.
Note: Two types of Sjögren *syndrome* are distinguished: a primary (isolated) type and a secondary type associated with another underlying autoimmune *disease* (*e.g.*, *rheumatoid arthritis, systemic lupus erythematosus, systemic sclerosis, primary biliary cirrhosis, autoimmune hepatitis, multiple sclerosis*, and *autoimmune thyroiditis*). Ro/SS-A and La/SS-B autoantibodies are used as classification criteria.
[ref. 3]

skeletal fluorosis

Sclerosis of the bones due to fluoride.
[After ref. 1]
See also *fluorosis*.

skin immune system (SIS)

Skin-associated *cells* that participate in an *immune response*, including *Langerhans cells, dendritic cells*, and *keratinocytes* (mainly responsible for the production of *cytokines*).
[ref. 3]

skin sensitization test

Any test used to study skin *hypersensitivity* such as the *guinea pig maximization test* or the *Buehler test*.
[ref. 3]

skin test

Procedure for evaluating *immunity* status, involving the introduction of a reagent into or under the skin.
[ref. 3]

slimicide

Substance intended to kill slime-producing organisms.
Note: Slimicides are used on, *e.g.*, paper stock, water-cooling systems, and paving stones.
[ref. 1]

slope factor

cancer slope factor

Value, in inverse *concentration* or *dose* units, derived from the slope of a *dose–response* curve; in practice, limited to *carcinogenic* effects with the curve assumed to be linear at low concentrations or doses.
Note: The product of the slope factor and the *exposure* gives a dimensionless quantity, sometimes called the potency factor, taken to reflect the probability of producing the related effect.
[After ref. 1]

slow-reacting substance of anaphylaxis (SRS-A)

Group of *leukotrienes* released by *mast cells* during *anaphylaxis*, which induces a prolonged *contraction* of smooth muscle.
[ref. 3]

sludge

Viscous, muddy *mixture* of liquid and solid waste, resulting from sewage treatment, dirty combustion of oil, or other industrial activity.
[*]
See also *activated sludge*.

small G protein

Any member of a family of monomeric *G proteins*, with molecular mass typically 20–40 kDa, that also binds guanine nucleotides and is involved in *signal transduction*.
[ref. 3]

small interfering RNA (siRNA) molecule

See *ribonucleic acid interference*.

small outer capsid (SOC) protein

Protein from the shell of the bacteriophage T4, commonly used in construction of *phage antibody libraries*.
[ref. 3]

smog

Mixture of smoke and fog.
Note: Smog is used to describe city fogs in which there is a large proportion of particulate matter and also a high concentration of sulfur and nitrogen oxides.
[ref. 2]

social interaction test

Behavioral test wherein a rodent stranger is placed in the cage of a domestic rodent and intensities and duration of interactions (*e.g.*, sniffing, aggression, avoidance) between the socially unacquainted animals are observed.
[ref. 4]

societal risk

See *risk, societal.*

soft acid

Lewis acid with an acceptor center of high polarizability.
Note: For further information on soft acids, see *hard acid.*
[*]
See also *class 'a' metal ion; class 'b' metal ion.*

soft tissue

Tissue surrounding bone and solid *organs*, including *connective tissue, nerves*, muscle, and *blood*.
[*]

soil

Naturally occurring, unconsolidated mineral and (or) organic material at the surface of the Earth that is capable of supporting plant growth.
Note 1: Where appropriate, soil may be taken to extend from the surface to 15 cm below the depth at which properties produced by soil-forming processes are detectable.
Note 2: Soil formation results from an interaction between climate, living organisms such as biologically active bacteria, mold and worms that provide nutrients, in addition to surface relief, acting on soil parent material.
Note 3: Unconsolidated material includes material cemented or compacted by soil-forming processes. Soil may have water covering its surface to a depth of 60 cm.
[ref. 2]

soil partition coefficient, soil K_d

Experimental ratio of a substance's *concentration* in the *soil* to that in the aqueous (dissolved) soil phase at *equilibrium*: it is valid only for the specific concentration and solid/solution ratio of the test.
[ref. 1]
See also *organic carbon partition coefficient.*

solute

Minor component of a *solution* that is regarded as having been dissolved by the solvent.
[ref. 8]

solution

Liquid or solid phase consisting of a homogeneous mixture of two or more components, the dominant component being called the solvent that dissolves the remaining *solutes*.
Note: The solvent itself may contain more than one component, *e.g.*, in the case of miscible liquids, such as a solution of an organic compound dissolved in an alcohol-water solvent.
[*]

solvent

See *solution*.

solvent abuse
solvent sniffing

Deliberate *inhalation* (or drinking) of volatile *solvents*, in order to become intoxicated (see *intoxication*).
[ref. 1]
See also *abuse*.

solvent drag

Movement of a *solute* (*e.g.*, a *contaminant*) along with the bulk movement of the *solvent*.
Note: *Osmotically* driven solvent-drag in water is a driving force for transport of substances through the space between adjacent *cells* (see *transport, paracellular*), *e.g.*, in the intestine and kidney.
[ref. 2]

solvent sniffing

See *solvent abuse*.

somatic

1. Pertaining to the body.
2. Describing *cells* that form the body, other than *germ line cells* or undifferentiated *stem cells*.

[ref. 5]

somatic death

Death of an individual organism.
[ref. 2]

somatic diversification theory

Theory that very few *immunoglobulins* are inherited, but that extensive *antibody* diversity arises from *mutations* in nonreproductive *cells*.
[ref. 3]
See also *somatic hypermutation; somatic recombination; V(D)J recombination*.

somatic gene conversion

Nonreciprocal exchange of nucleic acid sequences between *genes* in which part of the donor gene or genes is "copied" into an acceptor gene, but only the acceptor gene is altered.
Note: This exchange is a mechanism for generating a diverse *immunoglobulin* repertoire in many nonhuman species.
[ref. 3]

somatic hypermutation (SHM)

Programmed process of *mutation* affecting the *variable (V) regions* of *immunoglobulin genes* that affects only individual *immune cells*, and the mutations are not transmitted to *offspring*.
Note 1: Somatic hypermutation is part of the way the *immune system* adapts to new foreign substances.
Note 2: Mistargeted SHM is a likely mechanism in the development of *B-cell lymphoma*.
[ref. 3]

See also *somatic recombination.*

somatic recombination

Process giving rise to increased *antibody* diversity by cutting and splicing *immunoglobulin genes* during *lymphocyte* differentiation.
[ref. 3]
See also *combinatorial diversity; V(D)J recombination.*

somatomammotropin, human chorionic

human placental lactogen (hPL)

Placental hormone that affects maternal *metabolism* and supports *fetal growth* by making more glucose and fatty acids available to the fetus.
[ref. 5]

somatomedin

Any of a group of peptide *growth factors* produced by the liver following stimulation by *somatotropin.*
Note: Somatomedin acts directly on *cartilage cells* to stimulate skeletal *growth.*
[ref. 5]

somatotropin

growth hormone

Hormone produced in the *pituitary gland* that is essential for normal *growth* and stimulates the liver to produce *somatomedin.*
[ref. 5]

somite

One of bilaterally paired, segmented masses of *mesodermal tissue* lying along the *notochord* that gives rise to the *vertebrae* and associated muscle and *connective tissue.*
[ref. 5]

sonic hedgehog

Protein *morphogen* produced in the *notochord* that plays a critical role in early development, including *vertebrate organogenesis, brain* development and limb formation.
Note: Sonic hedgehog production in the *embryo* is dependent upon *secretion* of *fibroblast growth factors.*
[ref. 5]
See also *bone morphogenetic protein 4.*

soporific

Substance causing sleep.
[ref. 1]

sorbate

1. Noncommittal term used instead of *adsorbate* or *absorbate* when the *sorption* process is undefined.
   [ref. 2]
2. Salt of sorbic acid [(2*E*,4*E*)-hexa-2,4-dienoic acid].
   [*]

sorbent

Noncommittal term used instead of *adsorbent* or *absorbent* when the *sorption* process is undefined.
[ref. 2]

sorption

Process whereby a *solute* becomes physically or chemically associated with a *sorbent* regardless of the mechanism (*absorption, adsorption, chemisorption*).
Note: Sorption is sometimes used instead of adsorption or absorption when it is difficult to discriminate experimentally between these two processes.
[ref. 2]

sorption constant, K_d

Quantity describing the distribution of a substance between a *solvent* and a *sorbent*, typically water and *sediment*, at *equilibrium, e.g.*, $K_d = C(\text{sediment})/C(\text{water})$, where C denotes the concentration of the substance in the specified medium.
[ref. 2]

source-to-outcome pathway

Sequence of observable events from entry of a substance into the *environment* through *ecological* components to adverse outcomes.
Note: The source-to-outcome pathway includes *toxicity* pathways and *mode of action* information.
[*]

spawn

1. (v) Release *gametes* (of mature *adult* fish, frogs, molluscs, crustacea, *etc.*).
2. (n) Fertilized *eggs* of mature adult fish, *etc.*

[ref. 5]

spawning

1. (n) Release of *gametes* (*eggs* or *sperm*) from mature *adult* fish, frogs, molluscs, crustacea, *etc.*
2. (adj) Describing behavior related to the readiness of mature adult fish, *etc.*, to release gametes.

[ref. 5]

spasm

Sudden involuntary contraction of one or more muscles; includes *cramps* and *contractions*.
[ref. 4]

spasmolytic

Agent that relieves smooth muscle *spasms*.
[ref. 4]

spasticity (n)/spastic (adj)

Increased muscle tone at rest, characterized by resistance to passive stretch.
Note 1: Increased deep tendon *reflexes* and *clonus* are additional manifestations of spasticity.
Note 2: Spasticity may cause spastic *paresis*.
[ref. 4]

Spearman–Karber method

Nonparametric method to estimate the LC_{50}, EC_{50}, or LD_{50} when it is difficult or unnecessary to assume a specific *model* for the *dose-* or *concentration-effect* data.
[ref. 2]
See also *median effective concentration; median lethal concentration; median lethal dose.*

speciation

1. (in biology) Segregation of organisms into groups that are able to reproduce amongst themselves.
   [*]
2. (in chemistry) *Distribution* of an element among defined *chemical species* in a system.

[ref. 3]

speciation analysis (in chemistry)

Analytical activities of identifying and (or) measuring the quantities of one or more individual *chemical species* in a *sample*.
[ref. 3]

species (in biology)

Group of organisms of common ancestry that are able to reproduce only among themselves and that are usually geographically distinct.
[*]

species (in chemistry)

See *chemical species.*

species–area relationship

Common pattern in which the number of *species* on islands decreases as island area decreases.
[ref. 2]

species assemblage

Operationally defined subset of the entire *community*.
[ref. 2]

species-deletion stability

Tendency in a model *community* for the remaining *species* to remain at locally stable *equilibria* after a species is made extinct.
[ref. 2]

species differences in sensitivity

Quantitative or qualitative differences of response to the action(s) of a potentially *toxic* substance on various *species* of living organisms.
[ref. 1]

species diversity

Heterogeneity of an *ecological community*, considering both *species richness* and *species evenness*.
[ref. 2]

species evenness

Degree to which the individuals in the *community* are evenly or uniformly distributed among *species.*
[ref. 2]

species imbalance

Change in the *species* numbers or diversity in an *ecosystem,* or in their interactions, which results in change in *ecological* character and its functions and attributes.
[ref. 2]
See also *ecological imbalance.*

species richness index (*S*)

See *index, species richness.*

species sensitivity distribution (SSD)

Statistical relationship between *exposure concentration* and a defined *effect* derived from a combination of single-*species* test data to predict *concentrations* affecting only a certain percentage of the total number of species in a defined *community.*
Note 1: To produce an SSD, single-species data (*e.g., median lethal concentration* or *no-observed-effect concentration* values) for many species are fitted to a distribution relationship such as the *log-normal* or log-*logistic curve.* From this distribution of species sensitivities, a *hazardous concentration* is identified at which a certain percentage of all species is likely to be affected.
Not 2: The most conservative form of the SSD approach uses the lower 95 % tolerance limit of the estimated percentage to ensure that a desired level of protection is achieved
[ref. 2]

species-specific sensitivity

Quantitative and qualitative features of response to the action(s) of a potentially *toxic* substance that are characteristic for a particular *species* of living organism.
[ref. 1]

specific action concept

specific activity concept

Assumption made in radiotracer studies about the behaviour of a radionuclide used to trace or quantify the movement of a stable nuclide (*e.g.*, ^{14}C for stable C), implying that the radionuclide behaves identically in chemical and biological processes to its nonradioactive analog (*e.g.*, stable C).
Note: Sometimes the specific action concept is called the "specific activity concept", not to be confused with the specific activity (*e.g.*, dpm mol^{-1}) of a radioactive source.
[ref. 2].

specific death rate

See *death rate, specific.*

specific pathogen free (SPF)

Describing an animal *fetus* removed from its mother under *sterile* conditions just prior to term delivery, and subsequently reared and kept under sterile conditions.
[ref. 1]

specificity (of a screening test)

Proportion of truly unaffected (*e.g.*, non*diseased*) persons that are identified by a *screening* test, *i.e.*, the number of true positives as distinct from *false positives*).
[After ref. 1]
Compare *sensitivity*.

specimen

Specifically selected portion of any substance, material, organism (*e.g.*, tissue, *blood*, urine, or feces), or environmental medium assumed to be representative of the parent substance, material, *etc.* at the time it is taken.
Note: Such specimens are used for the purpose of diagnosis, identification, study, or demonstration.
[ref. 1]

spectral radiant power

Power of a radiant source at wavelength λ, per unit wavelength interval, thus typically given in units of Watt nm^{-1}.
[After ref. 1]

Spemann organizer

Group of cells in the amphibian *embryo* that is important in orientation of surrounding *cells* and facilitates development of the *central nervous system*.
Note: Cells on the *ventral* side of the ***Xenopus*** *blastula* secrete factors such as *bone morphogenetic protein-4* (BMP-4) to signal the overlying *ectoderm* to become skin. The Spemann organizer blocks the action of BMP-4 by secreting *chordin* and *noggin*, allowing the ectoderm to develop into the *brain* and *spinal cord* by default.
[ref. 5]

sperm

See *spermatozoon*.

sperm banking

Storage of frozen donor *sperm* for use in *artificial insemination*.
[ref. 5]

spermatid

Haploid cell in the late stage of developing into a *spermatozoon*, derived from the *secondary spermatocyte*.
[ref. 5]

spermatocide

spermicide

Agent intended to kill *spermatozoa*.
[ref. 5]

spermatocyte

Parent cell of a *spermatid*, derived by *mitotic* division from a *spermatogonium*.
Note: The primary spermatocyte gives rise to a pair of *haploid* secondary spermatocytes by *meiosis*.
[ref. 5]

spermatogenesis

Entire process by which *spermatogonial stem cells* divide and *differentiate* into *spermatozoa*.
[ref. 5]

spermatogenic cycle

Repetitive process underlying consecutive cell divisions of *spermatogonia* to produce *spermatocytes*.
[*]

spermatogenic wave

One of a sequence of waves of *spermatogenesis* that occur along the length of the *seminiferous tubules*, producing *spermatozoa* continuously, except for seasonal pauses that may occur depending on species.
[*]
See also *spermatogenic cycle*.

spermatogonial chromosome aberration test

Procedure in which rodents are exposed to a test substance and *chromosome abnormalities* are then studied microscopically in *germ cells*.
[ref. 5]

spermatogonium/spermatogonia (pl)

Primitive cell derived from *mitosis* of the *germ cell* that becomes the *diploid* primary *spermatocyte*.
[ref. 5]

spermatozoon/spermatozoa (pl)

sperm cell
Mature male *gamete*.
[ref. 5]

spermiation

Release of mature *spermatozoa* from the *Sertoli cells*.
[ref. 5]

spermicide

See *spermatocide*.

spermiogenesis

Maturation of an immature *spermatid* into a *spermatozoon*.
[ref. 5]

sphenoid bone

sphenoid

Irregular wing-shaped bone at the anterior base of the skull, forming part of the *orbit*, serving as an attachment site for muscles of mastication, and containing *foramina* for nerves and vessels of the head and neck.

Note: The complex structure, function, and development of the sphenoid bone have been linked with developmental *disorders* such as sphenoid *dysplasia* and *cystic* degeneration of the sphenoid.
[ref. 5]

sphincter

Ringlike muscle that maintains closure of a body passage or orifice by *contracting*, and opens the passage by relaxing.
[ref. 5]

sphingolipid

Member of a class of lipids containing the aliphatic amino alcohol *sphingosine*, or related structures, thus including *ceramide*.
Note: Abnormal sphingolipid *metabolism* is associated with lipid storage *diseases* such as *Tay-Sachs* and Niemann-Pick *diseases*.
[ref. 4]

sphingomyelin

One of a family of phospholipids found especially in the *central nervous system*, containing 1-phosphocholine bound to a *ceramide*.
[ref. 4]

sphingosine

2-aminooctadec-4-ene-1,3-diol

Major lipid component of cell *membranes*.
[ref. 4]
See also *sphingolipid, sphingomyelin*.

spiked bioassay (SB) approach

Procedure of placing test organisms in sediments spiked with different amounts of a *toxicant*, in order to generate a *concentration*-response model for effects on individuals, or to test hypotheses regarding the mechanism of previously observed effects.
[ref. 2]

spillover hypothesis (in metal toxicity)

Hypothesis that *toxic* effects of metals will begin to occur after the metal *concentration* exceeds the capacity of the amount of *metallothionein* present to bind the metal; the unbound metals then "spill over" to interact at sites of adverse action.
Note: The spillover hypothesis is based on an assumption that binding by metallothionein sequesters *toxic metals* from sites of action, but in fact, the metallothionein complex may itself be toxic, *e.g.*, the cadmium-metallothionein complex is toxic to the kidney.
[ref. 2]

spina bifida

Failure of the *neural tube* to close, resulting in the absence of part of the *vertebral* arch at the midline of the *spinal column* and exposure of the *spinal cord* and its covering *membranes*.
[ref. 5]

spinal column

See *vertebral column.*

spinal cord

Portion of the *central nervous system* outside the *brain* and inside the *vertebral column.*
[ref. 5]

spinal tap

See *lumbar puncture.*

spine (n)/spinal (adj)

See *vertebral column.*

spiral arteriole

spiral artery
spiral endometrial artery
corkscrew-like artery
coiled artery of the uterus

One of the corkscrew-like arterioles in pre*menstrual* or pro*gestational endometrium.*
[ref. 5]

splanchnic

Relating to the *visceral organs*, especially those of the *abdomen.*
[ref. 5]

spleen (n)/splenic (adj)

Largest of the *secondary lymphoid organs*, composed of *white pulp*, rich in lymphoid cells, and *red pulp*, which contains many *erythrocytes* and *macrophages.*
Note: The spleen traps and removes damaged erythrocytes carried in the *blood.*
[ref. 3]

splenic pulp

See *red pulp.*

splenocyte

Any *splenic* cell.
[ref. 3]

splicing

Processes through which *introns* are removed from a *messenger RNA* prior to *translation*, followed by joining of the *exons.*
[ref. 1]

split adjuvant technique

Test for *allergic contact dermatitis* in which guinea pig skin is exposed to repeated applications of a test substance and intradermal injections of complete *Freund's adjuvant* are administered separately.
[ref. 3]

spondylitis

Inflammation of the *vertebral column.*
[ref. 3]

spongioblast

Embryonic epithelial cell that develops into a neuro*glial cell.*
[ref. 5]

spontaneous autoimmune thyroiditis (SAT)

See *thyroiditis, autoimmune, spontaneous.*

spreader

Agent used in some *pesticide* formulations to extend the even disposition of the active ingredient.
[ref. 1]

stable age distribution

Relative *abundance* of age classes that a *population* approaches if it is allowed to grow exponentially (see *growth, exponential*).
[ref. 2]

stable population

Population with a zero *growth* rate and a constant distribution of individuals among its various age classes.
Note: Stable populations do not change in size over time if environmental conditions do not change.
[ref. 2]

stability half-life
stability half-time

Time required for the amount of a substance in a formulation to decrease, for any reason, by 50 %.
[ref. 1]
See also *half-life*; *half-time.*

staircase test

See *paw-reaching test.*

stalk (in anatomy)

Narrow connection with an *organ* or other structure.
[ref. 5]

stalk, allantoic

Narrow connecting tube between the intra- and extra-*embryonic* parts of the *allantois.*
[ref. 5]

standard

1. (general) That which is established as a measure or model to which others of a similar nature should conform.
   [ref. 1]
   See also *environmental quality standard.*
2. (in law or regulation)
   technical directive
   Technical specification, usually in the form of a document available to the public, drawn up with the consensus or general approval of all interests affected

by it, based on the consolidated results of science, technology, and experience, aimed at the promotion of optimum *community* benefits and approved by a body recognized on the national, regional, or international level.
[ref. 1]
3. (in analytical chemistry)
See also *reference material*.

standard morbidity ratio (SMR)
standardized morbidity ratio

Number of patients with a particular *disease* observed in a study group or *population* divided by the total number of people in the group or population, multiplied by 100.
Note: The standard morbidity ratio is usually expressed as a percentage.
[ref. 1]
See also *morbidity*.

standard mortality ratio (SMR)
standardized mortality ratio

Number of deaths observed in a study group or *population* divided by the number of deaths that would be expected if the study population had the same specific rates as the standard population, multiplied by 100.
Note: The standard mortality ratio is usually expressed as a percentage.
[ref. 1]

standardization

1. Making any substance, *drug*, or other preparation conform to type or precisely defined characteristics.
2. Establishment of precisely defined characteristics, or precisely defined methods, for future reference.
3. Definition of precise procedures for administering, scoring, and evaluating the results of a new method that is under development.

[ref. 1]

stannosis

Pneumoconiosis resulting from inhalation of tin dust.
[ref. 1]

startle reaction
startle response
startle part

Rapid physiological and psychological response to a sudden, unexpected *stimulus* that includes muscle *contraction* and avoidance posturing, with an increase in heart rate, respiration, skin conductance, and a negative affect.
Note: In the startle response test, types and intensities of reactions (*e.g., motor activity*) are evaluated.
[ref. 4]

startle reflex

The earliest *brainstem*-mediated part of the *reflex* reaction to a *stimulus* perceived as threatening.

Note: The *Moro reflex* in the newborn is a distinct response but related to the startle reflex, arising from a fear of falling, usually characterized by spreading of the arms and crying.
[ref. 4]

startle response test

See *startle reaction.*

startle response test, acoustic

Neurophysiological examination in which an animal is exposed to a brief (*e.g.*, 40 ms) acoustic *stimulus*, followed by measurement of the animal's *motor* reaction.
[ref. 4]
See also *startle reaction.*

static-renewal test

batch-replacement test
renewed static test
renewal test
semi-static test
static-replacement test

Modified aquatic *static-toxicity test* in which water is completely or partially replaced with new solutions at set periods during *exposures* or in which organisms are periodically transferred to new solutions.
[ref. 2]
See also *static-toxicity test.*

static-replacement test

See *static-renewal test.*

static-toxicity test

Aquatic *toxicity* test in which the *exposure* water is not changed during the test.
[ref. 2]
See also *static-renewal test.*

status epilepticus

Repeated or prolonged *seizure* lasting more than 30 min.
[ref. 4]

steady state

State of a system in which the conditions do not change with time, *e.g.*, because the system is in *equilibrium*, or the rates of forward and backward reactions or processes are equal.
[After ref. 1]

stem cell

Multipotent cell, with *mitotic* potential, that may serve as a precursor for many kinds of *differentiated* cells.
Note: *Embryonic* stem cells give rise to the embryonic *germ layers*, whereas adult stem cells are involved in tissue regeneration, repair processes and in *carcinogenesis*.
[ref. 5]

stem cell, adult

See *stem cell.*

stem cell, embryonic

See *stem cell.*

stem cell, hematopoietic

Self-renewing *stem cell* that is capable of giving rise to all of the formed elements of the *blood, i.e., leukocytes, erythrocytes*, and *platelets.*
[ref. 3]

stem cell, induced pluripotent (iPS cell)

Pluripotent stem cell that is generated from an *adult* cell by *genetic* reprogramming.
[ref. 5]

stem cell, lymphoid

Stem cell giving rise to the lineage of *lymphocytes.*
[ref. 3]

stem cell, myeloid

One of two groups of *stem cells* produced in the *bone marrow*. Myeloid stem cells may mature into several types of *blood cells*, including acidic *basophils, eosinophils, erythrocytes, macrophages, megakaryocytes*, and *neutrophils.*
[ref. 3]

stem cell, neural

Multipotent cell, with *mitotic* potential, that may serve as a precursor for *neuroprogenitor cells.*
Note: Adult neural stem cell refers to a cell localized in specific niches of the adult *central nervous* system, capable of generating new *neurons.*
[ref. 4]

stem cell, pluripotent

Self-replicating cell capable of developing into *cells* and *tissues* of the three primary *embryonic germ layers.*
[ref. 3]

stenosis

Abnormal narrowing of a passage or opening in the body, as of a blood vessel or muscular tube.
[ref. 4,5]

stereology (n)/stereological (adj)

Three-dimensional interpretation of two-dimensional cross sections of *tissue* and other materials.
Note 1: Stereology is often used for estimating the number of *neurons* or neuronal cell bodies in a volume of tissue.
Note 2: Stereology is different from *tomography*; the latter requires a complete set of planes to reconstruct the internal structure whereas stereology uses statistical methods to reconstruct the image from representative plane sections.
[ref. 4]

stereology, unbiased

Stereological method that uses systematic analysis of defined spatial fractions of a sample to estimate numbers of *neuronal* nuclei independent of changes in size and shape that may occur during tissue processing.
[ref. 4]

stereoselective synthesis

Chemical reaction (or reaction sequence) in which one or more new centers of chirality are formed in a substrate molecule and which produces the stereoisomeric (enantiomeric or diastereoisomeric) products in unequal amounts.
Note: Traditionally stereoselective synthesis has been called asymmetric synthesis.
[ref. 2]

stereoselectivity (n)/stereoselective (adj)

Specificity of chemical reactivity of stereoisomers based on their three-dimensional molecular structure.
[ref. 1]

sterility (n)/sterile (adj)

1. *Infertility*.
2. *Asepsis*.

[ref. 5]

sterilization

1. Process that makes an organism incapable of *fertilization* or reproduction, *e.g.*, *castration, vasectomy*, or *salpingectomy*.
2. Process that makes an object *aseptic*.

[ref. 5]

steroid (n)/steroidal (adj)

Naturally occurring compound and its synthetic analogues, based on the cyclopenta[*a*]phenanthrene carbon skeleton, partially or completely hydrogenated; there are usually methyl groups at C-10 and C-13, and often an alkyl group at C-17 and, by extension, one or more bond scissions, ring expansions, and (or) ring contractions of the skeleton, may have occurred.
Note: Natural steroids are derived by biogenesis from triterpenoids. They play important roles as *hormones* (sex hormones, cortisol), *membrane* components (cholesterol) and emulsifying agents (*bile* acids).
[ref. 5]

steroid 21-monooxygenase

Member (EC 1.14.14.16) of the *cytochrome P450* family of enzymes required for the synthesis of some *steroid hormones* including aldosterone and cortisol.
[ref. 5]

steroidogenesis assay

Procedure in which the effect of a test substance on *steroid* synthesis is studied, usually in a human adrenocortical *carcinoma* cell line.
Note: The steroidogenesis assay is part of the OECD framework for the "Testing and Assessment of Endocrine Disrupting Chemicals".
[ref. 5]

Stevens–Johnson syndrome

bullous erythema multiforme

Allergic reaction, often to a medication or *infection*, characterized by blistering of the skin and ulceration of *mucous membranes*.
[ref. 3]
See also *adverse drug reaction*.

stillbirth (n)/stillborn (adj)

Birth of a baby without any signs of life, at a time variously taken as 20-28 weeks of *pregnancy*.
Note: A stillborn baby may have died during pregnancy (called *intrauterine* death), *labor*, or *birth*.
[ref. 5]
Compare *miscarriage*.

stimulant

Agent that rouses or increases mental or physical activity.
[ref. 4]

stimulus

1. Anything that produces a reaction in an organism.
2. That which causes a response in an excitable tissue (see *excitation*) such as a *nerve*, muscle or gland.

[ref. 4]

stimulus, conditioned

Stimulus that comes to evoke a response after repetitive pairing with another stimulus that automatically elicits that response.
[ref. 4]
Compare *stimulus, unconditioned*.
See also *classical conditioning*.

stimulus, unconditioned

Stimulus that automatically elicits a paired response, such as food eliciting salivation in a hungry animal.
[ref. 4]
Compare *stimulus, conditioned*.

stochastic

Pertaining to, or arising by, chance random occurrence; hence, obeying the laws of probability but not precisely predictable.
[*]

stochastic effect

stochastic process
Opposite term: *deterministic effect*.

Phenomenon arising by chance or random occurrence, hence obeying the laws of probability but not precisely predictable.
Note: A *stochastic* model of *tumor* formation suggests that every individual exposed to a certain dose of a *carcinogen* has a probability of developing a tumor, but it is not predictable which individuals will be affected.
[*]

stochastic process

See *stochastic effect.*

stratification

1. (in epidemiology) Process of or result of separating a *sample* into several subsamples according to specified criteria, such as age groups or socioeconomic status.
2. (in geology) Process by which materials form or are deposited in layers, as in sedimentary rocks and some igneous rocks.
   Note: The atmosphere and the ocean also exhibit stratification, with the warmer air or water occupying the upper layers.

[ref. 1,2]

stratified sample

Subset of a *population* selected according to some important characteristic.
[ref. 1]
See also *stratification* (in epidemiology).

stress

1. (in ecology) Any condition that results in reduced growth of an organism or that prevents an organism from realizing its "genetic potential".
   [ref. 2]
2. (in physiology) Nonspecific response to severe, continuous or multiple demands or exposures.
   Note: Two forms of stress are sometimes distinguished; "distress" that reduces well-being and performance, and "eustress" that has beneficial effects.
   [*]

See also *stress, Selyean.*

stress, Selyean

Collective term for all the nonspecifically induced changes within a biological system following and during *environmental stress.*
[ref. 2]

stress protein

Any of several classes of proteins coded by *genes* transcriptionally activated (see *transcription*) by acute *stresses*, generally serving a protective or adaptive function.
Note 1: Stress proteins include chaperones such as the *heat shock proteins, enzymes* protective against *oxidative stress* such as *superoxide dismutase* (EC 1.15.1.1) and *glutathione peroxidase* (EC 1.11.1.9), and *metallothioneins.*
Note 2: Stressors inducing stress proteins include physical agents such as heat and radiation, processes such as infection and inflammation, oxidative stress and *hypoxia*, desiccation and starvation, metal species, and *xenobiotics.*
[ref. 2].

stress-protein fingerprinting

Proposed use of the patterns of *stress protein* induction seen in the field to suggest the particular *toxicant* inducing the response, after patterns from organisms sampled in the field are compared with those obtained with single-candidate toxicants in the laboratory.
[After ref. 2]

stress-response pathway

Signaling events induced when normal *cell* function or development is disrupted by *environmental* (physical or chemical) factors.
Note: Induction of stress-response pathways may lead to cellular repair and counteraction of *stress* effects, or to *adverse effects*.
[ref. 5]

stress theory of aging

See *aging, stress theory of.*

stressor (in ecotoxicology)

Any physical, chemical, or biological factor causing an adverse *response* in any component of an *ecosystem*.
[ref. 2]

striatum

Subcortical structure of striations of *gray matter* and *white matter* in the *forebrain* that serves as the major input to the *basal ganglia*, specifically the *caudate nucleus*, the *putamen* and the striated structure linking them.
[ref. 4]
See also *corpus striatum.*

stroke

Acute impairment of circulation to a part of the *brain*, lasting more than 24 h.
Note: Stroke may result from either a *hemmorhagic* or *thromboembolic* event.
[ref. 4]

stroma

Supporting *tissue* of an *organ*.
[ref. 3]
See also *connective tissue; extracellular matrix.*

stromal cell

Cell found in and producing the loose *connective tissue* (*stroma*) of an *organ* or other anatomical structure.
Note: Stromal cells include *immune* and *inflammatory* cells, pericytes, and *fibroblasts*.
[ref. 3,5]
See also *parenchymal cell.*

structural alert

Chemical grouping that is known to be associated with a particular type of *toxic* effect (*e.g.*, mutagenicity).
[ref. 1]

structural diversity

Range of types of physical structure in a *community* that may provide *habitats* for biological *species*.
[ref. 2]

structure–activity relationship (SAR)

Association between specific aspects of molecular structure and defined biological action.
[ref. 1]
See also *quantitative structure–activity relationship.*

structure–metabolism relationship (SMR)

Association between the physicochemical and (or) the structural properties of a substance and its route of *biotransformation.*
[ref. 1]

study (n)

1. Intensive attention to knowledge acquisition on a subject.
2. Detailed, systematic examination of a situation.

Note 1: General types of studies include

- *analytic study* (see *study, analytic*)
- *descriptive study*
- *feasibility study*
- *simulation study*

Note 2: In *epidemiology*, studies generally take the form of examining individuals, *cohorts*, or *populations* in a comparative manner, over suitable time periods and in comparison to suitable *control groups*, to reveal potential associations, causal relations or etiologies (*e.g.*, with *exposures* or *genetic makeup*) and specific outcomes (*e.g., adverse effects, disease*, or behaviors).
[*]
See also *validity of a study.*

study, analytic (in epidemiology)

Study designed to examine associations, commonly putative or hypothesized causal relationships, and to make causal inferences.
[After ref. 1]
See also *cohort study.*

study, association (in epidemiology)

Method of exploring novel genetic markers associated with a particular trait or the risk of developing a particular condition; the frequency of *alleles* or *genotypes* is compared between cases with the *disease* or trait under investigation and a group of individuals without that disease or trait (controls).
Note: An increase in the *genetic* marker between the two groups in an association study suggests that the marker may increase the likelihood of the trait or condition, or that it may be in linkage disequilibrium with an unrecognized genetic characteristic that does increase the likelihood.
[*]

study, case-base (in epidemiology)

Variant of the *case-control study* in which the controls are drawn from the same study base as the cases, regardless of their disease status. Cases of the disease of interest are identified, and a sample of the entire base population (cases and noncases) forms the controls.
Note: This design provides for estimation of the *risk ratio* or *rate ratio* without any rare disease assumption.
[*]
See also *case-cohort study.*

study, case-case (in epidemiology)

Case-only study in which cases of a given *disease* with a specific characteristic are compared with other cases with the same disease but without the characteristic. For example, this characteristic may be the result of an acquired (*somatic*) *genetic* alteration or an inherited genetic variant.
Note 1: The aim of a case-case study is to identify etiological or susceptibility factors specific to the subset of cases with the characteristic.
Note 2: A case-case study design is also used in investigating *infectious* diseases to detect different routes of transmission between subtypes of a disease.
[*]

study, case cohort (in epidemiology)

Variant of the *case control study* in which the *control group* is drawn from the same *cohort* as the cases but are identified before the cases develop; some of the controls may later become cases.
Note: This design provides an estimate of the risk ratio without any rare *disease* assumption.
[*]

study, case-control (in epidemiology)
case comparison study
case-compeer study
case-referent study

Observational *epidemiological* study of persons with a *disease* (or another outcome variable) of interest and a suitable *control group* of persons without the disease (*comparison group, reference group*).
Note: The potential relationship of a suspected risk factor or an attribute to the disease is examined by comparing the diseased and nondiseased subject groups with regard to how frequently the factor or attribute is present (or, if quantitative, the levels of the attribute) in each of the groups.
[*]

study, case-crossover (in epidemiology)

Type of case-only study in which each individual in the case group at one time period crosses over to become his own control at a later period.
Note: A requirement for a case-crossover study is that the effects (*e.g.*, of an exposure) are transient and do not effect the status or suitability of an individual case as a control at a later time.
[*]

study, cohort (in epidemiology)

Analytic study in which subsets (*cohorts*) of a defined *population* can be identified who are, have been, or in the future may be *exposed* or not exposed, or exposed in different degrees, to a factor(s) hypothesized to influence the probability of occurrence of a given *disease* or other outcome.
Note: The main feature of a cohort study is observation of a large population for a prolonged period (years), with comparison of *incidence rates* of the specified disease or outcome in groups that differ in *exposure* levels. The denominators used for analysis of the data obtained may be persons (*per capita*) or *person-time*.
[After ref. 1]
See also *study, longitudinal*; *study, observational*; *study, prospective*; *study, retrospective*.

study, concurrent cohort (in epidemiology)

Study in which the *cohort* is assembled now (in the present time) to be followed into the future.
Note: Such a study resembles a *prospective cohort study* in which the cohort is assembled at one time.
[*]

study, cross-sectional (in epidemiology)

Study in which groups (*cohorts*) of individuals of different types are combined into one large sample and studied at only a single time point (*e.g.*, a survey in which all members of a given *population*, regardless of age, religion, gender, or geographic location, are sampled for a given characteristic or finding in one day).
Note: Cross-sectional studies are used for examining phenomena expected to remain static through the period of interest, in contrast to *longitudinal studies* where change during the observation period may occur.
[*]

study, follow-up (in epidemiology)

Observation of a defined *population* over a period of time, chosen in order to observe changes in general *health* status or other health-related variables, in relation to recorded exposure conditions.
[*]

study, incidence (in epidemiology)

Observation of the number of new health-related events associated with recorded exposure conditions, in a defined *population* within a specified period of time; the *incidence* may be measured as a frequency count, *incidence rate*, or *incidence ratio*.
[*]
See also *incidence ratio, cumulative; study, longitudinal.*

study, intervention (in epidemiology)

Investigation designed to test a hypothesized cause–effect relationship by intentional change of a supposed causal factor in a *population*.
[ref. 1]

study, longitudinal cohort (in epidemiology)

Study in which groups of participants (*cohorts*), processes, or systems are studied over time, with data being collected at multiple intervals, or continuously where possible.
Note: The two main types of longitudinal study are the *prospective study* and the *retrospective study*.
[*]
Compare *cross-sectional study*.

study, mortality (in epidemiology)

Investigation dealing with *death rates* or proportion of deaths attributed to specific causes as a measure of response.
[ref. 1]

study, prospective cohort (in epidemiology)

Study in which groups of individuals (*cohorts*) are selected on the bases of factors that are to be examined, and followed over a period of time for possible effects on some outcome.
Note: The cohorts are followed in order to determine the *incidence rates* of the outcome being studied, and their relation to the exposure of concern.
[*]

study, retrospective cohort (in epidemiology)

Study in which the groups of chosen individuals are classified as either having an outcome of concern (cases) or lacking it (controls), and the subjects' histories are examined for factors that may be associated with *disease* occurrence.
Note 1: In retrospective studies, cases and controls are often matched for demographic or other variables.
Note 2. Retrospective studies have the drawback, when compared to *prospective studies*, that large *biases* may occur because of poor selection of controls, or because of inadequate recall of past exposure to risk factors.
Note 3. Advantages of retrospective studies are their potentially smaller scale, the short time required for their completion, and their applicability to rare diseases that would require study of very large *cohorts* in *prospective studies*.
[*]

stupor

State of impaired *conscious*ness showing diminution in response to environmental *stimulation*.
[ref. 4]

Sturm test

Biodegradation test based on the measurement of CO_2 production.
[ref. 2]

stygobiont

Organism that lives only in groundwater.
[ref. 2]

stygophile

Organism that lives in groundwater and in surface water.
[ref. 2]

subacute

Occurring over a period longer than an *acute effect*, but shorter than a *subchronic effect*.
Note: Subacute toxicity studies typically last 28 days.
[*]
Compare *subchronic*.

subacute cutaneous lupus erythematosus (SCLE)

Chronic remitting form of *dermatitis* characterized by severe photosensitivity and Ro/SS-A and La/SS-B *autoantibodies*.
[ref. 3]

subarachnoid

Underneath the *arachnoid membrane.*
[ref. 4]

subarachnoid hemorrhage

Entry of *blood* into the space between the *arachnoid membrane* and the *pia mater.*
[ref. 4]

subchronic

Repeated over a short period, usually about 10% of the life span; an imprecise term used to describe *exposure*s of intermediate duration between *acute* and *chronic.*
[ref. 1]
Compare *subacute.*

subchronic effect

Biological change resulting from an *environmental* alteration lasting about 10% of the lifetime of the test organism.
Note 1: In practice with experimental animals, a *subchronic* effect is usually identified as resulting from multiple or continuous *exposures* occurring over 90 days.
Note 2: Sometimes a subchronic effect is distinguished from a *subacute* effect on the basis of its lasting for a much longer time.
[ref. 1]

subchronic toxicity test

Animal experiment serving to study the effects produced by the test substance when administered in repeated *doses* (or continually in food, drinking water, air) over a period of up to about 90 days.
[ref. 1]

subclinical effect

Biological change with detectable, but not yet clinically relevant *symptoms* following *exposure* to an agent known to cause *disease,* either before symptoms of the disease occur or when they remain absent.
[ref. 1]

subcooled

Term applied to a substance that is a liquid at a temperature lower than the saturation temperature for the existing pressure (*i.e.*, the boiling point).
Note: Sometimes a subcooled substance is described as a "compressed" or "unsaturated" liquid since the existing pressure is greater than the saturation pressure for the given temperature.
[ref. 2]
See also *supercooled.*

subcooled liquid vapor pressure (P_L)

Vapor pressure of a *subcooled* liquid.
Note: This physicochemical property of subcooled liquid vapor pressure is an important factor in determining the fate of chemical substances in the *environment* and in allowing for the effects of environmental temperature variability.
[ref. 2]

subdural

Between the *dura mater* and the *arachnoid membrane*.
[ref. 4]

subfertility

Fertility below the normal range for a given *species*.
[ref. 1]

sublimation

1. (in chemistry) Direct transition of a solid to a vapor without passing through a liquid phase.
   [ref. 2]
2. (in psychology) Psychological defense mechanism whereby a socially unacceptable impulse is unconsciously converted into acceptable or productive activity.
   [*]

subjective environment
perceived environment

Surrounding conditions as perceived by persons living in these conditions.
[ref. 1]

substantia nigra

Component of the *basal ganglia* involved in production of the *neurotransmitter dopamine*.
[ref. 4]
See also *parkinsonism*.

substrate (in biology)

1. Substance upon which an *enzyme* acts to catalyze the formation of product.
2. Surface on which an organism grows or to which it is attached.

[ref. 1]

subthalamus

Part of the *diencephalon*, of which the major part is the *subthalamic nucleus*, and which connects to the globus pallidus, part of the *telencephalon*.
[ref. 5]

subthreshold dose

See *no-effect dose.*

succession

Orderly sequential progression of changes in *community* composition that occurs during development of new *populations* in any area, from initial colonization to the attainment of the *climax community* typical of a particular geographic area.
[ref. 2]
See also *succession, allogenic*; *succession, autogenic*; *succession, autotrophic*; *succession, heterotrophic*; *succession, primary*; *succession, secondary*.

succession, allogenic

Sequential appearance of biological *species* driven by external influences that alter local conditions.
Example: Silt deposition changing a marshland to a woodland.
[ref. 2]
See also *succession.*

succession, autogenic

Sequential appearance of biological *species* driven by processes operating within the *community environment* (compare *allogenic succession*).
Example: Primary and *secondary successions* that occur on newly exposed land.
[ref. 2]
See also *succession.*

succession, autotrophic

Sequential appearance of *autotrophic species* in a location, principally involving plants.
[ref. 2]
See also *succession.*

succession, heterotrophic

Temporal sequential appearance of different *heterotrophic species* at a location, most often decomposer organisms.
[ref. 2]
See also *succession.*

succession, primary

Sequential colonization by *species* that begin to colonize the bare ground and modify the *environmental* conditions after a region is completely denuded.
Example: Behind a retreating glacier, early colonizing organisms provide the *soils* needed by succeeding organisms.
[ref. 2]
See also *succession.*

succession, secondary

Sequential appearance of *species* following major changes to an established *ecosystem.*
Note: Catastrophic weather events, fire, or human activities all disturb the *environment* and may be followed by secondary succession. After such an event on land, well-developed *soil* remains, giving pioneer species an easy foothold; similar changes occur in abandoned agricultural areas.
[ref. 2]
See also *succession.*

sudorific

See *diaphoretic.*

sufficient evidence (in risk assessment)

Collection of facts and scientific references that is definite enough to establish that an *adverse effect* is caused by the agent in question.

Note 1: This definition of sufficient evidence is specified in the USEPA's Guidelines for *Carcinogen Risk Assessment*.
Note 2: In law, a distinction is often made between evidence that establishes a conclusion "beyond reasonable doubt" and "on the balance of probability". Evidence "beyond reasonable doubt" is usually required for a criminal law to be applied.
[ref. 1]

suggested no-adverse-response level (SNARL)

Maximum *dose* or *concentration* that on current understanding is likely to be tolerated by an *exposed* organism without producing any *harm*.
[ref. 1]

suicide reaction

Irreversible formation of molecular cleavage complexes (also referred to as "suicide complexes") that cause *cell* death.
[ref. 1]

sulcus

Any long, narrow groove, furrow or shallow depression, specifically referring to one of the fissures on the surface of the *brain*.
[ref. 5]

sulfotransferase

Enzyme activity (EC 2.8.2.x) involved in *phase II biotransformation* reactions, transferring sulfate from a donor (most commonly 3'-phosphoadenosine-5'-phosphosulfate, PAPS) to an alcohol or amine, forming the corresponding sulfonated product.
Note: The product of a sulfotransferase reaction is often a sulfonated *xenobiotic* with increased water-solubility that facilitates its excretion.
[*]

summary sheet

Two-to-four page summary of a *risk assessment*.
[ref. 1]

summation (in neurophysiology)

Process of addition of separate *postsynaptic* responses caused by *stimuli* that are adjacent in time and space.
Note 1: Summation may be spatial or temporal. *Excitation* of a *synapse* evokes a graded potential change in the postsynaptic membrane that may be below the *threshold* required to trigger an impulse, and if two or more such potentials are caused either nearly simultaneously, at different synapses on the same *neuron* (spatial summation), or in rapid succession at the same synapse (temporal summation), the summed response may be sufficient to trigger a postsynaptic impulse.
Note 2: Summation may occur between excitatory potentials, inhibitory potentials, or between an excitatory and an inhibitory potential.
[ref. 1]

superantigen

Antigen that reacts with all the *T-cells* belonging to a particular *T-cell receptor variable (V) region* family, and that therefore stimulates (or deletes) a much larger number of cells than does conventional antigen.
[ref. 3]

supercooled

Term describing a substance that persists as a liquid at a temperature below its freezing point without solidification or crystallization.
[ref. 2]
See also *subcooled*.

superfamily

Large group of proteins related by structural homology and function, or the *genes* that encode them.
[ref. 3]

superfecundation

Fertilization of two or more *ova* released in the same period of *ovulation*, either by different males or by the same male in separate acts of intercourse.
Note 1: If there are two or more different fathers, the state may be called heteropaternal superfecundation.
Note 2: Superfecundation is rare in humans, but heteropaternal superfecundation is common in some species, such as cats and dogs.
[ref. 5]

superfetation

Presence of two *fetuses* in the *uterus* at different stages of development, resulting from *fertilization* of *ova* released in two successive periods of *ovulation*.
[ref. 5]

Superfund

Program under federal authority, established by the U.S. Comprehensive Environmental Response, Compensation, and Liability Act (CERCLA) in 1980, to respond directly to releases or threatened releases (such as from landfills or waste disposal areas) of *hazardous* substances that may endanger *health* or welfare.
[ref. 1]

supernumerary

Exceeding the usual number; thus, in anatomy, anomalies such as a sixth finger on one hand or a third nipple in a human.
[ref. 5]

superoxide dismutase (SOD)

Antioxidant *enzyme* (EC 1.15.1.1) that removes potentially *toxic* superoxide ($O_2^{-\bullet}$) by catalyzing its disproportionation to dioxygen (O_2) and dihydrogen peroxide (H_2O_2).
[ref. 1]

superthreshold dose

See *toxic dose*.

suppression (in immunology)

Dominant immunological *tolerance*, a phenomenon that plays an active role in regulating *T-cell* and *B-cell* responses to both foreign *antigens* and *autoantigens*.
Note: Suppression producing the downregulation of responses to autoantigens is a major regulatory mechanism involved in the induction and maintenance of *self-tolerance*.
[ref. 3]

suppression, bystander

Suppression of an *immune response* to an *antigen* due to *tolerance* to an unrelated (hence bystander) antigen.
[ref. 3]
See also *effect, bystander.*

suppressor cell

suppressor T-cell
suppressor T-lymphocyte

T-cell that suppresses the *immune response* of *B-cells* and other T-cells to an *antigen*; in more current usage, classified as a *regulatory T-cell.*
[ref. 3]

supramolecular adhesion complex (SMAC)

Collection of molecules forming at the contact point of a *T cell* and an *antigen-presenting cell*, enriched in *T-cell receptor, adhesion molecules*, and signaling molecules.
[ref. 3]

supratentorial

1. *Intracranial* contents located above the *tentorium* of the *cerebellum*, notably the *white matter* of the *cerebrum.*
2. Often describing functional symptoms of *diseases* of the *white matter* that lead to physical and mental disability.

[ref. 4]

supratentorial herniation

See *herniation, supratentorial.*

surface layer

Molecular region of a bulk substance adjacent to another substance or another phase of the same substance, with physicochemical properties distinct from the bulk phase.
[*]
See also *interfacial layer.*

surfactant

surface-active agent

Substance that lowers the surface tension of the medium in which it is dissolved, and (or) the interfacial tension with other phases, and, accordingly, is enriched at the liquid/vapor interface and (or) at other interfaces.
Note: Surfactants facilitate dispersion of other substances in water.
[ref. 2]
See also *detergent.*

surfactant, pulmonary

Surface-active layer of phospholipids and proteins coating the *pulmonary alveoli* that increases lung compliance, facilitates lung expansion, and stabilizes *alveolar* volume.
Note: Lack of pulmonary surfactant is more common following *premature birth* than birth at full term, and is a cause of infant respiratory distress *syndrome.*
[ref. 5]

surrogate (in toxicology)

surrogate toxicant

Relatively well studied *toxicant* whose properties are assumed to apply to an entire chemically and toxicologically related class.
Example: Benzo[*a*]pyrene data may be used as toxicologically equivalent to those for all *carcinogenic* polynuclear aromatic hydrocarbons.
[ref. 1]

surrogate light chain

Light chain-like structure formed when the proteins encoded by the V_{preB} and λ_5 genes associate with each other.
Note: A surrogate light chain can form *immunoglobulin*-like complexes that are expressed on the surface of *pre-B-cells* at different stages of development.
[ref. 3]

surrogate organism

Test organism or *population* that is grown under laboratory conditions to serve as a substitute in *toxicity* testing for indigenous organisms, *communities*, or *populations*.
[ref. 2]

surveillance

Systematic ongoing collection, collation, and analysis of data, and the timely dissemination of information to those who need to know in order that action can be taken to initiate investigative or control measures.
[ref. 1]

survival curve

Graph of the proportion of a *population* surviving for incremental units of time after a defined starting point (*e.g.*, identification of an *exposure*, diagnosis of a *disease*, or institution of a treatment), plotted against time on the x-axis.
[*]
See also *product-limit method*.

survival time

Time interval between the beginning of a harmful *exposure* or a *disease*, and death of the organism.
[After ref. 2]

survivorship

Proportion of animals surviving between two specified ages.
[ref. 2]

survivorship curve

Graph showing how *survivorship* varies with age, starting from *birth*.
[ref. 2]

susceptible

Describing a group of organisms more vulnerable to a given *exposure* than the majority of the *population* to which they belong.
Note: *Susceptibility* may reflect gender, age, physiological status, or *genetic* constitution of the organisms at risk.
[ref. 1]

susceptibility

Condition of an organism or *ecological* system that makes it more vulnerable or lacking resistance to a given *exposure or disease* than expected for the majority of the *population* or group of ecological systems to which it belongs.
Note: Susceptibility is inversely proportional to the magnitude of the exposure required to cause a *toxic* effect.
[1,2]

susceptibility biomarker

See *biomarker of susceptibility.*

suspension feeder

filter feeder
Animal that feeds by straining suspended matter and food particles from water, typically by passing the water over a specialized structure, such as the baleen of baleen whales.
Examples: Clams, barnacles, krill, mysids, sponges, whale sharks, flamingoes.
[ref. 2]
See also *deposit feeder*; *fluid feeder*; *food-mass feeder.*

sweat

perspire (v)/perspiration (n)

1. (v) Excrete fluid released from sweat *glands* in the skin of mammals.
2. (n) Fluid released from sweat glands.

[*]
See also *diaphoretic.*

swimming test

forced swimming test
Porsolt forced swimming test
behavioral despair test

Procedure in which a test animal (rodent) is forced to swim to avoid drowning.
Note 1: Most often used to test *antidepressants*, which increase the time the animal spends in escape-directed swimming behavior.
Note 2: Interpretation is controversial, as cessation of swimming could be a learned response to hasten removal by the investigator.
[ref. 4]
See also *tail suspension test.*

switch region

See *switch sequence.*

switch sequence

Highly conserved repetitive sequence that mediates *class switching* in the *immunoglobulin heavy chain* gene locus.
[ref. 3]

sympathetic nervous system

Part of the *autonomic nervous system* originating in the *thoracic* and *lumbar* regions of the *spinal cord* that tends to inhibit or oppose the physiological effects of the

parasympathetic nervous system, as in tending to reduce digestive *secretions*, increase the heart rate, and contract blood vessels.
Note: Its major neurotransmitter is *noradrenaline*.
[ref. 1]

sympathetic ophthalmia

Autoimmune injury to one eye that occurs after penetrating injury or surgery to the other eye.
[ref. 3]

sympatholytic

anti-adrenergic

1. (n) Agent that blocks transmission of impulses from the *adrenergic* (*sympathetic*) post*ganglionic nerve* fibers to effector *organs* or *tissues*.
2. (adj) Having the property of producing such effects.

[ref. 4]

sympathomimetic

adrenergic

1. (n) Substance such as *noradrenaline* or a related compound, that produces *effects* resembling those of impulses transmitted by the post*ganglionic* fibers of the *sympathetic nervous system*.
2. (adj) Having the property of producing such effects.

[ref. 4]

symptom (n)/symptomatic (adj)

Any evidence of a *disease* or an effect induced by a substance as perceived by the affected subject (*e.g.*, dizziness, *pain*) or detected in a physical examination.
[ref. 1]
See also *asymptomatic; symptomatology*.

symptomatology (in toxicology)

General description of all of the *signs* and *symptoms* of *exposure* to a *toxicant*.
Note: Signs are the overt (observable) responses associated with exposure (such as *convulsions*, death, *etc.*), whereas symptoms are covert (subjective) responses (such as nausea, *headache, etc.*).
[ref. 1]

synapse (n)/synaptic (adj)

Functional junction between two *cells*, where an impulse is transmitted from one cell to another, by chemical or electrical signals.
[ref. 4]
See also *synapse, immunological*; *synapse, neuronal*.

synapse, chemical

Neuronal synapse using *neurotransmitters* to convey the signal.
[*]

synapse, electrical

Neuronal synapse where the two *neurons* are in electrical contact, enabling them to transfer signals from one to the other without chemical transmission.
Note: Electrical synapses are less frequent than *chemical synapses.*
[*]

synapse, immunological

Contact point between the *T-cell* and the *antigen-presenting cell* that is generated by reorganization and clustering of cell surface molecules in *lipid rafts.*
Note: The immunological *synapse* facilitates interactions between *T-cell receptor (TCR)* and *major histocompatibility complex molecules*, and between *adhesion molecules*, thereby potentiating a TCR-mediated activation signal.
[ref. 3]

synapse, neuronal

Functional junction between two *neurons*, where a *nerve* impulse is transmitted from one neuron to another.
[ref. 4]
See also *synapse, chemical*; *synapse, electrical.*

synapsis

syndesis

Point-wise pairing of *homologous chromosomes* during the *prophase* of *meiosis.*
[ref. 5]

synaptic cleft

Narrow gap between the *presynaptic* and *postsynaptic* regions of two communicating *neurons*, into which *neurotransmitters* are secreted to promote an *excitation.*
[ref. 4]
See also *synapse.*

synaptic inhibition

Suppression of *synaptic transmission.*
Note: Synaptic inhibition may occur *presynaptically* or *postsynaptically*, result from electrical or chemical effects, and be deliberately produced or part of a physiological process.
[ref. 4]
See also *inhibitory post-synaptic potential.*

synaptic plasticity

1. Ability of synapses to form and reform continually.
   Note: Synaptic plasticity is thought to contribute to learning and memory.
2. Malleability of signal strength arising at the level of *synaptic transmission.*

[ref. 4]
See also *augmentation*; *facilitation*; *long-term potentiation*; *potentiation.*

synaptic transmission

Neurotransmitter release, *diffusion*, and *receptor* binding, propagating an impulse across a *synapse.*
[ref. 4]

synaptonemal complex

Structure of *filamentous* proteins that forms between *homologous chromosomes* when they pair during *meiosis*.
Note: It may contribute to *synapsis* and *genetic recombination*.
[ref. 5]

syncephalus
monocephalus

Conjoined twins with two bodies and a fused head.
[ref. 5]

syncytiotrophoblast

Outer *syncitial* layer of *trophoblast* cells that invades the *endometrium* during *implantation*.
Note: The syncytiotrophoblast is the site of synthesis of *human chorionic gonadotropin* and is involved in *implantation*.
[ref. 5]

syncytium (n)/syncytial (adj)

Referring to a large multinucleated mass of cellular contents that arises from the fusion of originally individual *cells*.
[ref. 5]

syndactyly

Congenital occurrence of fusion or webbing of the fingers or toes.
[ref. 5]

syndrome

Group of *signs* and *symptoms* that frequently occur together, or a condition characterized by such a group.
[After ref. 5]

synergism (in toxicology)
synergistic effect
synergy (in toxicology)

Pharmacological or *toxicological* interaction in which the combined biological effect of *exposure* to two or more substances is greater than expected on the basis of the simple summation of the effects of each of the individual substances.
[ref. 1]

synergism (in pesticide use)

Action of a substance that is itself non*toxic*, but, when co-administered with a *pesticide*, increases the pesticide's efficacy or overcomes pesticide resistance in the target organism.
Note: Pesticide *synergists* often act by inhibiting *enzymes* involved in pesticide *metabolism*, typically *monooxygenases*.
[*]

synergist (n)/synergistic (adj) (in toxicology)

Substance that contributes more than additively to a mutual effect with another substance.
[ref. 1]

synergistic effect

See *synergism.*

synergy

See *synergism.*

syngeneic

Genetically identical, *e.g.*, a fully *inbred strain* of mice.
Note: A practical consequence of syngeneic identity is that *cells* can be transferred from one to other syngeneic animals without *rejection*.
[ref. 3]

syngenetic (in mineralogy)

Describing mineral deposits formed at the same time as the enclosing rocks; characterized by or pertaining to a formation contemporaneous with the enclosing or surrounding rock.
[ref. 2]

syngraft

See *isograft.*

synomone

Semiochemical that is produced by one organism inducing a response in an organism of another *species* that is favorable to both the emitter and the responding organism.
[ref. 1]
See also *allomone; kairomone.*

synophthalmia
cyclopia
monophthalmos

Congenital fusion of the *orbit*s in the midline; the resultant orbit then contains one eyeball.
[ref. 5]

synotia

Congenital malformation characterized by the union or approximation of the ears in front of the neck, often accompanied by the absence or defective development of the lower jaw.
[ref. 5]
See also *agnathia; megagnathia; otocephaly.*

synovium (n)/synovial (adj)

Membrane surrounding the fluid-filled space between the articulating *cartilaginous* surfaces of a joint, forming the inner layer of a joint capsule.
Note: The synovium can become thickened and *inflamed* in *rheumatoid arthritis* and other *arthroses*.
[*]

synteny (n)/syntenic (adj)

Property of *gene*s that reside on the same *chromosome*.
[ref. 1]

α-synuclein

Protein abundant in the human *brain*, thought to regulate the release of *dopamine*.
[ref. 4]

syringomyelia

syrinx

Cyst occurring within the *spinal cord* as a result of accumulation of *cerebrospinal fluid*.
[ref. 4]

systematic sample

Subset selected according to some simple rule such as specified date or alphabetic classification.
[ref. 1]

systematics (in biology)

Study of the classification and relationships of past and present living organisms based on their *evolutionary* relationships.
Note 1: Relationships in systematics are visualized in *cladograms.*
Note 2: Systematics is used to understand the evolutionary history of life on Earth.
[*]
See also *cladogram; evolution; evolutionary tree; phylogenetics; phylogeny; taxonomy*.

systemic

1. Relating to the body as a whole.
2. Occurring at a site in the body remote from the point of contact with a substance.

[ref. 1]

systemic autoimmune disease

See *autoimmune disease, systemic*.

systemic effect

Consequence that is either of a generalized nature or that occurs at a site distant from the point of entry of a substance.
Note: A systemic effect requires *absorption* and distribution of the substance in the body.
[ref. 1]

systemic lupus erythematosus (SLE)

Chronic *autoimmune disease* that is potentially debilitating and sometimes fatal, as the *immune system* attacks the body's *cells* and *tissues* with consequent *inflammation* and tissue damage.
Note 1: SLE can affect any part of the body, but most often harms the heart, joints, skin, lungs, blood vessels, liver, kidneys, and *nervous system*. The course of the disease is unpredictable, with periods of illness (called flares) alternating with remission.
Note 2: SLE can occur at any age, and is most common in women, particularly of non-European descent.
Note 3: SLE is very heterogeneous in clinical expression and serological factors. *Autoantibodies* directed against nuclear components (*antinuclear antibodies*) are typically

detected. Anti-dsDNA, anti-Sm, and antiphospholipid *antibodies* are used as classification criteria for different types of SLE.
[ref. 3]

systemic sclerosis (SSc)

Fibrosing disease of unclear etiology that affects multiple *organ* systems.
Note 1: The skin ("scleroderma") and blood vessels (arteries, small vessels) are most commonly affected by systemic sclerosis, but involvement of the lungs and *gastrointestinal tract* (esophagus) may also be observed.
Note 2: Anticentromere *antibodies* (ACA) as well as *autoantibodies* against DNA topoisomerase I (scl-70) (EC 5.99.1.2) and various nucleolar *antigens* are diagnostic and prognostic markers of systemic sclerosis and are often detectable years before disease manifestation. They are also detectable in individuals exposed to quartz *dust*.
[ref. 3]

systems biology

Study of the mechanisms underlying complex biological processes as integrated systems of many diverse, interacting components.
Note: Systems biology usually involves (1) collection of large sets of experimental data (by high-throughput technologies and (or) by mining the literature of molecular biology and biochemistry), (2) proposal of mathematical models that might account for at least some significant aspects of this data set, (3) accurate computer solution of the mathematical equations to obtain numerical predictions, and (4) assessment of the quality of the model by comparing numerical simulations with the experimental data.
[ref. 1]

$t_{1/2}$

See *half-life, half-time.*

T-cell

See *T-lymphocyte.*

α:β T-cell

Lymphocyte whose *T-cell receptor* is a heterodimer of an α chain and a β chain.
Note: α:β T-cells represent the majority of *thymocytes* in the *thymus* and *T cells* in the periphery.
[ref. 3]
See also α:β *T-cell receptor*; γ:δ *T-cell.*

γ:δ T cell

Lymphocyte whose *T-cell receptor* is a heterodimer of a γ chain and a δ chain.
[ref. 3]
See also γ:δ *T-cell receptor.*

T-cell, drug-specific

T-*memory cell* that is specific for a *drug allergen.*
[ref. 3]

T-cell, regulatory (Treg)

T-cell that controls the maintenance of normal *immune homeostasis.*
Note: Treg cells are involved in controlling (anergizing (see *anergy*) or counter-regulating) autoreactive cells (see *autoreactivity*) that have escaped from *thymic negative selection.*
[ref. 3]
See also *CD8+ T suppressor cell; CD4+CD25+ T-cell.*

T-cell-dependent antibody response (TDAR)

*Immunotoxic*ity test that evaluates the ability of animals to produce *antibodies* to a *T-dependent antigen* (*e.g., sheep red blood cells* or *keyhole limpet hemocyanin*).
[ref. 3]

T-cell receptor (TCR)

See *receptor, T-cell.*

α:β T-cell receptor

See *receptor, α:β T-cell.*

γ:δ T-cell receptor

See *receptor, γ:δ T-cell.*

Comprehensive Glossary of Terms Used in Toxicology
By John Duffus, Douglas M. Templeton and Michael Schwenk

Published by the Royal Society of Chemistry, www.rsc.org

TDP-43 transcription factor

Cleavage product (43 kDa) of the transactive response (TAR) *DNA* binding protein (TARDBP) that targets TAR DNA and transcriptionally represses HIV-1.
Note: Pathological accumulation of the *misfolded protein* cleavage product TDP-43 has been associated with *frontotemporal dementia* and *amyotrophic lateral sclerosis*.
[ref. 4]
See also *transcription factor*.

T-dependent antigen

See *antigen, T-dependent*.

TdT-dependent dUTP-biotin nick end labeling (TUNEL) assay

Method for detecting *apoptotic* cells in situ based on characteristic *DNA* fragmentation, exploiting the ability of *terminal deoxynucleotidyl transferase* to transfer a labeled deoxyuridine triphosphate to the terminal ends arising from DNA cleavage.
[ref. 3]

T helper cell

See *helper T-lymphocyte*.

Th0 cell

Helper T-lymphocyte with a less restricted *cytokine* profile than *Th1* and *Th2 cells*.
Note: Th0 cell-like responses are observed in patients with *rheumatoid arthritis, Sjögren syndrome*, and *Graves disease*.
[ref. 3]

Th1 cell

Helper T-lymphocyte producing mainly *interleukin*-2, *interferon*, and *tumor necrosis factor* β, and thereby responsible for *phagocyte*-dependent *host* responses.
Note 1: Th1-cell-dominated responses are seen in *autoimmune diseases* in which *cytotoxic T cells* and *macrophages* play a major role, *e.g., multiple sclerosis, diabetes mellitus type 1, Hashimoto thyroiditis*, and *Crohn disease*.
Note 2: Switching from a Th1- to *Th2*-cell response can prevent Th1-mediated tissue destruction in animal models.
[ref. 3]

Th2 cell

Helper T-lymphocyte found in mice producing *interleukins* IL-4, IL-5, IL-6, IL-9, IL-10, and IL-13.
Note 1: Besides other effects, Th2 cells provide optimal help for *antibody* responses.
Note 2: Th2 cell responses are also an important downregulatory mechanism for exaggerated *Th1* responses.
Note 3: A predominant Th2-cell *cytokine* profile is observed in patients with *atopic* disorders and *graft-versus-host disease*.
[ref. 3]

Th3 cell

Helper T-lymphocyte producing and responding to *transforming growth factor β* and helping *immunoglobulin A*-mediated *antibody* responses.
[ref. 3]

Th9 cell

Helper T-lymphocyte producing *interleukin* IL-9, which stimulates *mast cells.*
[ref. 3]

Th17 cell

T17

Helper T-lymphocyte, distinct from *Th1* and *Th2 cells*, that secretes the *interleukin* IL-17.
Note: T17 cells are thought to play an important role in *autoimmune disease.*
[ref. 3]

T-independent antigen

See *antigen, T-independent*

T-lymphocyte

Lymphocyte that matures in the *thymus* and has the ability to recognize specific peptide *antigens* through the *receptors* on its cell surface.
Note: T lymphocytes have *T-cell receptor* molecules that are specific for complexes comprising short peptides bound to and presented by *major histocompatibility complex molecules.*
[ref. 3]

T-maze

See *maze, T/Y.*

Tr1 cell

T-lymphocyte that regulates *Th1 cell* responses; it resembles the *regulatory T-cell* and is possibly related to the *Th3 cell.*
Note: Tr1 cells are abundant in the intestine and may be involved in *tolerance* to dietary *antigens.*
[ref. 3]

tachy-

Opposite term: *brady-*

Prefix meaning rapid, as in *tachycardia* and *tachypnoea.*
[ref. 1]

tachycardia

Opposite term: *bradycardia*

Abnormally fast heartbeat.
[ref. 1]

tachypnoea

Opposite term: *bradypnoea*

Abnormally fast breathing.
[ref. 1]

taeniacide

Substance intended to kill tapeworms.
[ref. 1]

tail flick test

Procedure in which the tail of a rodent is heated and the time taken for the animal to flick its tail (latency) is taken as a measure of the relative degree of *antinociception.*
[ref. 4]
See also *tail immersion test.*

tail bud

In the *vertebrate embryo*, mass of proliferating cells at the *caudal* end that arises from the *primitive node.*
[ref. 5]

tail immersion test

Procedure in which the tail of a rodent is placed in a hot water bath (typically between 54 °C and 58 °C) and the time it takes the animal to remove the tail from the water is interpreted as a measurement of the relative degree of *antinociception.*
[ref. 4]
See also *tail flick test.*

tail suspension test

Procedure in which a mouse is suspended by its tail and the time spent attempting to right itself is observed.
Note 1: Most often the tail suspension test is used to test *antidepressants*, which usually increase the time the animal spends in escape-directed righting behavior.
Note 2: Both the tail suspension test and the *swimming test* are sometimes referred to as behavioral despair tests.
[ref. 4]

talipes

See *clubfoot.*

tandem conjugate

Molecular construct with two fluorochromes where the first excites the second by its emission.
Note: Tandem conjugates are used in *flow cytometry* analysis.
[ref. 3]

tapping test

See *finger tapping test.*

target (in biology)

Any organism, *organ, tissue, cell,* or cell constituent that is subject to the action of an agent.
[ref. 1]

target cell (in immunology)

Cell killed by one of the body's *killer cells*, such as by a *cytotoxic T-lymphocyte* or *natural killer cell.*
[ref. 3]

target population (in epidemiology)

1. Collection of individuals, items, or measurements about which inferences are required.
   Note: The term "target population" is sometimes used to indicate the *population* from which a *sample* is drawn and sometimes to denote any *reference population* about which inferences are needed.
2. Group of persons for whom an intervention is planned.

[ref. 1]

tau protein

One of a class of proteins that stabilizes *microtubules*, particularly in *neurons*, *astrocytes*, and *oligodendrocytes* of the *central nervous system*.
Note 1: The various tau proteins are splice variants (see *splicing*) of the single *gene* microtubule-associated protein tau (MAPT).
Note 2: Defective tau proteins are associated with *dementias* such as *Alzheimer disease*.
[ref. 4]

tauopathy

One of a class of *neurodegenerative diseases*, including *Alzheimer disease*, associated with abnormal aggregation of *tau proteins*.
[ref. 4]
See also *paired helical filament; Western Pacific amyotrophic lateral sclerosis and parkinsonism-dementia complex.*

taxocene

Taxonomically defined subset of an entire *community*.
[ref. 2]

taxon/taxa (pl)
taxonomic unit

Name given to designate an organism or group of organisms.
Note: In biological nomenclature according to Carl Linnaeus, a taxon is assigned a *taxonomic* rank and can be placed at a particular level in a systematic hierarchy reflecting *evolutionary* relationships.
[ref. 2]

taxonomy (n)/**taxonomic** (adj)

Scientific approach to the allocation of biological names and the rules of naming organisms; the rank ordering of taxa according to presumptive *evolutionary* (*phylogenetic*) relationships.
[ref. 2]
See also *phylogeny; systematics.*

Tay-Sachs disease
infantile GM2 gangliosidosis

Autosomal recessive inheritance of *hexosaminidase A* deficiency leading to a *lysosomal storage disease* characterized by central and peripheral *neuronal* involvement and early death.
[ref. 5]

technical directive

See *standard.*

tegmentum

Floor of the midbrain.
Note 1: In the *embryo*, tegmentum refers more generally to the anterior portion of the *neural tube.*
Note 2: The tegmentum is the site of the nuclei of several cranial nerves.
[ref. 5]

Teleky's sign

See *wrist drop.*

telencephalon

Embryonic structure that develops into the *cerebrum.*
[ref. 5]

telomere

Structure that terminates the arm of a *chromosome.*
[ref. 1]

telophase

Final stage of both *meiosis* and *mitosis* in which distinct nuclei form in each daughter cell.
[ref. 5]

temperature sensitivity (n)/temperature-sensitive (adj)

1. Adverse responsiveness to heat or cold.
   Note: Temperature *sensitivity* is associated with a number of medical conditions, some physiologically well-defined (as in cold intolerance in hypothyroidism) and others less so (as in reported *chronic fatigue syndrome*).
2. *Phenotype* arising from engineered or selected gene mutations in experimental organisms, characterized by altered temperature dependency for optimal *growth* or survival.

[ref. 4]

temporal lobe

See *lobe, temporal.*

temporary acceptable daily intake

See *acceptable daily intake, temporary.*

temporary maximum residue limit

See *maximum residue limit, temporary.*

tentorium

tentorium cerebelli

Fold of the *dura mater* separating the *cerebrum* from the *cerebellum.*
[ref. 4]

teratocarcinoma

Malignant teratoma, occurring most often in the *testis*.
[ref. 5]

teratogen (n)/teratogenic (adj)

Chemical, physical, or biological agent that, when administered to a parent either prior to *conception* or before *birth* of the child, induces permanent structural *malformations* or *birth defects* in the *offspring*.
Note 1: Teratogens may act at vulnerable points in the development of *gametes* in parents or of *organ* development in the *embryo* and *fetus*.
Note 2: Modes of action of teratogens include mimicry of *morphogens* (thus interference with morphogenesis), modulation of *genes* and *gene expression*, and direct alterations in protein function.
[ref. 5]

teratogenesis

Process of development of *malformations* or *birth defects*.
[ref. 5]
See also *teratogen*.

teratogenetics

Study of how *genes* and *teratogens* interact to cause *birth defects*.
[ref. 5]

teratogenic index (TI)

Mortality of *eggs* expressed as a lethal concentration divided by the threshold concentration (*e.g.*, LC_{50}/TC_{50}) for production of abnormal *embryos* with nonheritable permanent structural *malformations* or defects, following exposure to a *teratogen*.
Note: The TI is thought to reflect the developmental *hazard* of a *contaminant*.
[ref. 5]

teratogenicity

Inherent ability to act as a *teratogen*.
[ref. 5]

teratology

Study of the causes, mechanisms and manifestations of developmental deviation of either structure or function.
[ref. 5]

teratoma

dermoid cyst
Benign *germ cell*-derived *tumor* containing *embryonic* elements of the three primary *germ layers*, such as skin, hair and muscle, occurring most frequently in the *ovary*.
[ref. 5]
See also *teratocarcinoma*.

terminal deoxynucleotidyl transferase (TdT)

Enzyme that inserts noncoded nucleotides at the junctions of *V, D*, and *J gene* segments of *immunoglobulin* and *T-cell receptor* locus DNA, thus increasing the diversity of *antigen*-specific recognition.

[ref. 3]
See also *TdT-dependent dUTP-biotin nick end labeling (TUNEL) assay*.

terrestrial

Relating to land, as distinct from air or water.
[ref. 2]

Tessier classification

Classification of bony and soft tissue *facial clefts* based on their anatomic location.
Note: In the Tessier classification, the facial clefts are numbered from 0-14, with 0 and 14 being in the midline.
[ref. 5]

testicular feminization

Type of male *pseudohermaphroditism* in which the individual has a male *karyotype* and has *testes* present within the *abdominal cavity*, but develops female *external genitalia* and female *secondary sexual characteristics*.
Note 1: Testicular feminization is due to an *androgen receptor mutation*, causing the *target tissues* to be insensitive to the *masculinizing* effects of *androgens*.
Note 2: Clinical presentation of testicular feminization is usually as a *phenotypic* female with primary *amenorrhea*.
[ref. 5]

testing of chemicals

1. (in toxicology) Evaluation of the potentially *toxic* effects of substances by their application through relevant routes of *exposure* to appropriate organisms or biological systems so as to relate effects to *dose* following application.
2. (in chemistry) Qualitative or quantitative analysis by the application of one or more fixed methods and comparison of the results with established standards.

[ref. 1]

testis (n)/testes (pl)/testicular (adj)

testicle

Gonad of a male animal, involved in secretion of *androgens* and the site of *sperm* production.
[ref. 5]

testis, undescended

cryptorchid testis
cryptorchidism

Testis that has failed to descend completely from its developmental origin in the lower *abdominal cavity* into the *scrotum*.
[ref. 5]

testosterone

Androgenic steroid hormone produced primarily in the *testis*, responsible for the development of the male sexual organs and male *secondary sexual characteristics*.
Note: The *ovary* also secretes testosterone, but circulating levels in the female are much lower than in the male.
[ref. 5]

tetanic

Pertaining to *tetanus*, characterized by tonic muscle *spasm*.
[ref. 4]

tetanus

1. Sustained muscle contraction.
2. Disease caused by *tetanus toxin* and characterized by painful, sustained muscle contraction with *spasticity* and *paralysis*.

[ref. 4]

tetanus toxin

tetanospasmin

Neurotoxin produced by the bacterium ***Clostridium tetani*** growing in anaerobic conditions, producing the disease *tetanus*.
Note: The action of tetanus toxin is in major part due to suppression of release of the inhibitory *neurotransmitter*, *γ-aminobutyric acid*.
[ref. 4]

tetanus toxin-binding ganglioside

See *ganglioside, tetanus toxin-binding*.

tetanus toxoid

Detoxified *tetanus toxin* used to produce active immunity (see *active immune response*) against tetanus.
[ref. 3]

tetany

Neurological syndrome characterized by muscle twitches, *cramps*, and *spasms*; and in severe forms, by spasm of the muscles of the *larynx* (*laryngospasm*) and *seizures*.
Note: Tetany is often a sign of irritability of the *central* and *peripheral nervous systems* resulting from a low concentration of ionized calcium in the serum.
[ref. 4]

tetracycline (INN)

(4*S*,4a*S*,5a*S*,6*S*,12a*S*)-4-(dimethylamino)-3,6,10,12,12a-pentahydroxy-6-methyl-1,11-dioxo-1,4,4a,5,5a,6,11,12a-octahydrotetracene-2-carboxamide

Broad-spectrum *antibiotic* of polycyclic polyketide structure.
Note: Tetracyclines are considered to be *teratogens* because they can deposit in, and cause discoloration of, the developing teeth, while also inhibiting the tooth development process.
[ref. 5]

tetradecanoyl phorbol acetate (TPA)

See *phorbol myristate acetate*.

tetralogy of Fallot

Set of four *congenital cardiac* defects involving (i) an opening in the wall that should separate the right and left *ventricles* (*ventricular septal defect*) allowing the *aorta* to receive venous as well as arterial *blood*, (ii) *stenosis* of the *pulmonary artery*, (iii) *hypertrophy* of the right ventricle, and (iv) displacement of the *aorta*.

Note 1: The constellation of anatomical defects in tetralogy of Fallot is understandable in terms of a flaw in the ordered sequence of events in the normal development of the heart and associated vessels.
Note 2: Tetralogy of Fallot is the most common cardiac cause of *cyanosis* in infants.
[ref. 5]

tetramer staining

Technique used for selective staining of *antigen*-specific *T-lymphocytes* in vitro or in situ, in which an antigen is presented to T-cells by *peptide tetramer* constructs of *major histocompatability class I molecules*.
Note: Tetramer staining is also used to isolate antigen-specific T-cell populations for *clonal expansion*.
[ref. 3]

tertiary lymphoid tissue/organ

Ectopic lymphoid aggregates that accumulate during the process of *chronic immune* stimulation, and exhibit characteristics usually associated with the *secondary lymphoid organs*.
[ref. 3]

tetrad test

Battery of tests, typically for the effects of cannabinoids in rodents, that includes hypomotility assessed by an *open field test, catalepsy* assessed by the *bar test*, hypothermia measured by rectal temperature, and *analgesia* measured by avoidance of heat, *e.g.*, in the *tail immersion test*.
[ref. 4]

tetrodotoxin (TTX)

(4*R*,4a*R*,5*R*,7*S*,9*S*,10*S*,10a*R*,11*S*,12*S*)-12-(hydroxymethyl)-2-iminooctahydro-5,9:7,10a-dimethano[1,3]dioxocino[6,5-*d*]pyrimidine-4,7,10,11,12-pentol

Neurotoxin that inhibits *action potentials* by blocking sodium *ion channels*.
Note: Tetrodotoxin is produced by bacteria living in symbiosis with fish of the order ***Tetraodontiformes***, including trigger fish and puffer fish.
[ref. 4]

tetrodotoxin (TTX)-insensitive

Denoting a class of sodium *ion channels*, found mainly in the heart, that is not blocked by *tetrodotoxin*.
Note: The significance of TTX-insensitive Na^+ channels lies in experimental characterization of channel subtypes in neuromuscular physiology, development, and *drug* design.
[ref. 4]

thalamus

Either of two paired midline masses of *grey matter*, the largest part of the *diencephalon*, lying between the *cerebral hemispheres* on either side of the third *ventricle*.
Note: The thalamus relays information on sensation, movement and spatial sense to the *cerebral cortex*, acts as a centre for *pain* perception, and plays a role in the regulation of wakefulness.
[4,5]

thalidomide (INN)

rac-2-(2,6-dioxopiperidin-3-yl)-2*H*-isoindole-1,3-dione

Teratogenic indole-based *drug* with *sedative* and anti-*angiogenic* properties.

Note 1: The introduction of thalidomide for alleviating nausea in *pregnancy* in some countries in 1957 was linked to severe *birth defects*, with *phocomelia* being highly characteristic.
Note 2: Currently, thalidomide is used successfully to treat and prevent the moderate-to-severe skin lesions caused by leprosy, and it is used together with dexamethasone to treat *multiple myeloma*.
[ref. 5]

theca

1. Covering or sheath
2. Also referring to the *theca* folliculi, a bilayer (thus theca interna and externa) connective tissue covering of the *ovarian follicles,* of which the theca interna is vascularized and involved in production of *androstenedione*.

[*]

theoretical maximum daily intake (TMDI)

See *maximum daily intake, theoretical.*

theranostic

Portmanteau word formed from the words "*therapeutic*" approaches and "diagnostic" methods; sometimes describing a single chemical entity, such as an *antibody*, that may be used both to identify *diseased tissue* and to treat it.
[*]

therapeutic

1. (n) Substance intended to restore or maintain *health.*
2. (adj) Referring to the treatment of *disease*, or promoting a sense of wellbeing.

[*]

therapeutic antibody

See *antibody, therapeutic.*

therapeutic cloning

See *cloning, therapeutic.*

therapeutic index

Toxic dose divided by the therapeutic dose; the higher the ratio, the greater the safety of the therapeutic dose.
[ref. 1]

therapeutics

Aspect of medicine concerned with the treatment of *disease* and the action of related *drugs*.
[*]

thermocline

Vertical zone in a body of water through which temperature drops rapidly.
[*]

thigmotaxis

Movement of an organism toward or away from a mechanical *stimulus*, physical contact, or spatial discontinuity, as in movement away from touch by a physical stimulus or when exploring close to a wall.
[ref. 4]

thoracic duct

Largest of the *lymphatic* vessels; it conducts *lymph,* transporting absorbed nutrients notably as chylomicrons, from its origin in the *abdomen* to the venous circulation at the junction of the left subclavian and jugular veins.
[ref. 5]

thoracic spine

Portion of the *vertebral column* of the upper back, between the *cervical spine* and *lumbar spine*, in humans consisting of 12 *vertebrae* designated T1 to T12.
[ref. 4]

thorax (n)/thoracic (adj)

1. Part of the body of a mammal between the neck and the *abdomen*, including the *cavity* enclosed by the ribs, breastbone, and *dorsal vertebrae*, and containing the chief *organs* of circulation and respiration.
2. Part of a bird, reptile, amphibian, or fish corresponding to the human thorax.
3. Section of the body of an insect, between the head and the abdomen, to which are attached the legs and wings.

[*]

three-dimensional quantitative structure–activity relationship (3D-QSAR)

Quantitative association between the three-dimensional structural properties of a substance and its biological properties.
[ref. 1]
See also *quantitative structure–activity relationship.*

threshold

Dose or *exposure concentration* below which a defined effect will not occur.
[ref. 1]
See also *critical effect.*

threshold concentration

See *threshold.*

threshold dose

See *threshold.*

threshold effect concentration (TEC)

threshold effect level (TEL)

Concentration calculated as the geometric mean of *no-observed-effect concentration* and *lowest-observed-effect concentration*.
Note 1: *'Chronic'* or *'subchronic'* may be added as qualifiers of TEC dependent on the duration of *exposure* in the test.

Note 2: The TEC is equivalent to the *maximum acceptable toxicant concentration* used in some countries, particularly for assessing water *pollution*.
[After ref. 2]

threshold effect level

See *threshold effect concentration*.

threshold limit value (TLV®)

Term reserved by the ACGIH for the maximum *concentration* of a substance to which a worker can be exposed daily during a working life without known *adverse effects*.
[*]

threshold limit value–ceiling (TLV®–C)

As defined by ACGIH, *concentration* of a potentially *toxic* substance that should not be exceeded during any part of the working *exposure*.
[ref. 1]

threshold limit value–short-term exposure limit (TLV®–STEL)

As defined by ACGIH, *concentration* to which it is believed that workers can be *exposed* continuously for a short period of time without suffering from either irritation or *chronic* or irreversible *tissue* damage; or experiencing an increased likelihood of accidental injury, impaired self-rescue, or materially reduced work efficiency; each of these provided that the daily *threshold limit value–time-weighted average* (TLV–TWA) is not exceeded.
Note: The TLV–STEL is not a separate, independent *exposure* guideline; rather, it supplements the TLV–TWA limit where there are recognized *acute* effects from a substance whose *toxic* effects are primarily of a chronic nature. TLV–STELs are recommended only where toxic effects have been reported from high short-term exposures in either humans or animals.
[ref. 1]

threshold limit value–time-weighted average (TLV®–TWA)

As defined by ACGIH, *time-weighted-average concentration* for a conventional 8-h workday and a 40-h workweek, to which it is believed nearly all workers may be repeatedly *exposed*, day after day, without *adverse effect*.
[ref. 1]

threshold of toxicological concern (TTC)

Human *exposure threshold* value for a group of chemical substances below which there should be no appreciable risk to human *health*.
[ref. 1]

threshold potential

Level of *depolarization* that must be reached to trigger an *action potential* in an *excitable cell*.
[ref. 4]
See also *excitation; hyperpolarization*.

threshold theory

Theory that, for a given substance, no *toxic* effect can occur below a defined *dose*.
[ref. 2]

thrombocyte

Same as *platelet*.

thrombocytopenia

Abnormally low concentration of *platelets* (thrombocytes) in the *blood*, sometimes specified as less than 150×10^9 L^{-1}.
Note 1: Thromocytopenia is an unwanted effect of some *drugs* (*e.g.*, heparin-induced thrombocytopenia) or may be mediated by antiplatelet *antibodies* (*e.g.*, *idiopathic thrombocytopenic purpura*), and carries an increased risk of spontaneous bleeding.
Note 2: Thromocytopenia is also frequently detected in patients with autoimmune diseases (*e.g.*, *systemic lupus erythematosus, Sjögren syndrome, mixed connective tissue disease*, or *antiphospholipid syndrome*).
[ref. 3,5]

thromboembolus (n)/thromboembolic (adj)

Sequential process of *thrombus* formation and *embolism*, leading to a medical event.
[*]

thrombosis

Coagulation or *clotting* of *blood* in a vessel of the blood circulatory system.
[*]

thromboxane

Any of several substances (predominantly thromboxanes A2 and B2), synthesized by *platelets* from arachidonic acid precursor, that cause *vasoconstriction* of *vascular* and bronchial smooth muscle and facilitate platelet aggregation.
[ref. 3]

thrombus

Clot anywhere in the *cardiovascular* system, formed from *blood* components, that may be attached to the vessel wall and (or) lead to occlusion.
[ref. 4]
See also *embolism, thromboembolism*.

thrush

Oral *infection* with ***Candida albicans***, often in patients with *immunosuppression*.
[ref. 3]

thymic atrophy

Involution of the *thymus gland* leading to a diminished capacity to generate new *T-cells*.
[ref. 3]

thymic education

Process by which *T-cells*, during development in the *thymus*, are screened for potentially harmful self-reactive cells that are removed and potentially beneficial T-cells are promoted.
[ref. 3]

thymocyte

See *pre-T-cell.*

thymoma

Rare, usually benign, tumor arising from tissue of the *thymus gland.*
Note: Thymoma is often associated with *myasthenia gravis.*
[ref. 3]

thymus (n)/thymic (adj)

Pyramid-shaped *organ*, found in the *thoracic* or cervical region of mammals, composed of *lymphatic tissue* in which minute concentric bodies (thymic corpuscles, the remnants of *epithelial* structures) are found.
Note 1: *Stem cells* in the outer cortex of the thymus develop into different kinds of *T-cells*. Some migrate to the inner *medulla* and enter the bloodstream; those that do not may be destroyed to prevent *autoimmune* reactions.
Note 2: The thymus is necessary for the development of thymus-derived *lymphocytes* (T-cells) and is the source of several hormones involved in T-cell maturation, for example, thymosin, thymopoietin, thymulin, and thymocyte humoral factor.
Note 3: If a newborn's thymus is removed, not enough T-cells are produced, the *spleen* and *lymph nodes* have little tissue, and the *immune system* fails, causing a gradual, fatal wasting *disease*. In contrast, removal of the thymus in adults has little effect.
[ref. 3]

thymus-dependent (TD) antigen

See *antigen, thymus-dependent.*

thymus-independent antigen

See *antigen, thymus-independent.*

thyroglobulin (TG)

Glycoprotein precursor of thyroid hormones, secreted by *thyroid* follicular cells.
Note: Thyroglobulin *autoantibodies* are found in patients with *autoimmune thyroiditis*, and *Graves disease*.
[ref. 3]

thyroglossal duct

Connection in the *embryo* between the site of initiation of development of the *thyroid gland* and its final location in the neck.
[ref. 5]

thyroid gland

Bilobar *endocrine gland*, located below the prominence of *cartilage* surrounding the *larynx* (the Adam's apple), that produces and secretes the *hormone*s triiodothyronine (T3), thyroxin (T4), and calcitonin.
Note: Thyroid gland function is disturbed in some *autoimmune diseases*, and also by substances that inhibit normal utilization of iodine by gland *cells*.
[ref. 5]

thyroid peroxidase (TPO)
thyroperoxidase

Thyroid enzyme (EC 1.18.1 8) that is a major *autoantigen* in *autoimmune diseases* of the *thyroid gland.*
[ref. 3]

thyroid tissue, accessory

Ectopic thyroid tissue arising from remnants of the *thyroglossal duct.*
[ref. 5]

thyroid-stimulating hormone (TSH)

Pituitary hormone that stimulates the *thyroid gland* to produce thyroxine (T4), and then triiodothyronine (T3).
[ref. 5]

thyroid-stimulating hormone receptor (TSHR)

See *receptor, thyroid-stimulating hormone.*

thyroiditis, autoimmune

Inflammatory destruction of the *thyroid gland* (ranging from a mild focal thyroiditis to extensive *lymphocytic* infiltration and scarring) often associated with *goiter* and hypothyroidism.
Note: The most common types of autoimmune thyroiditis are *Hashimoto thyroiditis* and atrophic thyroiditis.
[ref. 3]

thyroiditis, autoimmune, spontaneous (SAT)

Autoimmune thyroiditis that develops spontaneously (without any apparent cause or manipulation) in certain strains of mice and rats (*e.g., NOD mice*, BB and BUF rats) as well as in other animals [*e.g.*, obese strain (OS) chickens, marmoset monkeys, beagles].
[ref. 3]

thyrotoxicosis

Condition resulting from excessive concentrations of *thyroid hormones* in the *blood*, characterized by bulging eyes and rapid heart rate.
[ref. 1]

tic douloureux

See *neuralgia, trigeminal.*

tidal volume

Quantity of air or test gas that is displaced with maximum effort during one *respiratory cycle* of *inhalation* and *exhalation.*
[*]

tiered testing

Structured approach to assessing the fate and effects of substances, beginning with relatively simple tests to select substances of concern and describe their *toxicities.*

Note: If the information from initial low-tier tests is inadequate for regulatory decision-making, further more complex tests (higher tier tests) may be required.
Example: Under a tiered testing structure, testing might progress from *acute* studies to *chronic* laboratory studies, and then to field studies.
[ref. 2]

time-independent (TI) test

Acute toxicity test with no predetermined temporal endpoint.
Note 1: A time-independent test, sometimes referred to as a "threshold" or "incipient" lethality test, is allowed to continue until acute toxicity (mortality or some other defined sublethal effect) has ceased, or nearly ceased, in the test *population*.
Note 2: With most test substances, the endpoint in a time-independent test is reached within 7–10 d; but it may not be reached within 21 d, and practical or economic reasons may then dictate that the test be stopped and redesigned with a longer duration.
[ref. 2]

time-weighted-average exposure (TWAE)
time-weighted-average concentration (TWAC)

Concentration of a substance in an *exposure* medium (*e.g.*, air), measured during intervals over a specified time, the averaged measurement per unit time of all intervals then being multiplied by the total time of observation.
Note: For a TWAE in occupational exposure, a working shift of 8 h is commonly used as the averaging time.
[*]

tingling

Pricking type of *paresthesia*.
[ref. 5]

tinnitus

Continual perception of noise in one or both ears, such as ringing, buzzing, roaring, or clicking, in the absence of an external noise source.
[ref. 1]

tissue

Organization of *cells* of a common origin, their products, and *extracellular matrix* into a biological structure, intermediate between individual cells and an *organ* and having a specific function.
Note 1: It is often considered that there are four types of tissue: muscle, *epithelial*, nervous, and *connective tissue*, but *blood* may also be considered a tissue.
Note 2: Tissue samples, usually embedded, sectioned, and stained to detect specific structures, are a basis for *pathological* diagnosis.
Note 3: *Organs* are usually composed of different classes of tissues that interact to fulfill a higher level of function.
[*]

tissue culture

See *culture*.

tissue dose

Amount of a substance or physical agent (radiation) absorbed by a *tissue*.
[ref. 1]

tissue/plasma partition coefficient

See *partition ratio.*

tissue transglutaminase (tTG)

See *transglutaminase, tissue.*

titer (in immunology)

Reciprocal of the highest dilution of a titration of an *antigen* with an *antibody* that gives a measurable effect (*e.g., agglutination*), and thus an empirical measure of the *avidity* of an antibody.
Example: If the effect is seen down to a dilution of 1:1000, the antibody titer is 1000.
[ref. 3]

tolerable daily intake (TDI)

Estimate of the amount of a potentially harmful substance (*e.g.*, a *contaminant*) in food or drinking water that can be ingested daily over a lifetime without appreciable *health risk.*
Note 1: For regulation of substances that are consumed rarely, but then in TDI-exceeding amounts, a provisionally *tolerable weekly intake* may be applied as a temporary limit.
Note 2: *Acceptable daily intake* is usually used for substances not known to be harmful, such as *food additives.*
[ref. 1]
See also *tolerable weekly intake.*

tolerable risk

See *risk, tolerable.*

tolerable weekly intake (TWI)

Estimate of the amount of a potentially harmful substance (*e.g.*, a *contaminant*) in food or drinking water that can be ingested weekly over a lifetime without appreciable *health risk.*
[ref. 1]
See also *tolerable daily intake.*

tolerance (n)/**tolerant** (adj)

Adaptive state characterized by diminished effects of a particular *dose* of a substance; becoming less responsive to a *stimulus*, especially following continued exposure.
[After ref. 1,4]
Note: Tolerance may occur when a substance induces its own biotransforming (see *biotransformation*) *enzyme*(s).
[*]
See also *adaptation; tolerance, immunological.*

tolerance, central

Specific *immunological tolerance* due to the induction of *lymphocyte apoptosis* or *anergy* within the primary *lymphoid organs* (*bone marrow* in the case of *B-cell* tolerance and the *thymus* for *T-cells*).
[ref. 3]

tolerance, immunological

Persistent specific *immunological* unresponsiveness toward a substance that would normally be expected to elicit an *immune response*, resulting from previous non-sensitizing exposure to an *antigen*.
Note 1: Immunological tolerance to specific foreign antigens can be induced by the exposure to the foreign antigens during *embryonic* or *neonatal* life (depending upon species). In *adults*, tolerance (usually of shorter duration) can be induced by using particular routes of administration for the antigens or administration of agents that are particularly effective against *cells* proliferating in response to antigen.
Note 2: Mechanisms giving rise to immunological tolerance may include deletion of potentially reactive *lymphocytes* or their "inactivation" by immunological *suppression*.
[ref. 3]

tolerance, infectious

Continuing state of *tolerance* that can be transferred by *T-lymphocytes* from a tolerant animal.
Note: Infectious tolerance is involved in the maintenance of *transplantation* tolerance by the induction of *antigen*-specific *CD4+ regulatory T-cells*.
[ref. 3]

tolerance, neonatal

Tolerance to specific foreign *antigens* induced by the exposure of a bird or mammal to foreign antigens during *embryonic* or *neonatal* life, depending upon *species*.
[ref. 3]

tolerance index (TI)

Value of parameter measured under conditions of treatment with a potentially harmful substance, divided by the measured value of the same parameter in a control situation, multiplied by 100; *i.e.*, TI = (parameter treated/parameter control) × 100.
Note: The tolerance index was originally defined in terms of root *growth* in plants.
[ref. 2]
See also *tolerance index, air pollution; index*; *tolerance index, pollution; tolerance index, salt.*

tolerance index, air pollution (APTI) (in plant ecotoxicology)

Empirical *index* used to assess the *tolerance* of individual plants to *contaminated* air.
Note 1: The numerical value of the APTI is obtained by combining various quantities according to the formula $[A\ (T+P)+R]/10$, where A is the mass of ascorbic acid divided by the dry mass of a leaf, expressed as mg g^{-1}, T is the total mass of chlorophyll divided by the fresh mass, expressed as mg g^{-1}, P is the pH of a leaf extract, and R is the mass of water in the leaf divided by the wet mass, expressed as percent.
Note 2: In common usage, the equation for APTI is not formulated as a coherent equation, but requires the given units.
[ref. 2]

tolerance index, pollution (PTI)

Means of measuring *environmental* quality, usually water quality, by determining the presence of *indicator species*, classified into three groups—sensitive, facultative, and tolerant.
Note: To calculate a PTI, each group is assigned an *index* value 1, 2, or 3, with the sensitive group having the highest index value. The number of species present in

each group is identified in a representative environmental sample and multiplied by the group index, and the three scores are added together. The environmental quality is directly proportional to the value of the index.
[ref. 2]

tolerance index, salt (STI)

Measure of the ability of a plant or crop to tolerate growth in high-salt environments, calculated as total plant (shoot + root) dry mass after growth at different salt concentrations divided by the total plant dry mass obtained for nonsalt-stressed controls, according to the equation

$$S_{\mathrm{T}} = m_{\mathrm{d}}(\mathrm{s})/m_{\mathrm{d}}(\mathrm{c})$$

where S_{T} is the STI, m_{d} is the total dry mass, and s, c refer to defined salt-stress and control treatments, respectively.
[*]

tolerogen

Antigen used to induce *tolerance*.
Note: Induction of *immunological tolerance* depends on the circumstances of administration (*e.g.*, route and *concentration*) as well as on the molecular properties of the tolerogen.
[ref. 3]

toll-like receptor (TLR)

See *receptor, toll-like*.

tomography

Construction of a three-dimensional image of a structure from a series of planar sections obtained with penetrating waves.
Note: Wave sources used in tomography include light (optical tomography), X-rays, an electron beam producing X-rays [electron beam tomography (EBT)], and γ-rays [positron emission tomography (PET)].
[ref. 4]

tonic

1. (n) *Medicinal* preparation that increases or restores normal muscular tension.
2. (n) Medicinal preparation that gives a sense of wellbeing.
3. (adj) Characterized by tension, especially muscular tension.
4. (adj) Giving a sense of wellbeing.

[After ref. 1]

tonsil

Small, rounded mass of *tissue*, especially of *lymphoid tissue*; generally used alone to designate one of the paired palatine tonsils.
[ref. 3]

top-down ecotoxicological study

Approach to investigating ecotoxicological effects that starts with a determination of the presence and nature of any *adverse effects* via responses at *community* and *ecosystem* levels of organization, rather than at the level of the organism.
[ref. 2]
See also *bottom-up ecotoxicological study*.

topical (in medicine)

Applied directly to the surface of the body.
[ref. 1]

topical effect

Consequence of application of a substance to the surface of the body (*topical* application) at the point of application.
[ref. 1]

torsade de pointes

Potentially lethal form of ventricular *tachycardia* following *chronic abuse* of alcohol and mainly due to hypomagnesemia.
[ref. 1]

torticollis
wry neck

*Spasm*odic *contraction* of neck muscles drawing the head to one side with the chin pointing to the other side.
[ref. 4]

total diet study

1. Study designed to establish the pattern of *pesticide* residue intake by a person consuming a defined diet.
2. Study undertaken to show the range and amount of various foodstuffs in a typical diet or to estimate the total amount of a specific substance in a typical diet.

[ref. 1]

total organic carbon (TOC)

Organic matter content of *soil, sediment*, or water determined by measurement of organic carbon and calculated as the mass of organic carbon divided by the total mass of solid, or the mass of water.
Note 1: TOC is determined by oxidation of the organic matter to carbon dioxide after removal of inorganic carbon such as carbonate or hydrogen carbonate.
Note 2: TOC includes all the carbon atoms covalently bonded in organic molecules, both *dissolved organic carbon* (DOC) and particulate organic carbon.
Note 3: Much of the TOC in natural waters is composed primarily of nonspecific *humic materials*.
[ref. 2]
See also *dissolved organic carbon.*

total terminal residue (of a pesticide)

Sum of concentrations of a defined *pesticide* in form of the parent molecule, its metabolites and possible breakdown products in a food.
[ref. 1]
See also *residue.*

toxemia
blood poisoning

Condition in which the *blood* contains *toxins* produced by microorganism in the course of an *infection*.
[After ref. 1]

toxemia of pregnancy

See *pre-eclampsia.*

toxic

Able to cause injury to living organisms as a result of chemical or physicochemical interaction.
[ref. 1]

toxic chemical

See *toxic substance.*

toxic dose

superthreshold dose

Amount of a substance that produces *intoxication* without lethal outcome.
[ref. 1]

toxic epidermal necrolysis (TEN)

Lyell syndrome

Severe form of *Stevens–Johnson syndrome* with extensive detachment of the skin, often as a result of an *allergic adverse drug reaction.*
[ref. 3]

toxic material

See *toxic substance.*

toxic metal

Describing a metallic (or less accurately often a semi-metallic) *toxic substance*, usually other than an *essential nutrient.*
Note: *Speciation* of a toxic metal is critical in determining its biological properties.
[*]

toxic shellfish poisoning

See *shellfish poisoning.*

toxic shock syndrome

Systemic reaction produced by the *toxin* derived from the bacterium ***Staphylococcus aureus***; the toxin acts as a *superantigen* that activates a high proportion of *CD4+ T-lymphocytes* to produce *cytokines.*
[ref. 3]
See also *toxemia.*

toxic substance

toxic chemical
toxicant

Substance with the potential to cause *disorder, disease,* injury or death to living organisms as a result of chemical or physicochemical interactions.
Note 1: All substances are *toxic* above a certain *dose* (or *exposure*). Thus, the term 'toxic substance' is normally applied only to those substances causing *toxicity* at relatively low doses.
Note 2: Toxicity of any substance varies from organism to organism, so the term 'toxic substance' should be accompanied by the name of the organism to which it applies.

In common use, unless otherwise specified, the term refers to toxicity to humans and other mammals.
Note 3: In *ecotoxicology*, care should be taken in using the term 'toxic substance' because of the variation in *susceptibility* of different species, some of which may have adapted to survive, and even benefit from, exposure to substances that are very toxic to other species.
[After ref. 1,2]
See also *poison; toxicant; toxin.*

toxic unit (TU)

toxicity unit

Dose or concentration of a *toxicant* expressed in units of lethality, such as LD_{50} or LC_{50}.
Example: If TUs are based on the LC_{50}, a chemical with an LC_{50} of 20 mg L^{-1} would be present at 0.5 TU in a 10 mg L^{-1} solution.
Note: In combined *exposures*, the toxicities of the individual components can be expressed in TUs.
[ref. 1]
See also *median lethal concentration; median lethal dose.*

toxicant

Any *toxic substance.*
Note: Sometimes the term is meant to exclude *toxins*, differentiating them on the basis of their biological origin.
[*]

toxicity

1. Capacity of a substance to cause injury to a living organism, or the *adverse effects* of that substance, defined with reference to the quantity of substance administered or absorbed, the way in which the substance is administered and distributed in time (single or repeated *doses*), the type and severity of injury, the time needed to produce the injury, the nature of the organism(s) affected, and other relevant conditions.
2. Measure of incompatibility of a substance with life.
   Note: Taken in this second sense, toxicity may be expressed quantitatively as the reciprocal of the absolute value of *median lethal dose* ($1/LD_{50}$) or *median lethal concentration* ($1/LC_{50}$).

[ref. 1]

toxicity, acute

Opposite term: *toxicity, chronic*

1. *Adverse effects* of finite duration occurring within a short time (up to 14 d) after administration of a single *dose* (or *exposure* to a given *concentration*) of a test substance or after multiple doses (exposures), usually within 24 h of a starting point. (The starting point may be, *e.g.*, exposure to the *toxic substance*, loss of *reserve capacity*, or a developmental change.)
2. Ability of a substance to cause *adverse effects* within a short time of dosing or *exposure.*

[ref. 1]
See also *acute.*

toxicity, chronic
long-term toxicity
Opposite term: *toxicity, acute*

1. *Adverse effects* following *chronic exposure.*
2. Effects that persist over a long period of time, whether or not they occur immediately upon *exposure* or are delayed.

[ref. 1]
See also *chronic.*

toxicity, direct
Toxicity that results from, and is readily attributable to, substances acting at the sites of toxic action in and (or) on the exposed organisms that are exhibiting the adverse biological response in question.
[ref. 2]

toxicity, indirect
Adverse effect that results from agent(s) producing changes in the *environment* external to an organism under study.
Example: A decrease in the food supply for a *predatory species* due to direct *toxicity* from a substance to its prey may produce adverse effects in the predator species due to starvation, rather than producing any direct toxicity to the predator.
[ref. 2]

toxicity curve
Curve obtained by plotting, usually on a logarithmic scale, the median *toxic* responses or *survival times* of a group of test organisms against the *concentration* of a *toxic substance.*
[After ref. 2]

toxicity equivalency factor (TEF), f
Toxicity of one chemical substance divided by that of another structurally related substance (or *index* compound) chosen as a *reference toxicant.*
Note: The TEF is used in *risk assessment* to estimate the toxicity of a complex *mixture*, commonly a mixture of chlorinated dibenzo-*p*-dioxins [oxanthrenes], furans, and biphenyls, and in this case TEF is based on relative toxicity to 2,3,7,8-tetrachlorodibenzo-*p*-dioxin [2,3,7,8-tetrachlorooxanthrene] for which $f = 1$.
[ref. 2]

toxicity equivalent (TEQ), T_{xe}
Contribution of a specified component (or components) to the total *toxicity* of a *mixture* of related substances.
Note: The total toxicity equivalent of a mixture of components A, B . . . N with amount-of-substance *concentrations,* c_A, $c_B \ldots c_N$ is the sum of that for each of the components, *i.e.*,

$$T_{xe} = \sum_{i=A}^{N} (f_i c_i)$$

where the *toxicity equivalence factors,* f_i, are often expressed relative to the value for the *reference toxicant* 2,3,7,8-tetrachlorodibenzo-p-dioxin [2,3,7,8-tetrachlorooxanthrene] taken as 1.
[*]

toxicity exposure ratio (TER)

Measure of the *toxic* effect of a substance (*e.g.*, its LD_{50}, LC_{50}, NOEC) divided by the estimated *environmental exposure*, expressed in the same *concentration* units.
Note: The TER is the reciprocal of a *risk quotient* (*e.g.*, PEC/NOEC) or *hazard quotient* (*e.g.*, PEC/PNEC).
[After ref. 1]

toxicity identification (and) evaluation (TIE)

Fractionation designed to separate out defined substances, in order to identify the agent(s) primarily responsible for the *toxicity* of a complex *mixture*.
Note: TIE involves systematic treatment of a sample (*e.g.*, pH change, filtration, or aeration) to obtain defined fractions that are subsequently tested for their *toxicity*.
[After ref. 2]

toxicity pathway (TP)

Cellular or molecular effect pathway that, when sufficiently disturbed, is expected to cause an *adverse effect*.
[*]

toxicity test

Experimental study of the *adverse effects* of *exposure* of a living organism to a substance for a defined duration under defined conditions.
[ref. 1]

toxicity test, acute
short-term toxicity test
Opposite term: *toxicity test, chronic*.

Toxicity test in which organisms are observed during only a short part of their life span, and in which there is often only a single *exposure* to the test agent at the beginning of the study.
[ref. 1]

toxicity test, chronic
long-term toxicity test
Opposite term: *toxicity test, acute*.

Study in which organisms are observed during the greater part of their life span, and in which *exposure* to the test agent takes place over the whole observation time or a substantial part thereof.
[ref. 1]

toxicity value, T_x

Factor used to estimate a *hazard* that may be a *reference dose* or may be calculated from the equation

$$T_x = m\ C$$

where m is the slope of a published *dose–effect relationship* and C is the *concentration* of the *toxicant*.
[ref. 2]

toxicodynamics

Process of interaction of potentially *toxic substances* with *target* sites, and the biochemical and physiological mechanisms leading to *adverse effects*.
[ref. 1]

toxicogenetics

Study of the influence of hereditary factors on the effects of potentially *toxic* substances on individual organisms.
[ref. 1]

toxicogenomics

Scientific subdiscipline that combines *toxicology* with *genomics* to determine how an organism's *genetic* make-up influences its response to a *toxic substance*.
[ref. 1]
Note: Toxicogenomics uses technologies associated with *transcriptomics, proteomics*, and *metabolomics*.
[*]

toxicokinetics (n)/toxicokinetic (adj)

1. Overall process of the *absorption* by a living organism (*uptake*) of a potentially *toxic substance*, its distribution in *tissues* and *organs*, its *metabolism* (*biotransformation*) and the distribution of its *metabolites*, and the *elimination* of the substance and its metabolites from the organism.
2. Collection of data on absorption, distribution, metabolism and elimination, either as an integral component in the conduct of nonclinical toxicity studies, or in appropriately designed supportive studies, in order to assess systemic *exposure*.

[ref. 1]

toxicological data sheet

Document that gives in a standardized manner data relating to the *toxicology* of a substance, its production and application, its properties, and methods for its identification.
Note: A toxicological data sheet may also include recommendations on protective measures.
[ref. 1]

toxicologically based pharmacokinetic modeling (TBPK)

See *physiologically based pharmacokinetic modeling*.

toxicology

Scientific discipline involving the study of the actual or potential harmful effects of substances on living organisms and *ecosystems*, of the relationship of such harmful effects to *exposure*, and of the *mechanisms of action*, diagnosis, prevention, and treatment of *intoxications*.
[ref. 1]

toxicometry

Combination of investigative methods and techniques for making a quantitative assessment of *toxicity* and the *hazards* of potentially *toxic* substances.
[ref. 1]

toxicophobia

Morbid dread of *poisons*.
[ref. 1]
See also *phantom risk*.

toxicophore

toxicophoric group
toxogenic group
toxophoric group

Structural moiety known to be capable of exerting *toxic* effects.
Note: The presence of a toxicophoric group indicates only potential and not necessarily actual *toxicity* of a *drug* or other substance, and *metabolic activation* may be required to express its toxicity.
[ref. 1]

toxicophoric group

See *toxicophore*.

toxicovigilance

Active process of identification, investigation, and evaluation of various *toxic* effects of a substance or substances in the community, with a view to taking measures to reduce or control respective *exposure(s)*.
[ref. 1]

toxification

Metabolic conversion of a substance to a product that is more *toxic*.
[ref. 1]

toxin

Poison produced by a biological organism such as a microbe, animal, plant, or fungus.
Examples: Botulinum toxin, *tetrodotoxin*, pyrrolizine alkaloids, amanitin (1,8-anhydro-$C^{2,4}$,S^{8}-cyclo(L-asparaginyl-4-hydroxy-L-prolyl-(4*R*)-4,5-dihydroxy-L-isoleucyl-6-hydroxy-2-sulfanyl-L-tryptophylglycyl-L-isoleucyl-L-cysteine) (*R*)-*S*-oxide).
[ref. 4]
Note: As part of a compound word, toxin is sometimes used as any *toxic substance* affecting the indicated target, as in *immunotoxin* or *neurotoxin*.
[*]
See also *venom*.

toxinology

Scientific discipline involving the study of the chemistry, biochemistry, *pharmacology*, and *toxicology* of *toxins*.
[ref. 1]

toxogenic group

See *toxicophoric group*.

toxoid

Chemically or physically modified *toxin* that is no longer harmful but retains *immunogenicity*.
[ref. 3]

toxophoric group

See *toxicophoric group.*

toxoplasmosis

Infection with the parasite ***Toxoplasma gondii*** that, when acquired by the *fetus*, can lead to a variety of *congenital* abnormalities that may include *hydrocephalus* or *microcephaly*, intellectual disability, and problems with vision and hearing.
Note: Infection of the fetus with toxoplasmosis is via the mother, who may acquire it from contact with feces of the domestic cat or from undercooked meat.
[ref. 5]

traceability (n)/**traceable** (adj) (in metrology)

Property of a measurement result whereby the result can be related to a stated reference through a documented unbroken chain of calibrations, each potentially contributing to the measurement uncertainty.
[ref. 1]

trace element

See *element, trace.*

trace metal

See *trace element, trace nutrient.*

trace nutrient

See *nutrient, trace.*

tracer

1. That which allows something to be followed; *e.g.*, a radioactive isotope may replace a stable chemical element in a *toxic* compound enabling the *toxicokinetics* to be described.
2. Labeled or tagged member of a *population* used to measure certain properties of that population.

[After ref. 1]

tracer substance

Substance that can be tracked through one or more reactions or systems, often by detecting an incorporated isotope.
[ref. 1]
See also *tracer.*

trachea

Thin-walled, *cartilaginous* tube connecting the *larynx* to the bronchi and carrying air to the lungs.
[ref. 5]

trade-off (in population ecology)

Exchange of one advantageous character for another.
Example: Through *natural selection*, rapidly growing insects living in an agricultural area of *pesticide* use may, by natural selection, lose the capacity for rapid growth, with

some of the energy otherwise available for growth being diverted to degrade the *pesticide*. In this example, the trade-off may be at the cost of reduced *fitness*.
[ref. 2]

tranquilizer

Drug that calms and pacifies with minimal *sedating* or *depressant* effects.
Note 1: A tranquilizer decreases anxiety (*i.e.*, has anxiolytic properties) or agitation without necessarily decreasing awareness or wakefulness, although tranquilizers at higher dose may induce sleep.
Note 2: Minor tranquilizers are *sedatives*.
Examples: Benzodiazepines, antihistamines, alcohol, cannabis, chloral hydrate.
Note 3: Major tranquilizers include *antipsychotic* drugs and *neuroleptics*.
[ref. 4]

trans-acting element

See *trans-acting factor*.

trans-acting factor

Molecule such as a *transcription factor* or microRNA (see *ribonucleic acid interference*) coded by one *gene* that influences the *transciption* of a second gene.
Note: The *DNA* region that includes the gene coding a trans-acting factor, along with its regulatory sequences, is called a trans-acting element.
[*]
Compare *cis-acting element*.

transcellular

1. Passing through a *cell* or cells.
2. Passing from one cell to another.

[*]
Compare *paracellular*.
See also *transport, transcellular*.

transcription

Process by which the genetic information encoded in a linear sequence of nucleotides in one strand of *DNA* is copied into an exactly complementary sequence of *RNA*.
[ref. 1]
See also *transcription, reverse*.

transcription, reverse

Process by which an *RNA* molecule is used as a template to make a complementary single-stranded *DNA* copy.
[ref. 1]
See also *transcription*.

transcription factor

DNA-binding protein that is involved in regulating *gene expression*.
[ref. 5]

transcriptome

Total set of m*RNA* transcripts expressed in a *cell, tissue, organ* or organism at a given point in time.
[ref. 1]

transcriptomics (in toxicology)

gene expression profiling

Global analysis of *gene expression* to identify and evaluate changes in synthesis of m*RNA* after chemical *exposure*.
[ref. 1]
Note: Transcriptomics identifies which genes are active. Gene expression profiles obtained in this way may be clustered into a gene expression signature that is characteristic for the chemical used.
[*]
See also *transcriptome*.

transcutaneous electronic nerve stimulation (TENS)

Electrical *stimulus* applied across the skin to excite *nerves* for *therapeutic* purposes.
Note: TENS is most often used to control *pain*.
[ref. 4]

transcytosis

Vesicular transport of macromolecules from one side of a *cell* to the other, through the cell's interior.
[ref. 3]
Compare *transcellular*.

transfer RNA (tRNA)

See *ribonucleic acid, noncoding*.

transformation

1. Alteration of a *cell* by incorporation of foreign *genetic* material and its subsequent expression in a new *phenotype*.
2. Conversion of cells growing normally in *culture* to a state of rapid division resembling that of a *tumor*, especially applied to the capacity to initiate a *malignant* tumor if implanted into a test animal.
3. Change in biological form or structure, *e.g.*, of one cell or *tissue* type into another, such as ossification during *fetal* development or the transition of fat-storing hepatic stellate cells into *fibroblast*-like cells following hepatotoxic injury.
   Note: Sometimes "transformation" is used to describe a *metaplastic* transition.
4. Chemical modification of a substance in the *environment*.

[*]
See also *metamorphosis; metaplasia; transformation, environmental*.

transformation, abiotic

Process in which a substance in the *environment* is modified by nonbiological mechanisms.
[ref. 1]

transformation, environmental

Change in properties of substances resulting from interactions in the *environment*.
Examples: Methylation of *mercury* by marine organisms, sunlight-induced formation of ozone.
[ref. 1]

transformed cell

Cell in *culture* that has become *genetically* altered, either spontaneously or by incorporation of foreign *DNA,* to produce a culture with the capacity for an extended lifetime or passage number.
[After ref. 1]
See also *cell line; transformation.*

transformed cell line

See *cell line; transformed cell.*

transforming growth factor β (TGF-β)

Secreted member of the protein *superfamily* of the same name that functions in controlling the *cell cycle* and *apoptosis.*
Note 1: TGF-β is involved in several aspects of regulation of the *immune system* and blocks activation of *lymphocytes* and *macrophages.*
Note 2: TGF-β also plays key roles in *connective tissue* synthesis, *tissue* repair, and *fibrosis.*
[After ref. 3]

transfusion, blood

Transference of *blood* or blood-based products from one individual into the circulation of another.
[ref. 3]

transgene

Gene from one source that has been incorporated into the *genome* of another organism.
[ref. 1]

transgenic

Describing an organism that is genetically changed by the addition or deletion of *genetic* material or whose existing *genes* are altered by *gene targeting.*
[ref. 5]

transglutaminase, tissue (tTG)

Enzyme (EC 2.3.2.13) that catalyzes inter- or intra-protein crosslinks between the e-amino group of a lysine residue and the carboxamide group of glutamine.
Note: Tissue transglutaminase is the main target of *autoantibodies* in *celiac disease.*
[*]

translation

Process through which an amino acid chain (polypeptide) is generated as directed by a particular m*RNA* sequence.
[ref. 1]

translational toxicology

Process of extrapolation from toxicological data about an agent, obtained from studies of its effects on living nonhuman organisms, to the *hazard* and *risk assessment* of its potential for *toxicity* in humans.
[*]

translocation, chromosomal

Rearrangement involving transfer or exchange of *genetic* material between non-*homologous chromosomes* that may occur during *gametogenesis* or in *somatic* cells, potentially leading to *birth defects*.
[ref. 5]
See also *reciprocal translocation; Robertsonian translocation.*

transplacental carcinogen

See *carcinogen, transplacental.*

transplantation

Grafting solid *tissue* (*e.g.*, cornea) or *organ* (*e.g.*, kidney or heart), or *cells* (particularly *bone marrow*), from one individual to another.
[ref. 3]
See also *allograft; xenograft.*

transplant rejection

See *rejection.*

transport, active

Movement of a substance across a *cell membrane* against an electrochemical gradient, in the direction opposite to normal *diffusion* and requiring the expenditure of energy and involvement of a membrane *transporter* protein.
[ref. 1]

transport, environmental

Movement of *contaminants* from their point of release through the various *compartments* to locations where *exposure* is assumed to occur.
[ref. 2]

transport, facilitated

Passive *diffusion* down an electrochemical gradient, not requiring energy, but occurring at a rate faster than expected by simple diffusion alone.
Note 1: *Facilitated diffusion* may involve a *membrane* channel or a *carrier* molecule, often a protein. In the latter case, it may be referred to as facilitated transport.
Note 2: Both *facilitated diffusion* and facilitated transport exhibit ligand specificity and saturation kinetics.
[ref. 2]
See also *diffusion, exchange.*

transport, paracellular

Passage of a substance across a *cell* layer through the spaces between cells, without entry into any cell.
[*]
See also *transport, transcellular.*

transport, transcellular

Passage of a substance across a *cell* layer by uptake into, and subsequent elimination from, one or more cells.
[*]
See also *transport, paracellular.*

transporter

Transmembrane protein that drives the movement of an otherwise poorly permeating substance across a biological *membrane*.
[*]
See also *transporter, ABC; transport, active; transport, facilitated.*

transporter, ABC

Member of a family of ATP-dependent membrane *transporters* (derived from the initial letters of **A**TP-**b**inding **c**assette), located mainly in transporting *organs* such as liver, kidney and intestine.
Note 1: ABC-transporters are involved in *transcellular transport* of organic molecules, including many *drugs* and *xenobiotics*, modulating their intestinal absorption and favouring their *elimination* into *bile* and urine.
Note 2: ABC-transporters also play a role in the export of chemotherapeutic drugs out of targetted *tumor cells*, thus reducing local therapeutic *concentrations*, a phenomenon called *multidrug resistance*.
[*]

transporter associated with antigen processing (TAP-1, TAP-2)

Either of two molecules that carry *antigenic* peptides from the *cytoplasm* into the *lumen* of the *endoplasmic reticulum* for incorporation into *major histocompatibility class I molecules*.
[ref. 3]

transposition of the great arteries
transposition of the great vessels

Congenital cardiovascular malformation in which the position of the chief blood vessels of the heart (*aorta* and *pulmonary artery*) is reversed.
Note: Survival with transposition of the great arteries depends on a crossflow of *blood* between the right and left sides of the heart, as through a *ventricular septal defect*.
[ref. 5]
See also *conal growth hypothesis*.

transposon

Mobile nucleic acid element in a *genome*.
[ref. 1]

transsynaptic

Referring to an event, such as transmission of a nerve impulse, across a *synapse*.
[ref. 4]

transtentorial herniation

See *herniation, trianstentorial.*

Treacher Collins syndrome
Treacher Collins–Franceschetti syndrome
mandibulofacial dysostosis

Congenital deformity characterized by structural abnormalities of the head and face.

Note: *Autosomal dominant mutations* associated with Treacher Collins *syndrome* have been identified in several *genes* involved in early development of bone and the *tissues* of the face, the most frequently implicated being TCOF1.
[ref. 5]
See also *craniofacial.*

treadmill test

Procedure used to assess limb function and strength, often to evaluate models of peripheral neuropathy, in which a rodent is placed in an enclosed lane upon a surface that can be made to move at variable speed in a retrograde manner, thus allowing observation of the animal's gait dimension during a sustained attempt at forward motion.
Note 1: The treadmill test can be modified to provide a test of endurance in the animal, or to test *motor coordination* and gait.
Note 2: A treadmill test with humans is commonly used in a medical setting for assessment of cardiac performance and *pulmonary* function.
[ref. 4]

treatability

In relation to *waste* water, the amenability of substances to removal without adversely affecting the normal operation of biological treatment processes (such as in a sewage treatment plant).
[ref. 1]

tremor

Repetitive, often regular and usually involuntary oscillatory movement caused by alternating *contractions* of opposing muscle groups.
Note 1: There are many causes of tremor, some of them *benign.*
Note 2: A characteristic tremor originating in *cerebellar* pathways upon intentional fine movement ("intention tremor") can occur during alcohol *withdrawal.*
Note 3: A coarse rhythmic (3–5 Hz) tremor of the hands and forearms that appears when the muscles are relaxed ("resting tremor") is characteristic of *Parkinson disease.*
[ref. 4]

triage

1. Process of sorting people into groups based on their need for or likely benefit from immediate medical treatment.
   Note: Triage is used in hospital emergency rooms, on battlefields, and at disaster sites when limited medical resources must be allocated.
2. System used to allocate a scarce commodity, such as food, to those most likely to benefit from it.
3. Process in which things are ranked in terms of importance or priority.

[ref. 1]

trigeminal nerve

See *nerve, trigeminal.*

trigeminal neuralgia

See *neuralgia, trigeminal.*

trigger values

Criteria applied to results from tests (for fate or effects) that prompt further studies, *e.g.*, moving to the next tier of tests (see *tiered testing*), which are generally more complex.
[ref. 2]

trilaminar embryo

See *embryo, trilaminar*.

trimester

In *pregnancy*, one of three equal timed divisions of the normal human *gestation period*, each lasting approximately three months.
[ref. 5]

triple screen
triple test

Measurement of maternal serum levels of *α-fetoprotein, human chorionic gonadotropin*, and *estriol*, usually in the second *trimester* of *pregnancy*, used as an indicator of risk for certain *fetal chromosomal abnormalities* and *neural tube defect*s.
[ref. 5]

triploidy

Presence of three *haploid* sets of *chromosomes* in the *cell*.
Note: Triploidy is fatal in *fetal* or early *neonatal* life.
[ref. 5]
See also *diploid; euploid; ploidy*.

triptan

Member of a class of *drugs*, based on tryptamine, that act as *serotonin receptor agonist*s.
Note: Triptans are used for *pain* relief in the treatment of *migraine headache*.
[ref. 4]

trisomy

Condition of having three *homologous chromosome*s in each *somatic cell* instead of the normal pair.
[ref. 5]

trisomy 8
Warkany syndrome 2

Presence of an extra *chromosome* 8.
Note: Complete *trisomy* 8 is lethal, but most affected individuals show *mosaicism* with *craniofacial* abnormalities, a short wide neck, multiple joint defects, and deep creases in the palms and soles.
[ref. 5]

trisomy 13
Patau syndrome
trisomy D

Presence of part or all of an extra *chromosome* 13 from *nondisjunction* during *meiosis*.

Note 1: Trisomy 13 leads to multiple *congenital abnormalities* and intellectual disability, and is usually fatal in early childhood.
Note 2: Patau *syndrome*, in addition to complete trisomy 13, can also occur with an extra chromosome 13 attached to another chromosome as a result of a *Robertsonian translocation*.
[ref. 5]

trisomy 18

Edwards syndrome

Presence of part or all of an extra *chromosome* 18 from *nondisjunction* during *meiosis*.
Note: Trisomy 18 leads to multiple *congenital abnormalities* and intellectual disability, and is usually fatal in early childhood.
[ref. 5]

trisomy 21

Down syndrome

Presence of an extra *chromosome* 21.
Note 1: Trisomy 21 produces a characteristic constellation of physical abnormalities with delayed growth and mental development, but is compatible with life into *adulthood*.
Note 2: The terms mongoloid and mongolism, formerly used for trisomy 21, are now considered offensive.
[ref. 5]

trophectoderm

Outer layer of the *blastocyst* that contacts the *endometrium*, establishes nutrition for the *embryo*, and differentiates into the *trophoblast*.
[ref. 5]

trophic

Relating to feeding and nutrition.
[ref. 2]

trophic cascade

Situation arising when *predators* in a *food chain* decrease the abundance or impair the behavior of their prey, thereby lowering the level of predation experienced by the next lower *trophic level* in the chain (or level of herbivory if the intermediate trophic level is occupied by a *herbivore*).
Example: If the number of large *piscivorous* fish increases in a lake, their prey, *zooplanktivorous* fish, should decrease, large *zooplankton* should increase, and *phytoplankton biomass* should decrease.
Note: Trophic cascades may also be important for understanding the effects of removing top predators from *food webs*, as humans have done in many places through hunting and fishing activities.
[ref. 2]

trophic dilution

biodilution

Decrease in *contaminant* concentration as *trophic level* increases.
Note 1: Trophic dilution results when an increase in *biomass* at a lower trophic level (*e.g.*, algal biomass) reduces the concentration in the diets of those feeding on the species at that lower level.

Note 2: The extent of trophic dilution is affected by the rate of ingestion of the *pollutant* from food, as well as *biotransformation* and elimination processes in the higher level organism.
[After ref. 2]
Compare *bioconcentration*.

trophic enrichment

See *biomagnification*.

trophic level
trophic position

Position held by an organism in a *food chain*, sometimes assessed by the number of energy-transfer steps to reach that level.
Note: Organisms not needing organic food, such as plants, are said to be on a low trophic level, whereas *predator* species needing food of high energy content are said to be on a high trophic level.
[ref. 1,2]
See also *ecological energetics*.

trophic position

See *trophic level*.

trophic structure

Organization of an *ecological community* described in terms of energy flow through its various *trophic levels*.
[ref. 2]

trophic transfer

Transfer of a substance from one *trophic level* to another.
[ref. 2]

trophic transfer factor

Concentration of a substance in a *predator* divided by that in its prey.
[ref. 2]

trophoblast

Outer layer of the *blastocyst* that invades the *endometrium* and establishes nutrition for the *embryo*.
Note: Trophoblast cells do not form part of the *embryo*, but contribute to the development of the *placenta*.
[ref. 5]

trueness (in metrology)

Closeness of agreement between the average of a theoretically infinite number of replicate measured quantity values and the reference quantity value.
[ref. 1]

truncus arteriosus

Arterial trunk, opening from the *fetal* heart and developing into the *aorta* and *pulmonary artery*.
[ref. 5]

tryptophan
(2*S*)-2-amino-3-(1*H*-indol-3-yl)propanoic acid

Essential amino acid for humans, required for *T-cell* proliferation.
[ref. 3]
See also *indolamine-2,3-dioxygenase*.

tuberculin

Antigen found in extracts of ***Mycobacteria***, used in a *skin test* for tuberculosis *(Mantoux test)*.
[ref. 3]

tuberculin test

Diagnostic test in which *antigens* derived from the organism causing tuberculosis (***Mycobacterium tuberculosis***) are injected subcutaneously; individuals who have been exposed to the organism develop a *delayed-type hypersensitivity* response at the injection site 24 to 48 h later.
Note: The tuberculin test also shows a positive response in those who have been previously vaccinated with *bacille Calmette–Guérin*.
[ref. 3]

tuberoinfundibular pathway

Group of dopaminergic neurons in the *hypothalamus* involved in regulating *prolactin* secretion from the anterior *pituitary gland*.
[ref. 5]

tubular epithelium (in kidney)

Epithelial cell layer of the *renal* tubule (see *nephron*), involved in *tubular reabsorption*, secretion, and formation of urine from the high-volume *glomerular* filtrate.
[*]
See also *proximal tubule*.

tubular reabsorption

Transfer of water and *solutes* from the *lumen* of the renal tubule (see *nephron*) into the *blood*, via the tubular *epithelial cells* and peritubular fluid.
[*]

tumor
tumour

Any abnormal swelling or *growth* of *tissue*, whether *benign* or *malignant*.
[ref. 5]
Compare *neoplasm*.

tumor antigen

See *antigen, tumor*.

tumor immunology

Application of *immunology* to understanding *tumor* biology, *immune system* avoidance by tumors, and *immunotherapy* directed against tumors.
[ref. 3]

tumor-infiltrating lymphocyte (TIL)

See *lymphocyte, tumor-infiltrating.*

tumor necrosis factor (TNF)

cachectin
cachexin
TNF-α

Protein produced and secreted by several of the body's *cell* types, including *leukocytes.*
Note 1: TNF-α promotes the destruction of some types of *cancer* cells and is a *cytokine* involved in *systemic inflammation.*
Note 2: Activation of the TNF-α *receptor* may trigger *apoptosis* through the *extrinsic pathway.*
[ref. 3]

tumor necrosis factor β (TNF-β)

See *lymphotoxin.*

tumor necrosis factor (TNF) **receptor-associated factor** (TRAF)

Family of proteins involved in regulating *inflammation* and *apoptosis* through interaction with the *tumor necrosis factor receptor.*
[ref. 3]

tumor progression

Sequence of changes by which a *benign tumor* develops from the initial lesion to a *malignant* stage.
[ref. 1]

tumor rejection antigen (TRA)

See *antigen, tumor rejection.*

tumor-specific transplantation antigen (TSTA)

See *antigen, tumor-specific transplantation.*

tumor suppressor gene

See *gene, tumor suppressor.*

tumorigenic

Able to cause *tumors.*
[ref. 1]

tunica albuginea

Dense, *collagenous* fibrous coat surrounding an anatomical structure, and in particular surrounding the *ovaries, testicles*, and *corpora cavernosa* of the penis.
[ref. 5]

tunica vaginalis

Membranous sheath, derived from the *peritoneum*, surrounding the *testis* and *epididymis.*
[ref. 5]

turbidity, τ

Apparent absorbance of incident light due to light scattering.
Note: Water turbidity refers to the extent to which the clarity of water is reduced by the presence of suspended or other matter that causes light to be scattered rather than transmitted in straight lines through the sample.
[After ref. 2]

Turner syndrome

Ullrich-Turner syndrome

Phenotypic female lacking one *X chromosome*, the *genotype* being designated XO.
Note: Turner *syndrome* results in a number of developmental abnormalities including short stature, *webbed* neck, sexual immaturity, and *sterility*.
[ref. 5]

turnover time

See *mean life.*

twin-tracer technique

Experimental method for evaluating assimilation of a substance, *e.g.*, from the gut into the body or from the *blood* into a solid *tumor*, by introducing simultaneously a *tracer* (usually a radiotracer) of the substance being assimilated and a second inert tracer that will not be assimilated.
[After ref. 2]

two-compartment model

Outcome of a *compartmental analysis* utilizing two *compartments.*
[ref. 1]
See also *compartmental modeling; multicompartment model.*

two-generation reproductive toxicity study

Procedure using rodents wherein parents (P0 generation) and their *offspring* (*F1 generation*) are both exposed to a test substance and the second generation (F2) is examined for possible *toxic effects*.
[ref. 5]
See also *one-generation reproductive toxicity study.*

tympanic

In anatomy, relating to the resonant *cavity* and *membrane* of the inner ear.
[ref. 5]

type 1 diabetes mellitus

See *diabetes mellitus type 1.*

type 2 diabetes mellitus

See *diabetes mellitus type 2.*

type I hypersensitivity

See *Gell and Coombs classification; immediate-type hypersensitivity.*

type II hypersensitivity

See *Gell and Coombs classification.*

type III hypersensitivity

See *Gell and Coombs classification.*

type IV hypersensitivity

See *Gell and Coombs classification; hypersensitivity, delayed-type.*

type A organism (in relation to *sediment*)

Animal or plant living in contact with *sediments* but unable to ingest particulates.
Note: The classification of organisms into Types A and B implies that a Type A organism takes up substances from *interstitial water* but not from sediment-associated particulates.
Examples: Rooted *macrophytes, benthic algae.*
[ref. 2]
See also *type B organism.*

type B organism (in relation to *sediment*)

Animal or plant living in contact with *sediments* and capable of ingesting particulates.
Note: The classification of organisms into Types A and B implies that a Type B organism takes up substances from both *interstitial water* and from sediment-associated particulates.
Examples: Detritivorous organisms, *suspension feeders.*
[ref. 2]
See also *type A organism.*

tyrosine kinase

protein tyrosine kinase

Any *enzyme* that phosphorylates target proteins on tyrosine residues, thus playing a crucial role in *signal transduction.*
Note: Tyrosine kinases play a key role in *lymphocyte activation.* Major tyrosine kinases involved in *T-lymphocyte* activation are Lck, Fyn, and *ZAP-70*; those involved in *B-lymphocyte* activation are Blk, Fyn, Lyn, and Syk.
[ref. 3]
See also *kinase.*

ubiquitin

Highly conserved 76-amino acid peptide abundant in *eukaryotic cells* whose covalent attachment to a protein by a ubiquitin ligase complex targets that protein for destruction by the *proteasome*.
[ref. 3]

ulcer

Defect, often associated with bleeding and *inflammation*, occurring locally or at the surface of an *organ* or *tissue* owing to sloughing of *necrotic* tissue.
Note: Ulcers of the stomach and *duodenum* are common side effects of *nonsteroidal anti-inflammatory drugs.*
[ref. 1]

ultrafine particle

Airborne particle of *aerodynamic diameter* less than or equal to 100 nm.
Note: As a group, ultrafine particles are referred to as the PM0.1 fraction (derived from Particulate Matter 0.1 μm).
[ref. 1]
See also *nanoparticle*.

ultrasonography

Imaging technique that creates a picture of internal body structures from differentially reflected *ultrasound* waves.
Note: Using ultrasonography, the human *embryo* can be observed *in utero* as early as 5 1/2 weeks of *gestation*, and *fetal* monitoring by the technique (obstetric ultrasound) is standard.
[ref. 5]

ultrasound

1. Sound waves of frequency higher than the range audible to the human ear.
2. Imaging technique that uses such sound waves to create a picture of internal body structures.

[ref. 5]
See also *ultrasonography*.

umbilical

See *umbilicus*.

umbilical artery

Paired artery that, in the *fetus*, returns deoxygenated *blood* from each half of the *fetal* body to the *placenta*, via the *umbilical cord*.
Note: In the *adult*, part of the umbilical artery remains open as a branch of the internal *iliac artery*, and part ceases to be an artery and becomes the *medial umbilical ligament*.
[ref. 5]

Comprehensive Glossary of Terms Used in Toxicology
By John Duffus, Douglas M. Templeton and Michael Schwenk

Published by the Royal Society of Chemistry, www.rsc.org

umbilical cord

Cord-like structure connecting the *fetus* with the *placenta* and housing the *umbilical artery* and *umbilical vein* that carry nutrients from the mother and remove wastes from the fetus.
[ref. 5]

umbilical hernia

Protrusion of bowel or *omentum* through the *abdominal* wall at the *umbilicus.*
[ref. 5]

umbilical vein

left umbilical vein

Vessel within the *umbilical cord*, entering the *fetus* at the *umbilicus*, and carrying oxygenated *blood* from the *placenta.*
[ref. 5]

umbilicus (n)/umbilical (adj)

navel
belly button
omphalos

Feature marking the point in the *abdominal* wall where the *umbilical cord* entered the *fetus.*
[ref. 5]

uncertainty

1. (in metrology) Parameter characterizing the dispersion of the quantity values being attributed to a measurand, based on the measurements used.
   Note: The parameter used to express uncertainty may be, for example, a standard deviation, or the half-width of an interval having a stated coverage probability.
2. (in *risk management*) Consequence of information gaps regarding *hazard* and (or) extent of *exposure* to an agent, usually dealt with by introducing an *uncertainty factor.*

[ref. 1]

uncertainty factor (UF)

1. (in metrology) Confidence interval or *fiducial limit* used to assess the probable precision of an estimate.
2. (in *toxicology*) Value used in extrapolation from experimental animals to humans (assuming that humans may be more sensitive) or from selected individuals to the general population.
   Note 1: The uncertainity factor is used in extrapolation of experimental data to set safety values in regulatory practice to protect humans, including sensitive individuals; also known as a modifying factor.
   Note 2: An uncertainty factor in toxicology could be, for example, a value applied to the *no-observed-effect-level* (NOEL) or to the *no-observed-adverse-effect-level* (NOAEL) to derive an *acceptable daily intake* (ADI) or *tolerable daily intake* (TDI). In this example, the NOEL or NOAEL is divided by the uncertainty factor to calculate the ADI or TDI.

[ref. 1]

unconscious

1. Not in a *conscious* state.
2. In psychoanalytic theory, describing feelings and motivations of which one is unaware that nevertheless shape behavior.

[ref. 4]

uncoupling (n)/uncouple (v)

Process in the *mitochondrial membrane* whereby the proton gradient established by the *electron transfer chain* is dissipated, preventing productive interaction ('coupling') of ATP synthetase (EC 3.6.3.14) with its nucleotide substrate, and producing heat instead of making *ATP* from ADP.
Note 1: Endogenous uncoupling proteins (UCP) are proton channels that are active in brown fat, allowing that tissue to generate heat.
Note 2: *Poisons* (*e.g.*, 2,4-dinitrophenol) that interfere with *oxidative phosphorylation* by dissipating the proton gradient are called uncoupling agents.
[*]

uncus

Anterior projection of the *grey matter* surrounding the *hippocampus*, covered by a region of the *temporal lobe*, involved in *olfaction*.
Note 1: The uncus is a point of origin of *seizure*s accompanied by *hallucination*s and a sense of unpleasant odors.
Note 2: The uncus may *herniate* over the notch of the *tentorium* and compress the third *cranial nerve* (uncal herniation).
[ref. 4]

undescended testis

See testis, undescended.

unfolded protein response (UPR)

See *endoplasmic reticulum stress.*

unit risk

See *risk, unit.*

unresponsiveness (in immunology)

Inability to respond to an *antigenic stimulus*.
Note: Unresponsiveness may be specific for a particular antigen (see *tolerance*), or broadly nonspecific as a result of damage to the entire *immune system*, for example, after whole-body irradiation.
[ref. 3]

unsaturated liquid

See *subcooled.*

unscheduled DNA synthesis (UDS)

See *deoxyribonucleic acid (DNA) synthesis, unscheduled.*

upper boundary

Estimate of the plausible upper limit to the true value of a quantity.
Note: The upper boundary is usually not a statistical confidence limit.
[ref. 1]

upper motor neuron

See *neuron, upper motor*.

upstream water

See *water, upstream*.

uptake

Entry of a substance into the body; into an *organ*, a *tissue*, or a *cell*; or into body fluids.
Note 1: Uptake is often by passage through a *membrane*, but may also occur by other means.
Note 2: The term uptake may also be applied to *sorption* of a substance onto the outside of an organism, *e.g.*, onto the shell of a mollusc or the exoskeleton of an insect, without any of the substance entering the body or its cells.
[ref. 2]
See also *absorption* (in biology).

uptake rate constant

First-order one-compartment constant (see *one-compartment model*) to describe the *uptake* of a substance by an organism from water.
[ref. 2]

ureter

Duct by which urine is conveyed from the kidney to the urinary bladder.
[*]

urethra

Duct by which urine is conveyed out of the body from the urinary bladder, and by which, in male *vertebrates, semen* is also conveyed.
[ref. 5]

urogenital
genitourinary

Concerning the urinary and *genital organs*.
[ref. 5]

urogenital sinus

See *sinus, urogenital*.

urticaria (n)/urticarial (adj)

See *hives*.

urticaria, contact

Urticaria provoked by contact with inducing agents.
[ref. 3]

uterine crypt

Chamber on the interior surface of the *uterus* that serves as a site of *embryo homing* and *implantation*.
[ref. 5]

uterine cycle

Regular, periodic changes that occur in the *uterus* and, together with the *ovarian cycle*, constitute the *menstrual cycle* necessary for female *fertility*.
Note 1: The uterine *cycle* consists of three phases: i) *menstruation*, ii) a proliferative phase in which the uterine wall thickens under the influence of *estrogen*, and iii) a secretory phase in which the *corpus luteum* is producing *progesterone* and the *endometrium* becomes receptive to *implantation* of the *blastocyst*.
Note 2: The three phases of the uterine cycle correspond to the three phases of the ovarian cycle.
[ref. 5]

uterotrophic
uterotropic

Having an effect on the *uterus*.
Note: Uterotrophic usually refers to *estrogen*-like effects of uterine cell proliferation caused by some *drugs* and other substances with weak *estrogen*-mimetic properties.
[ref. 5]

uterotrophic assay

Procedure in which immature female rodents are treated for three days with a test substance. A resultant increase in *uterine* wet weight suggests an *estrogenic* activity of the substance.
[ref. 5]

uterus (n)/uterine (adj)
womb

Hollow muscular *organ* of the female reproductive system that receives the *fertilized ovum* (see also *implantation*) and supports the subsequent development of the *fetus*.
[ref. 5]

uterus, bicornate

Uterus that is divided into two lateral horns as a result of imperfect fusion of the paired *embryonic* tubes from which the uterus is formed.
Note: In humans bicornate uterus is a *malformation*, but in some mammalian species, including rodents and pigs, it is normal.
[ref. 5]

uvula
palatine uvula

Muscular projection from the posterior edge of the soft *palate*.
Note: The uvula contributes to the gag reflex and is involved in shaping some sounds of human speech.
[ref. 5]

Vα-Jα rearrangement

Preferential partnering of Jα gene segments with Vα gene segments during rearrangement in the *T-cell receptor* gene, possibly following deletion of the Vδ gene region.
[ref. 3]
See also *J gene; V gene.*

V(D)J recombination

Mechanism for generating *antigen*-specific *receptors* of *T-cells* and *B-cells*; it involves the joining of *V, D*, and *J gene* segments, mediated by a multi-*enzyme* complex, V(D)J recombinase, and products of the *recombination-activating genes.*
Note 1: The conventional syntax V(D)J indicates that V and J genes code the *light chain* and all three genes code the *heavy chain*, the processes being VJ and VDJ recombination, respectively.
Note 2: V(D)J recombination occurs only once in a cell's lifetime.
[ref. 3]
See also *somatic recombination.*

V domain

See *variable (V) region.*

V gene

See *variable (V) gene.*

V region

See *variable (V) region.*

vaccination

Immunization with a *vaccine* against a *pathogen* or *toxin.*
[ref. 3]

vaccination, deoxyribonucleic acid

DNA immunization
DNA vaccination

Injection of *DNA* into muscle, followed by its *transcription* and *translation* into a protein or proteins that elicit a specific *antibody* and *T-cell* responses.
[ref. 3]
See also *immunization; vaccination.*

vaccine

Antigen preparation, often consisting of a weakened or killed *pathogen*, such as a bacterium or virus, or of a portion of the pathogen's structure, intended to stimulate the *immune system* to provide future *tolerance.*
Note: Upon administration, the vaccine stimulates *antibody* production or *cellular immunity* against the pathogen, but is incapable of causing severe *infection.*
[ref. 3]
See also *vaccine, attenuated; vaccine, inactivated.*

Comprehensive Glossary of Terms Used in Toxicology
By John Duffus, Douglas M. Templeton and Michael Schwenk

Published by the Royal Society of Chemistry, www.rsc.org

vaccine, attenuated

Vaccine made from a live organism that targets cells of the *immune system* but has been engineered or weakened so as not to cause *disease*.
[ref. 3]
See also *vaccine, inactivated; vaccine, live attenuated*.

vaccine, inactivated

Vaccine formulated from the whole microorganism that has been rendered unable to reproduce or cause *disease*, often by *mutation* or heat denaturation.
[ref. 3]
See also *vaccine, attenuated*.

vaccine, live attenuated

Vaccine prepared from living attenuated organisms or from viruses that have been attenuated but can still replicate in the cells of the *host* organism.
Note: The live attenuated vaccine contains a version of living bacteria or viruses that have been weakened (attenuated) so they can no longer cause *disease*. Since they are very close to the actual infection, they can cause strong *cell* and *antibody* responses.
[ref. 3]
See also *vaccine, attenuated*.

vacuole

Membrane-bound *cavity* within a cell.
[ref. 1]

vagina (n)/vaginal (adj)

Fibromuscular *canal* passing between the *uterine cervix* and the opening to the *vulva*.
Note: The vagina permits sexual intercourse and delivery of babies.
[ref. 5]

vaginal cornification

Conversion of the normal *epithelium* of the *vagina* to a *keratinized* squamous (flattened) *epithelium*.
Note: The appearance of keratinized ("cornified") epithelial cells in a vaginal smear is an indication of increased *estrogen* levels.
[ref. 5]

vaginal patency

Referring to the opening of the *vagina* that usually occurs at *sexual maturity* and is maintained by *hormonal* influences pre-*menopausally*.
[ref. 5]

vaginal smear
vaginal wet mount

Preparation for examination by light microscopy of a sample of a *vaginal* discharge, used in the diagnosis of a vaginal *infection*.
Note: Vaginal smear should not be confused with a *Papanicolaou smear*.
[ref. 5]

vagus nerve

See *nerve, vagus*.

validity of a measurement

Expression of the degree to which a measurement measures what it purports to measure.
[ref. 1]

validity of a study

Degree to which the inferences drawn, especially generalizations extending beyond the *study sample*, are warranted when account is taken of the study methods, the representativeness of the study sample, and the nature of the *population* from which it is drawn.
[ref. 1]

variable (V) domain

See *variable (V) region.*

variable (V) gene

Gene, segment(s) of which rearrange together with *diversity (D) gene* and *joining (J) gene* segments, in order to encode the *variable (V) region* amino acid sequences of *immunoglobulins* and *T-cell receptors.*
[ref. 3]
See also *variable (V) region.*

variable (V) region

N-terminal portion of an *immunoglobulin* or *T-cell receptor* that contains the *antigen*-binding region of the molecule; V regions are formed by the recombination of V(D) and *J gene* segments.
Note: The V region consists of two V domains, VL and VH.
[ref. 3]
See also *somatic recombination; V(D)J-recombination.*

variation, developmental

Anatomical deviation that is not life-threatening.
[ref. 5]

vascular

Pertaining to vessels, such as the *blood* or *lymphatic systems.*
[*]
See also *cardiovascular.*

vascular addressin

See *addressin, vascular.*

vascular cell adhesion molecule (VCAM)

CD106

Molecule, expressed on the surface of *endothelial cells*, that functions in the adhesion of *lymphocytes, monocytes, eosinophils*, and *basophils* to the endothelium of the *vascular* surface.
[ref. 3]
See also *adhesion molecule.*

vasculitis/vasculitides (pl)

One of a group of *disorders* that share a common underlying problem of *inflammation* of a blood vessel or vessels.
Note 1: Vasculitis can lead to *necrosis, fibrosis*, or *thrombosis*.
Note 2: *Autoimmunity* plays an important role in some vasculitides (*e.g., ANCA-associated vasculitides, Goodpasture syndrome*, and *cryoglobulinemic vasculitis*).
[ref. 3]

vasculitis, antineutrophil cytoplasmic autoantibody-associated (ANCA)

One of a group of *autoimmune systemic* vasculitides associated with *antineutrophil cytoplasmic auto - antibodies, e.g., Wegener granulomatosis, microscopic polyangiitis*, and Churg–Strauss *syndrome*.
[ref. 3]

vasculogenesis

De novo development of blood vessel *endothelium* in the absence of preexisting vessels, *e.g.*, during *fetal* development or in connection with tissue repair, initiated by *migration* of *mesodermal* precursor cells.
[ref. 5]
Compare *angiogenesis; arteriogenesis.*

vas deferens
ductus deferens
spermatic duct

Secretory *duct* of the *testis* running between the *epididymis* and the *ejaculatory duct.*
[ref. 5]

vasectomy

Surgical removal of all or part of each *vas deferens*, typically as a means of *sterilization.*
[ref. 5]

vasoactive amine

Substance containing amino group(s) that increases vascular permeability and smooth muscle *contraction.*
Examples: Histamine, 5-hydroxytryptamine.
[ref. 3]

vasoconstriction
Opposite term: *vasodilation.*

Decrease of the caliber of the blood vessels (especially in the arteries and arterioles) as a result of contraction of smooth muscles in the vessel walls.
Note: Vasoconstriction results in an increase in *vascular* resistance followed by an increase in blood pressure.
[ref. 4]

vasodilation

See *vasorelaxation.*

vasodilator

Agent that induces *vasorelaxation*.
[ref. 4]

vasopressin

Pituitary hormone that acts to promote the retention of water by the kidneys and to increase blood pressure.
[ref. 5]

vasopressor
vasoconstrictor
pressor

Agent that induces *vasoconstriction*.
[ref. 4]

vasorelaxant

Agent having the property of reducing tension in the walls of a blood vessel, thus increasing the diameter of its *lumen* and decreasing vascular pressure.
[*]
See also *vasorelaxation*.

vasorelaxation
vasodilation
vasodilatation
Opposite term: *vasoconstriction*.

Increase in the diameter of the *lumen* of the blood vessels as a result of relaxation of smooth muscles in the vessel walls.
Note: Vasorelaxation results in a decrease in *vascular* resistance followed by a decrease of blood pressure.
[ref. 4]

vasospasm
angiospasm

Contraction of the muscular wall of blood vessels with sustained *vasoconstriction* possibly leading to *tissue ischemia*.
[ref. 4]

vector

See *cloning vector*.

vehicle (in pharmacology)

Substance(s) used to formulate active ingredients for administration or use.
Note: In this context, vehicle is a general term for, *e.g.*, solvents or suspending agents.
[ref. 1]

velopharyngeal insufficiency
velopharyngeal incompetence

Inability to achieve closure of the velopharyngeal *sphincter* (closure of the muscle of the *soft palate*) during speech, owing to muscular dysfunction, *cleft palate*, or other *disorders*.

Note: Velopharyngeal insufficiency often causes speech problems by allowing air to escape through the nose instead of the mouth.
[ref. 5]

vena cava

Large vein returning deoxygenated *blood* to the right heart.
Note: The vena cava has two branches in humans, the inferior vena cava (carrying blood from the lower body) and the superior vena cava (carrying blood from the head, arms, and upper body).
[ref. 5]

venom

Animal *toxin* generally used for self-defense or predation and usually delivered by a bite or sting.
[ref. 1]

venous shunt

See *shunt, arteriovenous.*

ventilation

1. Process of supplying a building or room with fresh air.
2. Process of exchange of air between the ambient atmosphere and the lungs; breathing.

[ref. 1]

ventral

Opposite term: *dorsal.*

Situated to the anterior side of the trunk; in humans, to the front of the body.
[ref. 5]

ventral thalamus

See *subthalamus.*

ventricle

Normal *cavity* within an organ, as in the *brain* or heart.
Note 1: In the brain there are two lateral ventricles and two midline (called the third and fourth) ventricles.
Note 2: The ventricles in the brain are filled with, and produce most of, the *cerebrospinal fluid*, and play a critical role in its circulation.
[ref. 4]
Note 3: The heart has two ventricles. The right ventricle pumps deoxygenated *blood* to the lungs via the *pulmonary artery* and the left ventricle pumps reoxygenated blood to the rest of the body via the *aorta.*
[*]

ventricular fibrillation

See *fibrillation, ventricular.*

ventricular septal defect (VSD)

Congenital defect with an opening in the wall separating the right and left *ventricle*s of the heart (see *ventricular septum*).
Note: A VSD allows reflux of *blood* back to the right ventricle during left ventricular *contraction*, producing varying degrees of *cyanosis*.
[ref. 5]

ventricular septum

See *septum, ventricular.*

ventriculo-atrial shunt

See *shunt, ventriculo-atrial.*

ventriculogram

Radiographic image of the *cerebral ventricles.*
[ref. 4]

ventriculomegaly

Enlargement of the *cerebral ventricle*s.
[ref. 4]
See also *hydrocephalus.*

ventriculo-peritoneal shunt

See *shunt, ventriculo-peritoneal.*

Verhulst equation

Algebraic model of *population growth*, expressed as

$$dN/dt = rN(1 - N/K)$$

where N is the population size, r is the population growth rate, and K is the environmental carrying capacity (the maximum population the *environment* can sustain with stability).
Note: The terms *r-strategy* and *K-strategy* are derived from the constants in the Verhulst equation.
[*]

vermicide

Substance intended to kill intestinal worms.
[ref. 1]

vermifuge

See *anthelmint(h)ic.*

vermis (in neuroanatomy)

vermis cerebelli
Narrow central part of the *cerebellum* between the two cerebellar hemispheres.
[ref. 4]

vertebra (n)/**vertebral** (adj)

One of the bony segments that together make up the bony column surrounding the *spinal cord*, including any such bone of the *cervical, thoracic* or *lumbar spine,* or the fused sacral and coccygeal bones.
[ref. 4,5]

vertebral arch

See *neural arch.*

vertebral column

spine
spinal column
backbone

Bony structure consisting of the *vertebra*e and enclosing the *spinal cord.*
[ref. 4]

vertebrate

Animal that has as part of its *nervous system* a *spinal cord* that is surrounded by a bony *vertebral* column.
[ref. 5]

vertigo

1. Illusion of movement as if the external world were revolving around one's self or as if one's self were revolving in space.
2. Dizziness, often associated with looking down from a height.

Note: Vertigo may be a result of malfunction of the inner ear or of the vestibular nerve.
[ref. 1]

very early activating antigen

See *antigen, very early activating.*

very late activation antigen (VLA)

See *antigen, very late activation.*

vesicant

1. (n) Substance that causes blisters on the skin.
2. (adj) Producing blisters on the skin.

Examples: Mustards, and the sap of the giant hogweed (***Heracleum mantegazzianum***) that contains furocoumarins that can cause phytophotodermatitis in humans.
[ref. 1]

vesicle (n)/**vesicular** (adj)

Small fluid-filled sac, bladder-like structure, or blister.
Note: The term "vesicle" may refer to an anatomic structure, a subcellular *organelle*, or a *liposome*-related particle.
[ref. 5]

vestigial

In anatomy, pertaining to a remnant of an *embryonic* or *fetal* structure persisting in the *adult*.
[ref. 5]

vetoing (in immunology)

Apoptotic elimination by a self-peptide-presenting (veto) cell of a *lymphocyte* that recognizes a self-peptide-*major histocompatibility complex molecule*.
[After ref. 3]

viability

Ability to continue living.
Note: *Fetal* viability refers to the ability of the *fetus* to survive outside the *uterus*.
[ref. 5]

viability selection

survival selection
Natural selection operating through the differential survival of individuals until they are able to reproduce.
[*]

vigilance

1. Ability to maintain concentration or sustain attention over prolonged periods of time.
2. Active process of detecting, investigating, and documenting unwanted effects of *drugs* (pharmacovigilance) or adverse effects of *toxic substances (toxicovigilance)*.

[ref. 5]

vigilance decrement

Decreased *vigilance* measured as a decline in the ability to maintain an accurate voluntary response to signals with time.
[ref. 5]

villus

1. Projection from a surface, typically the surface of a *mucous membrane*.
   Note: A *mucosal epithelial cell* may produce a large number of villi, thus increasing its surface area.
2. Elongated projection of the *dermis* into an *epidermal* space.

[ref. 5]

vimentin

Intermediate filament protein of the *cytoskeleton* that is expressed in *mesenchymal* cells and *endothelial cells*, and is indicative of cells undergoing an *epithelial-to-mesenchymal transition*.
Note: Vimentin *filaments* support cell *membranes*, keep some *organelles* in a fixed place within the *cytoplasm*, and transmit *membrane receptor* signals to the *nucleus*.
[After ref. 5]

virilization

Possession or acquisition of characteristics of a male body, especially by a female or *prepubescent* male.
[ref. 5]

virtually safe dose (VSD)

Dose of a *carcinogen* that, over a lifetime of human *exposure*, has been estimated, using mathematical modeling, to result in a very low *incidence* of *cancer*, somewhere between zero and a specified incidence (*e.g.*, 1 cancer in 10^6 exposed people).
[ref. 1]

virucide

See *antiviral.*

viscera (n)/visceral (adj)

Soft and (or) hollow *organs* of the body, in *vertebrates* particularly those found in the *thoracic* and *abdominal cavities.*
Note: The term viscera gives rise to the distinction between the visceral and *parietal serous membranes*, located respectively closest to the organ or to the body wall, *e.g.*, as applied to the *pericardium, peritoneal cavity* and *pleura.*
[ref. 5]

visual cortex

See *cortex, visual.*

vital stain

1. Stain tolerated by living *cells* that allows visualization of specific cell types, cellular structures or organelles, without damage or immediate loss of *viability.*
2. Stain that attaches to cells or parts of cells while they are still living, not entering them but allowing them to be clearly distinguished.

[*]

vital rate

Measure of how fast a *vital statistic* changes in a *population* (usually expressed per 1000 individuals).
Note: Vital rates are divided into two categories; crude rates referring to change in the whole population (*e.g.*, overall change in births and deaths per 1000), and refined rates, referring to change in a specific demographic characteristic (*e.g.*, age, sex, race).
[ref. 2]
See also *rate (in epidemiology).*

vital statistic

Recorded number of events affecting *population* size, such as live births, deaths, mariages or divorces, usually collected through civil registration.
[*]

vitellogenin (VTG)

Protein that forms part of the *yolk* of *egg*-laying *vertebrates*.
Note: Expression of VTG in male fish is used in *ecotoxicology* as an indicator of exposure to *environmental estrogenic endocrine disruptors*.
[ref. 5]

volatile organic chemical (VOC)

Any organic compound having, at 293.15 K, a vapor pressure of 0.01 kPa or more, or having a corresponding volatility under the particular condition of use.
Note: VOCs are parameters of indoor air quality.
[ref. 1]

voltage-gated ion channel

Ion channel that opens and closes in response to ion fluxes that change *membrane potential*.
[ref. 4]
Compare *ligand-gated ion channel*.

volume of distribution

Apparent (hypothetical) volume of fluid required to contain the total amount of a substance in the body at the same *concentration* as that present in the *plasma*, assuming *equilibrium* has been attained.
[ref. 1]

vulnerability (in toxicology)

Susceptibility to *harm* by *toxicants*.
[ref. 2]

vulva

External genitalia of the female.
[ref. 5]

Wahlund effect

Net deficit of *heterozygotes* observed when two *populations*, each in *Hardy–Weinberg equilibrium* but with different *allele* frequencies, are mixed and the *genotype* frequencies are quantified in a sample of the combined population.
Note 1: The Wahlund effect may be expressed as an overall reduction in heterozygosity in a population with subpopulations having different allele frequencies.
Note 2: A common cause of the Wahlund effect is separation of subpopulations caused by geographic barriers with segregation of alleles by *genetic drift*.
[After ref. 2]

waldsterben

Widespread and substantial decline in *health* and *growth* of forests (dieback), and the change in development of many softwood and hardwood *species* in forest *ecosystems* in central Europe in recent decades.
Note: The occurrence of a waldsterben phenomenon and the proposed triggering by air *pollutants* is not universally accepted.
[After ref. 2]

warm autoantibody type

See *autoantibody, warm type*.

wash-out

Removal of air *pollutants* by falling rain or snow.
See also *wet deposition*.
[ref. 2]

waste

Anything that is discarded deliberately or otherwise disposed of on the assumption that it is of no further use to the primary user.
[ref. 1]

waste-water

General term describing *effluents*, *leachate*, and *elutriate*s that enter the natural *environment*.
[ref. 2]

wasting syndrome

Disease, marked by weight loss and *atrophy* of muscular and other *connective tissues*, that is not directly related to a decrease in food and water consumption.
[ref. 1]

water, receiving

Surface water (*e.g.*, in a stream, river, or lake) that has received, or is about to receive, a discharged *waste* (*i.e.*, the surface water immediately around the discharge point).
[ref. 2]

Comprehensive Glossary of Terms Used in Toxicology
By John Duffus, Douglas M. Templeton and Michael Schwenk

Published by the Royal Society of Chemistry, www.rsc.org

water, reconstituted

See *reconstituted water.*

water, upstream

Water in a rivulet, river, or lake that is situated above a defined point, in a direction opposite to that of the current flow.
Note: Upstream water is not influenced by incoming *effluent* at or below the defined point because the effluent is carried away by the current.
[ref. 2]

water cycle

See *biogeochemical cycle.*

water maze test

Morris water maze test
water navigation test

Procedure in which a rat or mouse is placed in a pool of water and observed to swim, using visual environmental clues, to an invisible submerged platform that allows its escape from the water.
Note: The water maze is intended to test spatial memory and learning.
[ref. 4]
See also *maze; maze, Biel water.*

water potential (in physiology)

Difference in free energy or chemical potential (per unit molal volume) between water in, *e.g.*, physiological solutions or biological fluids, and pure water under reference conditions.
[After ref. 1]

watershed

See *drainage basin.*

weakest-link incongruity

Belief that protection of an organism during its most sensitive stage of life (see *critical life-stage testing*) will protect the organism throughout life.
Note: The weakest-link incongruity assumes that *exposure* of field *populations* to *concentrations* identified in laboratory testing as causing significant *mortality* at a critical stage of life will have a significant impact on the field population.
[After ref. 2]

wean

Accustomize a young mammal to independence from its mother's milk as a source of nutrition.
[ref. 5]

weathering

Degradation of materials by *abiotic environmental* forces and associated *biotic* processes.
Examples: Breakdown of rocks and other solid materials into progressively smaller fragments; combined effects of evaporation, dissolution, UV degradation, and bacterial activity on complex *mixtures* such as oil.
[ref. 2]

web (in anatomy)
webbing

Tissue or *membrane* present between adjacent structures.
Note: If a web occurs where it is not usually found, *e.g.*, in humans between the fingers or toes, or between the neck and shoulder, it represents a *congenital abnormality*.
[After ref. 5]

Wegener granulomatosis (WG)

Granulomatous inflammation involving the respiratory tract, and necrotizing *vasculitis* affecting small to medium-sized vessels (*e.g.*, capillaries, venules, arterioles, and arteries).
Note: Necrotizing *glomerulonephritis* is common in WG.
[ref. 3]
See also *granuloma*.

Weibull model

Construct based on a continuous probability distribution (Weibull distribution) used to model probability of an occurrence such as mechanical failure or adverse outcome.
Note: In one formulation of a Weibull model used to predict a dose-response outcome for *tumor* development, the probability $P(d)$ of a tumor developing from lifetime, continuous *exposure* at dose d is given by

$$P(d) = \gamma + (1 - \gamma)(1 - \exp[-\beta d^{\alpha}])$$

where γ is the background occurrence rate and α and β are fitted dose parameters.
[After ref. 1]

weight composition

Distribution of organisms among the various weight classes present in a *population*.
Note: The sum of individual weights over all weight classes equals the *population biomass*.
[ref. 2]

weight of evidence

1. (general) Quantitative, semiquantitative, or qualitative estimate of the degree to which the evidence supports or undermines a given conclusion.
2. (in toxicology) Estimate of the extent to which the available biomedical or *toxicological* data support the hypothesis that a substance causes a defined *toxic* effect, such as *cancer* in humans.

[ref. 2]

Weismannism

Theory of *evolution* and heredity propounded by the German biologist, August Weismann, especially in regard to the continuity of the hereditary lineage and the nontransmission of acquired characteristics, such that *natural selection* depends on the germ cells and is not affected by changes acquired by somatic cells.
Note: Weismannism is in contrast to Lamarckianism, which proposes the inheritance of acquired traits.
[*]

Wernicke aphasia

fluent aphasia
receptive aphasia
sensory aphasia

Type of *aphasia* associated with damage to *Wernicke's area*, or alternatively to the medial *temporal lobe* of the *brain*, characterized by preservation of speech but with loss of meaningful language and language comprehension.
[ref. 4]

Wernicke's area

Region of the *brain* in the superior temporal gyrus of the *dominant hemisphere*, associated with comprehension of written and spoken language.
[ref. 4]

Wernicke-Korsakoff syndrome

alcoholic encephalopathy

Co-existence of Wernicke *encephalopathy* (with gait, ocular and mental disturbances) and Korsakoff *psychosis* (severe memory loss, often with *aphasia, apraxia* or *agnosia*) caused by vitamin B1 (thiamine) deficiency in the context of chronic alcohol *abuse*.
[ref. 4]

western blotting

See *immunoblotting*.

Western Pacific amyotrophic lateral sclerosis and parkinsonism-dementia complex (ALS-PDC)

Neurodegenerative disease observed in the islands of Guam, Indonesia, Japan and Papua New Guinea, showing combinations of characteristics of *amyotrophic lateral sclerosis*, atypical *Parkinson disease* with *dementia*, or dementia alone that may present sequentially during life.
Note 1: *Neurotoxins* of the cycad plant (*e.g.,* ***Cycas micronesica***), such as β-*N*-methylamino-L-alanine (L-BMAA) produced by symbiotic cyanobacteria, and methylazoxymethanol (MAM), are suspected causative agents in ALS-PDC.
Note 2: Polyproteinopathy, notably *tauopathy*, is a common causative feature underlying the different clinical manifestations of ALS-PDC.
[ref. 4]

wet deposition

See *deposition, wet*

wetland

Area of land consisting of *soil* that is saturated with moisture, such as a swamp, marsh, or bog.
Note 1: Wetlands interface between truly terrestrial ecosystems and aquatic systems.
Note 2: Wetlands are *ecotones*; they often host considerable *biodiversity* and *endemism*.
Note 3: In many locations such as the United Kingdom and United States, wetlands are the subject of conservation efforts and *biodiversity action plans* (BAPs).
[ref. 2]
See also *conservation biology; conservation ecology*.

Wharton's jelly

Gelatinous substance that embeds the vessels of the *umbilical cord*.
Note: Wharton's jelly consists mainly of hydrated glycosaminoglycans such as hyaluronic acid and chondroitin sulfate.
[ref. 5]

wheal

Circumscribed papule or plaque of *edema* of the skin, occurring as an *urticarial* lesion.
[ref. 3]
See also *hives*.

wheal and flare

Dermatological reaction at a skin site where an *antigen* is injected into an *allergic* individual, characterized by a "flare" of *erythema* and a *wheal* produced by *serum* exuding into tissue, causing local *edema*.
[ref. 3]

white matter
substantia alba

Portion of the *brain* and *spinal cord* consisting mainly of *myelinated axons* and *glial cells*.
Note: *Neurons* of the *white matter* transmit signals between areas of *grey matter* within the *cerebrum*, to lower brain centers, and up and down the superficial aspect of the spinal cord.
[ref. 4]

white pulp

Collections of *lymphocytes* in the *spleen*, responsible for its *immune* function.
[ref. 3]
See also *red pulp*.

whole-effluent toxicity (WET)

Total *toxic* effect of an *effluent* measured directly in a *toxicity* test using aquatic organisms.
[ref. 5]

whole-embryo culture

Technique, used prior to *embryo* transfer during *in vitro fertilization*, in which *embryos* undergoing *organogenesis* are maintained in formulated medium outside the body.
Note: Whole embryo culture is a useful procedure for testing the *teratogenic* effects of a substance on organogenesis in rodent or chick embryos.
[ref. 5]

whole sediment

See *sediment, whole*.

wild type

Naturally occurring, unaltered, or most frequent variant of an *allele* or *phenotype*; if several alleles occur, the most frequent one is considered to be the wild type.
[ref. 5]

Williams syndrome
elfin facies syndrome

Congenital disorder with characteristic *facies* (described as elf-like), short stature, outgoing personality, and mild intellectual disability; associated with contiguous *gene deletions* on *chromosome* 7.
[ref. 5]

Wilson disease
hepatolenticular degeneration

Genetic defect in the copper transport protein ATP7B, resulting in copper overload, especially in the liver, leading to liver *cirrhosis*, and to neurotoxicity targeting the lenticular nucleus (consisting of the *globus pallidus* and *putamen*) of the *basal ganglia*.
[*]

Wisconsin card sorting test (WCST)

Procedure in which cards, depicting different arrangements, numbers, and colors of symbols, are presented to the test subject, who is asked to make the most appropriate match of a test card without further instructions.
Note: Successful performance of the WCST requires integration of higher level *cognitive* functions, and the procedure is sometimes referred to as a *frontal lobe* test.
[ref. 4]

Wiskott–Aldrich syndrome

eczema-thrombocytopenia-immunodeficiency *syndrome*
Condition characterized by chronic *eczema*, chronic suppurative otitis media, *anemia*, and *thrombocytopenic purpura* (accompanied by bloody diarrhea).
Note: Wiskott-Aldrich is an *immunodeficiency* syndrome transmitted as an *X-linked recessive* trait in which there is poor *antibody* response to polysaccharide *antigens* and dysfunction of *cell-mediated immunity*.
[ref. 3]

withdrawal

State in which cessation of exposure to a substance produces *symptoms*.
Note: The symptoms of withdrawal are usually adverse, and may be physiological or psychological in origin.
[ref. 4]
See also *addiction; withdrawal effect*.

withdrawal effect

Adverse event following *withdrawal*, from a person or other animal, of a *drug* to which they have been chronically *exposed,* or on which they have become dependent.
Examples: Symptoms of opiate discontinuation, rebound headache (see *headache, rebound*).
[After ref. 1]

Wnt

Describing a group of *signal transduction* pathways, the member proteins involved in those pathways, or the *genes* that encode those proteins.
Note 1: Wnt pathways are involved throughout *embryonic* development, regulating such processes as *cytoskeletal* dynamics, *cell* polarity, *proliferation, migration*, and body axis patterning.

Note 2: The Wnt proteins signal by binding to cell-surface *G-protein-coupled receptors* of the Frizzled family that signal to members of the Dishevelled (Dsh) family of *cytoplasmic* phosphoproteins.
Note 3: Wnt is derived from **W**ingless-related **int**egration site, originally identified in ***Drosophila***.
[ref. 5]

Wolffian duct

See *mesonephric duct*.

Wolfgram protein

Acidic proteolipid protein component of *central nervous system myelin*.
[ref. 4]

womb

See *uterus*.

working zone

Space that contains a worker's permanent or temporary station, usually extending up to 2 m above floor level.
[ref. 1]

wrist drop
radial nerve palsy

Inability to extend the wrist as a result of peripheral *nerve* damage, causing drooping of the hand.
Note: When associated with the effects of lead poisoning on the radial nerve, wrist drop is called Teleky's sign.
[ref. 4]
See also *peripheral neuropathy*.

X chromosome

Chromosome determining female sex in the absence of a *Y chromosome.*
[ref. 5]
See also *sex chromosome.*

x-disease

Hyperkeratotic *disease* (thickening of the outer layer of the *epidermis*), first reported in cattle, following *exposure* to chlorinated dibenzo-*p*-dioxins (oxanthrenes), naphthalenes, and related compounds.
[ref. 1]

X-linked

Carried by a *gene* located on the *X chromosome.*
[ref. 5]

X-linked agammaglobulinemia

See *agammaglobulinemia, X-linked.*

X-linked severe combined immunodeficiency

See *immunodeficiency, X-linked severe combined.*

xenobiotic

Substance with a chemical structure foreign to a given organism.
Note: The term xenobiotic is frequently restricted to man-made chemical structures.
[ref. 1]

xenogeneic

Exhibiting genetic differences between *species.*
[ref. 3]
Compare *allogeneic.*

xenograft

Tissue or organ *graft* between individuals of different *species.*
[ref. 3]

xenophagy

Autophagy selective for *degradation* of intracellular bacteria and viruses.
[ref. 3]

Comprehensive Glossary of Terms Used in Toxicology
By John Duffus, Douglas M. Templeton and Michael Schwenk

Published by the Royal Society of Chemistry, www.rsc.org

Y chromosome

Chromosome determining male sex.
[ref. 5]
See also *sex chromosome*.

Y-maze

See *maze, T/Y*.

yeast two-hybrid system

Experimental procedure for analyzing the interactions of proteins, involving *genetic* manipulation.
[ref. 1]

yolk

vitellus

Nutritive material stored in the *ovum* for the nourishment of the *embryo*.
[ref. 5]

yolk sac

Fluid-filled, *membrane*-bound pouch on the *ventral* side of the early *embryo* that provides nourishment until the circulatory system develops.
[ref. 5]

yolk stalk

Narrow *tubular* support that connects the *yolk sac* to the middle of the digestive tract of an *embryo*.
[ref. 5]

Comprehensive Glossary of Terms Used in Toxicology
By John Duffus, Douglas M. Templeton and Michael Schwenk

Published by the Royal Society of Chemistry, www.rsc.org

zebrafish

Tropical fish (***Danio rerio***) about 4 cm long, commonly used as a model organism in developmental biology.
Note 1: The zebrafish has been used in studies of neurodevelopment, *neuronal network* architecture, and the *blood brain-barrier*.
Note 2: The zebrafish is also used for alternative toxicity testing; multiple endpoints for developmental *neurotoxicity* are known.
[ref. 4]

zero-order kinetics

Kinetics of a reaction in which the *rate* is independent of the *concentration*(s) of the reactants.
[ref. 1]

zeta chain (TCR)-associated protein kinase-70 kDa (ZAP-70A)

T-lymphocyte-specific *tyrosine kinase* involved in T-lymphocyte *activation*.
[ref. 3]

zinc finger

Local tertiary structure of a protein typically containing cysteine and histidine residues, that binds a divalent zinc ion to form a loop or "finger", which in turn allows the protein to bind to DNA.
Note: Zinc fingers are present in many proteins, such as nucleases and *transcription factor*s, that regulate expression of eukaryotic *genes*.
[ref. 5]

zona pellucida

Acellular *glycoprotein*-rich *membrane* surrounding the mature *ovum*.
[ref. 5]

zoocide

Substance intended to kill animals.
[ref. 1]

zoonosis/zoonoses (pl)

Infectious *disease* that can be naturally transmitted between animals (usually vertebrates) and humans.
[*]
See also *epizootic*.

zooplanktivorous

Feeding on *zooplankton*.
[*]

Comprehensive Glossary of Terms Used in Toxicology
By John Duffus, Douglas M. Templeton and Michael Schwenk

Published by the Royal Society of Chemistry, www.rsc.org

zooplankton

Small floating or weakly swimming animals that drift with water currents and that, with *phytoplankton*, make up the planktonic (see *plankton*) food supply upon which almost all oceanic organisms ultimately depend.
[ref. 2]
See also *plankton*.

zygosis

Sexual union of two cells with fusion of their *nuclei*.
[ref. 5]

zygote (n)/zygotic (adj)

1. Cell such as a fertilized *egg* (*ovum* after *fertilization*) resulting from the fusion of two *gametes*.
2. Cell obtained as a result of complete or partial fusion of cells produced by *meiosis*.

[ref. 5]

zygote intrafallopian transfer (ZIFT)
tubal embryo transfer

Introduction of a *zygote fertilized in vitro* into one of the *Fallopian tubes*.
[ref. 5]
See also *in vitro fertilization*.
Compare *gamete intrafallopian transfer*.

zymosan

Crude preparation of yeast cell walls, consisting chiefly of polysaccharide, that activates the *alternative pathway* of the *complement system* in the presence of *properdin*, and is thus used in the *immunoassay* of properdin.
[ref. 3]

APPENDIX I

A Selection of Toxic Substances

This Appendix presents an alphabetical list of toxic substances with their various targets and modes of action. Some are specific drugs, toxins or other chemical structures, and some are more complex substances, mixtures or classes of compounds. Some information on sources, uses, mechanisms, targets, and effects is given in telegraphic style for each entry.

The format used is:

commonly used name

IUPAC name (when applicable)

sources and uses / mechanisms and actions

(PIN) denotes the Preferred IUPAC Name.
(INN) denotes the International Nonproprietary Name for a drug.

acetaminophen

paracetamol (INN)
N-(4-hydroxyphenyl)acetamide
4′-hydroxyacetanilide

analgesic / causes glutathione deficiency and at toxic doses glutathione depletion followed by liver necrosis.

2-acetylaminofluorene (2-AAF)

N-(9*H*-fluoren-2-yl)acetamide
common metabolite: *N*-(acetyloxy)-*N*-(9*H*-fluoren-2-yl)acetamide

experimental carcinogen / DNA-adduct forming agent, teratogenic in various laboratory studies.

Comprehensive Glossary of Terms Used in Toxicology
By John Duffus, Douglas M. Templeton and Michael Schwenk

Published by the Royal Society of Chemistry, www.rsc.org

acetylcholine

2-acetoxy-*N,N,N*-trimethylethanaminium

endogenous mediator / cholinergic neurotransmitter, effects increased by organophosphates and decreased by atropine.

acetylsalicylic acid

2-acetoxybenzoic acid
2-(acetyloxy)benzoic acid (PIN)

analgesic drug / prostaglandin synthesis inhibition, gastric mucosal damage.

acid anhydrides

group of industrial chemicals / reactive substances that tend to induce hypersensitivity reactions, such as dermatitis.

aconitine

8-(acetyloxy)-20-ethyl-3α,13,15α-trihydroxy-1α,6α,16β-trimethoxy-4-(methoxymethyl)-aconitan-14α-yl benzoate

monkshood plant poison / keeps neuronal sodium ion channels open, diarrhea, convulsions, arrhythmias, death.

acrylamide

prop-2-enamide

industrial monomer, cooking byproduct, food contaminant / decreased male and female fertility in experimental animals, fetotoxic but not teratogenic in experimental animals, nerve-terminal damage, peripheral and central neuropathy.

aflatoxin, aflatoxin B_1

(6a*R*,9a*S*)-4-methoxy-2,3,6a,9a-tetrahydro-4-methoxy-1*H*,11*H*-cyclopenta[*c*]furo[3′,2′:4,5]furo[2,3-*h*][1]benzopyran-1,11-dione

fungal product, food contaminant / suppression of antibody response, hepatotoxicity related to metabolic bioactivation, carcinogenic.

alcohol

See ethanol, methanol.

aldrin

(1*R*,4*S*,4a*S*,5*S*,8*R*,8a*R*)-1,2,3,4,10,10-hexachloro-1,4,4a,5,8,8a-hexahydro-1,4:5,8-dimethanonaphthalene

organochlorine pesticide (widely banned) / fetotoxic and teratogenic in experimental animals, decreased fertility in multiple species.

aluminium (Al)

metallic element / complex mechanism, speciation-dependent encephalopathy.

α-amanitin

1,8-anhydro-$C^{2.4}$,S^{8}-cyclo[L-asparaginyl-(4*R*)-4-hydroxy-L-prolyl-(4*R*)-4,5-dihydroxy-L-isoleucyl-6-hydroxy-L-tryptophylglycyl-L-isoleucyl-L-cysteine] (*R*)-*S*-oxide

plant product of ***Amanita*** mushrooms / heat-stable cyclic peptide, inhibits RNA-polymerases, accumulates in liver cells, causes liver failure.

γ-aminobutyric acid (GABA)

4-aminobutanoic acid

endogenous neurotransmitter / natural neurotransmitter at GABAergic synapse.

aminoglycosides

antibiotic drugs / accumulate in inner ear, hair cell damage, possible ototoxicity, deafness.

2-amino-3-(3-hydroxy-5-methyl-1,2-oxazol-4-yl)propanoic acid (AMPA)

agent used in experimental physiology / glutamate receptor (AMPA type) agonist, excitotoxic.

aminopterin (4-aminopteroic acid)

N-(4-{[(2,4-diaminopteridin-6-yl)methyl]amino}benzoyl)-L-glutamic acid

folic acid analog and antagonist / abortion, CNS- and craniofacial defects, growth retardation, and immunosuppressive effects.

amitriptyline (INN)

3-(10,11-dihydro-5*H*-dibenzo[*a,d*][7]annulen-5-ylidene)-*N,N*-dimethylpropan-1-amine

antidepressant drug / serotonin syndrome when given together with MAO-inhibitors

amitrole

1*H*-1,2,4-triazol-3-amine

herbicide / inhibits iodine uptake in thyroid, causes thyroid cancers in animals.

ammonia gas (NH_3)

industrial chemical, refrigerant / inhalation toxicant causing lung edema.

amphetamine

amfetamine (INN)

rac-1-phenylpropan-2-amine

therapeutic drug, drug of abuse / adrenaline analogue, central nervous stimulant, reduces hunger.

amphotericin B (INN)

(1*R*,3*S*,5*R*,6*R*,9*R*,11*R*,15*S*,16*R*,17*R*,18*S*,19*E*,21*E*,23*E*,25*E*,27*E*,29*E*,31*E*,33*R*,35*S*,36*R*,37*S*)-33-[(3-amino-3,6-dideoxy-β-D-mannopyranosyl)oxy]-1,3,5,6,9,11,17,37-octahydroxy-15,16,18-trimethyl-13-oxo-14,39-dioxabicyclo[33.3.1]nonatriaconta-19,21,23,25,27,29,31-heptaene-36-carboxylic acid

antifungal drug / kidney damage to glomerulus and nephron.

ampicillin (INN)

(2*S*,5*R*,6*R*)-6-[(2*R*)-2-amino-2-phenylacetamido]-3,3-dimethyl-7-oxo-4-thia-1-azabicyclo-[3.2.0]heptane-2-carboxylic acid

antibiotic / exanthema potentiated by ***Cytomegalovirus*** or mononucleosis infection.

amygdalin

(2*R*)-2-[(6-*O*-β-D-glucopyranosyl-β-D-glucopyranosyl)oxy]-2-phenyl-2-acetonitrile

glycoside in bitter almonds / glycosidases of intestinal bacteria release cyanide, inhibition of mitochondrial respiration.

angel dust

See phencyclidene (INN).

angiotensin converting enzyme (ACE) inhibitors

e.g. enalapril (INN), *N*-{*N*-[(1*S*)-1-(ethoxycarbonyl)-3-phenylpropyl]-L-alanyl}-L-proline
hypotensive drugs / fetal organ failures associated with hypotensive effect.

aniline

benzenamine
solvent and intermediate / may induce methemoglobinemia in the fetus, formerly considered a bladder carcinogen.

anti-androgens

hormone-active drugs and endocrine disrupters / disruption of sexual differentiation in various species.

anti-HIV drugs

therapeutic drugs / interaction with the cell cycle.

anticonvulsants

antiepileptic drugs / possible risks of developmental mental retardation and other growth abnormalities.

antihistamine, histamine H1 receptor antagonist

class of immunomodulating drugs / blocks a histamine receptor on cell surfaces, suppresses the effects of immunoglobulin E-induced histamine release from mast cells in allergy and inflammation.

antimycin A

fungal product from ***Streptomyces*** / inhibits electron transfer in mitochondrial electron transport chain.

antineoplastics

anticancer and antitumor drugs / interfere with DNA and cell cycle, possibly producing neoplasms and various reprotoxic effects.

arsenic (As)

semimetal element, geogenic contaminant of some drinking water and seafood / effects depend on the chemical species and condition, include immunostimulation or suppression, spontaneous abortion, stillbirth, carcinogenesis.

arsine (AsH_3)

arsane
hydrogen arsenide
arsenic trihydride
industrial gas, formerly chemical weapon / lethal at low dose, hemolytic.

asbestos

construction material, isolator / established lung carcinogen, characteristically producing mesothelioma.

ascomycin

immunomycin
FK 520
(3*S*,4*R*,5*S*,8*R*,9*E*,12*S*,14*S*,15*R*,16*S*,18*R*,19*R*,26a*S*)-8-ethyl-5,19-dihydroxy-3-{(1*E*)-2-[(1*R*, 3*R*,4*R*)-4-hydroxy-3-methoxycyclohexyl]-1-methylvinyl}-14,16-dimethoxy-4,10,12,18-tetramethyl-5,6,8,11,12,13,14,15,16,17,18,19,24,25,26,26a-hexadecahydro-3*H*-15,19-epoxypyrido[2,1-*c*][1,4]oxaazacyclotricosine-1,7,20,21(4*H*,23*H*)-tetrone

ethyl analogue of tacrolimus / inhibits degranulation of mast cells.

atropine

rac-8-methyl-8-azabicyclo[3.2.1]octan-3-yl-3-hydroxy-2-phenylpropanoate

poison of deadly nightshade, therapeutic drug / muscarinic acetylcholine receptor antagonist.

azathioprine (INN)

6-[(1-methyl-4-nitro-1*H*-imidazol-5-yl)sulfanyl]-7*H*-purine

immunomodulating drug / prodrug that is metabolized to an active species (purine-6-thiol), suppresses autoimmune reactions.

azidothymidine (AZT)

3′-azido-3′-deoxythymidine
ziduvudine (INN)
1-[(2*R*,4*S*,5*S*)-4-azido-5-(hydroxymethyl)oxolan-2-yl]-5-methylpyrimidine-2,4(1*H*,3*H*)- dione

antiviral drug / thymidine analogue, inhibits reverse transcriptase of human immunodeficiency virus.

barbiturates

e.g., phenobarbital (INN), 5-ethyl-5-phenyl-1,3-diazinane-2,4,6-trione

sedative drugs / GABA-A receptor modulators, causing sedation, sleep, anesthesia, coma.

barium (Ba)

metallic element, barium sulfate in medical contrast agents (virtually insoluble) / soluble salts block ion channels, causes cardiac arrhythmias.

batrachotoxin

family of toxic steroids of frogs, arrow poison / inactivator of sodium channels, cardiotoxic, neurotoxic.

benzene

industrial chemical / acutely narcotic, chronic exposure causes bone marrow cancer.

benzo[*a*]pyrene

benzo[*pqr*]tetraphene (PIN)

product of incomplete combustion / carcinogenic reactive metabolites, inducer of monoxygenase enzymes.

benzodiazepines

e.g., diazepam (INN)
7-chloro-1-methyl-5-phenyl-1,3-dihydro-2*H*-1,4-benzodiazepin-2-one

sedative drugs / GABA-A receptor modulators, inducers of sedation, anesthetics.

beryllium (Be)

metallic element, workplace exposure / speciation- and dose-dependent inducer of "chronic beryllium disease", a severe hypersensitivity of the airways; carcinogen.

bis(chloromethyl) ether

chloro(chloromethoxy)methane

formerly used as crosslinking agent / carcinogen.

bisphenol A

4,4′-(propane-2,2-diyl)diphenol

plasticizer / estrogen receptor-associated immune effects, fetotoxicity.

bongkrekic acid

(2*E*,4*Z*,6*R*,8*Z*,10*E*,14*E*,17*S*,18*E*,20*Z*)-20-(carboxymethyl)-6-methoxy-2,5,17-trimethyldocosa-2,4,8,10,14,18,20-heptaenedioic acid

food-borne bacterial product / inhibits mitochondrial ADP/ATP translocation and thus mitochondrial phosphorylation.

botulinum toxin

food-born protein toxin produced by ***Clostridium botulinum*** / powerful blocker of synaptic acetylcholine-release, muscle relaxing, paralytic.

brevetoxins

family of sea algae products / neurotoxic, affecting sodium channels.

bromoacetone

1-bromopropan-2-one

incapacitating agent ('tear gas') / mucosal irritation, neurogenic inflammation, lachrymation.

bromocriptine (INN)

2-bromo-12′-hydroxy-5′α-(2-methylpropyl)-2′-(propan-2-yl)ergotaman-3′,6′,18-trione

antiparkinson drug / dopamine-D2-agonist, may cause psychosis, dyskinesia.

bungarotoxins

snake venom proteins, used in experimental physiology / nicotinic acetylcholine receptor antagonists causing paralysis and respiratory failure.

busulfan (INN)

butane-1,4-diyl dimethanesulfonate

chemotherapeutic drug / alkylating agent, teratogenic, embryotoxic, fetotoxic, carcinogenic.

cadmium (Cd)

metallic element of both occupational and environmental importance / zinc-antagonistic, calcium-agonist, causing speciation-dependent suppressive effects, nephrotoxic, carcinogen, associated with placental necrosis.

caffeine

1,3,7-trimethyl-3,7-dihydro-1*H*-purine-2,6-dione

plant product, consumer good / CNS-stimulant, possible non-human teratogen.

cannabis, marijuana

See tetrahydrocannabinol.

capsaicin

(6*E*)-*N*-(4-hydroxy-3-methoxybenzyl)-8-methylnon-6-enamide

plant product, spice, topical analgesic / irritates, depletes nerve endings of neurotransmitter, causes neurogenic inflammation.

carbamates

insecticides / reversible acetylcholinesterase inhibition, symptoms of organophosphate poisoning.

carbamazepine

5*H*-dibenzo[*b*, *f*]azepine-5-carboxamide

antiepileptic drug / delayed-type hypersensitivity, including Stevens-Johnson syndrome, possible developmental disorders and risk of spina bifida.

carbaryl

1-naphthyl methylcarbamate

carbamate insecticide / inhibition of acetylcholinesterase in insects, much less in humans; possible alterations of immunoglobulin levels.

carbimazole (INN)

ethyl-3-methyl-2-thioxo-2,3-dihydro-1*H*-imidazole-1-carboxylate

thyroxin antagonistic drug / associated with risk of fetal hypothyroidism.

carbon dioxide (CO_2)

product of oxidative metabolism and combustion / narcotic agent, loss of consciousness, malformations in the offspring of experimental animals, male reproductive effects in experimental animals.

carbon disulfide (CS_2)

organic solvent / neurotoxic, associated with spontaneous abortion, premature birth.

carbon monoxide (endogenous) (CO)

cerebral gasotransmitter / natural neurotransmitter.

carbon monoxide (environmental) (CO)

incomplete combustion product / blocks hemoglobin oxygen-binding causing insufficient oxygen supply, unconsciousness, and death; possible chronic neural effects and neuropathological effects in offspring.

carbon tetrachloride (CCl_4)

organic solvent / reactive metabolites, hepatoxic, embryo- and fetotoxic.

carbonyl cyanide m-chlorophenyl hydrazone (CCCP)

[(3-chlorophenyl)hydrazinylidene]propanedinitrile

experimental agent / proton ionophore at the mitochondrial membrane, uncoupler, blocks ATP-formation.

chlorambucil (INN)

4-{4-[bis(2-chlorethyl)amino]phenyl}butanoic acid

chemotherapeutic drug / alkylating agent, cytotoxic, immunotoxic, fetotoxic.

chlorinated solvents

solvents (many are obsolete) / brain depression, substance-dependent organotoxicities, often related to biotransformation.

chlorination by-products

reaction products of chlorine with organic components in chlorinated water / some are irritants, some are mutagenic.

chlorine gas (Cl_2)

diatomic form of chemical element / inhalation causes serious or fatal lung edema.

2-chloroacetophenone

2-chloro-1-phenylethan-1-one

riot control agent / disabling tear gas having a sharp odor.

2-chloro-*N*-(2-chloroethyl)-*N*-methylethan-1-amine

anticancer drug, mustard / alkylating agent causing contact irritation, organ-failure, cancer.

chlorofluorocarbons

class of refrigerants / relevant in ecotoxicology, involved in gradual disappearance of the ozone layer.

chloroform ($CHCl_3$)

trichloromethane

organic solvent, anesthetic / causes brain depression, placental necrosis in experimental animals.

chlorohydrin

3-chloropropane-1,2-diol

industrial intermediate, food contaminant / irritant, pulmonary edema, various organ toxicities, adverse effects on male sperm production, potential chemosterilizer.

chlorotoxin

peptide toxin of the scorpion / chloride channel blocker causing muscle convulsions.

cholera toxin

exotoxin of cholera bacteria / opens ion-channels in colon epithelial cells, causes diarrhea and extreme water-loss.

chromium (Cr), chromium(II) chloride, chromium(III) chloride, chromium(VI) oxide (chromium trioxide)

industrial substances, environmental pollutants / speciation-dependent effects such as birth defects and fertility problems in experimental animals, hypersensitivity (*e.g.* chromium eczema), and carcinogenesis.

ciclosporin (INN)

cyclosporine
cyclosporin A
(3*S*,6*S*,9*S*,12*R*,15*S*,18*S*,21*S*,24*S*,30*S*,33*S*)-30-ethyl-33-[(1*R*,2*R*,4*E*)-1-hydroxy-2-methyl-hex-4-en-1-yl]-6,9,18,24-tetrakis(2-methylpropyl)-3,21-di(propan-2-yl)-1,4,7,10,12,15,19,25,28-nonamethyl-1,4,7,10,13,16,19,22,25,28,31-undecaazacyclotritriacontane-2,5,8,11,14,17,20,23,26,29,32-undecone

cyclic peptide from mold, immunosuppressive drug / T-cell-specific agent that binds to cyclophillin, inhibiting the production of IL-2, used to prevent graft rejection and treat some autoimmune diseases.

cigarette smoke (active)

active smoking / acute effects involve mucosal irritation and nicotinic neuronal effects; chronic smoking causes cardiovascular and pulmonary disorders, cancer of lungs and other organs.

cobalt (Co)

metallic element, ionic species in food and water, essential human nutrient / deficiency may cause a deficiency of vitamin B12 (cobalamin), essential for production of red blood cells and for normal nerve and brain function; speciation-dependent toxic effects include cardiomyopathy, tinnitus and deafness, thyroid problems, increased viscosity of the blood, and allergic contact dermatitis.

cocaine

methyl (1*R*,2*R*,3*S*,5*S*)-3-(benzoyloxy)-8-methyl-8-azabicyclo[3.2.1]octane-2-carboxylate

alkaloid of coca plant, recreational drug / reuptake-(noradrenalin, serotonin, dopamine) blocker leading to heightened awareness, local anesthesia, and in embryos possible mental retardation and withdrawal symptoms after birth.

colchicine

N-[(7*S*)-1,2,3,10-tetramethoxy-9-oxo-5,6,7,9-tetrahydrobenzo[*a*]heptalen-7-yl]acetamide

plant product, anti-gout drug / inhibitor of mitotic spindle formation, cell poison, teratogenic in mice, causes peripheral neuropathy.

concanavalin A

carbohydrate-binding protein (lectin) in Jack bean; experimental mitogen / like other lectins it binds to glycoproteins on cell surfaces, inducing physiological reactions at low doses and toxicity at high doses.

copper ions

metallic elemental species in food and water, essential human nutrient / deficiency is rare but can lead to myeloneuropathy and severe blood disorders; toxic effects include gastro-intestinal problems, tissue damage, hypotension, jaundice and coma, and underlie the pathogenesis of Wilson disease; highly toxic to dogs, may also be highly toxic to fish and other aquatic organisms, including algae.

corticoids

hormones and therapeutic drugs / support maturation of lungs in fetus, many effects on metabolism, immune reactions and stress.

croton oil

plant product containing phorbol, used to study pain, anti-irritation agents and carcinogenesis / causes painful skin and mucosa irritation, tumor promoter and cocarcinogen.

See also phorbol.

curare

(*e.g.*, tubocurarine)

7′,12′-dihydroxy-6,6′-dimethoxy-2,2,2′,2′-tetramethyltubocuraran-2,2′-diium

plant-derived poison, muscle relaxant / nicotinic acetylcholine receptor antagonist, causing flaccid muscle paralysis.

cyanotoxin

group of toxins (cyclic peptides, alkaloids, and others) of blue-green algae / hepatoxic, irritant, and neurotoxic, depending on algal species and exposure route.

cycasin

[(*E*)-methyl-*ONN*-azoxy]methyl β-D-glucopyranoside

cycad plant product / metabolized to reactive intermediates that are carcinogenic and neurotoxic.

cyclophosphamide (INN)

rac-2-[bis(2-chloroethyl)amino]-2λ^5-1,3,2-oxazaphosphinan-2-one

anticancer drug / alkylating agent with immunosuppressive features, used to treat some autoimmune diseases and as an experimental teratogen.

DDT

See 1,1,1-trichloro-2,2-bis(4-chlorophenyl)ethane

dendrotoxin

poison of the mamba snake / potassium channel blocker, leading to muscle convulsions.

2′-deoxycoformycin

See pentostatin.

dexamethasone (INN)

9-fluoro-11β,17,21-trihydroxy-16α-methylpregna-1,4-diene-3,20-dione

synthetic cortisol-related drug / relieves inflammation and inflammation-caused diseases, suppresses bone growth and repair, has many more side effects.

diazepam (INN)

7-chloro-1-methyl-5-phenyl-3*H*-1,4-benzodiazepin-2-one

sedative drug / modulator of GABA-receptor sensitivity, anesthetic, may cause dependency; during development may cause cleft lip and (or) cleft palate.

dibromochloropropane (DBCP)

1,2-dibromo-3-chloropropane

soil fumigant / testicular toxicant.

dichloroethyl sulfide

sulfur mustard

1-chloro-2-[(2-chloroethyl)sulfanyl]ethane

chemical warfare agent / nonspecific tissue destroying toxicant, blister-forming.

dichlorvos

2,2-dichlorovinyl dimethyl phosphate

2,2-dichloroethenyl dimethyl phosphate (PIN)

organophosphorus insecticide / teratogenic in pigs.

diclofenac (INN)

2-[(2,6-dichloroanilino)phenyl]acetic acid

antiinflammatory drug / prostaglandin synthetase inhibitor, often inducing gastric ulcers during chronic intake.

dieldrin

(1*R*,2*S*,3*S*,6*R*,7*R*,8*S*,9*S*,11*R*)-3,4,5,6,13,13-hexachloro-10-oxapentacyclo-[6.3.1.1^{3,6}.0^{2,7}.0^{9,11}]tridec-4-ene

{(1a*R*,2*R*,2a*S*,3*S*,6*R*,6a*R*,7*S*,7a*S*)-3,4,5,6,9,9-hexachloro-1a,2,2a,3,6,6a,7,7a-octahydro-2,7:3,6-dimethanonaphtho[2,3-*b*]oxirene}

organochlorine insecticide / reproductive and developmental effects in experimental animals.

diethyl ether

ethoxyethane

inhalation anesthetic / membrane destabilization, anesthesia.

di(2-ethylhexyl) phthalate

bis(2-ethylhexyl) phthalate

See phthalates.

diethylstilbestrol (DES)

4,4′-[(3*E*)-hex-3-ene-3,4-diyl]diphenol

synthetic estrogen / treatment of a pregnant woman with DES during the first trimester of pregnancy can cause clear cell adenocarcinoma of the vagina in her daughter at maturity.

dinitrotoluene

1-methyl-2,4-dinitrobenzene

organic chemical / methemoglobinemia in the fetus, male reproductive effects.

dinoseb

rac-2-butan-2-yl-4,6-dinitrophenol

herbicide / embryotoxic, may induce methemoglobinemia in experimental animals.

diphenylhydantoin

See phenytoin.

domoic acid

(2*S*,3*S*,4*S*)-4-[(2*Z*,4*E*,6*R*)-6-carboxyhepta-2,4-dien-2-yl]-3-(carboxymethyl)pyrrolidine-2-carboxylic acid

accumulates in shellfish that ingest red algae / the neurotoxic kainic acid analogue causes amnesic shellfish poisoning in a subsequent human consumer of the shellfish.

domperidone (INN)

5-chloro-1-{1-[3-(2-oxo-2,3-dihydro-1*H*-benzimidazol-1-yl)propyl]piperidin-4-yl}-1,3-dihydro-2*H*-benzimidazol-2-one

antinauseant / dopamine antagonist causing disorientation and dizziness.

dopamine (INN)

4-(2-aminoethyl)benzene-1,2-diol

endogenous neurotransmitter / when injected activates the cardiovascular system, counteracting low blood pressure.

drug of abuse

any recreational, often illegal and addictive drug / multiple neuropsychiatric effects, dependency, effects on sexual behavior and reproduction.

ecstasy

See 3,4-(methylenedioxy)methamphetamine.

enalapril (INN)

See angiotensin converting enzyme (ACE) inhibitors.

endocannabinoid

endogenous, lipid-derived neurotransmitter and mediator / released from the postsynaptic membrane, inhibits neurotransmission at the presynaptic membrane, decreases appetite.

endocrine disruptor

umbrella term for substances that disturb normal hormone activity / may induce hormonal imbalance, notably in the reproductive system.

endorphin

endogenous mediator / neuromodulator involved in pain reduction, mood improvement, and motility.

endosulfan

(5a*R*,6*S*,9*R*,9a*S*)-6,7,8,9,10,10-hexachloro-1,5,5a,6,9,9a-hexahydro-6,9-methano-2,4,3λ^4-benzodioxathiepin-3-one

organochlorine pesticide / effects on the reproductive systems of experimental animals.

endotoxin

bacterial lipopolysaccharide / pyrogenic substances, evoking a wide range of immune reactions and apoptosis and shock.

enkephalin

(*e.g.*, Met-enkephalin, Tyr-Gly-Gly-Phe-Met)
(*e.g.*, Leu-enkephalin, Tyr-Gly-Gly-Phe-Leu)

endogenous mediator / neuromodulator involved in pain reduction and mood improvement.

enzymes, proteolytic

class of enzymes / proteins that, when airborne, have the potential, like any other proteins, to cause hypersensitivity reactions (such as conjunctivitis, rhinitis, or asthma), but may cause additional tissue damage due to proteolysis.

ephedrine

rel-(1*R*,2*S*)-2-(methylamino)-1-phenylpropan-1-ol

natural plant product and drug / sympathomimetic effects in the periphery and brain.

epichlorohydrin

2-(chloromethyl)oxirane

industrial chemical / male reproductive toxicity seen in experimental animals.

ergotamine (INN)

(6a*R*,9*R*)-*N*-((2*R*,5*S*,10a*S*,10b*S*)-5-benzyl-10b-hydroxy-2-methyl-3,6-dioxooctahydro-2*H*-[1,3]oxazolo[3,2-*a*] pyrrolo[2,1-*c*]pyrazin-2-yl)-7-methyl-4,6,6a,7,8,9-hexahydroindolo[4,3-*fg*] quinoline-9-carboxamide)

ergot fungus alkaloid / interacts with neurotransmission of serotonin, epinephrine and dopamine, causing hallucination and vasoconstriction.

ethanol

recreational beverage, drug of addiction / acute: drunkenness, chronic: peripheral neuropathy, brain damage (neuronal loss), hepato- and cardiotoxicity, cancer in various organs, fetal alcohol syndrome associated with birth defects and cognitive deficits. therapeutic: antidote of methanol intoxication.

ethidium bromide

3,8-diamino-5-ethyl-6-phenylphenanthridin-6-ium bromide

agent used in DNA-research / DNA-intercalating agent, mutagenesis, cancer.

ethyl methyl ketone

butan-2-one

(often incorrectly called methy ethyl ketone (MEK))

solvent / potentiation of solvent neurotoxicity.

ethylene glycol

ethane-1,2-diol

antifreeze agent, wine adulterant / sweet tasting substance, metabolized to oxalic acid, neurotoxic, nephrotoxic.

ethylene oxide

oxirane industrial chemical / alkylating agent, irritant, mutagen.

ethylene thiourea

imidazolidine-2-thione

industrial chemical / teratogenic in rats.

ethylnitrosourea

N-ethyl-*N*-nitrosourea

alkylating agent / mutagenic, fetotoxic, teratogenic due to alkylation of DNA; also mutagenic and teratogenic in sperm stem cells.

etretinate (INN)

ethyl (2*E*,4*E*,6*E*,8*E*)-9-(4-methoxy-2,3,6-trimethylphenyl)-3,7-dimethylnona-2,4,6,8-tetraenoate

anti-psoriasis drug / teratogenic (see also vitamin A).

fentanyl (INN)

N-phenyl-*N*-[1-(2-phenylethyl)piperidin-4-yl]propanamide

opioid, used in anesthesia, misused as recreational drug, benzodiazepine antidote / pain relief, anesthesia, sedative, causes respiratory suppression.

filgrastim

synthetic protein / immunostimulating analogue of granulocyte colony-stimulating factor (G-CSF) pharmacologically used to stimulate the proliferation and differentiation of granulocytes.

fingolimod

FTY720
2-amino-2-[2-(4-octylphenyl)ethyl]propane-1,3-diol

sphingosine-1-phosphate analog, derived from the fungal product myriocin ((2*S*,3*R*,4*R*,6*E*)-2-amino-3,4-dihydroxy-2-(hydroxymethyl)-14-oxoicos-6-enoic acid) / inhibits migration of lymphocytes and dendritic cells.

FK-506

See tacrolimus.

flumazenil (INN)

ethyl 8-fluoro-5-methyl-6-oxo-5,6-dihydro-4*H*-imidazo[1,5-*a*][1,4]benzodiazepine-3-carboxylate

therapeutic benzodiazepine antagonist / GABA-A receptor antagonist, used to terminate benzodiazepine-action. Has various side effects such as anxiety.

flunarizine (INN)

1-[bis(4-fluorophenyl)methyl]-4-[(2*E*)-3-phenylprop-2-en-1-yl]piperazine

drug against headache / calcium-channel blocking agent, symptoms of depression and of parkinsonism.

5-fluorouracil

chemotherapeutic drug, experimental teratogen / embryotoxic, teratogenic.

folic acid

(2*S*)-2-[(4-{[(2-amino-4-hydroxypteridin-6-yl)methyl]amino}benzoyl)amino]pentanedioic acid

essential nutrient / deficiency leads to various types of malformations, neural tube defects, possible effects on sperm.

See also aminopterin

formaldehyde (CH_2O)

Industrial chemical, emissions from polyurethane cause indoor exposures / highly reactive substance which is an allergen in humans and can potentiate the allergenic effect of other substances, carcinogen.

gluten

wheat protein component / (auto)immunological reactions in sensitive persons induce intestinal mucosal damage, diarrhea and malnutrition.

glyphosate

N-(phosphonomethyl)glycine

widely used herbicide / controversially suspected carcinogen.

haloperidol (INN)

4-[4-(4-chlorophenyl)-4-hydroxypiperidin-1-yl]-1-(4-fluorophenyl)-butan-1-one

drug to treat schizophrenia / antagonist of dopamine and other neurotransmitters, depresses, may cause Parkinson-like symptoms.

halothane (INN)

2-bromo-2-chloro-1,1,1-trifluoroethane

inhalation anesthetic drug / may cause autoimmune and allergic hepatitis due to formation of neoantigen. Developmental delay and behavioral abnormalities in offspring.

heroin

morphine diacetate

17-methyl-4,5α-epoxymorphin-7-en-3,6α-diyl diacetate

drug of abuse / endorphin agonist with strong euphoric action and rapid onset of dependency.

hexachlorobenzene

fungicide, disinfectant / various unspecific organ toxicities, increased mass of lymphatic organs and various other immunotoxic effects in rodents.

hexane

solvent / metabolite hexane-2,5-dione is neurotoxic crosslinker, causing polyneuropathy.

histamine

2-(1*H*-imidazol-4-yl)ethanamine

endogenous mediator / vasoactive paracrine mediator, modulator of neurotransmission involved in pain, headache, anaphylaxis, gastric acid production.

hydralazine

(phthalazin-1-yl)hydrazine

antihypertensive drug / may cause autoimmunity, manifested as systemic lupus erythematosus-like syndrome, teratogenic in mice.

hydrazine ($H_2N\text{-}NH_2$)

industrial chemical, rocket fuel / irritant, toxic to many organs, carcinogen.

hydrogen cyanide (HCN)

industrial chemical, component of some plant seed glycosides / inhibits mitochondrial cytochrome c oxidase and thus blocks cellular respiration.

hydrogen fluoride (HF)

industrial chemical / on contacting moist tissue, rapidly converted to hydrofluoric acid that immediately destroys the tissue. Highly corrosive, toxic, and lethal.

hydrogen sulfide (H_2S)

endogenous mediator, emitted from gas wells / endogenous: neuro(gaso)-transmitter. environmental: inhibition of mitochondrial respiration, nausea, and apnea.

γ-hydroxybutyric acid (GHB)

4-hydroxybutanoic acid

therapeutic drug, general anaesthetic, drug of abuse / natural neurotransmitter at GHB-receptors, partial antagonist at GABA-A receptors, causing depression, anesthesia and amnesia.

ibuprofen (INN)

(2*RS*)-2-[4-(2-methylpropyl)phenyl]propanoic acid
See nonsteroidal antiinflammatory drugs.

immunocyanin

Drug derived from keyhole limpet hemocyanin (KLH) / immunostimulating.

indomethacin

indometacin (INN)
[1-(4-chlorobenzoyl)-5-methoxy-2-methyl-1*H*-indol-3-yl]acetic acid

nonsteroidal anti-inflammatory drug (NSAID) / inhibits prostaglandin synthesis, risk of gastric ulcer formation, risk of premature closure of ductus arteriosus, malformations and neonatal complications.

indoor smoke

open indoor fireplaces, passive smoking / risk of asthma, eye irritation and respiratory disease.

iodide (I^-)

essential nutrient / deficiency leads to goiter and cretinism, may provoke hypersensitivity.

isoflurane

rac-2-chloro-2-(difluoromethoxy)-1,1,1-trifluoroethane

inhalation anesthetic / anesthetic and muscle relaxant.

isotretinoin (INN)

13-*cis*-retinoic acid
(2*Z*,4*E*,6*E*,8*E*)-3,7-dimethyl-9-(2,6,6-trimethylcyclohex-1-enyl)nona-2,4,6,8-tetraenoic acid

drug used in treating acne / developmental toxicant, craniofacial, ear and cardiovascular malformations, intellectual deficits.

kainic acid

(2*S*,3*S*,4*S*)-3-(carboxymethyl)-4-(prop-1-en-2-yl)pyrrolidine-2-carboxylic acid

drug in experimental neurophysiology / glutamate (kainate) receptor agonist, excitotoxic.

kepone, chlordecone

1,2,3,4,6,7,8,9,10,10-decachloropentacyclo[5.3.0.$0^{2,6}$.$0^{3,9}$.$0^{4,8}$]decan-5-one

organochlorine insecticide (internationally banned) / depressed sperm count and motility, ecotoxic, appears in milk.

ketamine

(*RS*)-2-(2-chlorophenyl)-2-(methylamino)cyclohexanone

injection anesthetic / glutamate NMDA receptor antagonist.

keyhole limpet hemocyanin (KLH)

immunomodulating / large (8 to 32 MDa) multisubunit oxygen-transporting mollusc protein, used to stimulate immune response (cellular and humoral), also used as a carrier protein for haptens and in immunotherapy of bladder cancer. Smaller subunits are also used (*e.g.*, immunocyanin).

kolokol-1

incapacitating mixture, structure not revealed, potential chemical warfare agent / volatile mixture of endorphin agonist + anesthetic drug, induces unconsciousness.

lead (Pb)

metallic element, environmental contaminant / depending on its speciation, it is immunosuppressive and decreases resistance to infections in rodents: causes developmental neurotoxicity, abortion, growth retardation, and neurobehavioral deficits.

lectin

plant product *e.g.*, of beans / umbrella term for a class of glycoproteins that bind to sugar moieties of cell surfaces, potentially inducing harmful signals and cell death.

lidocaine (INN)

2-(diethylamino)-*N*-(2,6-dimethylphenyl)acetamide
2-(diethylamino)-2′,6′-dimethylacetanilide

local anesthetic / sodium channel blocker, inhibiting neuronal excitation and its propagation.

limonene

4-isopropenyl-1-methylcyclohexene

natural monoterpene in wood, slowly evaporating from indoor timber / allergen, causing sensitization in sensitive individuals.

lithium (Li) salts

antidepressant drug / associated with risk of malformations, notably of the heart (Epstein's anomaly).

lysergic acid diethylamide (LSD)

lysergide (INN)
N,N-diethyl-6-methyl-9,10-didehydroergoline-8β-carboxamide
(6a*R*,9*R*)-*N,N*-diethyl-7-methyl-4,6,6a,7,8,9-hexahydroindolo[4,3-*fg*]quinoline-9-carboxamide

drug of abuse / NMDA receptor antagonist, induces psychedelic experiences.

malathion

diethyl 2-[(dimethoxyphosphorothioyl)sulfanyl]succinate

organophosphate pesticide / neurotoxic insecticide exhibiting both immunosuppressive and immunoenhancing effects, effects on development and reproduction in several species of experimental animals.

manganese (Mn)

metallic element, occupational exposure / manganism, disease due to chronic manganese exposure, associated with mood changes and neurotoxicity, mechanism unresolved, speciation-dependent.

melamine

1,3,5-triazine-2,4,6-triamine

component of melamine resin, nitrogen-rich illegal milk adulterant / urinary calculi, unspecific disorders.

melatonin

N-[2-(5-methoxy-1*H*-indol-3-yl)ethyl]acetamide

hormone regulating circadian rhythm, anti jet-lag drug / possible gastrointestinal upset, headaches and dizziness when taken as a drug.

mepyramine (INN)

N^1-(4-methoxybenzyl)-N^2,N^2-dimethyl-N^1-(pyridin-2-yl)ethane-1,2-diamine

drug for relief of allergy symptoms / histamine H1 receptor antagonist, drowsiness.

mercury (Hg) (elemental form, inorganic compounds, and organomercury compounds)

metallic element used in industry and gold refining; organic mercury compounds are seafood pollutants; thimerosal [thiomersal; sodium ethyl(2-sulfido-κ*S*-benzoato)mercurate(1−)] is a preservative in vaccines; occurs in dental amalgams / speciation-dependent toxicity: chronic inhalation of mercury vapor causes tremor, personality disorder; mercury chloride induces autoantibodies and autoimmune disease in sensitive rat strains, immunosuppressive; methylmercury is highly toxic and lethal, teratogenic, and a developmental neurotoxicant.

mescaline

2-(3,4,5-trimethoxyphenyl)ethan-1-amine

product of peyote cactus / serotonin-agonist, hallucinations.

methamphetamine

metamfetamine (INN)
methylamphetamine
N-methyl-1-phenylpropan-2-amine

stimulant, drug of abuse, therapeutic drug, adrenalin analogue / central stimulation, increased energy and attentiveness, decreased hunger.

methane (CH_4)

formed by gastrointestinal bacteria in all mammals and in very large amounts in cattle / ecologically important as a "greenhouse gas".

methanol (CH_3OH)

possible side product of ethanol fermentation / after intake and oxidation to formic acid causes acidosis; damages the central nervous system and can cause blindness, coma and death.

methimazole

thiamazole (INN)
1-methyl-1*H*-imidazole-2-thiol
antithyroid drug / prematurity, intrauterine growth retardation, craniostenosis, cardiac failure, fetal hydrops, and intrauterine death.

methotrexate (MTX) (INN)

4-amino-10-methyl-4-deoxyfolic acid
N-(4-{[(2,4-diaminopteridin-6-yl)methyl](methyl)amino}benzoyl)-L-glutamic acid
antimetabolite and antifolate drug used in treatment of cancer and autoimmune diseases / abortifacient, teratogen, adversely affects male and female fertility, immunomodulator.

methoxsalen

See xanthotoxin.

methoxychlor

1,1′-(2,2,2-trichloro-1,1-diyl)bis(4-methoxybenzene)
organochlorine insecticide / male and female reproductive toxicity and developmental toxicity demonstrated in experimental animals.

methoxyethanol

organic solvent / causes low sperm count (oligospermia), teratogenic.

β-methylamino-L-alanine

(2*S*)-2-amino-3-(methylamino)propanoic acid
neurotoxin of bacteria and cycad plants / glutamate receptor excitotoxin, incorporation into proteins causes misfoldings, ALS-PDC disease.

N-methyl-D-aspartate (NMDA)

used in experimental neurophysiology / glutamate (NMDA) receptor agonist, excitoxic.

3-methylcholanthrene

3-methyl-1,2-dihydrocyclopenta[*ij*]tetraphene
experimental substance / activates aryl-hydrocarbon receptor, mutagenic, carcinogenic, reprotoxic.

methyldopa (INN)

α-methyldopa
(2*S*)-2-amino-3-(3,4-dihydroxyphenyl)-2-methylpropanoic acid
hypotensive drug / autoimmune reactions, hemolytic anemia and autoimmune hepatitis.

methylene blue

3,7-bis(dimethylamino)-5λ^4-phenothiazin-5-ylium chloride
dye, antidote in aniline poisoning / teratogenic, neurotoxic.

methylene chloride (CH_2Cl_2)

dichlormethane
organic solvent / unspecific neurotoxic signs, spontaneous abortion, low birth weight.

3,4-(methylenedioxy)methamphetamine (MDMA)

"ecstasy"
rac-1-(1,3-benzodioxol-5-yl)-*N*-methylpropan-2-amine
drug of abuse / releases serotonin, epinephrine and dopamine at brain synapses, heightens awareness and euphoria.

methylethylketone (MEK)

See ethyl methyl ketone.

N-methylformamide

chemical intermediate / teratogenic in several animal species.

methylmercury

See mercury.

N-methylpyrrolidone

1-methylpyrrolidin-2-one

solvent / fetotoxic and teratogenic in mice and rats at high doses.

methysergide (INN)

N-[(2*S*)-1-hydroxybutan-2-yl]-1,6-dimethyl-9,10-didehydroergoline-8b-carboxamide(6a*R*, 9*R*)-*N*-[(2*S*)-1-hydroxybutan-2-yl]-4,7-dimethyl-4,6,6a,7,8,9-hexahydroindolo[4,3-*fg*]quinoline-9-carboxamide

anti-headache drug / serotonin antagonist (partial), associated with cardiac valve dysfunction.

misoprostol (INN)

rac-methyl (13*E*)-11a,16-dihydroxy-16-methyl-9-oxoprost-13-en-1-oatemethyl *rac*-7-{(1*R*,2*R*, 3*R*)-3-hydroxy-2-[(1*E*,4*RS*)-4-hydroxy-4-methyloct-1-enyl]-5-oxocyclopentyl}heptanoate

synthetic prostaglandin drug / abortifacient, limb and neural tube defects.

mitomycin C

mitomycin (INN)

(4*S*,6*S*,7*R*,8*S*)-11-amino-7-methoxy-12-methyl-10,13-dioxo-2,5-diazatetracyclo[7.4.0.0^{2,7}.0^{4,6}]-trideca-1(9),11-dien-8-yl]methyl carbamate[(1a*S*,8*S*,8a*R*,8b*S*)-6-amino-8a-methoxy-5-methyl-4,7-dioxo-1,1a,2,4,7,8,8a,8b-octahydroazirino[2′,3′:3,4]pyrrolo[1,2-*a*]indol-8-yl]methyl carbamate

antibiotic, anti-tumor agent / may cause pancytopenia.

monoamineoxidase (MAO) inhibitors

antidepressant drugs / decreased degradation of ingested monoamines (*e.g.* tyramine) may cause high blood pressure and toxicities.

morphine

17-methyl-4,5α-epoxymorphin-7-en-3,6α-diol(4*R*,4a*R*,7*S*,7a*R*,12b*S*)-3-methyl-2,3,4,4a,7, 7a-hexahydro-1*H*-4,12-methanobenzofuro[3,2-*e*]isoquinoline-7,9-diol

analgesic drug / endorphin agonist, relieves pain, suppresses respiration.

MPPP

See MPTP

MPTP

1-methyl-4-phenyl-1,2,3,6-tetrahydropyridine

agent in experimental neurophysiology, contaminant from illicit synthesis of the opioid drug MPPP (1-methyl-4-phenylpiperidin-4-yl propanoate) / neurotoxin, destroys mitochondria in dopaminergic brain cells, causes parkinsonism.

muscarine

2,5-anhydro-1,4,6-trideoxy-6-(trimethylammonio)-D-*ribo*-hexitol

poison in ***Amanita muscaria*** mushrooms / agonist of muscarinic acetylcholine receptors, causes hallucinations.

muscimol

5-(aminomethyl)-1,2-oxazol-3-ol

poison in ***Amanita muscaria*** mushrooms / GABA-A agonist, causes hallucinations.

mustards, mustard gas

sulfur mustard
1-chloro-2-[(2-chloroethyl)sulfanyl]ethane)

chemical warfare agent / cytotoxic, vesicant.

See also dichloroethyl sulfide; 2-chloro-*N*-(2-chloroethyl)-*N*-methylethan-1-amine.

mycophenolate

(6*E*)-6-(4-hydroxy-6-methoxy-7-methyl-3-oxo-1,3-dihydro-2-benzofuran-5-yl)-4-methylhex-4-enoate

immunosuppressant drug / used to prevent rejection in organ transplantation and in treatment of autoimmune disease.

naloxone

17-allyl-3,14-diyhdroxy-4,5α-epoxymorphinan-6-one
(1*S*,5*R*,13*R*,17*S*)-10,17-dihydroxy-4-(prop-2-en-1-yl)-12-oxa-4-azapentacyclo $[9.6.1.0^{1,13}.0^{5,17}.0^{7,18}]$octadeca-7(18),8,10-trien-14-one

opiate antidote / endorphin antagonist, causing restlessness.

2-napthylamine

β-napthylamine
naphthalen-2-amine

dye precursor / bladder carcinogen.

narcotics

sedative and anesthetic drugs / substance-dependent effects on adult and fetal brain, potential withdrawal symptoms in the neonate.

nickel (Ni) and nickel compounds

speciation-dependent industrial and environmental pollutants from extraction and refining of nickel, and from nickel-containing products / common human contact sensitizer, speciation-dependent and biological species-dependent embryotoxicity, teratogenicity, and carcinogenicity.

nicotine

3-[(2*S*)-1-methylpyrrolidin-2-yl]pyridine

tobacco ingredient, insecticide / nicotinic acetylcholine receptor agonist, neurotoxic, may form carcinogenic nitroso-derivatives, associated with atherosclerosis.

nitrate (NO_3^-)

plant fertilizer, groundwater contaminant / reduced to nitrite in living organisms, nitrite converts hemoglobin to methemoglobin impairing oxygen transport in the blood, especially harmful in babies (blue baby syndrome); nitrite may also convert to potentially carcinogenic nitrosamines.

nitric oxide (NO)

nitrogen monoxide
nitrogen(II) oxide

endogenous mediator, atmospheric occurrence / neuro(gaso)transmitter, causes vasodilatation.

nitriles

industrial chemicals with a –CN group / neurotoxicity, axonopathy.

nitrogen dioxide (NO_2)

nitrogen(IV) oxide

combustion side product / airway irritant.

nitrosamine

class of substances with a –N(R)-NO structural feature, formed during *e.g.*, smoking, barbeque / most nitrosamines form reactive metabolites during biotransformation and are carcinogenic.

nitrous oxide (N_2O)

laughing gas
dinitrogen oxide
nitrogen(I) oxide

inhalation anesthetic / anesthesia.

nonsteroidal antiinflammatory drugs (NSAIDs)

synthetic antiinflammatory drugs such as acetylsalicylic acid (aspirin, [2-(acetoxy)benzoic acid]), indomethacin [2-{1-[(4-chlorophenyl)carbonyl]-5-methoxy-2-methyl-1*H*-indol-3-yl}acetic acid], diclofenac [[2-(2,6-dichloroanilino)phenyl]acetic acid] and ibuprofen [(*RS*)-2-(4-(2-methylpropyl)-phenyl)propanoic acid] / act by inhibiting cyclooxygenase, a key enzyme in prostaglandin synthesis, acute risk for gastric ulcers, chronic risk for renal damage, some have immunologically relevant adverse effects such as bone marrow depression, aspirin-induced asthma or "salicylate intolerance", a pseudoallergic reaction.

noradrenaline

norepinephrine (INN)
4-[(1*R*)-2-amino-1-hydroxyethyl]benzene-1,2-diol

endogenous mediator / neurotransmitter, inducing hypertension and tachycardia.

ochratoxin

(e.g., ochratoxin A)
N-{[(3*R*)-5-chloro-8-hydroxy-3-methyl-1-oxo-3,4-dihydro-1*H*-isochromen-7-yl]carbonyl}-L-phenylalanine

contaminant formed by molds of the genera ***Aspergillus*** and ***Penicillium*** on stored food / nephrotoxicity.

oligomycin A

natural product from streptomyces / blocks a mitochondrial proton channel, inhibits ATP synthesis.

oral contraceptives

contraceptive drugs / decreased fertility in females, possible association with developmental deficits of fetus is a matter of debate.

organophosphates

insecticides, chemical weapons / inhibit acetylcholinesterase, causing salivation, convulsions, and respiratory arrest.

organotins

pesticides, antifouling agents / tributyltin compounds and dioctyltin dichloride act on maturing and proliferating T-lymphocytes and are considered as prototypes of immunosuppressive chemical agents.

ouabain

See strophanthin.

oxalic acid

used industrially in cleaning and bleaching, also found in rhubarb / destructive of tissue if absorbed through the skin or in contact with the eyes; breathed in causes cough, wheezing, shortness of breath, spasm, inflammation and edema of the larynx and the bronchi; ingestion can cause formation of calcium oxalate kidney stones and resultant kidney failure.

oxalyldiaminopropionic acid

3-(oxaloamino)alanine
2-amino-3-(oxaloamino)propanoic acid

ingredient of the grass pea / glutamate receptor agonist, excitotoxin, neurotoxin, causes lathyrism.

oxidant gases

environmental air pollutants / ozone (O_3) and nitrogen oxides, when inhaled, impair functions of alveolar macrophages and augment pulmonary allergic reactions.

oxime antidote

antidote for organophosphate poisoning / reactivates inhibited acetylcholinesterase, no specific neurotoxicity.

ozone (O_3)

photochemical product in outdoor air / airway irritation and toxicity, eye irritation.

paclitaxel (INN)

4,10β-bis(acetyloxy)-13α-{[(2*R*,3*S*)-3-(benzoylamino)-2-hydroxy-3-phenylpropanoyl]oxy}-1,7β-dihydroxy-9-oxo-5β,20-epoxytax-11-en-2α-yl benzoate

anticancer drug extracted from the Pacific yew tree / influences microtubule dynamics, causing bone marrow suppression and thrombocytopenia.

paraquat

1,1′-dimethyl-4,4′-bi(pyridin-1-ium) dichloride

herbicide / liver, lung, heart, and kidney failure occur rapidly after ingestion and can lead to death after a few days; chronic exposure has similar consequences.

parathion

O,O′-diethyl *O″*-(4-nitrophenyl) phosphorothioate

organophosphate insecticide / acetylcholinesterase inhibitor, neurotoxin, suppresses the humoral and cell-mediated immune response. May reduce fertility in experimental animals, embryotoxic and fetotoxic.

penicillamine (INN)

3,3-dimethyl-D-cysteine
(2*S*)-2-amino-3-methyl-3-sulfanylbutanoic acid

chelating agent and antirheumatic drug / may cause disturbances of metal-metabolism and autoimmune disease such as myositis and connective tissue defects.

pentachlorophenol (PCP)

wood preservative, emitted into indoor air / exposure due to its emission from PCP-treated timber, unspecific neurological effects.

pentetrazol

6,7,8,9-tetrahydro-5*H*-tetrazolo[1,5-*a*]azepine

agent in anti-seizure research / GABA-A receptor ligand, causes seizures.

pentostatin (INN)

2′-deoxycoformycin
(8*R*)-3-(2-deoxy-D-erythro-pentofuranosyl)-3,6,7,8-tetrahydroimidazo[4,5-*d*][1,3]diazepin-8-ol

therapeutic drug for leukemia-forms / adenosine deaminase-inhibiting drug, cytotoxic, lymphotoxic and teratogenic.

persistent organic pollutants

umbrella term for long-living mostly chlorinated organic substances, such as PCB / tend to accumulate in the food-chain, high levels in seafood, substance-dependent toxic effects.

phalloidin

(1*S*,14*R*,18*S*,20*S*,23*S*,28*S*,31*S*,34*R*)-28-[(2*R*)-2,3-dihydroxy-2-methylpropyl]-18-hydroxy-34-[(1*S*)-1-hydroxyethyl]23,31-dimethyl-12-thia-10,16,22,25,27,30,33,36-octaazapentacyclo-[12.11.11.$0^{3,1}$1.$0^{4,9}$.$0^{16,20}$]hexatriaconta-3(11),4,6,8-tetraene-15,21,24,26,29,32,35-heptone

natural product of death cap mushroom (***Amanita phalloides***) / hepatotoxic, prevents depolymerization of actin.

pharmaceuticals in the environment

eliminated from drug-treated humans and animals into waste water / effects include antibacterial activity in wastewater treatment plants, hormonal activities affecting aquatic organisms, and tumorigenic activities.

phencylidine (INN)

"angel dust"
1-(1-phenylcyclohexyl)piperidine

drug of abuse / NMDA receptor antagonist, hallucinations.

phenol

industrial chemical / embryotoxic and fetotoxic in experimental animals.

phentolamine (INN)

3-{*N*-[(4,5-dihydro-1*H*-imidazol-2-yl)methyl]-4-methylanilino}phenol

antihypertensive / alpha-adrenergic antagonist, causing hypotension and tachycardia.

phenylalanine (in maternal hyperphenylalaninemia)

phenylalanine substitution in pregnant phenylketonuria (PKU) patients / possible mental retardation of newborn if maternal phenylalanine intake is too high.

phenytoin (INN)

diphenylhydantoin

5,5-diphenylimidazolidine-2,4-dione

antiepileptic drug / hypersensitivity reactions, similar to those caused by carbamazepine, craniofacial, limb, and cerebrovascular defects, growth and mental retardation, fetal loss.

phorbol

(1a*R*,1b*S*,4a*R*,7a*S*,7b*S*,8*R*,9*R*,9a*S*)-1,1a,1b,4,4a,7a,7b,8,9,9a-decahydro-4a,7b,9,9a-tetrahydroxy-3-(hydroxymethyl)-1,1,6,8-tetramethyl-5*H*-cyclopropa[3,4]benzo[1,2-*e*]azulen-5-one

plant-derived kinase activator / tumor promotor, various teratogenic effects, irritant.

See also croton oil.

phosgene ($COCl_2$)

carbonyl dichloride

industrial chemical / inhalation causes severe lung edema.

phthalates

esters of phthalic acid

plasticisers / teratogenic, fetotoxic, testicular toxicants in several animal species.

pimecrolimus (INN)

(3*S*,4*R*,5*S*,8*R*,9*E*,12*S*,14*S*,15*R*,16*S*,18*R*,19*R*,26a*S*)-{(1*E*)-2-[(1*R*,3*R*,4*S*)-4-chloro-3-methoxycyclohexyl]-1-methylvinyl}-8-ethyl-5,19-dihydroxy-14,16-dimethoxy-4,10,12,18-tetramethyl-5,6,8,11,12,13,14,15,16,17,18,19,24,25,26,26a-hexadecahydro-3*H*-15,19-epoxypyrido[2,1-*c*][1,4]oxaazacyclotricosine-1,7,20,21(4*H*,23*H*)-tetrone

immunomodulating drug structurally related to tacrolimus (fujimycin) / inhibits T-cell activation, used for treatment of atopic dermatitis and psoriasis.

piribedil (INN)

piprazidine

2-{4-[(1,3-benzodioxol-5-yl)methyl]piperazin-1-yl}pyrimidine

antiparkinson drug / dopamine agonist, enhancing dopamine activity.

platinum (Pt)

metallic element / platinum salts induce hypersensitivity reactions such as contact dermatitis and respiratory symptoms. Cisplatin (INN), a cytostatic compound, inhibits rapidly proliferating B-cells and T-cells.

polychlorinated biphenyls (PCB)

group of environmental contaminants, formerly with many applications, now widely banned / accumulate in food chain, toxicities are congener-dependent and include interference with thyroid hormones, growth retardation, hyperpigmentation, neurobehavioral deficit, lowered intelligence, and immunosuppression.

polychlorinated dibenzodioxins (PCDDs)

polychlorinated oxanthrenes

group of environmental contaminants, side products, accumulate in food chain / products of incomplete incineration and contaminants in 2,4,5-T [(2,4,5-trichlorophenoxy)acetic acid, formerly widely used as a herbicide and notoriously in Agent Orange in the Vietnam War], 2,3,7,8-tetrachlorodibenzo[*b,e*][1,4]dioxin (TCDD) is the most toxic representative of this group of chemicals. It causes thymic atrophy and suppression of cell mediated immunity in rodents, also chloracne.

polychlorinated dibenzofurans (PCDFs)

group of environmental contaminants, side products, accumulate in food chain / immunotoxic profile is similar to that of polychlorinated dibenzodioxins.

polycyclic aromatic hydrocarbons (PAH)

group of environmental contaminants, formed during incomplete combustion of fossil fuels, including benzo[*a*]pyrene, 7,12-dimethylbenzo[*a*]anthracene (7,12-dimethyltetraphene), and 3-methylcholanthrene (3-methyl-1,2-dihydrocyclopenta[*ij*]tetraphene) / some are human carcinogens, suppress humoral and cellular immunity, and are associated with reproductive disturbances, birth defects and cancer in laboratory animals.

polyisocyanates

group of industrial chemicals / reactive chemicals used in paints, which may induce asthma-like symptoms in workers, probably by forming neoantigens.

prednisone (INN)

17,21-dihydroxypregna-1,4-diene-3,11,20-trione

synthetic steroid with glucocorticoid action / used as an antiallergy and immunosuppressive drug and as an anti-inflammatory agent in the treatment of rheumatoid arthritis (RA), suppresses endogenous corticoid-production.

procainamide (INN)

4-amino-*N*-[2-(diethylamino)ethyl]benzamide

antiarrhythmic therapeutic drug / induces autoimmune disease, manifested as systemic lupus erythematosus-like syndrome.

progesterone (INN)

pregn-4-ene-3,20-dione

natural female hormone / possible masculinization of female fetus.

propylthiouracil (INN)

6-propyl-2-thioxo-2,3-dihydropyrimidin-4(1*H*)-one

therapeutic drug to treat hyperthyroidism / may induce hypersensitivity reactions, leading to agranulocytosis, hepatitis, or a lupus-like syndrome.

psilocybin

3-[2-(dimethylamino)ethyl]-1*H*-indol-4-yl dihydrogen phosphate

natural mushroom product / hallucinogen with a history as a recreational psychedelic substance, partial agonist at serotonergic receptors.

psychoactive drugs

include drugs to treat psychiatric disorders and addictive drugs / various substance-dependent effects on fetal neurological function. Possible withdrawal phenomena, notably in the newborn.

pyrrolizidine alkaloid

plant defense alkaloids containing a hydrogenated pyrrolizine skeleton / hepatotoxicity and liver cancer.

3-quinuclidinyl benzilate

1-azabicyclo[2.2.2]octan-3-yl 2-hydroxy-2,2-diphenylacetate

chemical warfare agent / acetylcholine antagonist at muscarinic receptors, causing confusion and incapacitation.

rapamycin

See sirolimus (INN).

retinoic acid

See retinoids, and 13-*cis*-retinoic acid under isotretinoin (INN).

retinoids

natural and synthetic (therapeutic) derivatives of vitamin A / individual members of this group may have teratogenic effects.

ricin

castor oil plant (***Ricinus communis***) seed protein product / highly toxic lectin, inactivating ribosomes after cellular uptake.

rimonabant (INN)

5-(4-chlorophenyl)-1-(2,4-dichlorophenyl)-4-methyl-*N*-(piperidin-1-yl)-1*H*-pyrazole-3-carboxamide

cannabinoid-receptor (CB1) antagonist / weight loss, feelings of anxiety.

rotenone

(2*R*,6a*S*,12a*S*)-8,9-dimethoxy-2-(prop-1-en-2-yl)-1,2,12,12a-tetrahydro[1]benzopyrano[3,4-*b*]furo[2,3-*h*][1]benzopyran-6(6a*H*)-one

natural plant product / inhibition of mitochondrial electron transfer.

sarin

rac-propan-2-yl methylphosphonofluoridate

chemical warfare agent / acetylcholinesterase inhibitor, typical symptoms of organophosphate poisoning.

saxitoxin

[(3a*S*,4*R*,10a*S*)-2,6-diamino-10,10-dihydroxy-3a,4,9,10-tetrahydro-1*H*,8*H*-pyrrolo[1,2-*c*]purin-4-yl]methyl carbamate

dinoflagellate poison / voltage-gated sodium channel blocker, causes paralytic shellfish poisoning.

selenium (Se)

nonmetal element, workplace exposure, overdosing of supplements / increased uptake causes selenosis, with various less specific symptoms, such as liver cirrhosis, cardiac insufficiency and hair loss.

selenium deficiency

insufficient selenium uptake, often due to low geogenic level / causes muscular dystrophy, neuropathy, Keshan-disease (cardiomyopathy).

D-serine

endogenous D-amino acid / excitatory co-neurotransmitter at the GABA (NMDA) receptor.

serotonin

5-hydroxytryptamine
3-(2-aminoethyl)-1*H*-indol-5-ol

endogenous neurotransmitter and mediator / involved in the regulation of many neuronal and somatic functions.

sertraline (INN)

(1*S*,4*S*)-4-(3,4-dichlorophenyl)-*N*-methyl-1,2,3,4-tetrahydronaphthalen-1-amine

therapeutic drug / selective serotonin reuptake inhibitor (SSRI), anti-depressant drug, used to treat panic disorders, toxic interaction with MAO-inhibitors occur, various side effects when overdosed.

silica (SiO_2)

silica gel
silicon dioxide

industrial chemical / inhaled dust particles of silica are toxic to lung macrophages and may depress immune parameters.

sirolimus (INN)

rapamycin
(3*S*,6*R*,7*E*,9*R*,10*R*,12*R*,14*S*,15*E*,17*E*,19*E*,21*S*,23*S*,26*R*,27*R*,34a*S*)-9,27-dihydroxy-3-[(1*R*)-2-[(1*S*,3*R*,4*R*)-4-hydroxy-3-methoxycyclohexyl]-1-methylethyl]-10,21-dimethoxy-6,8,12,14,20,26-hexamethyl-9,10,12,13,14,21,22,23,24,25,26,27,32,33,34,34a-hexadecahydro-3*H*-23,27-epoxypyrido[2,1-*c*][1,4]oxaazacyclohentriacontine-1,5,11,28,29(4*H*,6*H*,31*H*)-pentone

macrolide from ***Streptomyces***, immunosuppressive drug / used after organ transplantation to decrease the risk of rejection.

solanine

α-solanine
solanid-5-en-3β-yl 6-deoxy-α-L-mannopyranosyl-(1→2)-[β-D-glucopyranosyl-(1→3)]-galactopyranoside

(2*S*,3*R*,4*S*,5*S*,6*R*)-2-{[(2*R*,3*S*,4*S*,5*R*,6*R*)-3-hydroxy-2-(hydroxymethyl)-5-{[(2*S*,3*R*,4*R*,5*R*,6*S*)-3,4,5-trihydroxy-6-methyltetrahydro-2*H*-pyran-2-yl]oxy}-6-{[(2*S*,4a*R*,4b*S*,6a*S*,6b*R*,7*S*,7a*R*,10*S*,12a*S*,13a*S*,13b*S*)-4a,6a,7-trimethyl-1,2,3,4,4a,4b,5,6,6a,6b,7,7a,8,10,11,12a,13,13a,13b,14-icosahydro-9*H*-naphtho[2′,1′:4,5]indeno[1,2-*b*]indolizin-4-yl]oxy}tetrahydro-2*H*-pyran-4-yl]oxy}-6-(hydroxymethyl)tetrahydro-2*H*-pyran-3,4,5-triol

glycosylated alkaloid from ***Solanaceae*** plants / natural pesticide, cholinesterase inhibitor and mitochondrial toxin, causes dizziness, gastrointestinal upset, hallucinations, paralysis, and may be fatal at low doses.

solvents

used in industry and for hobbies / mechanism unresolved, headache, drunkenness, narcosis.

streptozocin (INN)

2-deoxy-2-{[methyl(nitroso)carbamoyl]amino}-β-D-glucopyranose

drug to treat insulinoma / specific uptake by pancreatic beta cells, followed by cleavage of nitrosourea which is cytotoxic, therefore an experimental diabetes-producing agent.

strophanthin

e.g., g-strophanthin (ouabain)
3β-[(6-deoxy-α-L-mannopyranosyl)oxy]-1β,5,11α,14,19-pentahydroxy-5β-card-20(22)-enolide

natural plant product, arrow poison / inhibits sodium/potassium pump, may increase cardiac output at low dose, causes arrhythmias at higher dose.

strychnine

strychnidin-10-one
(1*R*,11*S*,18*S*,20*R*,21*R*,22*S*)-12-oxa-8,17-diazaheptacyclo[15.5.2.$0^{1,18}$.$0^{2,7}$.$0^{8,22}$.$0^{11,21}$.$0^{15,20}$]tetracosa-2,4,6,14-tetraen-9-one

natural plant product / neurotoxic agent, blocks the action of the inhibiting neurotransmitter glycine, causes convulsions and finally respiratory arrest.

styrene

ethenylbenzene
vinylbenzene

industrial chemical / feeling of drunkenness, decreased color vision, vestibular effects.

succinylcholine

suxamethonium (INN)
2,2′-[(1,4-dioxobutane-1,4-diyl)bis(oxy)]bis(*N*,*N*,*N*-trimethylethan-1-aminium)

muscle relaxant drug / acetylcholine agonist at nicotinic receptor, muscle relaxation.

sucrose

saccharose
β-D-fructofuranosyl-α-D-glucopyranoside

carbohydrate nutrient / diabetogenic, notably in predisposed persons and pregnant women, causing increasing risk of complications of pregnancy and prenatal metabolic imprinting.

sulfamethoxazole

4-amino-*N*-(5-methyl-1,2-oxazol-3-yl)benzenesulfonamide
antibiotic drug / hypersensitivity reactions.

sulfite (SO_3^{2-})

food additive / pseudoallergic reaction (sulfite-intolerance) in sensitive individuals.

sulfur dioxide (SO_2)

combustion product of sulfur-containing fossils, outdoor pollutant / irritant of mucus membranes and respiratory tract.

suramin

8,8′-{carbonylbis[azanediyl-3,1-phenylenecarbonylazanediyl(4-methyl-3,1-phenylene)-carbonylazanediyl]}di(naphthalene-1,3,5-trisulfonic acid)
anti-protozoal drug / inhibits apoptosis is some tissues, reduces placental blood flow, retards fetal growth.

tabun

rac-ethyl N,N-dimethylphosphoramidocyanidate
chemical warfare agent / acetylcholinesterase inhibitor, typical symptoms of organophosphate poisoning.

tacrolimus (INN)

FK-506
fujimycin
(3*S*,4*R*,5*S*,8*R*,9*E*,12*S*,14*S*,15*R*,16*S*,18*R*,19*R*,26a*S*)-5,19-dihydroxy-3-{(1*E*)-2-[(1*R*,3*R*,4*R*)-4-hydroxy-3-methoxycyclohexyl]-1-methylethenyl}-14,16-dimethoxy-4,10,12,18-tetramethyl-8-(prop-2-en-1-yl)-5,6,8,11,12,13,14,15,16,17,18,19,24,25,26,26a-hexadecahydro-3*H*-15,19-epoxypyrido[2,1-*c*][1,4]oxaazacyclotricosine-1,7,20,21(4*H*,23*H*)-tetrone
immunosuppressive drug / used after allogenic organ transplantation to decrease the risk of rejection, inactivates T-lymphocytes by inhibiting signal transduction from the T-cell receptor; although its target (FK-506 binding protein) is different from that of ciclosporin (INN), it inhibits the same pathway and has similar effects on the immune system.

tetanus toxin

toxin of ***Clostridium tetani*** / GABA-release blocker, causes tetanic spasms.

tetrachlorodecaoxide (TCDO)

dioxygen tetrachlorite hydrate
dioxygen–dioxygen monochloride–water (1/4/*x*)
$O_2 \cdot 4O_2Cl \cdot xH_2O$
immunomodulating drug / chlorite-containing drug used for the dressing of wounds, immunomodulation, and as a protective agent against radiation. It forms a complex with hemoglobin and stimulates macrophages.

tetracycline (INN)

(4*S*,4a*S*,5a*S*,6*S*,12a*S*)-4-(dimethylamino)-3,6,10,12,12a-pentahydroxy-6-methyl-1,11-dioxo-1,4,4a,5,5a,6,11,12a-octahydro-2-tetracenecarboxamide

antibiotic drug / discolors (white to yellow, brownish or grey) growing teeth, may affect bone and tooth growth.

tetraethylammonium

agent in experimental neurophysiology / voltage-gated potassium channel blocker, causes muscle paralysis.

tetraethyllead

antiknock agent / volatile lipophilic liquid, neurotoxic and chronically causing lead-poisoning and lowered intelligence.

tetrafluoroethene

industrial chemical / kidney damage, kidney tumors; cysteine-conjugate as toxic species.

tetrahydrocannabinol

dronabinol (INN)

(6a*R*,10a*R*)-6,6,9-trimethyl-3-pentyl-6a,7,8,10a-tetrahydro-6*H*-dibenzo[*b,d*]pyran-1-ol

active cannabinoid of the hemp plant; therapeutic and recreational drug, classified as drug of abuse in many jurisdictions / cannabinoid receptor agonist, psychoactive effects, induces a state of relaxation, euphoria; anti-nausea and anti-anorectic effects; substance-specific neuroactivity or neurotoxicity possible.

tetrodotoxin

(4*R*,4a*R*,5*R*,7*S*,9*S*,10*S*,10a*R*,11*S*,12*S*)-12-(hydroxymethyl)-2-iminooctahydro-5,9:7,10a-dimethano[1,3]dioxocino[6,5-*d*]pyrimidine-4,7,10,11,12-pentol

poison of the puffer fish / voltage-gated sodium channel blocker causing paralysis.

thalidomide

rac-2-(2,6-dioxopiperidin-3-yl)-2*H*-isoindole-1,3-dione

drug used in treatment of certain cancers (multiple myeloma) and leprosy / teratogenic, particularly causing reduction defects of the limbs (phocomelia) and ears when mothers are treated on days 21-26 of pregnancy.

thiocyanate (SCN^-)

decay product of vegetable glycosides / inhibition of iodine uptake into the thyroid gland, may cause underactive thyroid.

tin (Sn)

metallic element, speciation-dependent biocide / neurotoxicity, endocrine modification, imposex.

tobacco smoke

recreational drug, tobacco smoke contains nicotine and many toxic substances / acute: nicotinic effects, irritation of eyes, chronic: cardiovascular disease, cancer. intrauterine exposure: growth retardation, prematurity, low birth weight.

toluene

methylbenzene

industrial chemical / sniffing results in "toluene embryopathy" with mainly neurological anomalies in the fetus.

toxaphene (chlorinated camphene)

1,2,2,3,3,4,7,7-octachloro-5,5-dimethyl-6-methylidenebicyclo[2.2.1]heptane

organochlorine insecticide / multiple reproductive and developmental effects in laboratory animals.

tri-*o*-cresyl phosphate (TCP, TOCP)

tris(2-methylphenyl) phosphate

plasticizer, misused as adulterant / acetylcholinesterase inhibitor, organophosphate-induced delayed neuropathy.

trichloroethene

industrial chemical / depression of the central nervous system, arrhythmias, carcinogenic in animals.

1,1,1-trichloro-2,2-bis(4-chlorophenyl)ethane

1′-(2,2,2-trichloroethane-1,1-diyl)bis(4-chlorobenzene)
dichlorodiphenyltrichloroethane
DDT

long-acting insecticide (now widely restricted in use) / associated with suppression of various types of inconsistent immune responses; causes thinning of egg shells and behavioral changes in birds, resulting in reproductive failure; found as a contaminant in human milk.

trifluoperazine (INN)

10-[3-(4-methylpiperazin-1-yl)propyl]-2-(trifluoromethyl)-10*H*-phenothiazine

antipsychotic drug / teratogenic.

trimethadione (INN)

3,5,5-trimethyl-1,3-oxazolidine-2,4-dione

anticonvulsant drug / craniofacial and cardiovascular defects, intellectual impairment.

trypan blue

tetrasodium 3,3′-[(3,3′-dimethylbiphenyl-4,4′-diyl)bis(diazenediyl)]bis(5-amino-4-hydroxynaphthalene-2,7-disulfonate)

dye, vital stain / experimental teratogen when injected into frogs.

tryptophan pyrolysis products

cooking side-products formed *e.g.* during barbecue / mutagenic.

tyramine

4-(2-aminoethyl)phenol

ingredient of some fermented foods / induces synaptic noradrenaline release, hypertension.

ultrafine particles

emissions *e.g.* from diesel engines / toxic to the lungs.

urushiol

(oily mixture of various 3-pentadecylbenzene-1,2-diol derivatives)

ingredient of poison ivy / contact dermatitis.

valinomycin

(3*R*,6*R*,9*S*,12*S*,15*R*,18*R*,21*S*,24*S*,27*R*,30*R*,33*S*,36*S*)-3,6,9,15,18,21,27,30,33-nonaisopropyl-12,24,36-trimethyl-1,7,13,19,25,31-hexaoxa-4,10,16,22,28,34-hexaazacyclohexatriacontane-2,5,8,11,14,17,20,23,26,29,32,35-dodecone

bacterial metabolite, used in membrane research / potassium-specific ionophore.

valproic acid (INN)

2-propylpentanoic acid

anticonvulsant drug / neural tube closure defects, mental retardation.

vinclozolin

rac-3-(3,5-dichlorophenyl)-5-ethenyl-5-methyl-1,3-oxazolidine-2,4-dione

fungicide / endocrine modifier, multigenerational epigenetic effects on the male reproductive system.

vinyl chloride

chloroethene

monomer for polyvinyl chloride (PVC) production / may cause a scleroderma-like syndrome, hepatotoxic, angiosarcoma in the liver.

vismodegib

2-chloro-*N*-[4-chloro-3-(pyridin-2-yl)phenyl]-4-(methylsulfonyl)benzamide

drug for basal cell carcinoma therapy / inhibits hedgehog signaling pathway that is involved in embryonic cell differentiation, teratogenic, enters the semen.

vitamin A

essential human nutrient, including retinol, retinoic acid and beta-carotene / excessive supplementation with liver-derived retinoids (not carotenes) is teratogenic, and can cause nausea, irritability, reduced appetite, vomiting, blurred vision, headaches, hair loss, muscle and abdominal pain and weakness, and drowsiness.

vitamin D_3

(5*Z*,7*E*)-9,10-secocholesta-5,7,10(19)-trien-3β-ol

physiological form of vitamin D / suppresses Th1 cytokines and increases Th2 cytokines.

vitamin E

essential human nutrient / deficiency associated with infertility.

voclosporin (INN)

(3*S*,6*S*,9*S*,12*R*,15*S*,18*S*,21*S*,24*S*,30*S*,33*S*)-30-ethyl-33-[(1*R*,2*R*,4*E*)-1-hydroxy-2-methylhepta-4,6-dien-1-yl]-6,9,18,24-tetraisobutyl-3,21-diisopropyl-1,4,7,10,12,15,19,25,28-nonamethyl-1,4,7,10,13,16,19,22,25,28,31-undecaazacyclotritriacontane-2,5,8,11,14,17,20,23,26,29,32-undecone

immunosuppressive drug / acts as a calcineurin inhibitor.

volatile organic compounds

umbrella term for organic substances, mostly solvents, found in indoor and outdoor air / nonspecific effects of solvents include dizziness and headache.

VX

S-{2-[bis(propan-2-yl)amino]ethyl} *O*-ethyl methylphosphonothioate

chemical warfare agent / acetylcholinesterase inhibitor, elicits typical symptoms of organophosphate poisoning.

warfarin (INN)

coumadin

rac-4-hydroxy-3-(3-oxo-1-phenylbutyl)-2*H*-1-benzopyran-2-one

anti-clotting drug, rodenticide / craniofacial defects, intrauterine growth retardation, central nervous system malformation, and stillbirth, inner bleeding.

xanthotoxin

methoxsalen

ammoidin

9-methoxy-7*H*-furo[3,2-*g*][1]benzopyran-7-one

herbal furanocoumarin, ingredient of giant hogweed and other related plants of the families ***Apiaceae*** and ***Rutaceae*** / photosensitizing agent, skin contact with the plant in sunlight results in blisters of the skin, used for phototherapy of psoriasis.

xenon (Xe)

gaseous chemical element, inhalation anesthetic, cardioprotectant, neuroprotectant / induces anesthesia.

xylene

dimethylbenzene

solvent / eye and skin irritation, narcotic, behavioral changes, enhances drunkenness.

zinc (Zn) ions

metallic elemental species in food and water, essential human nutrient / deficiency may cause birth defects; zinc ion toxicity is commonly fatal in dogs through severe hemolytic anemia and liver or kidney damage; highly toxic to plants and invertebrates.

APPENDIX II

Abbreviations used in this Glossary

2,4-D	2,4-dichlorophenoxyacetic acid
2,4-DB	2,4-dichlorophenoxybutyric acid [4-(2,4-dichlorophenoxy)-butyric acid]
2,4,5-T	2,4,5-trichlorophenoxyacetic acid
5-HT	5-hydroxytryptamine
AAE	acquired angioedema
ACA	anticentromere antibody
ACE	angiotensin converting enzyme
ACh	acetylcholine
AChE	acetylcholinesterase
ACR	acute-to-chronic toxicity ratio
ACTH	adrenocortocotropic hormone
AD	autonomic dysreflexia
Ad4BP	adrenal 4 binding protein
ADA	adenosine deaminase
ADAM	a disintegrin and metalloproteinase domain-containing protein
ADCC	antibody-dependent cellular cytotoxicity
ADH	antidiuretic hormone
ADHD	attention deficit hyperactivity disorder
ADI	acceptable daily intake
ADME	absorption, distribution, metabolism, excretion
ADMET	absorption, distribution, metabolism, excretion, toxicokinetics
AEC	adenylate energy charge
AF	accumulation factor; application factor; assessment factor
AFP	α-fetoprotein
AGD	anogenital distance
AGE	advanced glycation endproduct
AGM region	aorta-gonad-mesonephros region
AHH	aryl hydrocarbon hydroxylase
AHR	aryl hydrocarbon receptor
AIC	Akaike Information Criterion

Comprehensive Glossary of Terms Used in Toxicology
By John Duffus, Douglas M. Templeton and Michael Schwenk

Published by the Royal Society of Chemistry, www.rsc.org

AID	activation-induced cytidine deaminase
AIDS	acquired immunodeficiency syndrome
AIF-1	allograft inflammatory factor 1
AIF	apoptosis-inducing factor
AIH	autoimmune hepatitis
AIRE	autoimmune regulator
ALAD	aminolevulinic acid dehydrase; 5-aminolevulinate dehydrase; porphobilinogen synthase
ALARA(P)	as low as reasonably achievable (practicable)
ALL	acute lymphoblastic (lymphocytic) leukemia
ALS	amyotrophic lateral sclerosis
ALS-PDC	amyotrophic lateral sclerosis and parkinsonism–dementia complex
AMA	antimitochondrial antibody
AMH	anti-Müllerian hormone
AML	acute myelogenous leukemia
AMPA	2-amino-3-(3-hydroxy-5-methyl-1,2-oxazol-4-yl)propanoic acid
ANA	antinuclear antibody
ANCA	antineutrophil cytoplasmic autoantibody
ANF	antinuclear factor
ANS	autonomic nervous system
AOP	adverse outcome pathway
APC	antigen-presenting cell
APECED syndrome	autoimmune polyendocrinopathy–candidiasis–ectodermal–dystrophy syndrome
APR	acute-phase response
APS	antiphospholipid syndrome
APTI	air pollution tolerance index
AR	androgen receptor
ARDS	acute (or adult) respiratory distress syndrome
ARND	alcohol-related neurodevelopmental disabilities
ARNT	aryl hydrocarbon receptor nuclear translocator protein
ASA test	active systemic anaphylaxis test
ASD	atrial-septal defect
ASP	amnesic shellfish poisoning
AT	ataxia telangiectasia
ATCN	asymptotic threshold concentration
ATM	ataxia telangiectasia-mutated
ATP	adenosine triphosphate
AUC	area under the concentration–time curve
AUMC	area under the moment curve
AV	arteriovenous
AVM	arteriovenous malformation
AVP	arginine vasopressin
AVS	acid-volatile sulfide
AZT	azidothymidine
B	biomagnification factor
BAC	bacterial artificial chromosome; blood alcohol concentration
BAF	bioaccumulation factor
BAL	British anti-Lewisite
BALT	bronchus-associated lymphoid tissue
BAP	biodiversity action plan

BBB	blood-brain barrier
BCC	bioaccumulative chemicals of concern
BCF	bioconcentration factor
BCG	bacille Calmette–Guérin
BCR	B-cell receptor
BCR gene	breakpoint cluster region gene
BDNF	brain-derived neurotrophic factor
BEI	biological exposure index
BEM	biological effect monitoring
BF	bioaccumulation factor
BI	bioavailability index
BLIMP-1	B-lymphocyte-induced maturation protein 1
BLM	biotic ligand model
BLNK	B-cell linker protein
BMC	benchmark concentration
BMCL	confidence limit for BMC
BMD	benchmark dose
BMDL	benchmark dose confidence limit
BMDS	benchmark dose at a given standard deviation
BMMA	β-*N*-methylamino-L-alanine
BMP	bone morphogenetic protein
BMR	basal metabolic rate; benchmark rate
BNT	Boston naming test
BOD	biochemical oxygen demand; biological oxygen demand
BSAF	biota-sediment accumulation factor
BSF	B-cell stimulatory factor; biota-sediment factor
BSID	Bayley scales of infant development
b.w., b.wt.	body weight
CALT	conjunctiva-associated lymphoid tissue
CAR	conditioned avoidance response
CAT	computerized axial tomography
CBA	cost–benefit analysis
CBR	critical body residue
CD	cluster determinant; cluster of differentiation
CD40L	CD40 ligand
cDNA	complementary DNA
CDR	complementarity-determining region
CEA	carcinoembryonic antigen
CF	concentration factor
CFC	chlorofluorocarbon
CGD	chronic granulomatous disease
ChE	cholinesterase
CLA	cutaneous lymphocyte antigen
CLL	chronic lymphocytic leukemia
CMA	chaperone-mediated autophagy
CMI	cell-mediated immunity
CML	chronic myelogenous leukemia
CMPP	2-(4-chloro-2-methylphenoxy)propionic acid
CMR	carcinogenic mutagenic reprotoxic
CMV	cytomegalovirus
CNS	central nervous system
COD	chemical oxygen demand
CoMFA	comparative molecular field analysis
ConA	concanavalin A

COMT	catechol-*O*-methyltransferase
COPC	compound of probable concern; contaminant of potential concern
CPT	continuous performance test
CRA	cytokine release assay
cRBC	chicken red blood cell
CREST	calcinosis, Raynaud phenomenon, esophageal dysfunction, sclerodactyly, and telangiectasias
CRM	certified reference material
CRP	C-reactive protein
CSAF	chemical specific adjustment factor
CSE	chronic solvent-induced encephalopathy
CSF	cerebrospinal fluid
CSF	colony-stimulating factor
CSM	conceptual site model
CT	computed tomography
CTD	common technical document (drug registration)
CTEV	congenital talipes equinovarus
CTL	cytotoxic T lymphocyte
CTLA-4	cytotoxic T-lymphocyte antigen-4
CTS	carpel tunnel syndrome
CV	ceiling value
CWC	Chemical Weapons Convention
CYP	cytochrome P450
Cyt	cytochrome
D	absorbed dose of radiation
DAF	decay-accelerating factor
DAT	direct antiglobulin test
DDT	1,1,1-trichloro-2,2-bis(4-chlorophenyl)ethane
p,p′-DDT	*p,p′*-dichlorodiphenyltrichloroethane [1,1,1-trichloro-2,2-bis(4-chlorophenyl)ethane]
DEB	dynamic energy budget
DES	diethylstilbestrol
DGS	Di George syndrome
DME	drug metabolizing enzyme
DNA	deoxyribonucleic acid
DNEL	derived no-effect level
DNOC	dinitro-orthocresol [3,5-dinitrobenzene-1,2-diol]
DNT	developmental neurotoxicity testing
DO	dissolved oxygen
DOC	dissolved oxygen content; dissolved organic carbon
DOM	dissolved organic matter
DSP	diarrheal shellfish poisoning; diarrheic shellfish poisoning
DSST	digit symbol substitution test
DT	depuration time
DTH assay	delayed-type hypersensitivity assay
DU	Dobson unit
EA	environmental assessment
EAE	experimental allergic encephalomyelitis
EBI	ergosterol biosynthesis inhibitor (fungicide)
EBT	electron beam tomography
EBV	Epstein–Barr virus
EC	effective concentration; Enzyme Commission; European Community
EC_{50}	median effective concentration to 50 % of a population

ECF-A	eosinophil chemotactic factor of anaphylaxis
ECM	extracellular matrix
EC*n*	median effective concentration to *n* % of a population
ECT	electroconvulsive therapy
eCTD	electronic common technical document (drug registration)
ED	effective dose
ED_{50}	median effective dose to 50 % of a population
EDC	endocrine-disrupting compound
EDI	estimated daily intake
ED*n*	median effective dose to *n* % of a population
EEC	estimated (expected) environmental concentration
EEC	estimated environmental exposure concentration; estimated exposure concentration; expected environmental exposure concentration
EED	estimated exposure dose
EEG	electroencephalography
EEL	environmental exposure level
EFcrust	enrichment factor (for the Earth's crust)
EGF	epidermal growth factor
EIA	environmental impact assessment
EIS	environmental impact statement
ELISA	enzyme-linked immunosorbent assay
ELISPOT assay	enzyme-linked immunospot assay
ELS	early life stage
EMDI	estimated maximum daily intake
EMG	electromyography
EMT	epithelial-to-mesenchymal transition
ENO2	enolase 2
EPSP	excitatory post-synaptic potential
EQO	environmental quality objective
EqP	equilibrium partitioning
EQS	environmental quality standard
ER	endoplasmic reticulum
ERG	electroretinogram
Erk	extracellular regulated kinase
ERL	extraneous residue limit
EROD	ethoxyresorufin *O*-deethylase [7-ethoxyphenoxazin-3-one *O*-deethylase]
ES cell	embryonic stem cell
EST	expressed sequence tag
ET	effective time
ETS	environmental tobacco smoke
F	fraction of dose absorbed; bioavailability
f	toxicity equivalency factor
FACB	Fertility Assessment by Continuous Breeding
FACS	fluorescence-assisted (or activated) cell sorting
FAS	fetal alcohol syndrome
FASD	fetal alcohol spectrum disorder
FATS	fish acute toxicity syndrome
FAV	final acute value
FCAS	familial cold autoinflammatory syndrome
FCV	final chronic value
FET	fish embryo test
FETAX	frog embryo teratogenesis assay Xenopus
FGF	fibroblast growth factor

FHL	familial hemophagocytic lymphohistiocytosis
FIAM	free ion activity model
FITC	fluorescein isothiocyanate
FLD	fatty liver disease
fMLP	formyl-methionyl-leucyl-phenylalanine
FND	frontonasal dysplasia
FONSI	finding of no significant impact
FS	feasibility study
FSH	follicle-stimulating hormone
FSH-RH	follicle-stimulating hormone releasing hormone
FTD	frontotemporal dementia
FTLD	frontotemporal lobular degeneration
FUS	fused in sarcoma (transcription factor)
G-CSF	granulocyte colony-stimulating factor
GABA	γ-aminobutyric acid (IUPAC name 4-aminobutanoic acid)
GABAergic neurons	γ-aminobutyric acid-responsive neurons
GAD	glutamic acid decarboxylase
GALT	gut-associated lymphoid tissue
GAP	good agricultural practice
GAS	general adaptation syndrome
GBS	Guillain–Barré syndrome
GCP	good clinical practice
GDNF	glial-derived neurotrophic factor
GEM	genetically engineered microorganism
GFAP	glial fibrillary acidic protein
GFR	glomerular filtration rate
GH	growth hormone
GHRF	growth hormone releasing factor
GHRH	growth hormone releasing hormone
GHS	global harmonization system for classification of hazardous substances
GIFT	gamete intrafallopian transfer
GIS	geographic information system
GIT	gastrointestinal tract
GLP	good laboratory practice
GM-CSF	granulocyte–macrophage colony-stimulating factor
GMO	genetically modified organism
GMP	good manufacturing practice
GnRH	gonadotropin-releasing hormone
GPCR	G-protein-coupled receptor
GPMT	guinea pig maximization test
GRAS	generally regarded as safe
GRH	gonadotropin-releasing hormone
GSH	glutathione (reduced)
GSSG	glutathione (oxidized)
GVH(D)	graft-*versus*-host (disease)
HAART	highly active antiretroviral therapy
HAE	hereditary angioedema
HAL	health advisory level
HAZOP	hazard and operability study
HCB	hexachlorobenzene
HCG	human chorionic gonadotropin
HC*p*	hazardous concentration (producing an effect)
HCS	hazardous concentration (of a substance)
HEDSET	harmonized electronic data set

HEQ	human equivalent dose
HEV	high endothelial venule
hGH	human growth hormone
HGP	Human Genome Project
HI	hazard index
HIGM	hyper immunoglobulin M syndrome
HIT	heparin-induced thrombocytopenia
HIV	human immunodeficiency virus
HLA	human leukocyte antigen
HMGB	high-mobility group box protein
HMI	humorally mediated immunity
HMO	hepatic microsomal monooxygenase
4-HNE	4-hydroxy-2-nonenal
HOX	heme oxygenase
hPL	human placental lactogen
HPS	hypersensitivity pneumonitis
HPVC	high production volume chemical
HQ	hazard quotient
HSG	Health and Safety Guide (IPCS)
hsc70	heat shock cognate 70 protein
HSP	heat shock protein
Ia	immune response-associated antigen or protein; I region-associated
IAT	indirect antiglobulin test
Iba-1	ionized calcium-binding adapter molecule 1
IBD	inflammatory bowel disease
i.c.	intracutaneous
IC	inhibitory concentration
ICA	islet cell antibodies
ICAM	intercellular adhesion molecule
ICE	interleukin-1β converting enzyme
IC*n*	inhibitory concentration to *n* % of a population
ICOS	inducible co-stimulatory protein
ICOSL	ligand of inducible co-stimulatory protein (LICOS)
ICP	intracranial pressure
ICSI	intracytoplasmic sperm injection
i.d.	intradermal
ID	inhibitory dose
IDDM	insulin-dependent diabetes mellitus
IDLHC	immediately dangerous to life and health concentration
ID*n*	inhibitory dose to *n* % of a population
IDO	indolamine-2,3-dioxygenase
IDR	idiosyncratic drug reaction
IED	individual effective dose
IEL	intraepithelial lymphocyte
IF	intermediate filament
IFN-γ	interferon gamma
Ig	immunoglobulin
IL	interleukin
i.m.	intramuscular
inhl	by inhalation
INN	international nonproprietary name
i.p.	intraperitoneal
IPAF	interleukin-1β converting enzyme (ICE) protease-activating factor

IPD	individual protective device
IPEX	immunodysregulation, polyendocrinopathy, enteropathy, X-linked
iPS	induced pluripotent stem cell
IPSP	inhibitory post-synaptic potential
IQ	intelligence quotient
IRIS	integrated risk information system
ISCOM	immunostimulating complex
IT50	median inhibitory time
ITAM	immunoreceptor tyrosine-based activation motif
I-TEF	international toxicity equivalency factor
ITIM	immunoreceptor tyrosine-based inhibitory motif
ITP	idiopathic (or immune) thrombocytopenic purpura
IUGR	intrauterine growth restriction (retardation)
i.v.	intravenous
IVCCA	in vivo cytokine capture assay
IVF	in vitro fertilization
JAK	Janus-family tyrosine kinase
JAM test	"just another method" test
JNK	c-Jun protein kinase
K cell	killer cell
KAR	killer cell activatory receptor
K_d	soil partition coefficient
K_D	partition ratio
KE	key event
KIR	killer cell inhibitory receptor; killer cell immunoglobulin-like receptor
KLH	keyhole limpet hemocyanin
KLR	killer lectin-like receptor
K_M	Michaelis constant
K_{OA}	octanol/air partition coefficient
K_{OC}	organic carbon partition coefficient
K_{OW}	octan-1-ol/water partition coefficient
KS	Kaposi sarcoma
LADD	lifetime average daily dose
LAK	lymphokine- (lymphocyte-) activated killer cells
LALT	larynx-associated lymphoid tissue
LBA	lymphocyte blastogenesis assay
LBB	lethal body burden
LC	lethal concentration
LC_{50}	median lethal concentration
LCA	leukocyte common antigen
LC_{min}	minimum lethal concentration
LC_n	median concentration lethal to n % of a test population
LD	lethal dose
LD_{50}	median lethal dose
LDL	low-density lipoprotein
LD_{min}	minimum lethal dose
LD_n	median dose lethal to n % of a test population
LED	lowest effective dose
LED_x	lowest effective dose for a biological effect in x % of the individuals in the test population
LEL	lowest-effect level (same as LOEL)
LEMS	Lambert–Eaton myasthenic syndrome
LFA	leukocyte functional antigens

LFA-1	lymphocyte function-associated antigen-1
LFER	linear free energy relationship
LGL	large granular lymphocyte
LH	luteinizing hormone
LHRH	luteinizing hormone-releasing hormone
LICOS	ligand of inducible co-stimulatory protein
LKM	liver–kidney microsomal antibody
LLE	loss of life expectancy
LLNA	(murine) local lymph node assay
LOAEL	lowest-observed-adverse-effect level
LOC	lab-on-a-chip
LOD score	logarithm (base 10) of odds score
LOEC	lowest-observed-effect concentration
LOEL	lowest-observed-effect level
LPS	lipopolysaccharide
LPT	lymphocyte proliferation test
LQT syndrome	long QT syndrome
LRR	leucine-rich repeat
LSD	lysergic acid diethylamide
LSER	linear solvation energy relationship
LT	lethal time; lymphotoxin
LT_n	median time for death of *n* % of a test population
LTRE	life-table response experiment
LTT	lymphocyte transformation test
LV	limit value
M cell	microfold cell
Mab	monoclonal antibody
MAC	maximum allowable concentration; membrane attack complex
MAdCAM-1	mucosal addressin cell adhesion molecule-1
MAK	Maximale Arbeitsplatz Konzentration (German)
MALT	mucosa-associated lymphoid tissue
MAM	methylazoxymethanol
MAO	monoamine oxidase
MAPC	multipotent adult progenitor cell
MAPK	mitogen-activated protein kinase
MAPT	microtubule-associated protein tau (gene)
MASP	mannan-binding lectin serine peptidase; mannose binding-protein associated serine protease
MAT	mean absorption time
MATC	maximum acceptable toxicant concentration
MBL	mannose-binding lectin
MBP	mannose-binding protein
MCAD	mast cell activation disorder
MCAS	mast cell activation syndrome
MCL	maximum contaminant level
MCLG	maximum contaminant level goal
MCPA	2-methyl 4-chloro-phenoxyacetic acid [2-(4-chloro-2-methylphenoxy)propionic acid]
MCS	multiple chemical sensitivity
MCTD	mixed connective tissue disease
MDMA	3,4-methylenedioxy-methamphetamine
MEL	maximum exposure limit
MEST	mouse ear-swelling test
MET	mesenchymal-to-epithelial transition

MF	modifying factor
MFO	mixed function oxidase
MHC	major histocompatibility complex
MIC	minimum inhibitory concentration
MIE	molecular intiating event
MIF	Müllerian inhibiting factor
MIGET	mouse IgE test
MIH	Müllerian-inhibiting hormone
miRNA	microRNA
MIS	Müllerian-inhibiting substance
MIT	median inhibitory time
MLE	maximum likelihood estimation
MLR	mixed lymphocyte reaction; mixed lymphocyte response
MMPI	Minnesota multiphasic personality inventory
MMR	macrophage mannose receptor
MN	micronucleus
MND	motor neuron disease
MO	monooxygenase
MOA	mode of action (in toxicology)
MOE	margin of exposure
MOS	margin of safety
MPA	microscopic polyangiitis
MPC	maximum permissible concentration
MPL	maximum permissible level
MPO	myeloperoxidase
MPPP	1-methyl-4-phenyl-4-propionoxypiperidine
MPS	mononuclear phagocytic system
MPTP	1-methyl-4-phenyl-1,2,3,6-tetrahydropyridine
MPT(P)	mitochondrial permeability transition (pore)
MPTP	1-methyl-4-phenyl-1,2,3,6-tetrahydropyridine
MRI	magnetic resonance imaging
MRL	maximum residue limit; minimal risk level (ATSDR)
mRNA	messenger ribonucleic acid
MRT	magnetic resonance tomography; mean residence time
MS	multiple sclerosis
MSAFP	maternal serum α-fetoprotein
MSD	minimum significant difference
MSDS	material safety data sheet
MSG	monosodium glutamate
MSH	melanocyte-stimulating hormone
MT	metallothionein
MTC	maximum tolerable concentration
MTD	maximum tolerable dose; maximum tolerated dose
MTEL	maximum tolerable exposure level
mTOR	mammalian target of rapamycin
MTTD	median time to death
MTX	methotrexate
MVP	minimum viable population
NAA	natural autoantibodies
NACHT domain	(protein domain derived from several other acromyms not included in this glossary, namely, NAIP, CIITA, HET-E, and TP1)
NADP(H)	nicotinamide adenine dinucleotide phosphate (reduced)
NAFL(D)	nonalcoholic fatty liver (disease)
NAG	*N*-acetyl-D-glycosaminidase

NALP3	NACHT domain-, leucine-rich repeat-, and PYD-containing protein 3 (same as NLRP3)
NALT	nasal-associated lymphoid tissue
NC_n	median concentration narcotic to *n* % of a population
ncRNA	non-coding RNA
NCTB	neurobehavior core test battery
ND_n	median dose narcotic to *n* % of a population
NED	no-effect dose; normal equivalent deviation
NEL	no-effect level, same as NOEL
NFAT	nuclear factor of activated T cells
NGF	nerve growth factor
NK cell	natural killer cell
NKT cell	cell-type intermediate between NK cell and T lymphocyte
NLR	NOD-like receptor
NLRP	NOD-like receptor protein; nucleotide-binding domain, leucine-rich repeat-containing protein
NLRP3	NOD-like receptor protein 3 (same as NALP3)
NMDA	*N*-methyl-D-aspartic acid
NMJ	neuromuscular junction
NMRI	nuclear magnetic resonance imaging
NOAEL	no-observed-adverse-effect level
NOD	nucleotide-binding oligomerization domain-containing protein
NOD mouse	non-obese diabetic mouse
NOEC	no-observed-effect concentration
NOED	no-observed-effect dose
NOEL	no-observed-effect level
NOG	noggin protein
NRAMP	natural resistance-associated macrophage protein
NRL	allergen natural rubber latex allergen; no-response level
NSAID	nonsteroidal anti-inflammatory drug
NSC	normalized sensitivity coefficient
NSE	neuron-specific enolase
NSP	nanosized particle; neurotoxic shellfish poisoning
NTE	neuropathy target esterase; neurotoxic esterase
OC	organic carbon, organochlorine compound
OEL	occupational exposure level
OES	occupational exposure standard
OP	organophosphorus compound
OPIDN	organophosphate-induced delayed neuropathy
OR	odds ratio
ORF	open reading frame
PADI	pseudo-acceptable daily intake
PAF	platelet-activating factor
PAH	polycyclic aromatic hydrocarbon
PALS	periarteriolar lymphoid sheath
PAMP	pathogen-associated molecular pattern
PAPS	3′-phosphoadenosine-5′-phosphosulfate
PBA	pseudobulbar affect
PBB	polybrominated biphenyl
PBC	primary biliary cirrhosis
PBL	peripheral blood leukocyte; peripheral blood lymphocyte
PBMC	peripheral blood mononuclear cell
PBPD	physiologically based pharmacodynamic modeling
PBPK	physiologically based pharmacokinetic modeling

PBT	persistent, bioaccumulative, and toxic
PBTK	physiologically based toxicokinetic modeling
p.c.	per cutim (Latin) = through the skin
PCA	test passive cutaneous anaphylaxis test
PCB	polychlorinated biphenyl
PCC	population critical concentration
PCDD	polychlorinated dibenzodioxin
PCDF	polychlorinated dibenzofuran
PCR	polymerase chain reaction
PCT	proximal convoluted tubule
PD	population density
PDGF	platelet-derived growth factor
PEC	predicted environmental concentration; predicted exposure concentration
PEL	permissible exposure limit
PET	positron emission tomography
PF	platelet factor
PFC	plaque-forming cell
PFOA	perfluorooctanoic acid
PFOS	perfluorooctane-1-sulfonate
PHA	phytohemagglutinin
PHF	paired helical filament
PIC	prior informed consent
PICT	pollution-induced community tolerance
PIN	preferred IUPAC name
PIP	persistent inorganic pollutant
PKC	protein kinase C
PKU	phenylketonuria
PLC	phospholipase C
PLNA	popliteal lymph node assay
$PM_{0.1}$	ultrafine particles in air with a maximum aerodynamic diameter <0.1 μm
$PM_{2.5}$	particles in air with a maximum aerodynamic diameter of 2.5 μm
PM_{10}	particles in air with a maximum aerodynamic diameter of 10 μm
PMA	phorbol 13-acetate 12-myristate (same as TPA)
PMN	pre-manufacture notification
PMR	proportionate mortality rate; proportionate mortality ratio
PNEC	predicted no-effect concentration
PNI	psychoneuroimmunology
PNS	peripheral nervous system
p.o.	per os (Latin) = by mouth
P_{OA}	octanol/air partition coefficient
POC	particulate organic carbon
POM	particulate organic matter
POMS	profile of mood state
POP	persistent organic pollutant
P_{OW}	octan-1-ol/water partition coefficient
PPAR	peroxisome proliferator-activated receptor
PPD	personal protective device; purified protein derivative
PPE	personal protective equipment
PR3	proteinase 3
pre-BCR	pre-B cell receptor
PRL	prolactin

PRR	pattern recognition receptor
PSC	primary sclerosing cholangitis
PSD	prevention of significant deterioration
PSP	paralytic shellfish poisoning
PTI	pollution tolerance index
PTWI	provisional tolerable weekly intake
PWM	pokeweed mitogen
PYD	pyrin (N-terminal homology) domain
Q	quality factor (radiation)
QSAR	quantitative structure–activity relationship
3D-QSAR	three-dimensional quantitative structure–activity relationship
QSMR	quantitative structure–metabolism relationship
QT interval	interval between the Q and T waves in an electrocardiogram
RA	rheumatoid arthritis
RACB	Reproductive Assessment by Continuous Breeding
RADS	reactive airways dysfunction syndrome
RAG	recombination-activating gene
RAGE	receptor for advanced glycation endproduct
RANTES	regulated upon activation normal T-cell expressed and secreted
RAR	retinoic acid receptor
RaRF	Ra-reactive factor
RAST	radioallergosorbent test
RD	rate difference
REL	recommended exposure limit (NIOSH)
RER	relative excess risk
RES	reticuloendothelial system
RfC	reference concentration
RfD	reference dose
RfDdt	developmental reference dose
RFLP	restriction fragment length polymorphism
Rh factor	rhesus factor
RI/FS	remedial investigation and feasibility study
RIA	radio-immunoassay
RME	reasonable maximum exposure
RNA	ribonucleic acid
RNAi	ribonucleic acid interference
RNS	reactive nitrogen species
ROCF test	Rey–Osterrieth complex figure test
ROI	reactive oxygen intermediates
ROS	reactive oxygen species
RR	rate ratio; relative risk
rRNA	ribosomal RNA
RSD	reflex sympathetic dystrophy
RSS	recombination signal sequence
RSV	respiratory syncytial virus
RXR	retinoid X receptor
S	salinity
S9	"supernatant 9000 *g*" rat liver microsome preparation
SALT	skin-associated lymphoid tissue
SAM	standardized aquatic microcosm
SAPK	stress-activated protein kinase
SAR	standard absorption rate; structure–activity relationship
SAT	spontaneous autoimmune thyroiditis

SB	spiked bioassay
s.c.	subcutaneous
SCA	single-chain antibody
SCAS	semi-continuous activated sludge
SCE	sister chromatid exchange
SCID	severe combined immunodeficiency
SCLE	subacute cutaneous lupus erythematosus
SCNT	somatic cell nuclear transfer
SCOB	schedule-controlled operant behavior
SD	standard deviation
SDN	sexually dimorphic nucleus
SDS	safety data sheet
SE	standard error
SF	safety factor
SHM	somatic hypermutation
shRNA	short hairpin ribonucleic acid
SIgAD	selective immunoglobulin A deficiency
SIGLEC	signaling lectins
siRNA	small interfering ribonucleic acid
SIS	skin immune system
SLA	soluble liver antigen
SLE	systemic lupus erythematosis
SLUDDE	salivation, lacrymation, urination, defecation, dyspnea, emesis
SLUDGE	salivation, lacrymation, urination, defecation, gastrointestinal upset, emesis
SMAC	supramolecular adhesion complex
SMR	standard morbidity ratio; standard mortality ratio; structure–metabolism relationship
SNARL	suggested no-adverse-response level
SNP	single-nucleotide polymorphism
SOC protein	small outer capsid protein
SOD	superoxide dismutase
SPF	specific pathogen-free
SRBC	sheep red blood cell
SRY protein	sex-determining region Y protein
SSc	systemic sclerosis
SSD	species sensitivity distribution
SSRI	selective serotonin reuptake inhibitor
STAT	signal transducer and activator of transcription
STEL	short-term exposure limit
STH	somatotropic hormone
STI	salt tolerance index
STP	sewage treatment plant
STR	short tandem repeat
$t_{1/2}$	half life; half time
T3	triiodothyronine
T4	thyroxin
TAP	transporter associated with antigen processing
TARDP	transactive response (TAR) DNA binding protein
TBPK	toxicologically based pharmacokinetic modeling
TBT	tributyl tin
TBTO	tributyltin oxide
TC	teratogenic concentration; threshold concentration

TCDD	2,3,7,8-tetrachlorodibenzo-*p*-dioxin [2,3,7,8-tetrachlorooxanthrene]
TCDO	tetrachlorodecaoxide
TCP	tri-*o*-cresyl phosphate
TCR	T-cell receptor
TD antigen	thymus-dependent antigen
TDAR	T-cell-dependent antibody response
TDF	testis-determining factor
TDI	tolerable daily intake
TdT	terminal deoxynucleotidyl transferase
TEC	threshold effect concentration
TEL	threshold effect level
TEF	toxicity equivalency factor
TEL-ARNT	translocated ETS leukemia-ARNT fusion protein (where ARNT is defined above and ETS refers to the E twenty-six transformation-specific family of transcription factors)
TEN	toxic epidermal necrolysis
TENS	transcutaneous electronic nerve stimulation
TEQ	toxicity equivalent
T_{eq}	toxicity equivalent
TER	toxicity exposure ratio
TG	thyroglobulin
TGF-β	transforming growth factor β
TI	teratogenic index; time independent
TIE	toxicity identification and evaluation
TIL	tumor-infiltrating lymphocyte
TL	threshold level, tolerance limit
TL_m (TL_{50})	median tolerance limit
TL_n	see LT_n
TLR	toll-like receptor
TLV®	threshold limit value
TLV®-C	threshold limit value – ceiling
TLV®–STEL	threshold limit value – short-term exposure limit
TLV®–TWA	threshold limit value – time-weighted average
TMDI	theoretical maximum daily intake
TNF	tumor necrosis factor
TOC	total organic carbon
TOCP	tri-*o*-cresyl phosphate
TPA	tetradecanoyl phorbol acetate (same as PMA)
TPO	thyroid peroxidase
TRA	tumor rejection antigen
TRAF	TNF receptor-associated factor
tRNA	transfer RNA
TSH	thyroid-stimulating hormone
TSHR	thyroid-stimulating hormone receptor
TSTA	tumor-specific transplantation antigen
TTC	threshold of toxicological concern
tTG	tissue transglutaminase
TTX	tetrodotoxin
TU	toxicity unit
TUNEL	TdT-dependent dUTP-biotin nick end labeling
TWA	time-weighted average
TWAC	time-weighted average concentration
TWAE	time-weighted average exposure

TWI	tolerable weekly intake
*T*x	toxicity value
UCP	uncoupling protein
UDP	uridine diphosphate
UDP-GA	uridine-5′-diphosphoglucuronic acid
UDS	unscheduled DNA synthesis
UF	uncertainty factor
UGT	uridine diphosphate (UDP)-glucuronosyltransferase
UPR	unfolded protein response
VCAM	vascular cell adhesion molecule
VLA	very late activation antigen
V_{max}	maximum velocity
VNTR	variable number tandem repeat
VOC	volatile organic compound
vPvB	very persistent and very bioaccumulative
VSD	ventricular septal defect; virtually safe dose
VTG	vitellogenin
WCST	Wisconsin card sorting test
WET	whole-effluent toxicity
WG	Wegener granulomatosis
WHAM	Windermere humic aqueous model
WWTP	waste-water treatment plant
ZAP-70	zeta chain (TCR)-associated protein kinase-70 kDa
ZIFT	zygote intrafallopian transfer

APPENDIX III

Abbreviations and Acronyms of Toxicological Organizations, Legislative Terms and Regulatory Bodies

ABT	American Board of Toxicology
ACGIH	American Conference of Governmental Industrial Hygienists
AFNOR	Association Française de Normalisation
APHA	American Public Health Association
ASTM	American Society for Testing and Materials
ATS	Academy of Toxicological Science
ATSDR	Agency for Toxic Substances and Disease Registry
BCR	Bureau Communautaire de Reference (Bruxelles)
BIBRA	British Industrial Biological Research Association
CCFA	Codex Committee on Food Additives
CCPR	Codex Committee on Pesticide Residues
CDC	Centers for Disease Control and Prevention
CEC	Commission of the European Communities
CEN	Committee Européen de Normalisation
CEQ	Council on Environmental Quality
CERCLA	Comprehensive Environmental Response, Compensation, and Liability Act (USA)
CHIP	Classification, Hazard Information, and Packaging (UK)
COSHH	Control of Substances Hazardous to Health Regulations (UK)
CPL	Classification, Packaging, and Labeling
CTD	Common Technical Document [Note: for Pharmaceuticals for Human Use for submission to the FDA and ICH]
DFG	Deutsche Forschungsgemeinschaft (German Research Council)
EC	European Community; European Commission
EAC	European Agency for Chemicals
ECB	European Chemicals Bureau
ECETOC	European Centre for Ecotoxicology and Toxicology of Chemicals
ECHA	European Chemicals Agency

Comprehensive Glossary of Terms Used in Toxicology
By John Duffus, Douglas M. Templeton and Michael Schwenk

Published by the Royal Society of Chemistry, www.rsc.org

EEA	European Environmental Agency
EEC	European Economic Community
EFSA	European Food Safety Authority
EINECS	European Inventory of Existing Chemical Substances
ELINCS	European List of New Chemical Substances
EMEA	European Medicines Agency
EMPA	Eidgenössische Materialprüfungs- und ForschungsAnstalt (Swiss Federal Laboratories for Materials Testing and Research)
EPA	Environmental Protection Agency (USA) (same as USEPA)
EPPO	European and Mediterranean Plant Protection Organization
EU	European Union
EUROTOX	European Society of Toxicology
EUSES	European Uniform System for Evaluation of Substances
FAO	Food and Agricultural Organization
FDA	Food and Drug Administration (USA) (same as USFDA)
FIOH	Finnish Institute of Occupational Health
HSE	Health and Safety Executive (UK)
IAEA	International Atomic Energy Agency
IARC	International Agency for Research on Cancer
ICCA	International Council of Chemical Associations
ICH	International Conference for Harmonization (Pharmaceuticals)
ICRP	International Commission on Radiological Protection
ICSU	International Council of Scientific Unions (since 1998, International Council of Science)
IFCC	International Federation of Clinical Chemists
ILO	International Labor Organization
IPCS	International Program on Chemical Safety, UNEP, ILO, WHO
IRIS	Integrated Risk Information System (USA)
IRPTC	International Register of Potentially Toxic Chemicals, now UNEP Chemicals
ISEAAA	International Society for Exposure Assessment and Analysis
ISO	International Organization for Standardization
IUCLID	International Uniform Chemical Information Database
IUPAC	International Union of Pure and Applied Chemistry
IUTOX	International Union of Toxicology
JECFA	Joint FAO/WHO Expert Committee on Food Additives
JMPR	Joint FAO/WHO Meeting on Pesticide Residues
MHRA	Medicines and Healthcare Products Regulatory Agency (U.K.)
NAS	National Academy of Sciences (USA)
NBS	National Bureau of Standards (USA), now NIST
NIH	National Institutes of Health (USA)
NIOSH	National Institute of Occupational Safety and Health (USA)
NIST	National Institute of Standards and Technology (USA), formerly NBS
NRC	National Research Council (USA)
OECD	Organization for Economic Cooperation and Development
OEHHA	Organization of Environmental Health Hazard Assessment (USA)
OMS	Organisation Mondiale de la Santé (same as WHO)
OSHA	Occupational Safety and Health Administration (USA)
OSPAR	Commission for the OSLO and Paris Conventions
RCPath	Royal College of Pathologists
REACH	Registration, Evaluation, Authorisation and Restriction of Chemicals
RIVM	Rijksinstituut voor Volksgezondheid en Milieu
RSC	Royal Society of Chemistry

SARA (US)	Superfund Amendment and Reauthorization Act
SCOPE	Scientific Committee on Problems of the Environment (ICSU)
SOT	Society of Toxicology (USA)
STP	Sewage treatment plant
TOSCA (TSCA)	Toxic Substances Control Act (USA)
UNCED	United Nations Conference on Environment and Development (held in Rio de Janeiro, Brazil, 1992)
UNEP	United Nations Environment Program
USEPA	United States Environmental Protection Agency (same as EPA)
USFDA	United States Food and Drug Agency (same as FDA)
WHMIS	Workplace Hazardous Materials Information System (Canada)
WHO	World Health Organization (same as OMS)